Ophthalmic Echography

Documenta Ophthalmologica Proceedings Series

Ophthalmic Echography

Proceedings of the 10th SIDUO Congress,
St. Petersburg Beach, Florida, U.S.A.,
November 7–10, 1984

Edited by K.C. Ossoinig

Department of Ophthalmology, University of Iowa
Hospitals and Clinics, Iowa City, Iowa, U.S.A.

1987 **MARTINUS NIJHOFF/DR W. JUNK PUBLISHERS**
a member of the KLUWER ACADEMIC PUBLISHERS GROUP
DORDRECHT / BOSTON / LANCASTER

Distributors

---

for the United States and Canada: Kluwer Academic Publishers, P.O. Box 358, Accord Station, Hingham, MA 02018-0358, USA·
for the UK and Ireland: Kluwer Academic Publishers, MTP Press Limited, Falcon House, Queen Square, Lancaster LA1 1RN, UK
for all other countries: Kluwer Academic Publishers Group, Distribution Center, P.O. Box 322, 3300 AH Dordrecht, The Netherlands

Library of Congress Cataloging in Publication Data

```
SIDUO Congress (10th : 1984 : Saint Petersburg, Fla.)
  Opthalmic echography.

  (Documenta ophthalmologica.  Proceedings series)
  Includes index.
  1. Ultrasonics in opthalmology--Congresses.
I. Ossoinig, K. (Karl)  II. Title.  III. Series.
[DNLM: 1. Eye--pathology--congresses.  2. Ultrasonic
Diagnosis--congresses.   W3 D0637 / WW 141 S569 1984o]
RE79.U4S5  1984     617.7'07543      87-1704
```

ISBN-13: 978-94-010-7988-4   e-ISBN-13: 978-94-009-3315-6
DOI: 10.1007/978-94-009-3315-6

Copyright

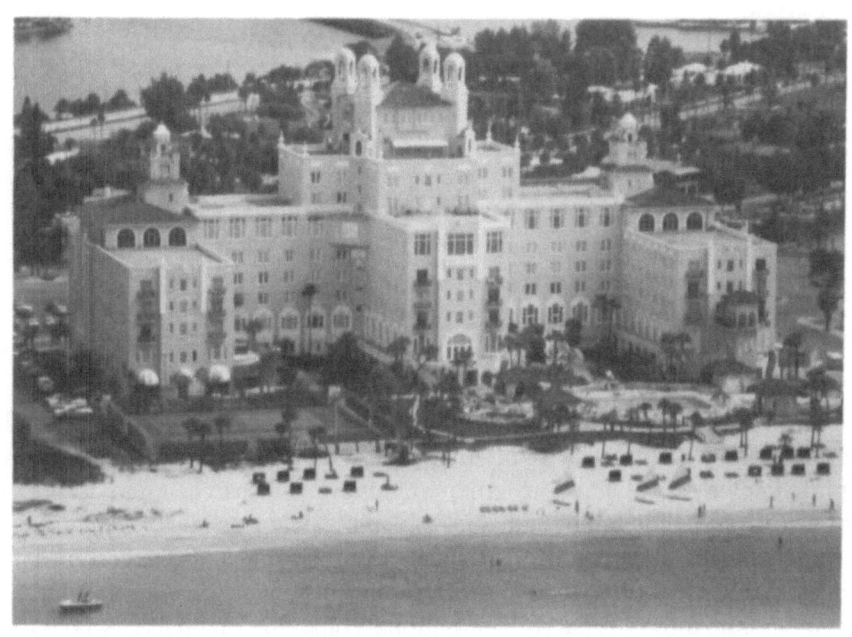

Don CeSar Beach Resort, St. Petersburg Beach, Florida, USA.
Place of the 10th Biennial SIDUO Congress

Preface

Two decades of intensive and fruitful international cooperation, through and within SIDUO, have clearly left their mark on Diagnostic Ultrasound in Ophthalmology. Evolving from an experimental and research oriented laboratory test Ophthalmic Echography has become a mature clinical examination method offering a variety of approaches to a multitude of diagnostic challenges. SIDUO X set out to celebrate this successful growing up and to commemorate those 20 years of international collaboration; in fact, SIDUO X became the sofar largest congress of SIDUO with a record participation and a record program.

This book presenting the proceedings of SIDUO X testifies to that by containing 103 scientific contributions delivered by 173 authors from 17 countries throughout the world. These contributions range from educational reviews to pioneering original work, from technological and methodological novelties to papers on fascinating clinical applications, from reports of the influence of the examiners' manual skills to the impact of computer evaluation of echographically obtained data; they cover virtually all facets of Diagnostic ultrasound in ophthalmology including: Biometry for intraocular lens calculations, for measurements of microscopically thin layers such as the retina and the choroid as well as the most accurate in-vivo measurements of the optic nerve and of the extraocular muscles that are possible; the Diagnosis of posterior segment lesions of the eye and most of the aspects of orbital and periorbital diseases.

While reflecting the state of the art of ophthalmic echography in the 1980's, this book promises to remain an indispendable, important and extremely useful companion for future generations of ophthalmic echographers providing them with an abundant source of educational, historical and inspirational information and allowing them, God willing, an ever better utilization of the tremendous diagnostic potential of echography as a powerful tool in the continuing struggle to fight the causes of blindness and human suffering.

In this spirit I would like to pay tribute to all who through their hard work, idealistic gift of their time and talents, through sacrifice and through willingness to share their knowledge and skills with their colleagues have contributed so much to make SIDUO X and this book such a successful venture. I would like to thank those great ophthalmologists who through their foresight and leadership, for all these years, have given tremendous support to Ophthalmic Echography and to SIDUO X: in particular, Frederick C. Blodi, President of the Academia Ophthalmologica Internationalis, Edward W.D. Norton, the honorary Guest of SIDUO X, and Jules Francois, previous President of the International Council of Ophthalmology, who was looking forward so much to be one of the leaders of the SIDUO X celebration, but who by fate was called from this life only a few months before the congress and whose unforgotten support of SIDUO was remembered in the Eulogy given by our President Pier-Enrico Gallenga during SIDUO X.

These men like the many pioneers of echography including the two first and most prominent ones, Gilbert Baum and Arvo Oksala, who were so fittingly honored with the Siduo Pioneer Award at SIDUO X, deserve our all gratitude and appreciation for what Ophthalmic Echography now is.

Thanks are due to our Sponsors who have made SIDUO X possible, in particular to Biophysic Medical who, to a large extent financed these Proceedings.

I would also like to thank our Scientific and Congress Secretaries Sandra F. Byrne, Ronald L. Green, Deborah A. Hatz and James L. Queen for their enormous help in organizing SIDUO X. Last but not least I wish to express my particular thanks and appreciation to my wife Inge who not only signed responsible for an outstanding social program during the congress, but was instrumental and of invaluable help in every phase of preparing and accomplishing SIDUO X and these Proceedings.

Table of contents

PART THREE: DIAGNOSTIC ULTRASOUND – ORBITAL AND
PERIORBITAL DISEASES

10. Orbital and periorbital tumors

11. Orbital inflammation

12. Vascular disorders

13. Lacrimal-system disorders

APPENDIX: THERAPEUTIC ULTRASOUND

List of contributors

Abrams, Gary W., M.D., Milwaukee Eye Institute, 8700 W. Wisconsin Avenue, Milwaukee, WI 53226, U.S.A.

Avitabile, Dott. Teresio, Clinica Oculistica, Università di Bari, Piazza Giulio Cesare, Bari, Italy

Baba, Yukio, M.D., Dept. of Ophthalmology, Miyazaki Medical College, 5200 Kihara, Kiyotake, Miyazaki 889–16, Japan

Bartolomei, Dott. M.P., Via L Il Magnifico 24, Firenze, Italy

Berlin, Louise A., Director, Ophthalmic Sonography, Cleveland Clinic, 9500 Euclid Ave, Cleveland, OH 44106, U.S.A.

Binkhorst, Richard D., M.D., 718 Park Avenue, New York City, NY 10021, U.S.A.

Blackshear, W.M., M.D., University Professional Center, 3500 Fletcher Avenue, Suite 520, Tampa, FL 33612, U.S.A.

Boerrigter, R.M.M., M.D., Katholieke Universiteit, Kliniek voor Oogheelkunde, Philips van Leydenlaan 15, Nijmegen, The Netherlands

Bourgeois, K.A., M.D., Hermann Eye Center, University of Texas Health Science Center at Houston, 1203 Ross Sterling Avenue, Houston, TX 77030, U.S.A.

Boyer, David S., M.D., Suite 1620, 1127 Wilshire Boulevard, Los Angeles, CA 90017, U.S.A.

Burton, T.C., M.D., The Eye Institute, 8700 West Wisconsin Avenue, Milwaukee, WI 53226, U.S.A.

Buschmann, Prof. Dr. Werner, Universitätsklinik, Röntgenring 12, 8700 Würzburg 1, West Germany

Byrne, Barry M., Dept. of Ophthalmology, University of Texas Medical Center, 7703 Floyd Curl Drive, San Antonio, TX 78284, U.S.A.

Byrne, Sandy Frazier, Director of Echography Service, Bascom Palmer Eye Institute, 900 NW 17th St., Miami, FL 33101, U.S.A.

Cascio, Dott. Giovanni, Istituto Clinica Oculistica Università di Palermo, Via L. Giuffré 13, I-90172 Palermo, Italy

Caya, J.G., Ophthalmic Echography Services, 4508 SE 6th Place, Cape Coral, FL 33904, U.S.A.

Cennamo, Prof. Dott. Giovanni, Università Degli Studi di Napoli, II Facolta di Medicina e Chirurgia, Clinica Oculistica, Nuovo Policlinico: 80131 Napoli, Italy

Clemens, Dr. S., Univ. Augenklinik, Domachstr. 15, D-4400 Münster, West Germany

Cody, K., 539 Acacia Avenue, Bakersfield, CA 93305, U.S.A.

Coleman, D. Jackson, M.D., Head, Cornell Ophthalmology Associates, The New

York Hospital, Cornell Medical Center, 515 East 71st St., New York, NY 10021, U.S.A.

Colliac, Dr. J.P., Centre National d'Ophthalmologie des Quinze-Vingts, 28, rue de Charenton, F-75571 Paris Cedex 12, France

Cutcomb, J., Dept. of Ophthalmology, University of Iowa Hospitals, Iowa City, IA 52242, U.S.A.

De Vries-Knoppert, W.A.E.J., M.D., Dept. of Ophthalmology, Free University, De Boelelaan 1117, Amsterdam, The Netherlands

Di Liberto, Dott. A., Istituto Clinica Oculistica Universitá di Palermo, Via L Giuffré 13, I-90172 Palermo, Italy

Dixon, Penny A., Ophthalmic Echography Services, 4508 SE 6th Place, Cape Coral, FL 33904, U.S.A.

Doro, Dott. Daniele, Clinica Oculistica Universitá di Padova, I-35138 Padova, Italy

Drysdale, A.M., M.D., 212–597 Parliament St., Toronto, Ontario M4X 1W3, Canada

Ellsworth, Robert M., M.D., Cornell Ophthalmology Associates, The New York Hospital, Cornell Medical Center, 515 East 71st St., New York, NY 10021, U.S.A.

Falco, Dott. Leonardo, Medico Chirurgo, Via L Il Magnifico 24, Firenze, Italy

Fiore, Dott. D., Dept. Neuroradiology, University of Padova, I-35100 Padova, Italy

Fishman, Marcy L., R.D.M.S., Ultrasound Laboratory, 800 Westwood Blvd., Los Angeles, CA 90024, U.S.A.

Fishman, Martin L., M.D., 431 Monterey Avenue, P.O. Box 95, Los Gatos, CACA 95031, U.S.A.

Fledelius, Hans, M.D., Eye Dept., Frederiksborg Amts Centralsygehus, DK-3400 Hillerod, Denmark

Folk, James C., M.D., Director of Vitreo-Retinal Service, Dept. of Ophthalmology, University of Iowa Hospitals, Iowa City, IA 52242, U.S.A.

Foxman, Scott, M.D., Ultrasound Lab., Jules Stein Eye Institute, 800 Westwood Plaza, Los Angeles, CA 90024, U.S.A.

Frank, Kay Ellen, M.D., University Ophthalmologists, Inc., 2065 Adelbert Rd., Cleveland, OH 44106, U.S.A.

Freese, Manfred, Ph.D., Director of Research, Radionics Medical Division, 1240 Ellesmere Rd., Scarborough, Ontario M1P 2X4, Canada

Frieling, Dr. Elisabeth H., Augenabteilung des Bundeswehrkrankenhauses, 7900 Ulm, West Germany

Gallenga, Prof. Dr. Pier Enrico, Direttore Clinica Oculistica Universitá, Piazza Dei Templi Romani 3, I-66100 Chieti, Italy

Galli, Dott. Gloria, Clinica Ocul. Univ. di Ferrara, Via Don Sturzo 14, 40135 Bologna, Italy

Gallie, B.L., M.D., 212–597 Parliament St., Toronto, ONT M4X 1W3, Canada

Gangemi, Dott. M., Dept. of Neurosurgery, II School of Medicine, University of Naples, Naples, Italy

Giuliano, Dott. S., Istituto Clinica Oculistica Universitá di Palermo, Via L Giuffré 13, I-90172 Palermo, Italy

Goes, Dr. Frank J, Akademisch Consulent, Oogchirurgie, Van Eycklei 5 (Bus 2), B-2018 Antwerpen, Belgium

Goleminova, Dr. R., Inst. Med. Superieur de Sofia, Clinique d'Ophtalmologie, Sofia, Bulgaria

Gragoudas, E., M.D., Massachusetts Eye & Ear Infirmary, 243 Charles St., Boston, MA 02114, U.S.A.

Green, Ronald L., M.D., Estelle Doheny Eye Foundation, 1355 San Pablo St., Los Angeles, CA 90033, U.S.A.

Greenall, Dr. P., Milton Cottage, Main Street, Forest Hills, Oxford, OX9 WY, England

Grizzard, W. Sanderson, M.D., 2655 Swann Avenue, Suite 100, Tampa, FL 33609-4060, U.S.A.

Guerriero, Dott. Silvana, Clinica Oculistica, Universitá di Bari, 70100 Bari, Italy

Haigis, Dr. D.W., Kopfklinikum Würzburg, Universitätsklinik und Poliklinik für Augenkranke, Josef-Schneider-Strasse 11, D-8700 Würzburg, West Germany

Haik, Barrett G., M.D., Cornell Ophthalmology Assoc., The New York Hospital, Cornell Medical Center, 515 East 71st. St., New York, NY 10021 U.S.A.

Harrie, Roger P., M.D., Salt Lake Clinic, Dept. of Ophthalmology, 333 S. 9th East, Salt Lake City, UT 84102, U.S.A.

Hasenfratz, Dr. Gerhard C., Direktor der Echographie, Univ. – Augenklinik, Mathildenstr. 8, 8000 München 2, West Germany

Hawkswell, Dr. A., Dept. of Ophthalmology, St. James's University Hospital, Leeds LS9 7TF, England, UK

Hayashi, Dr. Hideyuki, Dept. of Ophthamology, Fukuoka University, School of Medicine Nanakuma, Jonan-Ku Fukouka 814–01, Japan

Hayashida, Dr. Tadashi, Miyazaki Medical College, Kiyotake, Miyazaki 889–16, Japan

Hays, C., M.D., Cirujano Oftalmologo, Vicente Garcia Torres #46, Coyoacan, Mexico 21 D.F., Mexico

Hernandez, E., M.D., Cirujano Oftalmologo, Vicente Garcia Torres #46, Coyoacan, Mexico 21 D.F., Mexico

Hildenbrand, Dr. G., Institut für experimentelle Ophthalmologie der Univ. Bonn, Sigmund-Freudstr. 25, D-5300 Bonn 1, West Germany

Hillman, Mr. Jeffrey S., FRCS, Dept. of Ophthalmology, St. James's Hospital, Leeds LS9 7TF, England, UK

Holasek, Ed, Case Western Reserve University, School of Medicine, Cleveland, OH 44022, U.S.A.

Holladay, Jack T., M.D., Hermann Eye Center, University of Texas Health Science Center at Houston, 6411 Fannin Street, Houston, TX 77030, U.S.A.

Horikoshi, Jun, M.D., Dept. of Ophthalmology, St. Marianna Univ. School of Med., 2095 Sugao, Miyamae-Ku Kawasaki 213, Japan

Hughes, J. Randall, Bascom Palmer Eye Institute, 900 N.W. 17th St., Miami, FL 33101, U.S.A.

Irion, Dr. K.M., Institut für experimentelle Ophthalmologie der Univ. Bonn, Sigmund Freudstr. 25, D-5300 Bonn 1, West Germany

Islas, Gilberto, M.D., Platon 318, Polanco Mexico, DF 11560, Mexico

Itani, K.M., M.D., Dept. Ophthal., Echography Service, Univ. Iowa Hospitals, Iowa City, IA 52242, U.S.A.

Itoh, M., M.D., Ophthalmology Dept., Tokyo Univ. of Agriculture & Technology, Tokyo, Japan

Japp, B., M.D., 212–597 Parliament St., Toronto, Ontario M4X 1W3, Canada

Jennings, W.D., University Ophthalmologists, Inc., 2065 Adelbert Rd., Cleveland, OH 44106, U.S.A.

Kardon, R.H., M.D., Dept. of Ophthalmology, University of Iowa Hospitals, Iowa City, IA 52242, U.S.A.

Kerman, Barry M., M.D., Ultrasound Lab, Jules Stein Eye Institute, UCLA Center for the Health Sciences, Los Angeles, CA 90024, U.S.A.

Kitagawa, Y., M.D., Dept. of Ophthalmology, Fukuoka University, School of Med. Nanakuma, Jonan-Ku Fukouka 814–01, Japan

Kiumura, Y., M.D., Ophth. Dept., St. Marianna Univ., 2095 Sugao, Takatsu-Ku, Kawasaki, Japan

Kodama, Dr. Yoshihisa, Dept. of Ophthalmology, Miyazaki Medical College, Kiyotake, Miyazaki 889–16, Japan

Koester, Charles J., Ph.D., Department of Ophthalmology, Columbia University, 635 West 165th Street, New York, NY 10032, U.S.A.

Kohno, J., M.D., Ophthalmology Department, St. Marianna University, 2095 Sugao, Takatsu-Ku, Kawasaki, Japan

Komatsu, A., M.D., Ophthalmology Department, St. Marianna University, 2095 Sugao, Takatsu-Ku, Kawasaki, Japan

Kreissig, Prof. Dr. Ingrid, Direktor, Univ-Augenklinik, Schleichstr 12, D-7400 Tübingen, West Germany

Kroll, Prof. Dr. P., Univ. Augenklinik, Domackstr 15, D-4400 Münster, West Germany

Kyono, S., M.D., Dept. of Ophthalmology, Fukuoka University, School of Medicine Nanakuma, Jonan-Ku Fukouka 814–01, Japan

Lamb, S., University Professional Center, 3500 Fletcher Avenue, Suite 520, Tampa, FL 33612, U.S.A.

Lepper, Dr. Rolf-Dieter, Paul Kleestr. 17, D5309 Mechenheim, West Germany

Lewis, John W., M.D.; 2017 Oceanview, Seabrook, TX 77586, U.S.A.

Lieb, Dr. W., Augenklinik/Klinikum der Johannes Gutenberg Univ., Postfach 3960, Langenbeckstr. 1, 6500 Mainz, West Germany

Lizzi, F.L., Ph.D., Riverside Research Institute, 330 W. Forty Second Street, New York, NY 10036, U.S.A.

Long, S.A., Ph.D., University of Houston, Department of Electrical Engineering, Houston, TX 77004, U.S.A.

Lorusso, Dott. Vincenzo, Clinica Oculistica, Universitá di Bari, 70100 Bari, Italy

Lueneborg, Dr. H.G., Universitäts-Augenklinik, Sigmund Freudstr. 25, D-5300 Bonn, West Germany

Maberley, Alan L., M.D., F.R.C.S., UBC/VGM Eye Care Center, 2550 Willow St., Vancouver, B.C. V5Z 3N9, Canada

MacNeill, James R., M.D., F.R.C.S., 7031 Fielding Ave., Halifax, Nova Scotia B3 L2H1, Canada

Massin, Dr. Marcel, Centre National d'Ophthalmologie des Quinze-Vingts, 28, rue de Charenton, F-75571 Paris Cedex 12, France

Masuyama, Dr. Yoshimasa, Dept. of Ophthalmology, Miyazaki Medical College, Kiyotake, Miyazai 889–16, Japan

Mazzeo, Dott. Vincenzina, Clinica Oculistica Universitá di Ferrara, Corso Giovecca 202, 44100 Ferrara, Italy

Meyer-Schwickerath-Schiweck, Dr. B., Univ.-Augenklinik, Sigmund-Freud-Str. 25, D-5300 Bonn 1, West Germany

Miller, J.B., M.D., Suite 1620, 1127 Wilshire Boulevard, Los Angeles, CA 90017, U.S.A.

Moragrega Adame, Eduardo, M.D., Cirujano Oftalmologo, Vicente Garcia Torres #46, Coyoacan, Mexico 21 D.F., Mexico

Moro, Prof. Dr. F., Director, Ophthalmology Clinic, Univ. of Padova, Via Giustiniani #2, Padova, Italy 35138

Mudrov, Dr. N., Inst. Med. Supérieur de Sofia, Clinique d'Ophtalmologie, Sofia, Bulgaria

Nardi, Dott. M., Via L Il Magnifico 24, Firenze, Italy

Nasr, Amin Marwan, M.D., King Khalid Eye Spec. Hospital, P.O. Box 7191, Riyadh, Saudi Arabia

Nover, Prof. Dr. Arno, Direktor, Univ. Augenklinik, Langenbeckstr 1, D-65 Mainz, West Germany

Ohashi, Kohji, M.D., Dept. of Ophthalmology, St. Marianna University, School of Medicine, 2095, Sugao, Miyamae-ku, Kawasaki-shi 213, Japan

Oshima, K., M.D., Dept. of Ophthalmology, Fukuoka University, School of Medicine Nanakuma, Jonan-Ku Fukouka 814–01, Japan

Ossoinig, Karl C., M.D., Director, Echography Service, Dept. of Ophthalmology, University of Iowa Hospitals, Iowa City, IA 52242, U.S.A.

Packer, A.J., M.D., Suite B, 2020 Gravier Street, New Orleans, LA 70112, U.S.A.

Passani, Dott. Franco, Via Galilei 138, 54036 Marina di Carrara, Italy

Pautler, S.E., M.D., 2655 Swann Avenue, Suite 100, Tampa, FL 33609, U.S.A.

Pavlin, Charles J., M.D., 212–597 Parliament St., Toronto, ONT M4X 1W3, Canada

Payne, D.G., M.D., 212–597 Parliament St., Toronto, ONT M4X 1W3, Canada

Perri, Dott. P., Clinica Ocul. Univ. di Ferrara, Via Don Sturzo 14, 40135 Bologna, Italy

Perrone, Dott. S., Dept. of Ophthalmology, Univ. of Padova, I-35100 Padova, Italy

Prager, Tom, Ph.D., Herman Eye Center, University of Texas Health Science Center at Houston, 6411 Fannin Street, Houston, TX 77030, U.S.A.

Prahs, Dr. Berndt, Augenklinik, Josef-Schneiderstr. 11, 8700 Würzburg, West Germany

Purnell, Edward W., M.D., Professor & Chief, Dept. of Ophthalmology, Case Western Reserve University, 2074 Abington Rd., Cleveland, OH 44106, U.S.A.

Rabie, Dr. E.P., Dept. of Ophthalmology, Royal Eye Hospital, Oxford Road, Manchester M13 9WH, England UK

Ravalli, Dott. Luca, University Eye Clinic, Corso Giovecca 203, I-44100 Ferrara, Italy

Reibaldi, Prof. Dott. Alfredo, Director, Clinica Oculisticá Universitá di Catania, Catania, Italy

Reinert, Dr. S., Institut für experimentelle Ophthalmologie der Univ. Bonn, Sigmund Freudstr. 25, D-5300 Bonn 1, West Germany

Reshef, Daniel, M.D., Dept. of Ophthalmology, Hadassah Univ. Hospital, P.O. Box 9483, Jerusalem, Israel

Reuter, Dr. Reinhold, Univ. Augenklinik, Sigmund Freudstr. 25, D-5300 Bonn-Venusberg, West Germany

Rochels, Prof. Dr. Rainer, Augenklinik/Klinikum der Johannes Gutenberg Univ., Postfach 3960, Langenbeckstr 1, 6500 Mainz, West Germany

Rondeau, Mark E., Department of Ophthalmology, Cornell University Medical College, 1300 York Avenue, New York, NY 10021, U.S.A.

Rosa, Dott. N., Istituto di Clinica Oculistica, Il Facoltá di Medicina e Chirurgia, Universitá degli Studi di Napoli, Via Pansini No. 5, I-80131 Napoli, Italy

Rosenberg, N.T., M.D., Eye Dept., Frederiksborg Amts Centralsygehus, DK-3400 Hillerod, Denmark

Rossi, Prof. Dr. Antonio, Director, Clinica Oculistica/Univ. di Ferrara, Corso Giovecca 203, I-44100 Ferrara, Italy

Rothe, Dr. Robert, Univ. Augenklinik Bonn, Abbestrasse 12, D-5300 Bonn-Venusberg, West Germany

Saint-Louis, Leslie S., M.D., 650 1st Avenue, New York, NY, 10016, U.S.A.

Sawada, Prof. Dr. Atsushi, Head, Ophthal. Dept., Miyazaki Med. College, 5200 Kihara, Kiyotake, Miyazaki 889–16, Japan

Scherer, Dr. Udo, Mathildenstr 11, 6500 Mainz, West Germany

Scorrano, Dott. Rita, Clinica Oculistica, Universitá di Ferrara, I-44100 Ferrara, Italy

Scuderi, Prof. Dott. G. Clinica Oculistica, Univesitá di Bari, Piazza Giulio Cesare, 70124 Bari, Italy

Seddon, Johanna, M.D., Mass. Eye & Ear Infirmary, 243 Charles St., Boston, MA 02114, U.S.A.

Shammas, H. John, M.D., 3737 E. Century Blvd. #340, Lynwood, CA 90262, U.S.A.

Silverman, Ronald H., M.S., Department of Ophthalmology, Cornell University Medical College, 1300 York Avenue, New York, NY 10021, U.S.A.

Sjarov, M., M.D., Inst. Med. Supérieur de Sofia, Clinique d'Ophtalmologie, Sofia, Bulgaria

Skalka, Harold W., M.D., 1720 University Blvd., Birmingham, AL 35233, U.S.A.

Smith, Mary, Tulane Medical Center School of Medicine, Department of Ophthalmology, 1430 Tulane Avenue, New Orleans, LA 70112–2699, U.S.A.

Soriano, Dr. Horacio M., Rio Bamba 72-4, P DTAS 4YT, 1025 Buenos Aires, Argentina

Spettoli, Dott. Marisa, Via Battara 38, 44100 Ferrara, Italy

Stanowsky, Dr. Alexander, Augenklinik/Zentral-klinikum Augsburg, Stenglinstr., D-8900 Augsburg, West Germany

Stella, Dott. L., Dept. of Neurosurgery, II School of Medicine, University of Naples, Naples, Italy

Sterns, Gwen K., M.D., Dept. of Ophthalmology, Rochester General Hospital, 1425 Portland Ave., Rochester, NY 14621, U.S.A.

Stone, Robert D., M.D., 400 Parnasssus Ave., A-704, San Francisco, CA 94143, U.S.A.

Storey, Dr. J.K., Central Manchester Health Auth., Manchester Royal Eye Hospital, Oxford Rd., Manchester M13 9WH, England UK

Sugata, Yasuo, M.D., Dept. of Ophthalmology, Komagome Hospital, Honkomagome 3–18–22, Bunkyo-Ku Tokyo, Japan

Susal, Alan, M.D., 93 Arch St., Redwood City, CA 94062, U.S.A.

Suzuki, Jun, M.D., Dept. of Ophthalmology, St. Marianna University, School of Medicine, 2095, Sugao, Miyamae-ku, Kawasaki-shi, Kanagawa-ken, 213 Japan

Takahashi, N., M.D., Ophthalmology Dept., St. Marianna Univ., 2095 Sugao, Takatsu-Ku, Kawasaki, Japan

Takao, Yuhei, M.D., Dept. of Ophthalmology, Fukuoka Univ. 45–1, 7-Chome, Nanakuma Jonan-Ku, Fukuoka 814–01, Japan

Tamayo, Gustavo, M.D., Fundacion Oftalmologica Nacional, Calle 50 No. 13–22, Bogota, Colombia, South America

Tamburrelli, Ciro, M.D., Clinica Oculistica-Universitá Cattolica, S.C: Policlinico A. Gemelli, V. Della Pineta Sacchetti 644, 00186 Roma, Italy

Tane, Prof. Dr. Sadanao, Ophthalmology Dept., St. Marianna Univ., 2095 Sugao, Takatsu-Ku, Kawasaki, Japan

Tanev, Dr. V., Inst. Med. Supérieur de Sofia, Clinique d'Opthalmologie, Sofia, Bulgaria

Thijssen, J.M., Dr., Katholieke Universiteit, Kliniek voor Oogheelkunde, Philips van Leydenlaan 15, Nijmegen, The Netherlands

Tomita, M., M.D., Opthalmology Dept., Metropolitan Komagome Hospital, Honkomagome 3–18–22, Bunkyo-Ku Tokyo, Japan

Torii, Dr. Hideo, Dept. of Ophthalmology, Miyazaki Medical College, Kiyotake, Miyazaki 889–16, Japan

Torpey, Joan, M.D., Department of Ophthalmology, Lennox Hill Hospital, 100 E. 77th Street, New York, NY 10021, U.S.A.

Trier, Prof. Dr. Hans-Georg, Institut für experimentelle Ophthalmologie der Univ. Bonn, Sigmund Freudstr. 25, D-5300 Bonn 1, West Germany

Uva, Dott., M.G., Clinica Oculistica, Universitá di Bari, Piazza G. Cesare, I-70124 Bari, Italy

Van Der Heijde, Dr. G.L., Free University of Amsterdam, Laboratory of Medical Physics, Van der Boechhorststraat 7, 1081 BT – Amsterdam, The Netherlands

Van Heuven, W.A.J., M.D., Head of Dept. of Ophthalmology, Univ. of Texas Health Science Center, 7703 Floyd Curl Drive, San Antonio, TX 78284, U.S.A.

Verbeek, Dr. A.M., Weezenhof 20-24, Nijmegen 6536 HM, The Netherlands

Verhey, L., Ultrasound, Massachusetts Eye & Ear Infirmary, 243 Charles St., Boston, MA 02114, U.S.A.

Wallner, Dr. B., Universitätsklinik, Röntgenring 12, 8700 Würzburg 1, West Germany

Warner, Laura, Dept. of Ophthalmology, Echography Service, Univ. of Iowa Hospitals, Iowa City, IA 52242, U.S.A.

Weingeist, Thomas A., M.D., Ph.D., Prof. and Head of Dept. of Ophthalmology, University of Iowa Hospitals, Iowa City, IA 52242, U.S.A.

Weyer-Haak, Nancy, Ultrasound Lab, Massachusetts Eye & Ear Infirmary, 243 Charles St., Boston, MA 02114, U.S.A.

Winn, T.L., M.D., P.O. Box 48126, Wichita, KS 67201, U.S.A.

Yamamoto, Dr. Yukio, Ophthalmology Dept., Metropolitan Hiroo General Hospital, Tokyo, Japan

Young, F.A., Ph.D., Director, Primate Research Center, Washington State University, Pullman, WA 99164, U.S.A.

Zakov, Z. Nicholas, M.D., Cleveland Clinic Foundation, 9500 Euclid Ave., Cleveland, OH 44106, U.S.A.

Societas Internationalis pro Diagnostica Ultrasonica in Ophthalmologia

SIDUO SOCIETY 1980–84

OFFICERS:

President
H.G. Trier (Bonn)

Vice-President
P.E. Gallenga (Chieti)

EXECUTIVE BOARD:

A. Bertenyi (Budapest)
F. Bigar (Zürich)
N.R. Bronson (Southampton)
W. Buschmann (Würzburg)
S.F. Byrne (Miami)
G. Cennamo (Naples)
D.J. Coleman (New York)
R.L. Dallow (Boston)
P.E. Gallenga (Chieti)
F. Goes (Gent)
J.S. Hillman (Leeds)
B.L. Hodes (Tucson)
H. Hughes (Sidney)
L. Kolozsvary (Debrecen)
M. Massin (Paris)
K.C. Ossoinig (Iowa City)
J. Poujol (Paris)
E.W. Purnell (Cleveland)
R. Sampaolesi (Buenos Aires)
A. Sawada (Miyazaki)
H.W. Skalka (Birmingham)
S. Tane (Kawasaki)
J.M. Thijssen (Nijmegen)
P. Till (Wien)

Secretary-Treasurer
J.M. Thijssen (Nijmegen)

Deputy Treasurer (North America)
B.L. Hodes (Hershey)

Deputy Treasurer (Eastern Europe)
A. Bertenyi (Budapest)

H.G. Trier (Bonn)
M. Wainstock (Detroit)

PAST PRESIDENTS:

J. Vanysek (Brno) 1964–1967
A. Oksala (Turku) 1968–1971
H. Gernet (Münster) 1972–1976
K.C. Ossoinig (Iowa City)
1977–1980

PAST HONORÀRY
PRESIDENTS:

J. Böck (Wien)
A.H. Keeney (Louisville)
J. Vanysek (Brno)
K. Velhagen (Berlin)

HONORARY MEMBERS:

G. Baum (New York)
H. Gernet (Münster)
A. Oksala (Turku)
K.C. Ossoinig (Iowa City)
J. Vanysek (Brno)

SIDUO X Congress November 6–10, 1984

SPONSORS:

Department of Ophthalmology
and College of Medicine
The University of Iowa

SIDUO (Societas Internationalis
de Diagnostica Ultrasonica in
Ophthalmologia)

AIUM (American Institute of
Ultrasound in Medicine)

Bascom Palmer Eye Institute
University of Miami

ORGANIZING COMMITTEE:

Congress President:
   Karl C. Ossoinig (Iowa City)

Scientific Secretaries:

   Sandra F. Byrne (Miami)
   Ronald L. Green (Los Angeles)

Congress Secretaries:

   Deborah A. Hatz (Iowa City)
   James L. Queen (Iowa City)

INTERNATIONAL SCIENTIFIC PROGRAM COMMITTEE:

Chairman:
   H.G. Trier (Bonn)

Members:
   D.J. Coleman (New York)
   P.E. Gallenga (Chieti)
   K.C. Ossoinig (Iowa City)
   E.W. Purnell (Cleveland)
   J.M. Thijssen (Nijmegen)

REGIONAL ADVISORY COMMITTEE:

Societas Internationalis pro Diagnostica Ultrasonica in Ophthalmologia

SIDUO SOCIETY 1985–1988

OFFICERS:

President
P.E. Gallenga (Chieti)

Vice-President
B.L. Hodes (Tucson)

EXECUTIVE BOARD:

A. Bertenyi (Budapest)
F. Bigar (Zürich)
W. Buschmann (Würzburg)
S.F. Byrne (Miami)
R.M. Calderon (Boston)
D.J. Coleman (New York)
V. Dorn (Zagreb)
Y.L. Fisher (New York)
D.G. Fuller (Dallas)
P.E. Gallenga (Chieti)
H. Gernet (Münster)
J.S. Hillman (Leeds)
B.L. Hodes (Tucson)
H. Hughes (Sidney)
J. Poujol (Paris)
E.W. Purnell (Cleveland)
R. Sampaolesi (Buenos Aires)
A. Sawada (Miyazaki)
J. Shammas (Lynwood)
H.M. Soriano (Buenos Aires)
S. Tane (Kawasaki)
J.M. Thijssen (Nijmegen)
P. Till (Wien)
H.G. Trier (Bonn)
W.A.J. Van Heuven

Secretary
J.M. Thijssen (Nijmegen)

Treasurer
J.S. Hillman (Leeds)

(San Antonio)
A.M. Verbeek (Nijmegen)

HONORARY MEMBERS:

G. Baum (New York)
H. Gernet (Münster)
A. Oksala (Turku)
K.C. Ossoinig (Iowa City)
J. Vanysek (Brno)

PAST PRESIDENTS:

J. Vanysek (Brno) 1964–1967
A. Oksala (Turku) 1968–1971
H. Gernet (Münster) 1972–1976
K.C. Ossoinig (Iowa City)
1977–1980
H.G. Trier (Bonn) 1981–1985

PAST HONORARY
PRESIDENTS:

J. Böck (Wien)
A.H. Keeney (Louisville)
J. Vanysek (Brno)
K. Velhagen (Berlin)

Opening of SIDUO X by Professor Dr. Hans-Georg Trier, President of SIDUO

Professor Ossoinig, Ladies and Gentlemen:

It is with great pleasure that I welcome you, the members and guests of SIDUO, as you convene to participate in the 10th congress of our society. I am particularly pleased to greet our Honorary Members present in the audience – Professor Gilbert Baum and Professor Hermann Gernet.

It has now been 20 years since the first International Symposium for Diagnostic Ultrasound in Ophthalmology – SIDUO I – was held in Berlin, East Germany in 1964 under the scientific chairmanship of Werner Buschmann. As a consequence of this meeting, SIDUO as a scientific society was founded during the second symposium, SIDUO II, which was held in Brno, Czechoslovakia, in 1967. Thus, the 10th SIDUO Congress here in St. Petersburg is also an anniversary for the 20-year existence of the SIDUO concept. This is a good reason for inviting you to relive the history of SIDUO in a brief review.

In 1953, echo-cardiography and echo-encephalography originated from the University of Lund in Sweden. The following year, Howry in Denver, Colorado used intensity-modulated scanning techniques for the body. In 1956, Mundt and Hughes in Chicago were the first ones to describe an ultrasonic reflection technique for diagnostic use in ophthalmology; after that, ophthalmic diagnostic ultrasound became another rapidly developing field. At that time, the American Institute of Ultrasound (AIUM) already existed, but most of its members were engaged in work on ultrasonic therapy. In founding SIDUO, scientists in ophthalmology became the first group to constitute an international society for diagnostic ultrasound. At the same time, ophthalmology became the first medical discipline to have its own ultrasonographic society. During the next fifteen years, rapid technological and technical advances made diagnostic ultrasound a fascinating and sophisticated non-invasive examination of the eye and orbit. SIDUO contributed considerably to the rapid development of diagnostic ultrasound in ophthalmology, particularly through its biennial meetings. These conferences were characterized by an intensive and fruitful exchange of scientific and clinical information between ophthalmologists and scientists with a background in physics and engineering. After the first symposium in Berlin, the series of SIDUO conferences continued in different countries. Each conference added specific qualities to this scientific exchange.

I wish to review these SIDUO meetings briefly: SIDUO II in Brno, Czechoslovakia was organized by Jan Vanysek and Juliana Preisova in 1967. As I mentioned before, our Society was founded at this occasion.

SIDUO III was organized by Karl Ossoinig in Vienna in 1969. The scope of this meeting was greatly extended by inviting representatives of all medical disciplines engaged with ultrasonic diagnosis, thus forming the First World Congress on ultrasound. Arvo Oksala was SIDUO president at that time. SIDUO III had historical consequences by giving rise to the foundation of the World Federation of Ultrasound in Medicine and Biology – today a society of 15,000 members.

SIDUO IV, held in Paris in 1971, was organized by Marcel Massin and Jacques Poujol. SIDUO V, organized by Jules Francois and Frank Goes, took place in Ghent, Belgium in 1973. At that time, our president was Hermann Gernet. The next conference, SIDUO VI, in San Francisco in 1976, was again co-organized with the World Federation, whose chairman was Gilbert Baum. SIDUO VII, held in Muenster in West Germany in 1978, was directed by Hermann Gernet. President of SIDUO at that time was Karl Ossoinig.

The 1980 meeting, held in Nijmegen, The Netherlands, was presided over by Han Thijssen; and, last but not least, Jeffrey Hillman and the City of Leeds in Great Britain hosted SIDUO IX in 1982. While during the last few years technical progress in ultrasonography has slowed down, questions of education, effectiveness and quality assurance have, as in other medical disciplines, become more and more important. The same is true of the validation of ultrasonic findings in comparison to other non-invasive diagnostic methods.

I am convinced that in the future SIDUO will remain both valuable and necessary if the Society succeeds in dealing with these actual problems adequately. SIDUO X, finally, was convened in the United States because a significant number of our members live in this country. We have tried to enlist the support of all the important specialists in the country to cover during the meeting the full spectrum of advances made in our field. Additionally, a step toward the selection of more specific scientific topics in the various sessions has been made for this meeting.

On behalf of SIDUO, I thank all of you who have contributed so much toward making this meeting a success. We are particularly indebted to Professor Ossoinig who has taken over the burden of organizing this meeting with his well-known energy and skill, and also wish to heartily thank the organizational and advisory committees. I do hope that the extensive scientific program presented at this Congress will not diminish the pleasure the social program is intended to provide for you. I am sure that this meeting will consolidate the international contacts of the Society, and our personal ties and friendships. I feel very privileged to open the SIDUO X Congress.

Presentation of pioneer awards

Today's extensive application of diagnostic ultrasound in ophthalmology is based on the initial results of A- and B-mode echography. The names of two of our members particularly stand for pioneering work in the development of these techniques: that of ARVO OKSALA for A-mode, and of GILBERT BAUM for B-mode echography. SIDUO earlier recognized the merits of these men by bestowing Honorary Memberships upon both of them.

The SIDUO Executive Board decided to emphasize the important aspects of their work in the history of diagnostic ultrasound by bestowing upon them the SIDUO PIONEER AWARD.

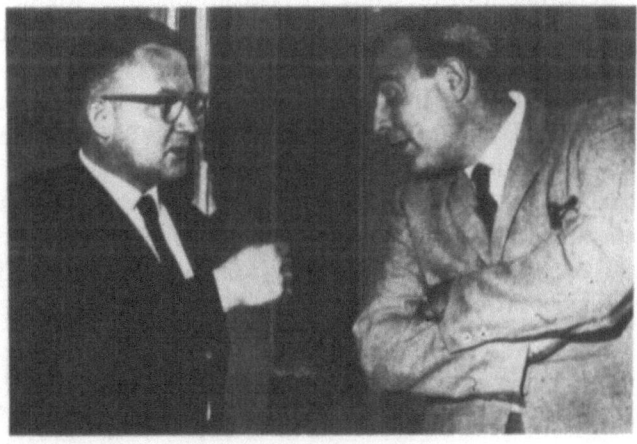

Arvo Oksala and Gilbert Baum at the International Symposium on Diagnostic Ultrasound in Ophthalmology, Italy 1968 (by courtesy of P.E. Gallenga).

Presentation to Gilbert Baum

Gilbert Baum was born in 1922 in New York City. After having studied at the University of Wisconsin and at the Long Island College of Medicine, he graduated as a Medical Doctor in 1945. He specialized in ophthalmology, and is a Diplomate of the American Board of Ophthalmology and the National Board of Medical Examiners, as well as a Fellow of the American Academy of Ophthalmology and Otolaryngology. He has been engaged in ultrasonic research since 1951.

His fundamental studies of the ultrasonic effects on ocular tissues are well known. His work, printed in numerous publications, also concerns the research and development of intensity-modulation techniques for ophthalmology. He demonstrated the feasibility of B-mode scanning of the eye, analyzed the influence of various equipment parameters, and developed optimized mechanical, ultrasonic and electronic equipment for high-resolution B-mode imaging with the potential of repeatable quantitative results. Professor Baum likewise developed new display techniques, such as video-inversion and deflection-modulation, and worked on three-dimensional documentation of B-mode results.

The image quality he achieved in his early work on several applications of B-mode echography of the eye has not been surpassed by later commercial techniques. His work has been generally accepted as being the basis for ophthalmic B-mode echography. It was summarized in his important book, 'Fundamentals of Medical Ultrasonography', published in 1975. Professor Baum likewise covers related fields, such as holography and ultrasonic mammography. Most of his work was done while director of the Ultrasound Service in the Eye Department of the Albert Einstein College of Medicine in New York City. His work has always been characterized by scientific accuracy and innovative thinking.

Gilbert Baum is an Honorary Member of SIDUO and of AIUM, as well as a past President of the WFUMB and of AIUM, and a Senior Member of the Institute of Electrical and Electronics Engineers. He was honored with several awards, including the AIUM Recognition Award in 1973, and the Honor Award of the American Academy of Ophthalmology in October, 1984.

Professor Baum, on behalf of the Society, I take great pleasure in presenting to you this Pioneer Award.

H.G. Trier
President of SIDUO

Presentation to Arvo Oksala

Mr. President, Members of the Executive Board, Ladies and Gentlemen:

It is with great pleasure that I fulfill my task to honor one of the most outstanding members of our Society: Professor Dr. Arvo Oksala. For those of you unfamiliar with the history of ultrasound in ophthalmology, I will note a few landmarks in the work of Professor Oksala. He started a 5-year cooperation with the physicist Annti Lehtinen in 1957. They published their first results on A-mode echography in 1957. Professor Oksala was at that time able to detect non-radiopaque foreign bodies, retinal detachments, subretinal tumors, and to peer behind a cataractous lens. Later on he performed experiments to investigate the potential of using A-mode echography to detect vitreous opacities, vitreous hemorrhages and vitreous detachments. In 1958 he demonstrated the detection of a scleral rupture, and in 1960 he published a paper regarding the differentiation of subretinal hemorrhage from solid tumor. The total results of his cooperation with Lehtinen amounted to 23 publications in 4 years.

His approach was, and still is, to differentiate pathologies by using the quantitative aspects of A-mode echo patterns. In 1962 he introduced the term 'selective echography' for this approach, and he has inspired many others to follow this route beyond mere detection to a differential diagnosis of ocular pathology. The work of Professor Oksala was appreciated by many ophthalmological societies, and our Society bestowed upon him an Honorary Membership in 1971.

At the occasion of this 10th biennial Congress and the 20th anniversary of SIDUO, the Executive Board has decided to bestow upon Professor Arvo Oksala the SIDUO PIONEER AWARD.

J.M. Thijssen
Secretary of SIDUO

Instrumentation and techniques for biometry

J.M. THIJSSEN
Nijmegen, The Netherlands

Introduction

The explosive spread of intraocular lens implantations has brought about an impressive development of instruments dedicated to ultrasonic biometry of the eye. The high accuracy of digitized electronics has enabled industry to construct equipment which meets the accuracy limits set by the demands for the prospective calculation of the implant lens power. Furthermore, the on line addition of the arithmic facilities of microcomputers has enhanced the accuracy of the biometry further by statistical processing and analysis of the biometric data.

Measurement techniques

The various methods to apply the ultrasound transducer to the eye, that are presently employed, are (cf. Fig. 1):
1. Direct application, either manually, or by using a slit lamp gantry.
2. Manual application of the transducer in an open scleral shell which is filled with a saline solution.
3. Direct application of the transducer equipped with a membrane-closed water stand-off, either manually, or by using a slit lamp gantry.

The advantages and disadvantages of these techniques are (cf. Table 1):

Ad 1. The direct application is rather simple, but two decisive disadvantages of it have to be mentioned: the cornea may be impressed by the rigid surface of the transducer to an unknown degree and therefore the biometry may be very inaccurate. The second problem arises from the overloading of of the receiver circuitry by the high voltage transmitting pulse. The location of anterior surface of the cornea cannot be accurately estimated and the biometry suffers from a considerable zero point error.

Ad 2. The scleral shell method is somewhat more laborious than the other

K.C. Ossoinig (editor), Ophthalmic Echography, ISBN 978-94-010-7988-4

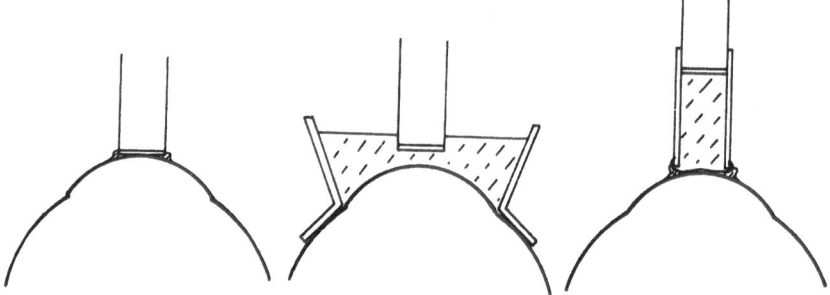

Fig. 1. Left: direct application of transducer on to cornea. Center: water filled scleral shell. Right: water filled closed water stand-off.

techniques, but it has the advantage that the skilled examiner can optimally align the sound beam along the optical axis of the eye.

Ad 3. The alignment is more difficult, especially in patients with a dense cataract and even more when the retinal projection is wrong, if the transducer is fixed in a slit lamp gantry. Furthermore, since contact is made between the membrane of the water stand-off and the cornea, the corneal echospike is of minor usefulness in the alignment procedure, and finally, indentation of the cornea may easily occur as well. The major advantage of the employment of a slit lamp gantry is the simplicity of the whole biometric procedure.

Estimation techniques and equipment (Tables 2, 3)

The estimation techniques employed in ocular biometry with ultrasound are the following:

1. The introduction of fully digitized signal processing of A-mode, or B-mode, echograms enables the measurement of the ocular dimensions after storage in a memory and subsequent display on a screen ('freeze frame'). Mostly calipers are then manually set and the distance between two points in

Table 1. Survey of advantages and disadvantages of measurement techniques.

Disadvantage		Advantage	
1.	Zero point error, corneal indentation	1.	Simple operation
2.	Laborious operation	2.	Optimal alignment
3.	Alignment, (indentation)	3.	Simple operation

Table 2. Survey of estimation techniques and equipment.

---

1. Frozen A-mode
2. Hard copied A-mode
3. Electronic systems
   3.1. Two gates manual level crossing, A-mode ('succesive')
   3.2. Multi gates, automatic, A-mode, ('segmented')
   3.3. Multi gates, automatic, histogram, ('segmented')
   3.4. Two gates, automatic, no display

---

the image displayed. Otherwise the dimensions have to be read directly from the screen, which introduces errors because of line thickness and parallax.

2. The other possibility to estimate the ocular dimensions is to make a hard copy of the A-mode echogram (either or not after freezing) e.g. by taking a picture. The equipment is often calibrated in micro seconds through a quartz controlled oscillator and a calibration signal derived from it is preferrably documented simultaneously with the echogram. The copied echogram is then employed to measure the dimensions.

3. Electronic devices are mostly integrated in the echographic equipment and provide an automatic measurement of the time between echospikes. This measurement is started by either manually or automatically setting so-called gates (Fig. 2), which are electronic square wave voltages during which electronic counters can be controlled. The level is sometimes variable by manual control, in order to adapt to the amplitude level of the echogram. When the leading edge of an echospike surpasses the level this event starts or halts a counter, or a counter is just read out. The oscillator is working at a very high frequency, e.g. 40 MHz, which yields technically a high measuring accuracy (0.08 mm).

Table 3. Survey of advantages and disadvantages of estimation techniques and equipment.

Disadvantage	Advantage
1. Line thickness, parallax, (calibration)	1. Optimal A-mode, (calipers)
2. Line thickness, (calibration)	2. Optimal A-mode, optimal (peak) level
3.1. Laborious operation	3.1. Interactive search
3.2. Echo identification	3.2. High accuracy
3.3. Worse alignment control	3.3. Indication of accuracy
3.4. Bad alignment control	3.4. Simple, cheap

4

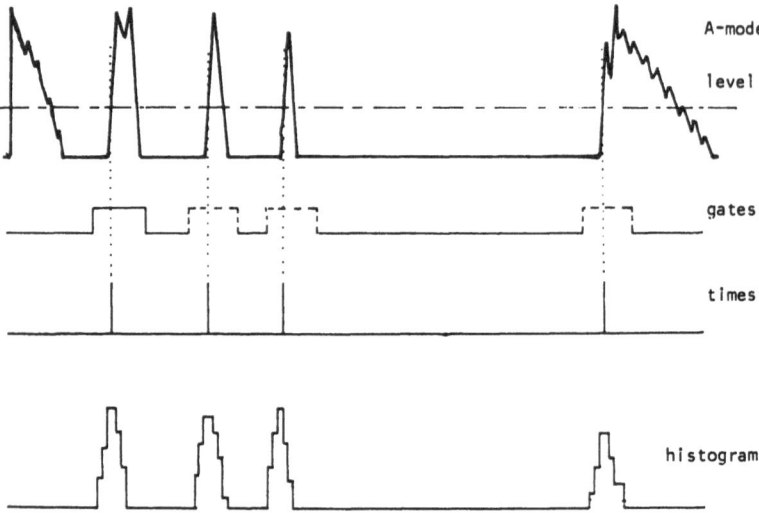

Fig. 2. Scheme of principles of electronic system to evaluate A-mode for biometry: Level crossings of echo spikes within gates yield time events which are employed to read-out an electronic counter. Lower trace: histogram display of time measurements.

The electronic devices can be divided in the following categories (cf. Tables 2, 3).

3.1. The equipment may employ just two gates, which can be set around two selectable echopeaks. If the dimensions of the various eye media have to be estimated several measurements have to be performed in succession.

3.2. An alternative is the employment of four gates simultaneously, which can be termed an automatic gate setting and segmented estimation of the axial length from the measured times between the various echo spikes. It is very important to have the A-mode echogram, as well as the position of the gates, available on the display in order to be able to align the sound beam through optimization of the echospikes, but also to detect any mistakes made by the level detection, due to false echoes (e.g. nuclear cataract echoes).

3.3. Another kind of equipment employing multi gates displays the histograms of the various distances instead of the A-mode echogram. The display is obtained after statistical processing of many subsequent echograms (e.g. 60) acquired in a short time (e.g. 50 ms). The advantage of averaging the measurements is obvious, but the displayed histograms cannot substitute the A-mode echogram.

3.4. A rather simple device is developed from thickness gauges used for non-destructive testing. It consists of two gates and the counter information is numerically displayed either in microseconds, or in millimeters. Although some pattern recognition may be built in to enhance the reliability of the measurement, no real adequate control of the beam alignment is present.

Conclusion

From the surveys of the pros and cons of the measurement techniques and estimation techniques the following 'ideal' system for ultrasonic biometry of the eye can be conceived:

    1. Transducer:
- broadband, high frequency, focussed
- both applicable with open and with closed water stand-off
- A-mode display

    2. Equipment:
- automatic, multi gates which are visible at A-mode screen
- rapid multiple measurements (within 0.1 s)
- statistical analysis
- (print out)
- (lens calculation)

'Simultaneous' versus 'successive' measurement of ocular segments in axial biometry. A statistical study on biometric data from cataractous eyes

H.G. TRIER, B. MEYER-SCHWICKERATH-SCHIWECK,
G. HILDENBRAND and R.D. LEPPER
Bonn, West-Germany

Introduction

Today, axial biometry is of great importance prior to IOL-surgery. This application justifies technical refinements in ultrasonic biometry, if these contribute significantly to the accuracy of IOL-calculations.

Table 1 gives a classification of the different available techniques regarding their key features.

Axial *segmental* biometry of the eye is characterized by separate measurement of ultrasonic transit-time for the three ocular segments: cornea and anterior chamber, lens, vitreous compartment. Segmental biometry can be carried out by *electronic measuring devices,* using digital interval counters or digital calipers in stored echograms (frozen A-mode). This study compares the two basic strategies of *simultaneous* or *successive* measurement, using a real-time electronic oculometer.

Table 1. Key features of different techniques for axial biometry of the eye.

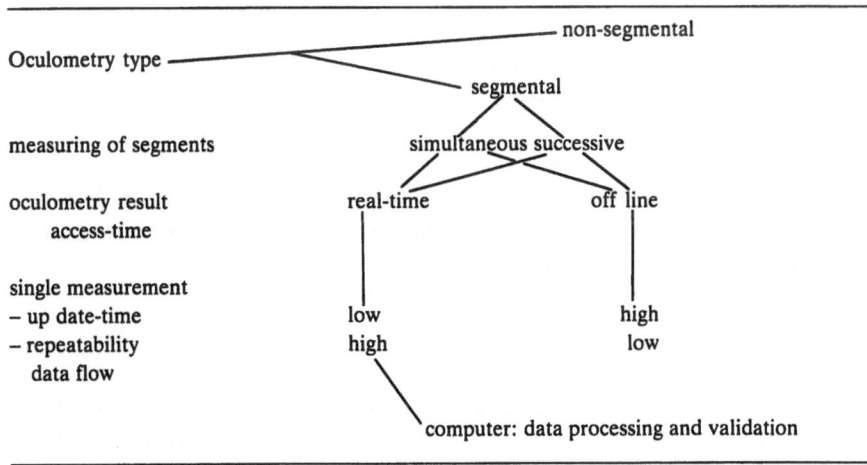

K.C. Ossoinig (editor), Ophthalmic Echography, ISBN 978-94-010-7988-4
© 1987, Martinus Nijhoff/Dr W. Junk Publishers, Dordrecht.

The features of the two strategies are as follows:

– *Successive* measuring of the segments is characterized by threefold setting and adjustment procedures for one electronic gate, thus leading to extended data collection time.
– *Simultaneous* measurement of the segments means that data collection, comprising measurement of all 3 segments, is completed during one single sound wave transit, that is during about 30 μs only.

The aim of this study was to clarify, if the two strategies lead to different results in axial biometry of cataractous eyes.

Methods

Strategy

300 cataractous eyes have been examined using a prototype of the real-time simultaneous-type oculometer RESSOURCE* developed by Lepper, Trier & Reuter [2]. This system provides computerized data collection, data reduction, storage and processing. Not only the final values of the ocular segments have been documented, but also the preceding reduced data, describing for each examined eye a sample of about 300–500 segmental single measurements by statistical parameters.

The basic idea was to understand the available simultaneous results as a special combination out of several measurements successively performed on the eye. It was assumed that by the successive procedure of measuring, single values for segmental lengths are obtained which belong somehow to the distribution curve of simultaneous-type segmental values. However, without using adequate data collection the user of a normal successive-type device does not know whether the measured value represents a maximal, minimal, or a nearly average value of the distribution. Basically, successive oculometry therefore involves the risk that three separate segmental length values create an artificial combination not really existing in the eye, which might be greater or smaller than the true axial-length value.

The structure of simultaneous-type data proved suitable to simulate different kinds of successive-type measurement, thus enabling a comparison of both techniques from the same sample.

---

* RESSOURCE-method = *R*eal-Time *S*imultaneous *S*egmental *O*culometry by *U*ltrasound with Data *R*ecording with *C*omputerized *E*valuation. Biometric System manufactured by Grieshaber & Co AG, Winkelriedstr. 52, 8203 Schaffhausen (Switzerland).

Measurement conditions and structure of original data

The patients were examined in supine position using the fellow-eye for fixation as far as vision decrease by cataract allowed. The examiner inserted a contact eye cup between the lids, filled it with saline, and held it in position by one hand. Then, an 8 Mhz-transducer of 5 mm crystal diameter with slight focusing was dipped into the cup using the other hand, without touching the eye. The transducer was perpendicularly adjusted to the echo giving interfaces, while looking at the A-mode display of the RESSOURCE system.

Data collection. Data structure is described in Table 2. For each eye a data array including a total of 5 ... 18 samples were taken, consisting of n = 32 data groups for each sample. Each data group, thus, included first 32 data for the segment cornea (C) + anterior chamber (A.C.), characterized by the calculated mean, the standard deviation, and histogram; second, 32 data for the lens; third, for the vitreous, and fourth, for the axial length, each one with the same statistical measures.

Features extracted from the simultaneous data array

From the total of simultaneous-type data, we selected in clinical routine the one sample that combined the highest frequency of distribution and the lowest standard deviation for all three segments. This sequence of data was considered the optimal result for the individual axial-length measurement and was utilized for IOL-calculation. In addition, the samples with the minimal and maximal axial length value were extracted (Table 3).

Table 2. Structure of a data array including K samples (K = 5 ... 18). C = cornea, A.C. = anterior chamber.

Sample 1.1	Data Collection Time 1/30 sec
n data groups (n = 22 ... 32), consisting of	
n data C + AC	$\bar{X}_a \pm 2s_a$ (μsec) (mm)
n data lens	$\bar{X}_b \pm 2s_b$
n data vitreous	$\bar{X}_c \pm 2s_c$
n data axial length	$\bar{X}_d \pm 2s_d$
Sample 1.2	
Sample 1.K	

Table 3. Features derived from RESSOURCE data, describing simultaneous type.

Feature	No. 4	AL 'optimal'	$\bar{x}_a + \bar{x}_b + \bar{x}_c)$
	No. 5	AL minimal[1]	Min $(\bar{x}_a + \bar{x}_b + \bar{x}_c)$
	No. 6	AL maximal[1]	Max $(\bar{x}_a + \bar{x}_b + \bar{x}_c)$

1 = based on mean values.

Simulation of successive-type data

A number of different combinations (features) were selected from the original simultaneous-type data in each eye in order to simulate different possible results of successive-type measurement (Table 4).

The features 19–22 simulate the worst case of successive measurement. However, in practice not a combination of extreme values, but of random values must rather be expected. Therefore, segmental values were selected from the distribution at random and were combined to a random axial-length value in feature 26. The different results of successive-type simulation were then compared with the results of the simultaneous type.

Results and discussion

Numerical results and tests of significance

Table 5 gives part of the numerical results, including mean, median, standard deviation s, variance s^2, minimum, maximum, and range of the features for axial length. (Results on segments alone are not considered here).

As an example, Fig. 1 shows the relative frequency distribution of the axial length composed at random, successive type (continuous line), and the 'optimal' axial length, simultaneous type (dotted line). For part of the features tests

Table 4. Features derived from RESSOURCE data, describing successive type.

Feature		
No. 19	AL minimal[2]	Min $(\bar{x}_a - 2s) + \text{Min}(\bar{x}_b - 2s) + \text{Min}(\bar{x}_c - 2s)$
No. 20	AL maximal[2]	Max$(\bar{x}_a + 2s) + \text{Max}(\bar{x}_b + 2s) + \text{Max}(\bar{x}_c + 2s)$
No. 21	AL minimal[1]	Min $\bar{x}_a + \text{Min } \bar{x}_b + \text{Min } \bar{x}_c$
No. 22	AL maximal[1]	Max $\bar{x}_a + \text{Max } \bar{x}_b + \text{Max } \bar{x}_c$
No. 26	AL random[2]	Zu $(\bar{x}_a \pm 2s) + \text{Zu } (\bar{x}_b \pm 2s) + \text{Zu } (\bar{x}_c \pm 2s)$

1 = based on mean value
2 = based on ± 2s ranges

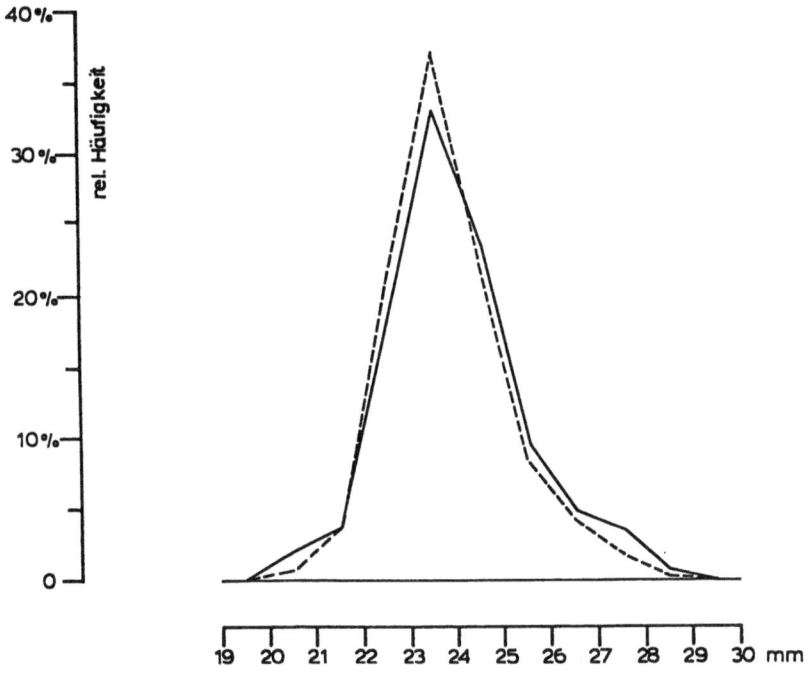

Fig. 1. Relative frequency distribution (smoothed). Continuous line = axial length values, combined from segments by random (successive type, feature 26; $\bar{X} = 23{,}91$ mm). Dotted line = axial length values, 'optimal' value, (simultaneous type, feature 4, $\bar{X} = 23{,}82$ mm).

Table 5. Numerical results. Simu = simultaneous type, succ = successive type, Ft = feature, $\bar{x}$ = mean, $\tilde{x}$ = median, s = standard deviation, s^2 = variance, min = minimal value, max = maximal value, R = range of values.

	Ft	$\bar{x}$	$\tilde{x}$	s	s^2	min	max	R
Simu min[1]	5	23.75	23.60	1.26	1.60	20.65	28.10	7.45
Simu max[1]	6	24.04	23.90	1.32	1.75	20.74	28.35	7.61
Succ min[2]	19	23.04	23.02	1.45	2.12	17.28	27.54	10.26
Succ max[2]	20	24.77	24.49	1.56	2.46	20.98	29.63	8.65
Succ min[1]	21	23.57	23.42	1.31	1.72	17.55	27.78	10.23
Succ max[1]	22	24.22	24.03	1.38	1.93	20.84	28.71	7.87
Simu opti	4	23.82	23.65	1.27	1.62	20.73	28.10	7.37
Succ random	26	23.91	23.74	1.44	2.10	20.31	28.72	8.41

1 = based on mean value, 2 = based on ± 2s ranges.

of significance were performed:
- the Kolmogoroff-Smirnov-test in order to prove normal data distribution
- the Wilcoxon-test for paired differences for features 4 vs. 26
- the Friedman-test and Wilcoxon-Wilcox-test for a number of features (see Table 6).

The comparison of
- feature 4: axial length, simultaneous-type, 'optimal' value vs
- feature 26: axial length, simulated successive type, composed at random, gave the following results:

The evaluation proved a significant difference on the 5%-level of error probability between the two distributions. The difference of means is 0.09 mm. In an eye of normal length this corresponds to ≈0.27 diopters of IOL power, which seems clinically significant. For successive-type measurements both the range of data (1.04 mm) and the variance (0.48 mm) are greater than those obtained by simultaneous measurements.

Discussion

The results prove that by the simulated successive method, even at the best, the axial length is measured less accurately than by the simultaneous method (features 4 vs 26). The comparison of the other features proves that in unfavourable cases successive measurement may cause very fargoing errors, thus leading to strong deviations from the optimal axial-length value.

Table 6. Test of significance in simultaneous type/successive type data. AL = axial length.

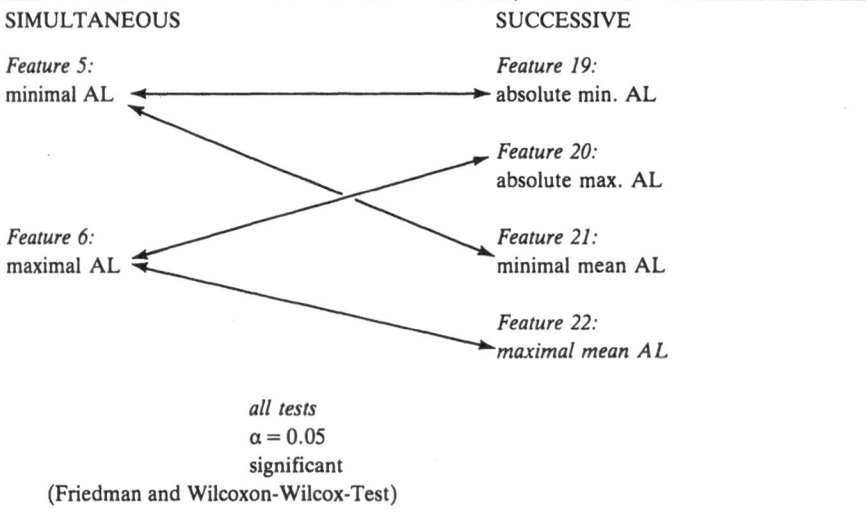

all tests
α = 0.05
significant
(Friedman and Wilcoxon-Wilcox-Test)

The observed differences between the methods point to the role of two factors:

- Superiority of *simultaneous* technique in segmental biometry. For the simultaneous method only corresponding segments combine, thus balancing each other with regard to the total axial length.
- *Computer data averaging*. This technique improves the results with the successive-type data gradually (compare features 20/22).

The analysis of distribution suggests that both factors are involved in the observed differences.

References

1. Meyer-Schwickerath-Schiweck B. Ultraschallmessung der Achsenlänge menschlicher Augen mit Katarakt. Eine statistische Analyse zum Meßergebnis mit zwei verschiedenen Verfahren. Thesis, University of Bonn, Med. Faculty 1984.
2. Lepper R-D, Trier HG, Reuter R. 1980. Neuartige Ultraschallbiometrie. Klin. Mbl. Augenheilk. 177: 101–108.

The results of this study were taken from thesis [2]; the statistical evaluation was advised by PD Dr. med. Gisela Hildenbrand.

Immersion ultrasonography and axial length measurements: a comparison of errors*

ROBERT DUDLEY STONE
San Francisco, USA

Introduction

In spite of the widespread availability and use of contact applanation instruments for the determination of axial length for IOL calculations, we have persisted in using the formal immersion-method of ultrasonography [3] for the procedure of axial length determination. Immersion axial length determination has several theoretical advantages [1, 4, 5, 6, 8], although a large clinical series utilizing this technique has not been available for comparison. We wanted to attempt to demonstrate that immersion ultrasonographic axial length determination was actually superior to the applanation technique. However, we were compromised by the multiple variables involved in the clinical setting, and have settled for a comparison of errors. Immersion ultrasonography does have certain advantages in that it allows for the simultaneous performance of serial scanned B-mode tomography in every eye sent for axial length determination. There were 26 patients in whom we discovered concomitant intraocular pathology that was unsuspected by the referring physician.

Methods and materials

We researched the cross reference files of the Ophthalmic Ultrasound Laboratory at the University of California, San Francisco, and noted those patients who were sent for an examination for the presence of a cataract or for an axial length determination and IOL power calculation. From a total of 515 patients who received immersion A-scan biometry from 5/14/79 to 12/16/83 in our laboratory, we were able to identify 268 patients from the University of California Eye Clinic and the University of California full time faculty for this

* Supported in part by an unrestricted grant from Research to Prevent Blindness, Inc., New York, New York.

K.C. Ossoinig (editor), Ophthalmic Echography, ISBN 978-94-010-7988-4

study. In attempting the review of these 268 patient records, we discovered that 151 eyes actually received an implant using our predicted value as a guideline for IOL implantation (128 patients received one implant, 15 patients received two implants), 34 patients did not receive the implant, 10 patients received the implant but not enough information was available in the record for this study, five implants were actually aborted during surgery, and 68 charts were not found. We, therefore, studied the 151 eyes receiving implants and for whom we had adequate information available. We had preoperative immersion axial length measurements using our technique, and preoperative keratometry (autokeratometry in 90%) from our laboratory records. The powers of lenses actually implanted were obtained from the patients' medical records. Using the powers of lenses actually implanted, the appropriately modified theoretical formula (Colenbrander) [9] used *pre*operatively for the predicted implant power, the *pre*operative immersion biometry and *pre*operative keratometry, we predicted a postoperative refractive error for each lens power actually implanted. We then compared the predicted postoperative refractive error to the actual postoperative refractive error obtained from the patients' actual records.

The controllable variables in this study consisted of the preoperative keratometry which was performed by the technicians in the Ultrasound Laboratory itself. Autokeratometry (Humphrey) was obtained in most (90%) and manual keratometry (B & L) was obtained in the remainder or whenever there was a question about the autokeratometry. The immersion A plus B scanning was done simultaneously using the Sonometrics Model 150 with the DBR 300 module. A 10 MHz weakly focused B-scan transducer was utilized in all cases for the simultaneous axial length determination and immersion tomography. Positioning of the sound path was done visually utilizing the B-scan oscilloscope screen. We therefore felt we were able to better position the sound beam along the most appropriate axis for measurement. The same modified theoretical formula [9] was utilized for all calculations with assumed anterior chamber depths of 3.50 mm for all anterior chamber lenses and 4.00 mm for all posterior chamber lenses. All preoperative predictions were for emmetropia.

The uncontrolled variables in this study consisted of K-readings which were supplied by the referring physician, the lens actually chosen for implantation (manufacturer, style) and the surgical technique utilized. During this study, over 30 different surgeons were involved in the actual operation and implantation utilizing our prediction. This is because the majority of these patients came from our Clinic Teaching Service.

Our comparison of errors, therefore, consisted of calculating predictions for the postoperative error (Rx spherical equivalent) for emmetropia using the preoperative keratometry, preoperative axial length, and the lens power actually implanted (from the records). We then made a comparison of the predicted postoperative error (Rx spherical equivalent) for emmetropia with the actual postoperative refraction (from the records).

Results and discussion

Our intraocular lens power prediction technique, therefore, utilizing immersion axial eye length determination, keratometry, and a theoretic formula (Colenbrander) produces satisfactory results for our purposes in a large teaching university hospital setting (Table 1). While a regression formula technique [10] might have certain advantages in the hands of one surgeon who is able to control all of the variables, we have felt that a regression calculation technique would be too cumbersome in our teaching university hospital setting. During the course of this particular study, for example, approximately 30 different surgeons of all degrees of expertise were involved. 21 different styles of lenses were implanted. These and other factors make the regression formula technique too cumbersome to be used accurately to its full advantage in our physician/patient population. We feel that while immersion ultrasonography has certain minor disadvantages in setting up the water bath for each case, it has a high degree of accuracy. All 151 eyes available for this study are included in this data summary. The final visual acuity range from 20/200 to 20/15. The average best final visual acuity was approximately 20/40 (39.80). The average predicted IOL implant power was +18.40 diopters. The average IOL power actually used for implantation was +19.19 diopters. The average predicted postoperative refractive error by the technique we described was −0.66 diopters (spherical equivalent). The average actual postoperative refractive error found in the patients' chart upon review was −0.63 diopters (spherical equivalent). The average actual difference between the predicted postoperative refractive error and the actual postoperative refractive error was 0.01 diopters

Table 1. Summary of data for 151 eyes reviewed by the method described in the text. Please refer to the results and discussion in the text for comments.

151 Eyes available for this study						
	Pred. Powr.	Powr. Used	Pred. Rx	Postop. Rx	Diff. Rx	VA
AVG	18.40	19.19	− 0.66	− 0.63	0.01	39.80
STD	3.41	2.63	1.28	1.42	1.03	33.30
VAR	11.64	6.90	1.64	2.02	1.06	
MIN	6.83	10.00	− 6.50	− 7.25	− 3.63	15.00
MAX	28.05	27.00	4.60	5.00	4.27	200.00

(spherical equivalent) using our technique. The standard deviation of this difference in predicted versus postoperative refractive error was 1.03. This is sometimes called the Standard Error of Estimate or S.E.E. [7]. The calculated deviation, using the method recommended by Sanders, et. al [10], for this series averaged -0.09 diopters. The deviation, using the method recommended by Binkhorst [2] averaged -0.01 diopters on the other hand.

Our intraocular lens power prediction technique, therefore, utilizing immersion axial eye length determination, keratometry, and a theoretic formula (Colenbrander) produces satisfactory results for our purposes in a large teaching university hospital setting.

Acknowledgements

Sharon Humphrey, R.D.M.S., Marvin Zielinski, C.O.T., Jane Rubatzky, B.S., and Larry Wong, were technicians in the Ultrasound Laboratory during this study. Nancy King typed the manuscript. The statistics were prepared utilizing an IBM PC XT computer and Lotus 123 and DBase III software programs. Hyo J. Kim, M.D., provided Computer Sciences consultation in the analysis of data and preparation of graphic materials.

References

1. Binkhorst RD. 1975. The optical design of intraocular lens implants. Ophthal Surg 6: 17–31.
2. Binkhorst RD. 1976. Pitfalls in the determination of intraocular lens power without ultrasound. Ophthalmic Surg 7: 69.
3. Coleman DJ, Lizzi FL, Jack RL. 1977. Ultrasonography of the eye and orbit. Lea & Febiger, Philadelphia, p. 353–357.
4. Dallow RL (ed). 1979. Ophthalmic Ultrasonography: Comparative techniques. Int Ophthal Clin 19 (4): 1–310.
5. Dallow RL. 1983. The eye. In Goldberg BB, Wells PNT (eds) Ultrasonics in clinical diagnosis. Churchill Livingstone, p. 167–179.
6. Gernett H, Franceschetti A. 1967. Ultrasonic biometry of the eye. In Oksala, A, Gernett H. (eds) Ultrasonics in ophthalmology. Karger, Basel, p. 175–200.
7. Hoffer KJ. 1982. Preoperative cataract evaluation: Intraocular lens power calculation. Int Ophthalmol Clin 22 (2): 37–75.
8. Jansson F. 1963. Measurements of intraocular distances by ultrasound. Acta ophthal 74 (suppl): 1–51.
9. Kollarits CR, Little J, Kollarits FJ. 1978. Calculation of intraocular lens power using the Texas instruments ti programmable 59 calculator. Am Intra-ocular Implant Soc J. 4 (July): 90–98.
10. Sanders D, Retzlaff J, Kraff M, et. al. 1981. Comparison of the accuracy of the Binkhorst, Colenbrander, and SRK implant power prediction formulas. Am Intra-ocular Implant Soc J 7 (fall): 337–340.

Biometry with the echo-memory of the ophthason A 11 equipment

V. TANEV and N. MUDROV
Sofia, Bulgaria

Ultrasound biometry is widely applied in ophthalmology. Most frequently the A-scan is made use of.

The ophthason A 11 equipment secures prompt and easy ophthalmometry for the purposes of routine ophthalmological practice. It allows the measurement of elements of the globe along its anatomical axis, as well as clinical echometry, including the measurement of the thickness of the choroid, the optic nerves, extraocular muscles, etc.

To measure the separate areas of the globe along its anatomical axis – cornea, anterior chamber, lens, and vitreous, ophthason A 11 is equipped with an adapter for ultrasonic biometry, designed by V. Tanev (Fig. 1). This adapter allows the coupling of the echographic probe to the patient's eye.

The adapter is made of three parts. The lowermost one is a scleral ring, with a radius (r) between 10,4 and 13,2 mm, and with a length [1] of 2 to 5 mm. This part of the adapter rests upon the eye. Higher up the cylindrical part of the adapter is situated, corresponding to the dead zone of the probe. The upper

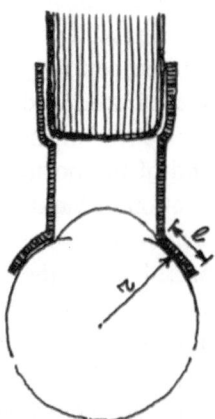

Fig. 1. Biometry with the echo memory of the Ophthason A 11.

K.C. Ossoinig (editor), Ophthalmic Echography, ISBN 978-94-010-7988-4

part of the adapter varies in shape, depending on the employed probe. It secures fixation of the probe. This construction enables a stable coupling of the probe to the eye. Good visualization of the corneal echo is provided. The adapter does not touch the cornea and thus avoids any deformation of the cornea.

Now coupling is effected with the sclera, the device being adapted to its radius. Stable contact between probe, adapter and eye as well as fixation of the globe are secured; thus the ultrasonic beam passes along the anatomical axis of the eye independent of the visual acuity or whether the ocular media are transparent.

The adapter may be easily sterilized with mercury oxycyanate or hibitane. Disposable adapters may be used too.

In routine practice the examination of various age groups (from newborn to elderly patients) may be performed using a kit of three adapters whose radius of curvature (r) and scleral ring lengths [1] vary as follows:

r (mm)	1 (mm)
10,4	2
12,0	4
13,2	5

To facilitate biometry, a digital memory with a 1 kbyte capacity is incorporated into the apparatus. Preliminary analog-to-digital conversion is accomplished with an equivalent frequency of 20 MHz. The electronic markers used to measure the distances are mobile on the screen and may be fixed upon desired points of the displayed image.

Biometry is accomplished in the following manner: after conventional local anesthesia of the eye, the adapter is placed underneath the lid directly upon the sclera. The cornea remains free centrally. The adapter is filled with physiological saline and the probe is introduced into it.

On the oscilloscope display the echoes of the cornea, of the anterior and posterior capsule of the lens, and of the posterior ocular wall should have maximal amplitude. Thus propagation of the ultrasonic beam along the ana-tomical axis is secured. With the help of the manual 'memory' knob or a foot switch, the echogram is memorized. Now the adapter and the probe are removed from the patient's eye.

During biometry, amplification is accomplished with a linear or a log-arithmic amplification. However, with linear amplification, the echoes are more conspicuous. Then the markers are moved on the screen and are fixed on the desired points of the displayed memorized signals.

Of special importance is the alignment of the marker to the signal of the ocular posterior wall which is concave. Initially several minor echo signals appear in front of the main signal as a result of the ultrasonic beam hitting a concave surface. The main echo corresponds to the center of the concave surface of the posterior wall. To measure very small distances (e.g., the thickness of the cornea) the electronic markers are set on the peaks of the echo signals.

To achieve greater accuracy, the memorized echogram may be stretched out with a special dial. To approximate the peaks of the echoes to the marker peaks, the decibel memory regulator or the vertical dark lines of the oscilloscope screen may be used. Distances are automatically plotted in microseconds or mm and are displayed on the oscilloscope screen. The variable velocity of the ultrasonic propagation in various parts of the globe has been considered. For the anterior chamber and the vitreous a velocity of 1534 m/ sec., and for the lens a velocity of 1647 m/sec., were applied in the calculations.

For other clinical applications of biometry, such as the measurement of choroidal thickness, the height of intraocular lesions, measurements of muscle and optic-nerve thicknesses, etc., the ultrasonic probe is positioned directly on the globe; again, the memorizing possibilities of the ophthason A 11 are used.

With this equipment, one measurement does not take more than three minutes and measurements of high accuracy are obtained.

The accuracy of ultrasonic biometry of the eye in dependence on the examiner's skill

R.-D. LEPPER and H.G. TRIER
Bonn, FRG

Since 1978 more than 10.000 patients in the Bonn university eye clinic have been measured by means of computerized biometry with ultrasound for the purpose of determining an individual intraocular implant lens (Lepper et al., 1980). In 1981 (Lepper & Trier, 1984a) we developed an improved computerized biometric system (BMS 811 ECHOCOMP, now GBS, Grieshaber). These systems can be described by the word RESSOURCE (which means: 'RE'al time 'S'imultaneous 'S'egmental 'O'culometry by 'U'ltrasound with data 'R'ecording and 'C'omputerized 'E'valuation). The system consists of: a personal computer, ultrasonic transceiver, 4 electronic clocks, and an evaluation logic (Fig. 1).

A special feature of the biometric system is the permanent function check especially the time base check of the clocks. This check is performed without user intervention as a background job. Electronic malfunction is indicated promptly. Therefore, the user can be sure the instrument is functioning correctly.

The electronic accuracy of our RESSOURCE-system is +/− 0.02 mm (clock frequency 40 MHz). The question arose, whether this precision meets the needs in daily routine determination of intraocular implant lens power. The answer to this question could not (solely) be given in terms of pre- and postoperative 'refractive balance' (Lepper & Trier, 1984b). As we wanted to

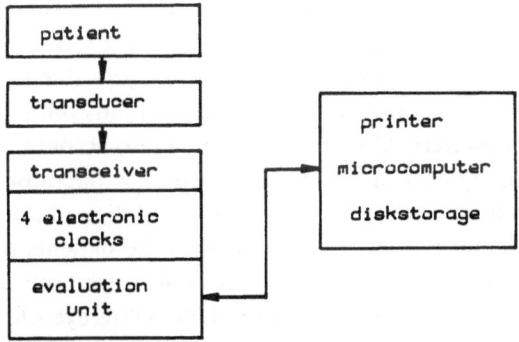

Fig. 1. Functional block diagram of the RESSOURCE-system used. The electronic resolution corresponds to .02 mm (BMS 811 ECHOCOMP, Ruck Opthalm Syst and GBS, Grieshaber).

K.C. Ossoinig (editor), Ophthalmic Echography, ISBN 978-94-010-7988-4

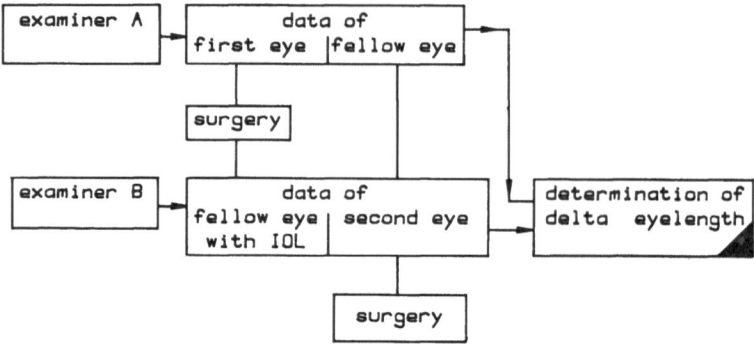

Fig. 2. Measurement strategy for the determination of an individual intraocular lens power, patient and examiner 'flow'.

exclude surgical effects we decided to look for the differences of the axial length of actual cataract patients being measured twice.

Material and methods

The routine measurements in our laboratory are performed by physicians. The patient is placed in a supine position and a small funnel placed under his lids. After filling the funnel with water, the physician manually adjusts a hand held transducer coaxially to the patients eye, thus compensating for individual exophoria problems.

The use of aiming devices was experimentally tried, too. However, as cataract patients often have fixation problems, this method proved not to be very useful in daily routine.

Our RESSOURCE-system usually displays several sets of eye length data. Each set represents 32 single measurements which are evaluated according to statistical measures by the computer. The eye length value is the sum of the three axial distances (anterior chamber, lens, vitreous body). The different velocities in different parts of the eye are taken into account.

According to the quality of the measurements the operator decides which data set he wants to accept for the following calculation of the IOL. The two selected sets of data are printed and kept with the patients record. For the purpose of minimizing aniseiconia we always measure both eyes of our patients. Many patients return for treatment of the fellow eye a few months later enabling us to measure the fellow eye a second time with the same system. In many cases the second measurement is performed by a different examiner, as the physicians rotate every 3 months. Figure 2 demonstrates the measurement strategy.

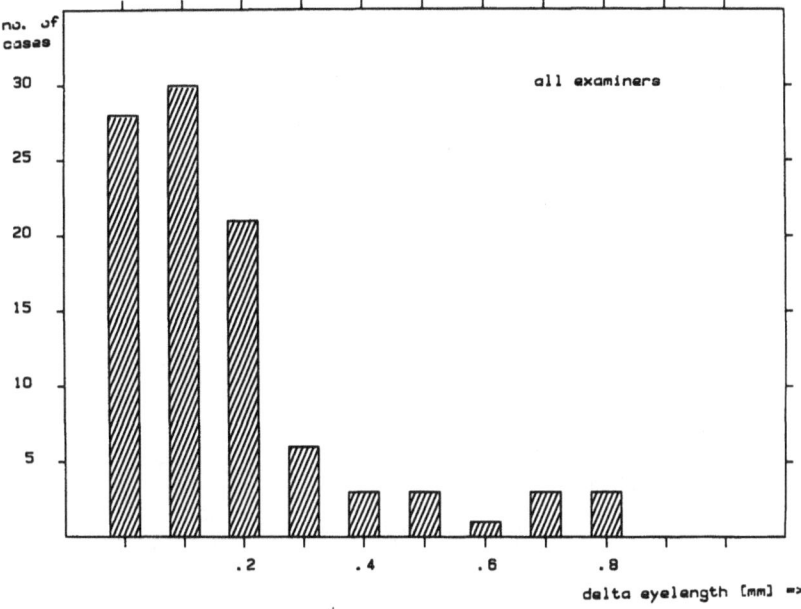

Fig. 3. Measurement differences of the axial length in 98 patients with the same eye measured twice at different times (all examiners).

Results

We collected 98 patients where we measured the fellow eye twice. In Fig. 3 the distribution of the differences of the axial length values is shown. It should be noted that a major part (86.7%) of the measurements agree to 0.3 mm. This roughly corresponds to a refractive error of one diopter. However, some major measurement errors need explaining, as electronic malfunction can be excluded.

The larger discrepancies are most likely due to pathological conditions of the eye. This was the result of a study made by Meier & Haefliger (1984). They showed that a pathological change of the shape of the posterior pole e.g. tilted disk or posterior staphyloma can cause several millimeters uncertainty of the eye length value. In these cases an additional B-scan examination seems necessary to improve accuracy of the biometry. As the measurements were performed by several examiners there must be a correlation of the accuracy with the examiner, too. Figure 4 a) and b) demonstrate the measurement differences for two examiners.

To get a rough idea in how far an examiner acts onto a patients eye Table 1 demonstrates the percentage of cases in which an individual examiner tended to measure the eye as 'shorter'.

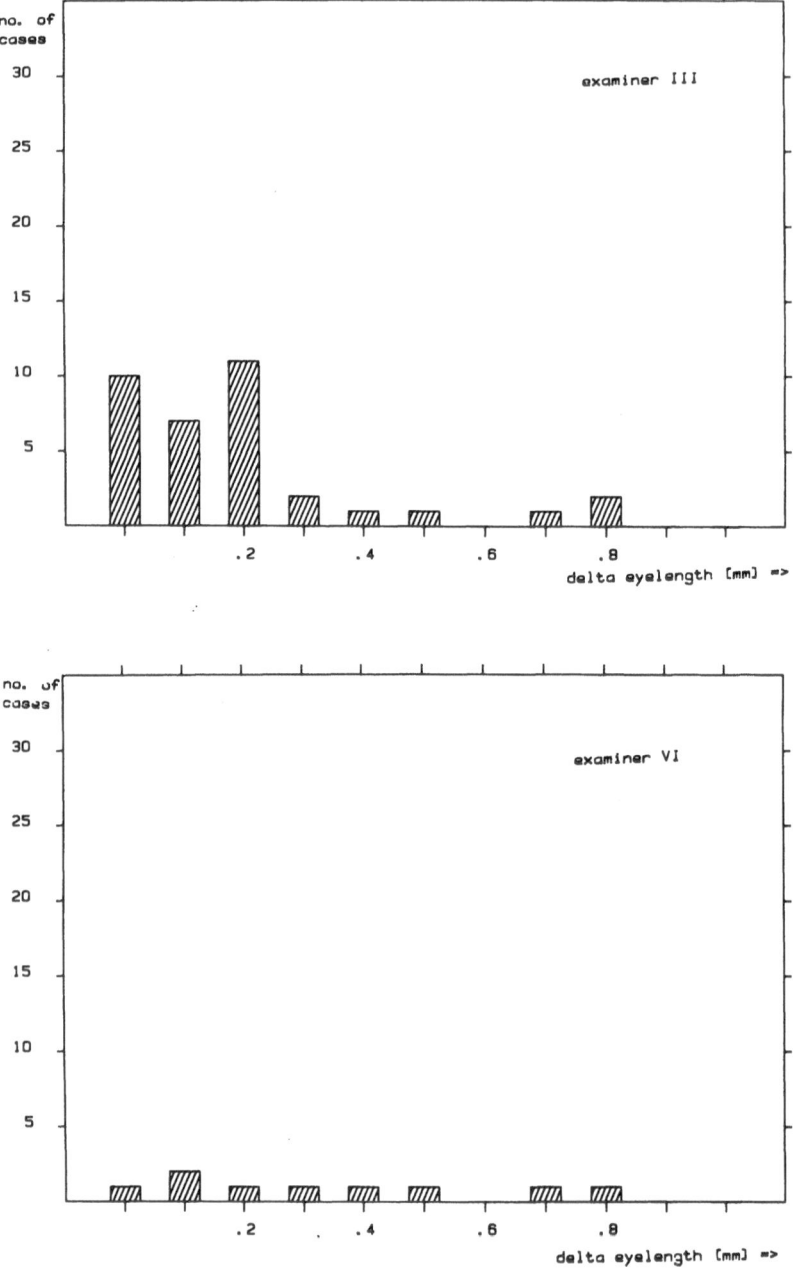

Fig. 4 a) and b). Measurement differences of the axial length of patients measured by two examiners against the values measured by others (or the same).

examiner	no. of. examinations	globe compression % of cases
I	22	36
II	10	40
III	41	41
IV	17	41
V	16	50
VI	11	55
VII	30	63
VIII	34	71

Table 1. Percentage of measuring a 'shorter eye' by a single examiner with respect to the second measurement of the same eye by a different (or the same) examiner. Not included are examiners with less than 10 measurements.

Discussion

Evidently the average measurement discrepancy of 0.17 mm exceeds by far the electronic precision of our instrument. When excluding apparative malfunction we must conclude that the measurement was not performed optimally in every case.

As the physicians use water to fill the funnel there is a leakage problem sometimes. In order to overcome this leakage problem the newcomer tends to press the funnel onto the globe thus compressing the eye. This results in a 'shorter eye'. Table I demonstrates globe compression. The differences between different examiners are remarkable. If e.g. all were equally good they all would have a chance of 50% to compress.

Optimal transducer position is adjusted by the examiner. The criterion most often used is a steep corneal echo combined with a steep echo from the posterior pole of the eye. This criterion implies a relatively precise prealignment of the transducer to the optical axis of the eye by means of visual inspection. If the transducer is adjusted as described, the lens echoes are usually measurable in the same position, too.

However there are some cases where it is impossible to achieve a steep backwall echo with the transducer aligned on-axis. This is very often the case in high myopia and with posterior staphyloma. Being trained to adjust the transducer for a steep backwall echo the examiner readjusts the transducer in these cases giving more or less erroneous results. In these cases we recommend to align the transducer to the optical axis by means of visual inspection and select the shortest axial length value measured with the highest sound intensity available (Gernet, 1984).

Conclusions

Ultrasonic biometric devices have been improved to the extent that measurement errors are due to the unskilled examiner. Even trained examiners sometimes have difficulties obtaining correct measurements in cases of severe cataract or pathological conditions at the posterior pole. We have to conclude that a further increase in electronic accuracy is of no use in practical terms of IOL determination. On the other hand the biometric system used should have a minimum resolution which corresponds to 0.25 dpt. IOL power: This is 0.08 mm resolution of axial length or at least 10 MHz counting frequency.

The variability of the data demonstrates that no automatic system is capable of deciding whether the transducer is aligned properly or not as sometimes even the examiner is not able to decide on this correctly.

References

Gernet H. 1984. Private communication.

Lepper R-D, Trier HG & Reuter R. 1980. Neuartige Ultraschallbiometrie Klin Mbl Augenheilk 177: 101.

Lepper R-D & Trier HG. 1984. Computerized ocular biometry: a newly developed compact system. Proc SIDUO IX, Leeds U.K. 1982; Ophthalmic Ultrasonography, Hillman, J.S. & M.M. Le May eds. pp. 237–241 (W Junk Publ, The Hague).

Lepper R-D & Trier HG. 1984. Refraction after intraocular lens implantation: Results with a computerized system for ultrasonic biometry and for implant lens power calculation Proc. SIDUO IX, Leeds U.K. 1982; Ophthalmic Ultrasonography, Hillman, J.S. & M.M. Le May eds, pp. 243–248 (W. Junk Publ., The Hague).

Meier U & Haefliger E. 1984. Die Fundus-Asymmetrie-Supertraktion der Papille und hinteres Sklerastaphylom – als Fehlerquelle bei der Berechnung intraokularer Linsen Klin Mbl Augenheilk 185 (1984): 259–262 (F. Enke, Stuttgart, 1984).

Measuring intraocular lens power within the eye

T.C. PRAGER, J.T. HOLLADAY, S.A. LONG, J.W. LEWIS, C.J. KOES-
TER, K.A. BOURGEOIS and T.L. WINN
Houston, USA

Abstract

Although various methods exist for confirming the power of an intraocular lens (IOL) prior to implantation, few clinicians perform this step due to the improved quality control by manufacturers, 5, 6, 7, the risk of contamination and the increased surgical time. After the lens has been implanted, however, there has been no method described for directly measuring the power. We present a method using slit lamp photography which measures with an average error of only 0.25 D the IOL power within the eye.

A method is described for determining the power of an intraocular lens (IOL) within the eye by measuring the horizontal dimension of the corneal reflected image (Purkinje-Sanson I) and the anterior IOL reflected image (Purkinje-Sanson III) as seen through a standard slit lamp with a target approximately 68 mm in front of the cornea. The horizontal K-reading (180 degrees) and the anterior chamber depth are the two other parameters necessary to calculate the exact power of the IOL. Seven tables have been provided which utilize these four measurements, eliminating the need for complex calculations.

To determine the accuracy of his technique, ten implanted IOL's ranging from 9 D to 27 D were chosen, their power calculated and compared to the actual IOL power. The largest error was 0.5 D and the average error was 0.25 D.

K.C. Ossoinig (editor), Ophthalmic Echography, ISBN 978-94-010-7988-4

Postoperative computer refraction of implant patients

RICHARD D. BINKHORST
New York, USA

The formula used to calculate the intraocular lens (IOL) power for emmetropia contains the following variables: the refracting power of the cornea, the axial length, and the anterior chamber depth. The formula was expanded to contain a fourth variable, the desired refraction, to calculate the IOL power required to achieve this refraction [1]. The latter formula is more useful in preoperative IOL power calculation than the formula for emmetropia because emmetropia is usually not the goal. One may aim at a different refraction, e.g. to match a fellow eye with good vision, while in general one aims at a small amount of myopia to compensate for the lack of accommodation in the artiphakic eye and to avoid an error on the hyperopic side.

Since pre- an postoperative astigmatism are usually different, one uses the average of the refracting power of the cornea in the principal meridians for preoperative IOL power calculation. The postoperative refractive state one aims at is thus actually the spherical equivalent of the postoperative refraction.

The same formula can be used for a different application by solving the equation for the refraction rather than for the IOL power. Thus the formula can be used to calculate the refraction of implant patients postoperatively given the refracting power of the cornea, the axial length, the IOL power used, and the anterior chamber depth. Moreover, one can now make the calculation separately for the two principal meridians of the cornea. The difference in the refractions of these meridians is then the spectacle cylinder, either in plus cylinder form or in minus cylinder form, depending on which meridian is used for the sphere.

A program was developed for Texas Instruments 58 and 59 calculators [1], no longer manufactured but still widely used, and their replacement, the Texas Instruments Compact Computer (CC-40) [2]. This program determines the postoperative refraction of implant patients. Since it is based on ultrasonic measurement of the axial length and external K-readings, the results are not dependent on clarity of the media and size of the pupil, as is the case with retinoscopy and automated refractors. It is only necessary, at each postopera-

K.C. Ossoinig (editor), Ophthalmic Echography, ISBN 978-94-010-7988-4

32

```
IOL Power, Pgm 4
Postop Refraction
[C] Copyright Dr.R.D.Binkhorst 1984

K-reading 1    45.25
Axis K1            75
K-reading 2    43.50
Axis K2           165
Axial length   23.57
AC depth        4.20
IOL power      19.00


REFRACTION
 -1.90 +1.78 x 165
 -0.12 -1.78 x  75
Vertex dist    12.00
Spher equiv    -1.01
```

Fig. 1. Printout of computer refraction of artiphakic eye.

tive visit, to take the K-readings. One may use the preoperative axial length throughout the postoperative period. Further required are the IOL power used and the anterior chamber depth or an estimation thereof (Fig. 1).

This study analyzes the results of this program for computer refraction for 198 eyes of 146 implant patients referred for a visual problem. The K-readings were obtained with a duly calibrated Haag-Streit keratometer. The axial lengths were measured with a Sonometrics Digital Biometric Ruler, model DBR-300, an A-scan ultrasonic instrument the accuracy of which has been established previously [3].

Table 1 shows a comparison between the computed refractions and the manifest refractions of 134 eyes with a visual acuity of 20/40 or better. The sphere of the computed refraction was within 0.50 D in 70% and the cylinder was within 0.50 D in 87%. The cylinder axes were within 5 degrees in 87%. These findings are in good agreement with previously reported results [4].

The standard deviations would be the measure of accuracy of the computed refractions. However, the manifest refractions were used as a basis for comparison. Assuming the accuracy of the manifest refractions to be 0.25 D it was calculated from the respective variances that the accuracy of the computed

```
IOL Power, Pgm 4
Postop Refraction
[C] Copyright Dr.R.D.Binkhorst 1984

K-reading 1  45.00
Axis K1         90
K-reading 2  42.75
Axis K2        180
Axial length 23.45


REFRACTION
+10.60 +1.64 x 180
+12.24 -1.64 x  90
Vertex dist  12.00
Spher equiv +11.42
```

Fig. 2. Printout of computer refraction of aphakic eye.

refractions was 0.27 D for the sphere and 0.14 D for the cylinder. The greater accuracy for the cylinder is explained by the fact that the cylinder depends mostly on the difference between the K-readings rather than on the K-readings and the axial length [5].

The 64 eyes with visual acuity less than 20/40 were excluded from the study because the manifest refractions were felt to be less accurate. In fact, the poorer the visual acuity, the more the computed refraction was relied on. When visual acuity was 20/200 or less, it was rarely possible to improve on the

Table 1. Comparison between computed refractions and manifest refractions in 134 artiphakic eyes.

	sphere	cylinder
Average error in diopters	−0.12	−0.01
Average deviation in diopters	0.41	0.21
Standard deviation in diopters	0.37	0.21

computed refraction. Yet, subjectively, the patients felt often that the computed refraction was of considerable help to them.

In conclusion it can be stated that computer refraction is a valuable time-saver in the postoperative management of all implant patients, and that it is especially useful in arriving at an accurate correction of implant patients with poor visual acuity.

The program is equally useful for aphakic refractions. Only the K-readings and the axial length are then required [3] (Fig. 2).

References

1. Binkhorst RD. 1978. Intraocular Lens Power Calculation Manual – A Complete Guide to the Author's TI-59 Programs. New York, Binkhorst.
2. Binkhorst RD. 1984. Intraocular Lens Power Calculation Manual – A Guide to the Author's TI CC-40 Programs, 3rd ed. New York, Binkhorst.
3. Binkhorst RD. 1981. The accuracy of ultrasonic measurement of the axial length of the eye. Ophthal Surg 12 (5): 363–365.
4. Banfiel RA, Pallin SL, Walman GB. 1981. A-scan/keratometry post-op refraction. Am Intra-Ocular Implant Soc 7: 272.
5. Binkhorst RD. 1979. The cause of excessive astigmatism with intraocular lens implants. Ophthalmology 86: 672–674.

Ultrasonic biometry for lens implantation: analysis of systematic errors

J.M. THIJSSEN and R.M.M. BOERRIGTER
Nijmegen, The Netherlands

Summary

Systematic errors in the echographic biometry of the eye are discussed: correction applied to the thickness of the retina, deviation of the visual axis from the optical axis of the eye and the errors arising from the employment of a single average ultrasound velocity in the eye media. The effects of the systematic errors on the results of the optical calculation of the emmetropizing power of implant lenses are investigated. The effects on the SRK calculation method are indicated and appear to be of the same order of magnitude as those on the optical method. The optical method yields unbiased lenspowers, whereas the SRK method produces refraction errors which systematically depend on the implant lens power.

Introduction

The preoperative estimation of lens implants is generally based on data obtained from the ultrasonic biometry of the axial length of the eye and the keratometry. The estimation is derived from a calculation based on geometrical optics, while using the refractive indices of the eye media. However, many assumptions are still to be made: the effective refractive index of a simplified cornea, the postoperative location of the implanted lens, and the thickness of the retina. Moreover, for practical reasons the echograms are evaluated often by taking into account a single average sound velocity of the eye media. So, even if it is taken for granted that the optical calculations are correct several sources of systematic errors are to be expected. Added to this category of errors additional inaccuracy is caused by the echographic measurement itself, because apart from the instrumental read-out the exactness of the alignment of the sound beam through the center of the eye ball may also cause substantial errors in the estimation of the axial length.

K.C. Ossoinig (editor), Ophthalmic Echography, ISBN 978-94-010-7988-4

We recently undertook a study to evaluate the findings of 200 eyes with an implanted posterior chamber lens (Boerrigter et al. 1984). Three questions had to be answered:

1. Does the preoperative clinical information (refractive error, keratometry) allow an accurate prediction of the emmetropizing implant lens?
2. What is the quality of ultrasonic biometry when combined with an optical calculation of the lens power (Thijssen, 1975)?
3. What is the quality of ultrasonic biometry when combined with a regression formula (Sanders and Kraff, 1980; Retzlaff, J., 1980).

The answer to the first question was negative because an adequate prediction based on clinical information was accurate (+ 2D limits for the refractive error) in only 62% of the cases. The optical calculation was correct in 76% and the regression approach in 90% of the cases. It must be concluded that the regression formula (SRK-formula), when adequately estimated, for the considered measurement set-up is superior.* In this contribution the possible improvements on the systematic errors involved in the optical method will be discussed.

The optical method: systematic error analysis

The formula employed in the optical calculations to obtain the emmetropic implant lens (cf. Thijssen, 1975):

$$P_e = n_v/(L - d_a - d_l \, n_v/n_l) - n_a/(\, n_a/K - d_a - d_l) \tag{1}$$

with P_e = emmetropizing power of implant lens (D)
  n_v; n_a; n_l = refraction index of vitreous; acqueous, implant lens
  L   = axial length   (m)
  d_a = anterior chamber depth   (m)
  d_l = thickness implant lens   (m)
  K   = keratometry reading   (D)

A thickness of 0.2 mm was added to the echographically estimated retina. If however the axial length differs from the average the retina will be thicker, or thinner depending on whether the eye is short, or long, respectively. The real thickness of the retina was calculated while assuming that the total retinal volume is constant during life. In order to be able to find an indication of the systematic error caused by the variable thickness the relation of corneal power to the axial length was investigated (Fig. 1) and the regression line was taken as a first approximation for this relation. The formula in Eq. [1] was then employed to find the change in lenspower per millimeter change of axial length

---

* This result is not surprising, because a regression line yields the best retrospective fit to the data. Therefore, the prospective value of the SRK formula still has to be proven.

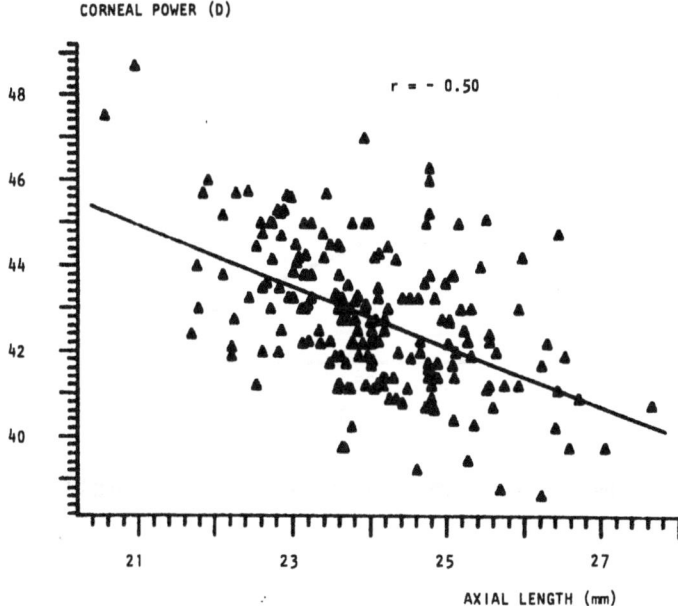

CORNEAL POWER (D)

r = - 0.50

AXIAL LENGTH (mm)

Fig. 1. Correlation plot of corneal power K vs. axial length L (n = 201). Correlation coefficient r = 0.50, regression line: K = 60 − 0.71 L.

for the range of axial lengthes from 20 to 30 millimeter (Fig. 2). This change in lenspower per millimeter was taken into consideration to investigate the systematic error which arises if the axial length would have been corrected by a fixed value of 0.2 millimeters. The result of these calculations is shown in Fig. 3. It appears that particularly in short eyes a substantial error is caused by the fixed addition.

A second source of systematic error is the alignment of the sound beam through the center of the eye ball, i.e. along the optical axis of the eye media. The visual axis is however deviating from this axis by a 5°. The effect of this deviation is that the measured axial length is longer than the visual axis by an amount that is depending on the axial length itself. This effect was systematically calculated and its effect on the implant lens power was then estimated while taking into account the change in lenspower per millimeter vs. axial length (Fig. 2). The addition to the lenspower needed to correct for this effect is shown in Fig. 3.

The total systematic error (i.e. the dioptric addition needed when a fixed addition of 0.2 mm to the axial length would have been made) is also shown in Fig. 3. It will be evident that for long eyes as well as short eyes corrections are substantial. The necessity to perform a correction is depending on the magnitude of the measurement errors. In the population of cases studied (cf.

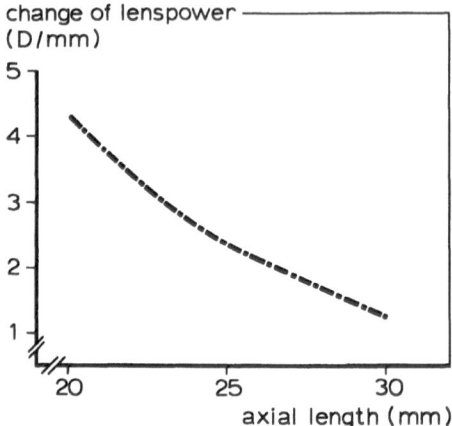

Fig. 2. Variation of power of emmetropic implant lens per millimeter axial length vs. axial length.

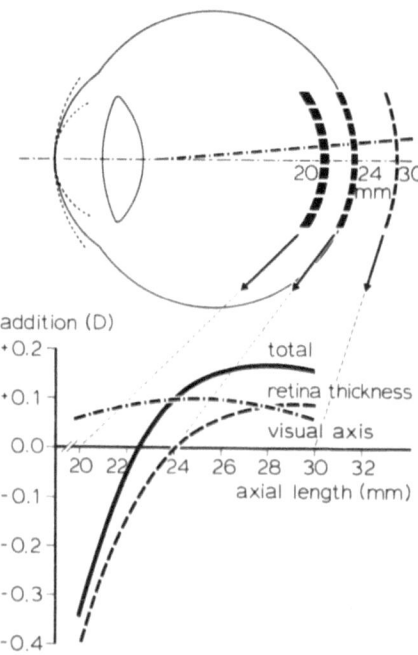

Fig. 3. Addition to be made to the emmetropic lenspower calculated by the optical method as a function of axial length. Effects of thickness change of retinal thickness and the deviation of the visual axis of the eye from the optical axis, as well as the total effect.

Boerrigter et al. 1984) it appeared that only a minor effect was obtained: the lens predictions would have been accurate in 80%, if the limits of +2 D were employed (as compared to 76% without the correction).

Another even more important source of systematic errors is caused by the employment of echographic equipment based on a simple echographic axial length measurement and in which a single, average, sound velocity of 1550 m/s for the eye media is implemented. The average velocity is derived from the known sound velocities in the eye media while considering an average healthy human eye, i.e. axial length 24 mm, lens thickness 4 mm. However, when either the axial length or the thickness of the retina differ considerably from the average a systematic error will be made. E.g. if the lensthickness equals 7 mm the optical calculation of the power of the implant lens would be +0.6 D in error (i.e. −0.6 D of myopia). If the axial length is different from the average the error in the lens power that results is negligeable. It has to be stressed from this evidence that only biometry which takes the eye media separately into account, can be considered adequate and will completely prevent the occurence of this kind of systematic error.

The SRK method: systematic errors

The formula found in the regression analysis (cf. Boerrigter et al. 1984) was almost identical to the SRK formula:

$$P_s = 118.2 - 2.51L - 0.92K \tag{2}$$

P_s = emmetropizing lens power	(D)
L = axial length	(mm)
K = keratometer reading	(D)

The systematic errors connected to the axial length, as discussed before for the optical method, are of a comparable order of magnitude for the SRK method. This can be understood from the Eq. (2) where the axial length is multiplied by a factor 2.51, which means that the addition of 1 millimeter changes the outcome, i.e. the lenspower, by a 2.5 D. As can be seen in Fig. 2 this change per millimeter is found in the optical method only in the range of axial lengthes just above the average of 24 mm. So the effects on the lens power, by systematic errors in the axial length measurement will be underestimated for short eyes and overestimated for long eyes.

Comparison of optical and SRK methods

The postoperative refraction error of the patients multiplied by a factor of 1.1 (cf. Boerrigter et al. 1984) was added to the implanted lenspower, thus yielding

40

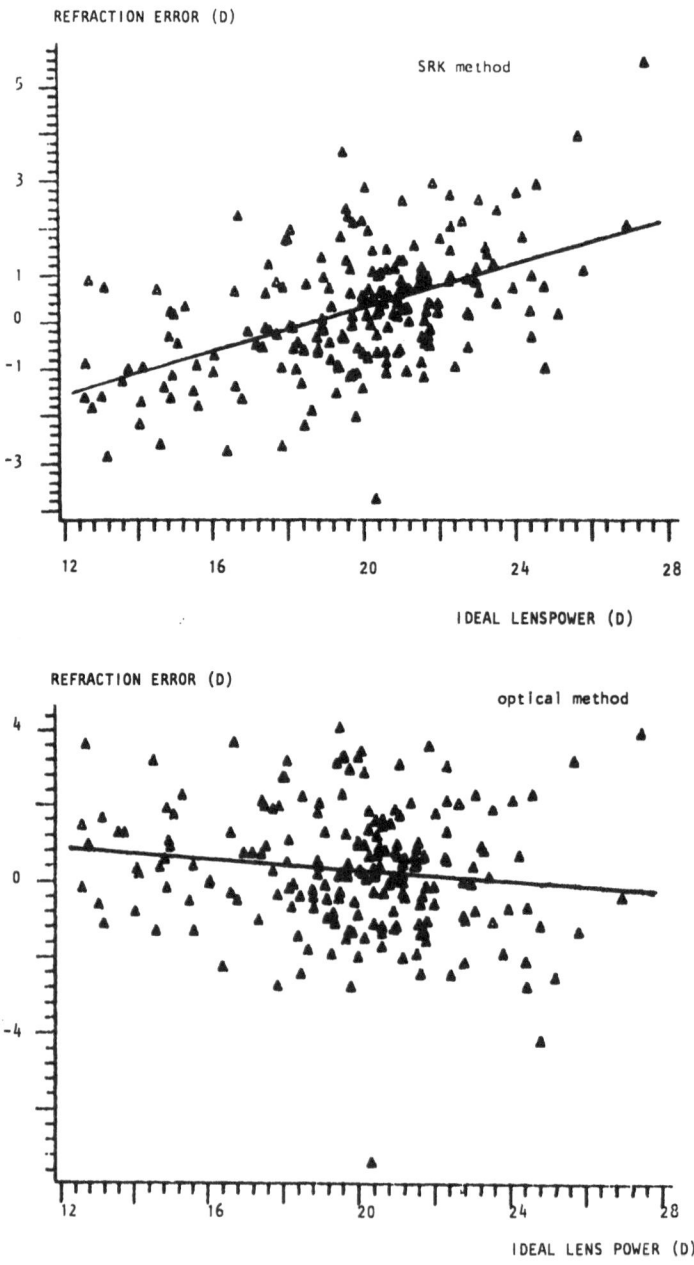

Fig. 4a. Correlation plot of retrospective refraction error vs. emmetropic implant lens power for the data obtained by the SRK method.

Fig. 4b. Same as in Fig. 4a for the data obtained by the optical method.

what was called the 'ideal lens', i.e. the real emmetropizing implant lens power. This ideal lens power was then subtracted from the calculated lens-power obtained with either one of the two methods. The results are shown in Fig. 4. It will be evident that the regression line through the SRK data (Fig. 4a) is significantly negative (slope = + 0.23, correlation coefficient 0.507), in other words weak lenspowers are overestimated, and strong lenspowers are underestimated. The data for the optical method are almost unbiased, i.e. a flat regression line is observed (slope = 0.07, correlation coefficient −0.13), after the systematic errors in the axial length measurement have been corrected for.

Acknowledgements

The authors are very much indebted to prof. dr. A.F. Deutman and his clinical staff, who performed the surgery and made the clinical data available, and to A.M. Verbeek, M.D. who performed the echographic biometry.

Bibliography

Boerrigter RMM, Thijssen JM, Verbeek AM. 1984. Intraocular lens power calculations: the optimal approach. Subm Brit J Ophthalmol.

Retzlaff J. 1980. Posterior chamber implant power calculation: regression formulas. Amer Intraocul Implant Soc J 6: 268–270.

Sanders DR, Kraff MD. 1980. Improvement of intraocular lenspower calculation using empirical data. Amer Intraocul Implant Soc J 6: 262–267.

Thijssen JM. 1975. The emmetropic and the iseikonic implant lens: computer calculation of the refractive power and its accuracy. Ophthalmol (Basel) 1971: 467–486.

Intraocular lenses: which formula for the mini-computer?

M. MASSIN and J.P. COLLIAC
Paris, France

To appreciate the intraocular optics, we have used the matricial calculation since it appeared to us the most appropriate for optical systems containing more than 2 diopters. Also, it was easily realized with our mini-calculators.

At first we defined a theoretical mean emmetropic eye from our own measurements as well as from the literature. Its statistical values are:

Indexes of refraction

Cornea	:	1.377
Aqueous	:	1.337
Lens	:	1.42
Vitreous	:	1.336

Distances

Corneal thickness	:	0.52 mm
Depth of the A.C.	:	2.80 mm
Lens thickness	:	4 mm

The axial length is directly related to the refraction according to the following formula providing the optical anterior system is constant:

$$1 = \overline{S1S7} = n8 \frac{a + b\,Rs}{c + d\,Rs}$$

where 1 is the distance between the summit of the cornea and the posterior pole of the lens; n8 is the refractional index of the vitreous; $Rs = \dfrac{1}{S1\,R}$; $R =$ punctum remotum; a, b, c and d are the Gauss coefficients needed by the matricial calculation.

We can now use a new formula indicating the power of the emmetropizing lens for an eye whose corneal power is 42.7 diopters, the depth of the A.C. is 3.32 mm, and the thickness of the implant is 0.5 mm:

$$D5 = \frac{n8\,(a2 - c2\,6) - c21}{n8\,a2\,6 + a2\,1'} \qquad \text{Where } 6 = \frac{16}{n6}$$

K.C. Ossoinig (editor), Ophthalmic Echography, ISBN 978-94-010-7988-4
© 1987, Martinus Nijhoff/Dr W. Junk Publishers, Dordrecht.

length and refractional index of the lens of the patient.

We gathered several formulas from the literature and applied them to our theory – the Gernet formula:

$$DI = \frac{1.336 - a\, Dc}{(a-d)\,(1 - \dfrac{a\, Dc}{1.336})} , \text{ the Binkhorst formula:}$$

$$DI = \frac{1.336\,(4r - a)}{(a-d)\,(4r-d)} , \text{ the Colenbrander formula:}$$

$$DI = \frac{1.336}{a - d - 0,0005} - \frac{1.336}{\dfrac{1.336}{Dc} - d - 0.0005}$$

the Shammas formula:

$$DL = \frac{1.336}{a - 0.1\,(a-23) - d - 0,05} - \frac{1}{\dfrac{1.0125}{Dc} - \dfrac{d + 0.05}{1.336}}$$

All these formulas were obtained through mathematical calculations from a theoretical point of view. The abbreviations have the following meanings: a: axial length; d: anterior chamber (from the anterior surface of the cornea to the anterior face of the implant); Dc: corneal power; r: mean radius of the cornea (mm.).

We introduced a fifth formula – the SRK. This formula is not theoretical, but statistical, and was obtained from many observations:

$$Di = A - 2.5a - 0.9\, Dc,$$

where a is the axial length, Dc is the corneal power, and A is constantly changing with the pattern of the implant.

We could then calculate the emmetropizing implant for each power of our theory, with our own matricial formula, and then with each of the others; the results could then be plotted on a graph.

The result is that the Colenbrander and the Binkhorst formulas look like ours, except that they are a little myopic. The Gernet formula is close to our formula for the hyperopic eyes, and 1 diopter less than ours for the myopic eyes. The Shammas formula coincides with our own. Most interesting is the SRK. It is close to the matricial formula between 10 and 0, and far from it above and below.

We have then programmed a CASIO 720 P with the Binkhorst formula and compared the results with the true ocular refraction measured at least 3 months after the operation. For the time being we have only 7 patients: it is not enough to make inferences. Yet we have found that 5 patients were over-

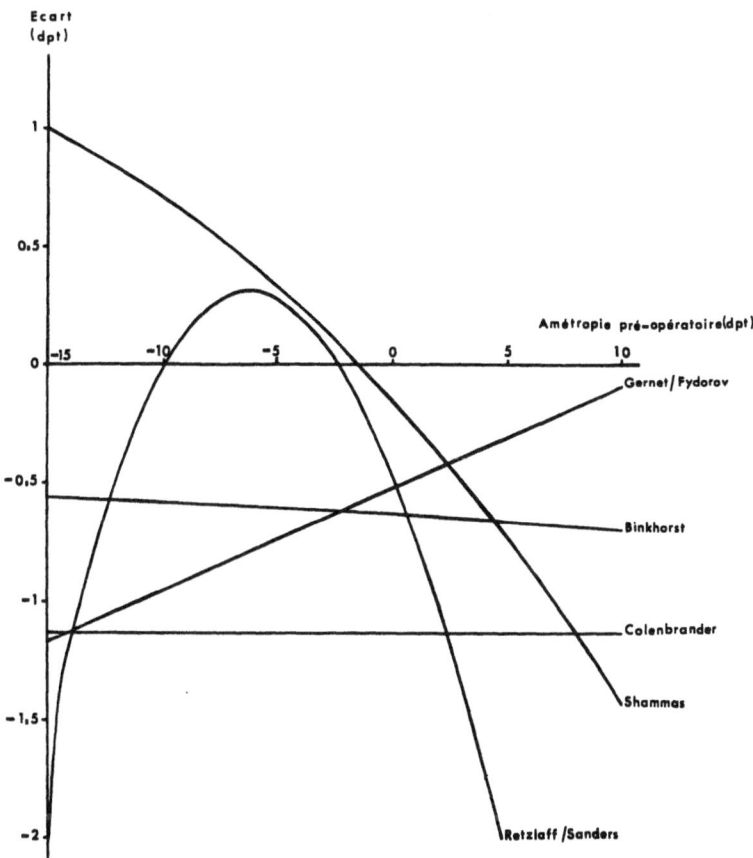

Fig. 1.

corrected 1 diopter when the theory stated a difference of $^1/_2$ diopter. All these eyes were emmetropic or very weakly ametropic. But the difference was greater for 2 hyperopic eyes: 1.75 and 3.75 diopters. It may be that our theory pattern with a constant anterior segment and a variable length is incorrect, and that the S.R.K. formula is closer to reality.

We intend now to introduce the S.R.K. formula into our mini-calculator together with the Binkhorst so that we will be able to compare the results on a greater number of patients.

Individual A-constant determination in IOL power calculation with the SRK-formula

B. PRAHS
Würzburg, FRG

Introduction

The accuracy of all implant calculations is dependent on the implant manufacturer, implant style, measuring equipment, measuring methods and the surgeon's technique. Main error sources are to be found in individual biometric methods and surgical techniques. They can only be detected and eliminated by a postoperative refraction control. In most of the cases it is not possible to determine whether a systematic prediction error is caused by a systematic error of biometry, by surgical technique or by both of them. Since the SRK-formula (1) is linear, every constant systematic measurement error is expected to cause a constant systematic deviation from the desired postoperative refraction. On the other hand every kind of systematic postoperative prediction error can simply be corrected in future calculations by a changed A-constant.

$$P = A - BL - CK \tag{1}$$

(P: implant power for emmetropia; L: axial length; K: average keratometer reading (diopters); A, B, C: constants derived from linear regression analysis).

The constants $B = 2.5$ and $C = 0.9$, which were originally derived from more than 2500 implant cases by linear regression analysis, remain unchanged. As only the A-constant has to be individualized, the minimum number of evaluated cases necessary to obtain significant results is relatively small. The authors of the SRK-formula advise an individualizing of the A-constant with a calculation sheet. A routine check in this way is hardly possible; therefore we propose a computerized error analysis.

Methods

The IOL calculations are done with a personal computer. The biometric data

K.C. Ossoinig (editor), Ophthalmic Echography, ISBN 978-94-010-7988-4

are not deleted after the lens is calculated, but stored in some data file. Only the additional input of the postoperative refraction and the power of the actual implant are necessary to check the A-constant. It takes only some basic lines to program the formulas below. The goal-refraction has to be compared with the postoperative refraction. Differences between the calculated and the actually implanted lenses have to be taken into account. The prediction error (Dev) in each case is:

$$Dev = Rp - Rg + (Pi - Pc) * 0.8 \qquad (2)$$

(Rp: postop. refraction; Rg: goal refraction; Pi: power of the implant; Pc: calculated implant power).

The systematic deviation is:

$$Dev = (Dev)/n \quad (n = number\ of\ cases) \qquad (3)$$

This systematic prediction error (Dev) may be corrected by a changed A-constant A':

$$A' = A + Dev * 1.25 \qquad (4)$$

With such a program, together with appropriately stored patient data, a routine and automatic control of the IOL-calculations is possible at any time. The cumulative refraction errors and the standard deviation are additionally calculated from the input data to make the prediction error more transparent. A t-test helps to decide whether the newfound individual A-constant differs significantly from the designated one; in other words, whether a correction of the A-constant for future IOL-calculations should be done or not.

Error analysis of 150 posterior chamber lens implantations

population
evaluated operation period (mm/dd/yy) : 11/11/83–11/11/84
visual acuity better than : 0.4
IOL-type : Kratz 10° angulated loops
surgeon : Pr
remarks : phako/running suture

results
systematic deviation from the calculated postoperative refraction: Dev = +0.58 dpt
corrected A-constant : A' = 115.9
standard deviation : SD = +/−1.2 dpt

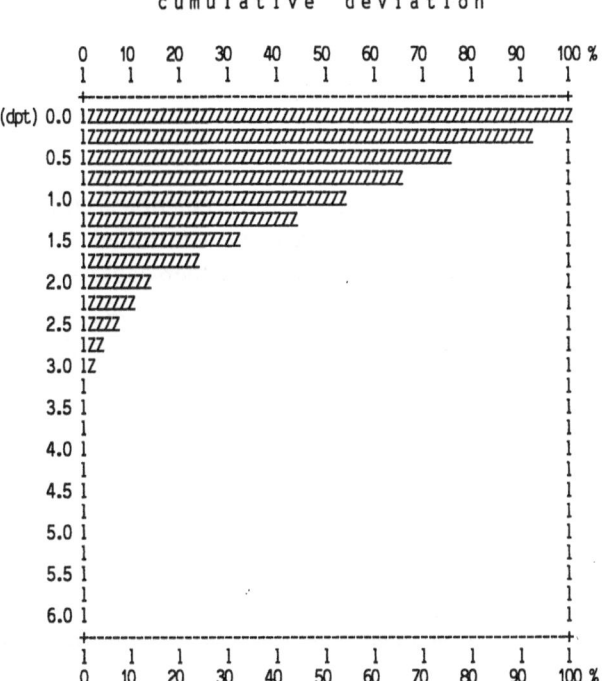

Fig. 1. Cumulative deviations from the predicted postoperative refraction (n = 150).

Discussion

The systematic deviation from the predicted postoperative refraction is generally small, though systematic prediction errors up to 3 diopters and more may
occur by improper calibration and measuring technique. If possible, the cause
of error should be corrected. Only errors of unknown origin are to be corrected by a changed A-constant. The study population is determined by the
operation period, visual acuity, IOL-type, surgeon(s), and other specified
criteria such as suture technique, etc. The choice of the population is essential
for the question in mind. If only an individualized A-constant is requested,
rarely occurring large prediction errors and cases with poor post-operative
visual acuity should be excluded from the evaluation. If one is interested,
however, in the general prediction accuracy, all cases should be evaluated.

The result of the evaluation is a printout of the systematic and cumulative
deviations from the predicted postoperative refraction, the corrected A-constant and the standard deviation. A corrected A-constant for future calculations is only printed out if the t-test is positive on a 5% level.

A standard deviation larger than 1.5 dpt requires a critical check of the biometry and the surgical technique.

Conclusions

A routine quality control improves not only the prediction accuracy; biometry methods and surgical techniques may also be controlled. Regarding the method of individualizing the A-constant with the 'personal A-constant calculation sheet', the proposed routine quality control using a pc-program does not require a large expenditure since only the IOL power, post-operative refraction, surgeon and surgical technique have to be stored additionally. With the patient's data stored, only the study population must be defined, and all calculations are performed automatically.

References

Gills JP. 1980. Minimizing postoperative refractive error. Contact lens 6, 56.

Gruber PF. 1982. Fehlerpropagation bei der Berechnung von intraokularen Linsen. Klin Mbl Augenheilk 180, 432.

Prahs B. 1982. Correction of ultrasonic distance measurements for the calculation of IOLs. Docum Ophthal Proc Series, Vol 30.

Prahs B, Duzanec Z. 1983. Déviations de la Refraction de but calculées après l'implantation de lentilles intra-oculaires. Bull et Mem S.F.O., 207–209.

Sanders J, Sanders D, Kraff M. 1982. A Manual of Implant Power Calculation, 17a–17b.

Biometry of lens implantation in the capsular bag

F. GOES
Antwerp, Belgium

In this study all pre- and postoperative measurements as well as the surgery were done by the author. Eye-length measurements were performed with the Ocuscan 400 equipment using the contact method (V 1550 m/sec 20 MHZ probe) in 250 eyes (Fig. 1). Anterior chamber depth measurements were done with the same Bausch and Lomb keratometer.

The operation technique was characterized by conservation of the anterior capsule until the end of the procedure. It consisted of primary implantation of a Galand style posterior chamber lens in the capsular bag. After a corneal incision, an anterior capsulotomy from 2 to 10 o'clock was done. Then after cortical clean-up, the lens was vertically inserted in the capsular bag, convex surface forward. Afterwards the lens was rotated 90° so that the superior loop was placed in the capsular bag and that the lens was horizontally positioned within the bag. Finally a U-shaped anterior capsulectomy was performed with two scissor cuts and the wound was closed with five 10 0 nylon sutures (Galand et al., 1984). A Galand lens has prolene loops and an overall length of 10.5 mm.

Anterior chamber depth

Because a postoperative difference of lens position of 1 mm will affect the refraction by 1 D in myopic eyes (>25 mm), by 1.5 D in emmetropic eyes and by up to 2.5 D in hyperopic eyes (≤21 mm), it is important to predict the postoperative position for any particular type of implanted lens.

The existence of a correlation between pre-and postoperative A.C. depth is denied by most authors because the cataract influences the A.C. depth. However, Oguchi and Van Balen (1974), and Hoffer (1979) mentioned some correlation.

In our series, the mean eye-length was 22.90 (Standard Deviation (S.D.) = 1.15: extremes 19.50 and 27.60). Preoperatively the mean value for the anterior segment was 3.20 mm (S.D. = 0.49: extremes 1.8 and 4.2), and post-oper-

K.C. Ossoinig (editor), Ophthalmic Echography, ISBN 978-94-010-7988-4

52

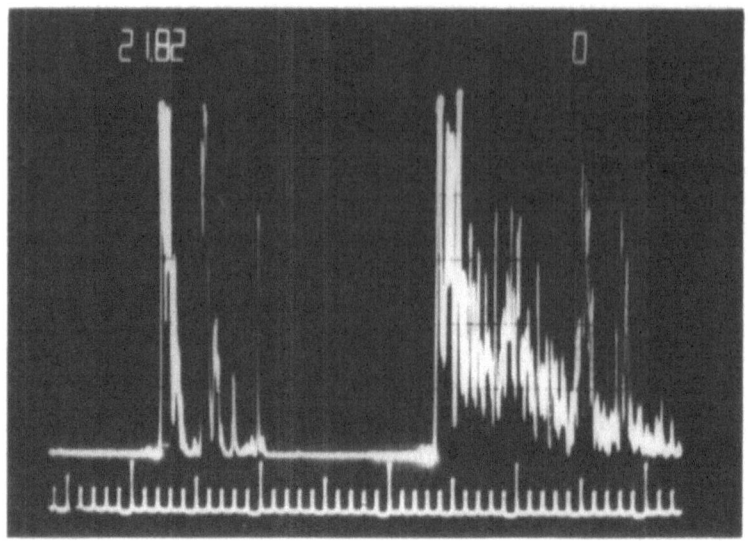

Fig. 1. Ocuscan oculometry with the 20 MHz transducer.

atively the mean value was 4.09 mm (S.D. = 0.23: extremes 3.50 and 4.70).

In 16 eyes the lens was positioned with the convex surface backwards and here the mean value for the postoperative anterior segment was 4.6 mm (4.35–5.0 mm). Fourteen of the 23 eyes, where preoperatively the anterior segment measured less than 2.5 mm, were glaucomatous eyes.

Postoperatively the anterior segment was equal to, or less than, 3.8 mm in 12 eyes, and seven of these eyes had also a very short preoperative measurement. The anterior segment measured at least 4.40 mm postoperatively in 20 cases: six of these eyes had an eye-length of more than 25 mm but the mean preoperative value of the anterior segment in this group was normal (3.40 mm).

Shorter eyes had preoperatively a shorter anterior eye-segment: L −1 S.D.: mean 2.56 mm, L −2 S.D.: mean 2.50 mm. These eyes also had a shorter postoperative anterior eye-segment: L −1 S.D.: mean 3.88 and L −2 S.D.: mean 3.68 (Table 1).

Longer eyes had a longer anterior eye segment preoperatively: L = +1 S.D.: mean 3.51 mm, and L +2 S.D.: mean 3.81 mm. These eyes had also a longer

Table 1. Pre-op and post-op. anterior eye segment according to the eye-length mean value (mm).

L: 22.90 (1.15)	+1 S.D.	+2 S.D.	−1 S.D.	−2 S.D.
A.S. pre-op: 3.20 (0.49)	3.51	3.81	2.56	2.50
A.S. post-op. 4.09 (0.23)	4.25	4.44	3.88	3.68

postoperative anterior eye-segment: L +1 S.D.: mean 4.25, and L +2 S.D.: mean 4.44 mm. It is important to consider these factors because it means that we have to implant a stronger lens in highly myopic eyes, and a weaker lens in hyperopic eyes because the refractive value will be less in the former and more in the latter.

Corneal curvature

An error of 0.1 mm in the measurement of corneal radius corresponds to a postoperative error of about 0.5 D. Accurate preoperative readings are, therefore, essential and this is possible to within 0.05 mm (0.25 D), but the corneal curvature may also change postoperatively. According to most authors, the average K will not change in an important way or will become steeper after surgery (Lindstrom 0.11 mm steepening: Shammas, 1982). We checked the postoperative astigmatism and the eventual change of the corneal radius 3 months after surgery in 180 eyes with uncomplicated surgery and preoperative astigmatism of not more than 1.5 D. Postoperatively, the mean corneal refractive power increased only by 0.101 D (extreme changes between −0.75 and +1.25 D). An important postoperative change of the corneal radius was only present in one case, the change being ≤0.25 D in 50% (92/180) of the eyes. A postoperative decrease of the corneal refractive value was also rare (41/180 eyes). In our series, the mean postoperative astigmatism was 1.40 D. It was more than 1.5 D in 25%, and more than 2.5 D in 10%.

Refractive error

In the calculation of the postoperative refractive error, only eyes with an acuity of 20/30 or more were included. In order to obtain emmetropia in 217 Galand lens implantations with a postoperative VA of at least 20/30, a 21 D lens was needed in 19% and a 20 D lens in 17%. A lens of less than 21 D was needed in 45% and a lens of more than 21 D was needed in 36%. We calculated the IOL power using the Binkhorst formula without retinal correction (but with correction for the anterior chamber), the Shammas fudged formula, the SRK formula and a simple nomogram proposed by Binkhorst.

In our series of *66 standard lenses* (42 iris fixated – 24 posterior chamber) the mean refractive error was ± 1.60 D. The error was ≥3 D in 8%, ≥2 D in 30% and only 33% of the eyes were within a 1 D error range. For this type of lens implant in the capsular bag, we determined an *A constant of 117.83*. Using this factor in the *S.R.K. formula*, the postoperative refractive error was >1 D in 16% (21/128), and >2 D in 4% (5/128: 2 total cataract, 1 important astigma-

54

Table 2. Mean and standard deviation of residual refractive error after prediction according to different formulas.

S.R.K.	:	0.73 (0.58)
Shammas	:	0.91 (0.85)
B.K.	:	0.95 (0.81)
Nomogram	:	0.92 (0.76)

tism). It never exceeded 3 D. The mean postoperative refractive error was ± 0.73 D (S.D. = 0.58) and the mean algebraic residual refractive error was +0.0009 D (Table 2).

Using the *Shammas* fudged formula, the mean residual error was ± 0.91 D (S.D. = 0.85). The refractive error was >1 D in 25% (31 cases), >2 D in 6% (8 cases) and >3 D in 1.5% (2 cases). This formula gave a mean algebraic refractive error of +0.03 D. We compared the refractive error obtained with the S.R.K. and with Shammas' formula. Both formulas gave exactly the same average algebraic refractive error, but there were differences from +3.60 to −1.70 D. In very short eyes, Shammas' formula predicted too high.

When we used the simple *nomogram* by Binkhorst, we came out with a mean refractive error of ± 0.92 D (S.D. = 0.76: extremes −2.75 and +2.25). The mean algebraic refractive error was +0.01 D. The error was >1 D in 23% (28/128), and >2 D in 7% (8 cases) (Table 3).

In the *Binkhorst formula,* the calculated anterior segment according to the eye length did not correspond with the reality because we found differences from −0.45 to +0.45 mm. With this formula, the mean refractive error was ± 0.95 D (S.D. = 0.81: extremes +4.20 and −3.10). The error was >3 D in 2%, >2 D in 7% and >1 D in another 28% of the cases. The mean algebraic error using this formula was +0.03 D.

In another series of 100 Galand lens implants that we could examine in Ghent, we obtained similar results (Table 4) (Goes et al., 1984).

Table 3. Residual refractive error according to different formulas.

	>1 D	>2 D	>3 D
S.R.K.	16%	4%	0%
Shammas	25%	6%	1.5%
B.K.	27%	7%	2%
Nomogram	23%	7%	0%

Table 4. Mean and standard deviation of residual refractive error after prediction according to different formulas. (Goes et al, 1984).

	S.R.K.	Shammas	B.K.
S.D.	0.59	0.74	0.73
Mean	0.84	0.91	0.92

Conclusion

1. With the Galand lens implant placed in the capsular bag (convex surface forward), the mean value for the postoperative anterior segment is 4.09 mm (0.23).

2. We could not find any significant correlation between pre- and postoperative anterior segment dimensions. There was, however, a significant correlation between the preoperative anterior eye segment and the eye length and, more importantly, between the postoperative anterior eye segment and eye length.

3. With our measurement technique, we obtained the highest accuracy of prediction using the S.R.K. formula with an A constant of 117.83.

References

Galand A, Van Oye R, Budo C, Goes F, Foets B. 1984. Results of implantation in the capsular bag. A short-term review of 1588 cases. Congress European Implant lens Council, Harrogate.

Goes F, Allewaert R, Riems D, Van Oye R. 1984. Biometry in Lens implantation in the capsular bag. (In press).

Hoffer KJ. 1979. Postoperative measurement of anterior chamber depth. Intraocular lens Symposium. L.A.

Oguchi Y, Van Balen ATM. 1974. Ultrasonic study of the refraction of patients with pseudophakos. In 'Ultrasound in Medicine and Biology'. London Pergamon Press: 267–273.

A-scan biometry of 1000 cataractous eyes

H. JOHN SHAMMAS
Los Angeles, USA

Abstract

We reviewed the axial length measurements of 1000 cataractous eyes ranging from 20.9 mm to 29.4 mm with an average value of 23.45 mm. Average measurements were 3.4 mm for the anterior chamber depth, 4.43 mm for the lens thickness and 15.62 mm for the vitreous cavity. Comparative studies revealed that an increase in axial length is due to an increase in the anterior chamber and vitreous cavity's depth and a concommitant decrease in the lens thickness.

Introduction

The ocular components have been extensively measured in normal adults [1–4]. Hoffer [5] recently reported on axial length and anterior chamber depth measurements in cataractous eyes. The purpose of this study is to review the axial length measurements of 1000 cataractous eyes. The anterior chamber depth, lens thickness and vitreous cavity's depth were also measured and evaluated in relation to the eye length.

Material and methods

We reviewed the axial length measurements of 1000 eyes scheduled for cataract surgery. All eyes were measured electronically [5] with the Kretz 7200 MA ultrasound unit and the Digital Ocular Computer (DOC) using an immersion technique [7]. The measurement was taken between the leading edges of the corneal spike (C) and the retinal spike (R) (Fig. 1).

The ocular components were measured manually from the polaroid pictures. The anterior chamber depth was measured between the peaks of the anterior corneal spike (C) and the anterior lens surface spike (L 1); the lens

K.C. Ossoinig (editor), Ophthalmic Echography, ISBN 978-94-010-7988-4

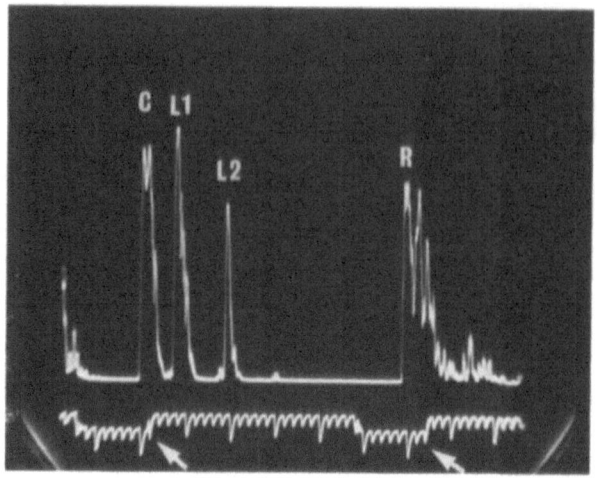

Fig. 1. Axial length is measured from the anterior surface of the cornea ('C') to the anterior surface of the retina ('R'). 'L₁' and 'L₂' represent the anterior and posterior surfaces of the lens respectively. Note the presence of gates (arrows) in the scale for electronic measurement of the axial length.

thickness was measured between the peaks of the anterior (L 1) and posterior (L 2) lens spikes. The readings were taken in microseconds from the unit's electronic scale and converted to millimeters using an average velocity of 1532 m/s for the anterior chamber depth and 1641 m/s for the lens thickness [8]. The vitreous cavity's depth was obtained by substracting the anterior chamber depth and lens thickness from the axial length.

The 1000 cases were then divided into five categories according to the axial length:

Category	Axial length
very short eyes	less than 22.0 mm
short eyes	22.0–22.9 mm
average eyes	23.0–23.9 mm
long eyes	24.0–24.9 mm
very long eyes	25.0 mm and over

The anterior chamber depth, lens thickness and vitreous cavity's depth were measured in each of these categories.

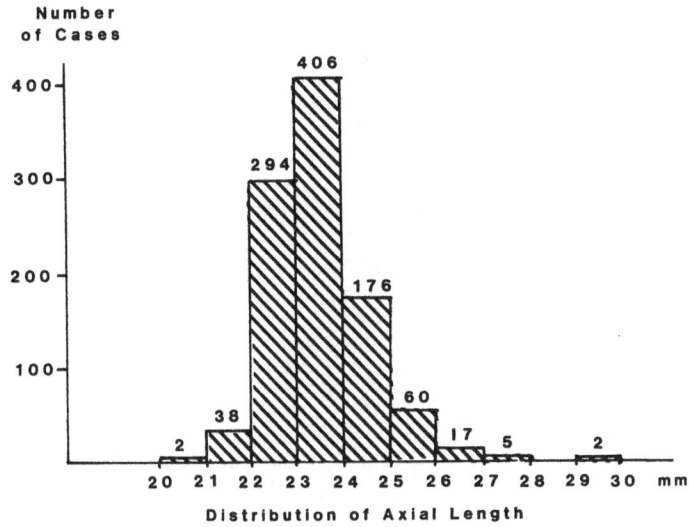

Fig. 2. Distribution of axial length.

Results

The axial length ranged from 20.9 to 29.4 mm with an average value of 23.45 mm ± 1.48. Figure 2 shows the distribution.

The anterior chamber depth ranged from 2.4 to 5.3 mm with an average value of 3.40 mm ± 0.35. Figure 3 shows the distribution. Table 1 shows the mean, standard deviation and range of the anterior chamber depth in the five categories. The mean anterior chamber depth was 3.02 mm in very short eyes and increased to 3.68 mm in very long eyes.

The lens thickness ranged from 3.2 to 5.7 mm with an average value of

Table 1. Mean, standard deviation (S.D.) and range of anterior chamber depth.

Axial length in mm	Number	Anterior chamber depth in mm		
		Mean	S.D.	Range
20.9–21.9	40	3.02	± 0.38	2.4–3.5
22.0–22.9	294	3.27	± 0.33	2.5–3.7
23.0–23.9	406	3.43	± 0.29	2.6–4.3
24.0–24.9	176	3.56	± 0.36	2.9–4.8
25.0 – and over	84	3.68	± 0.31	3.2–5.3
All eyes	1000	3.40	± 0.35	2.4–5.3

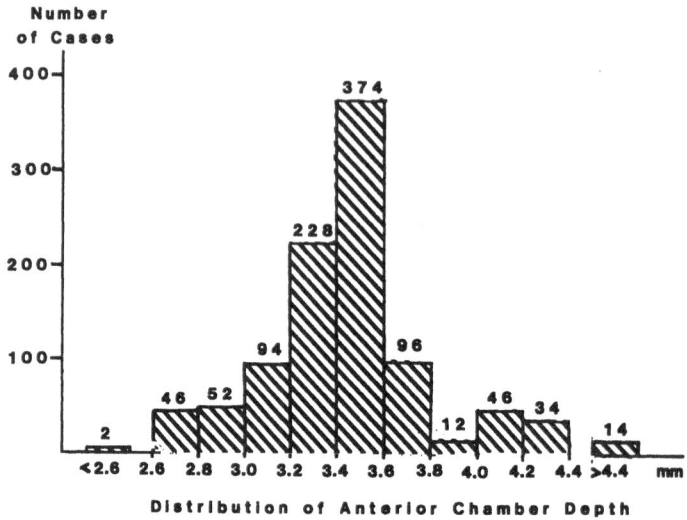

Fig. 3. Distribution of anterior chamber depth.

4.43 mm ± 0.46. Figure 4 shows the distribution. Table 2 shows the mean, standard deviation and range of the lens thickness in the five categories. The mean lens thickness was 4.78 mm in very short eyes and decreased to 4.26 mm in very long eyes.

The vitreous cavity's depth ranged from 12.0 to 21.1 mm with an average value of 15.62 mm ± 1.09. Figure 5 shows the distribution. Table 3 shows the mean, standard deviation and range of the vitreous cavity's depth in the five categories. The mean vitreous cavity's depth was 13.81 mm in very short eyes and increased to 17.87 mm in very long eyes.

Table 2. Mean, standard deviation (S.D.) and range of lens thickness.

Axial length in mm	Number	Lens thickness in mm		
		Mean	S.D.	Range
20.9–21.9	40	4.78	± 0.66	3.8–5.7
22.0–22.9	294	4.55	± 0.42	3.7–5.3
23.0–23.9	406	4.36	± 0.47	3.4–5.2
24.0–24.9	176	4.41	± 0.44	3.2–5.2
25.0 and over	84	4.26	± 0.35	3.2–5.0
All eyes	1000	4.43	± 0.46	3.2–5.7

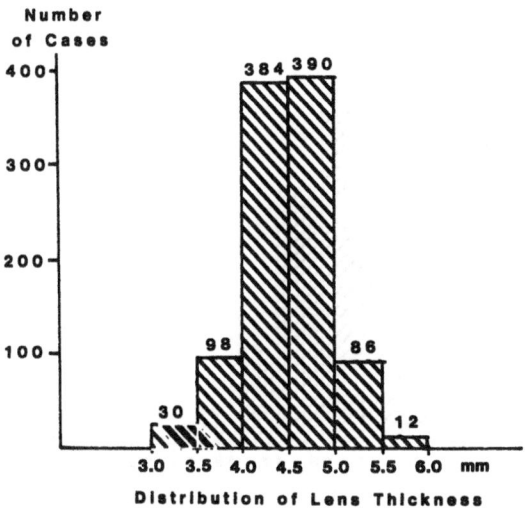

Fig. 4. Distribution of lens thickness.

The correlation coefficient between the axial length and each of the anterior chamber depth, lens thickness and vitreous cavity's depth was very high r = 0.9 (p<0.001).

Discussion

The average anterior chamber depth in our series was 3.40 mm which is similar to the findings of Jansson [2], Sorsby [3] and Flidelius [4] in normal eyes. The anterior chamber is relatively shallow in short eyes and deeper in longer eyes.

Table 3. Mean, standard deviation (S.D.) and range of vitreous cavity's depth.

Axial length in mm	Number	Vitreous cavity's depth		
		Mean	S.D.	Range
20.9–21.9	40	13.81	±0.61	12.0–15.1
22.0–22.9	294	14.73	±0.48	13.2–15.9
23.0–23.9	406	15.60	±1.11	13.6–17.8
24.0–24.9	176	16.35	±0.45	15.2–17.9
25.0 – and over	84	17.87	±0.62	16.4–21.1
All eyes	1000	15.62	±1.09	12.0–21.1

62

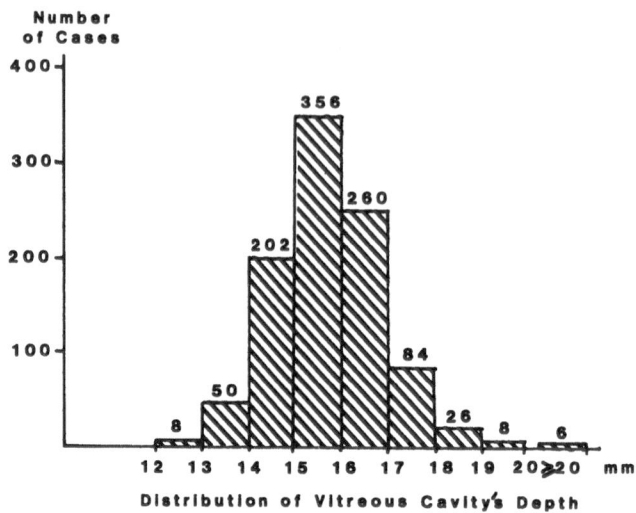

Fig. 5. Distribution of vitreous cavity's depth.

This deepening of the anterior chamber with increased axial length is also noted by Hoffer [5].

The lens is thick in short eyes and thin in long eyes. The decrease in lens thickness when the axial length is longer is in favor of an emmetropizing relationship between these two factors.

The average axial length was 23.45 mm which is very similar to the 23.43 mm reported by Jansson [1] in 36 healthy eyes and slightly lower than the 23.65 mm reported by Hoffer [5]. A-scan biometry is a reliable method for determining the axial length [7] and can be performed with either a contact or an immersion technique. In a previous study [9] we found that measurements obtained with the contact technique were shorter than those obtained with the immersion technique. We routinely use an immersion technique for axial length measurement prior to cataract and implant surgery and we obtain a high accuracy in our intraocular lens calculations [10].

References

1. Jansson F. 1963. Determination of the axis length of the eye roentgenologically and by ultrasound. Acta Ophthalmol 41: 1–11.
2. Jansson F. 1963. Measurement of intraocular distances by ultrasound and comparison between optical and ultrasonic determination of the depth of the anterior chamber. Acta Ophthalmol 41: 25–61.
3. Sorsby A. 1971. Epidemiology of refraction. Int Ophthalmol Clin 11: 1–18.

4. Fledelius H, Alsbirk PH. 1975. Comparative ultrasound oculometry. TAU-measurements of thirty eyes with three standard equipments. Bibl Ophthal 83: 263–268.
5. Hoffer KJ. 1980. Biometry of 7500 cataractous eyes. Amer J Ophthalmol 90: 360–368.
6. Shammas HJ. 1983. Manual versus electronic measurement of the axial length. In Ultrasonography in Ophthalmology, Proceedings of the 1982 Ninth SIDUO Congress. Documenta Ophthalmol. 38: 225–229.
7. Shammas HJ. 1984. Atlas of Ophthalmic Ultrasonography and Biometry, pp. 273–285. St. Louis. The C.V. Mosby Co. Publishers.
8. Jansson F, Kock E. 1962. Determination of the velocity of ultrasound in the human lens and vitreous. Acta Ophthalmol 40: 420–433.
9. Shammas HJ. Immersion versus contact technique for axial length measurement. Amer Intra-Ocular Imp Soc: In print.
10. Shammas HJ. 1982. The fudged formula for intraocular lens power calculations. Amer Intra-Ocular Impl Soc 8: 350–352.

Factors in emmetropization

ROGER P. HARRIE
Salt Lake City, USA

It is an accepted fact that the values of the components of refraction are associated in an individual eye to produce emmetropia (Sorsby, 1957 and Stromberg, 1936). In fact, the number of emmetropes in the general population is three times greater than that predicted from the normal statistical distribution curve (Duke-Elder, 1969). Various authors have concluded that the axial length of emmetropic eyes (Stenstrom, 1948) can vary randomly over a fairly wide range and the major factor in emmetropization is the refractive power of the anterior segment (corneal curvature and lens dioptric power) (Franceschetti, 1965). There is some controversy over whether the greater force is the cornea or the lens in emmetropization power (Francois, 1977). The refractive components have also been studied in non-emmetropic (ametropic) eyes.

The refractive state of ametropia raises several questions (Hartridge, 1950). What happens to the refractive components either individually or in association to produce a non-emmetropic state?) (Michaels, 1980). Is one component consistently responsible for the progressive deviation from 'normal' as an eye becomes more and more nearsighted or farsighted? Are ametropic eyes predictable as a group in regards to the deviation of the various refractive components or are there subgroups which behave differently? Do any of the refractive components act as a modulator to oppose the increasing 'abnormality' of a group of eyes higher in ametropic values? The purpose of this study is to analyze a group of ametropic (especially myopic eyes) with regard to these questions. Measurements (manifest and retinoscopic refraction, keratometry, and standardized A-scan axial length) were made on 141 eyes of an office patient population.

Materials and methods

141 eyes were randomly measured in an office patient population. Refraction

K.C. Ossoinig (editor), Ophthalmic Echography, ISBN 978-94-010-7988-4
© 1987, Martinus Nijhoff/Dr W. Junk Publishers, Dordrecht.

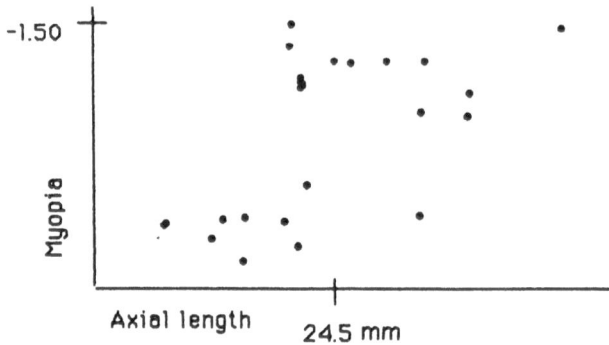

Fig. 1.

was performed both subjectively by manifest refraction and objectively by retinoscopy. The spherical equivalent value was obtained from these measurements. Keratometry was performed by means of a Bausch and Lomb keratometer. The horizontal and vertical measurements were averaged. Axial length was measured with a standardized Kretz A-scan (using the immersion technique (Ossoinig, 1979). A corrected axial length was obtained by measuring for lens thickness and including this in the final calculation of cornea to retina distance.

Results

141 eyes were analyzed of which 118 were myopic and 23 were hyperopic. The results were analyzed by dividing the eyes into different subgroups under both the myopia and hyperopic categories. In the myopic group it was found that the eyes seemed to cluster into the following subgroups: 1) −0.25 to −1.49, 2) −1.50 to −2.49, 3) −2.50 to −3.99, 4) −4.0 to −10.0, 5) −10.1 and above. Scattergrams were calculated for each subgroup. The first group is illustrated in figure 1 and consists of 21 eyes. Analysis of this group illustrates that within the group the eyes with lower degree of myopia were also those with shorter axial length and as the axial length increases there is an abrupt increase in the degree of myopia. This is a rather distinct separation of these two categories as seen in the graph. Figure 2 illustrates the scattergrams from the second group consisting of 22 eyes and there is a random distribution of myopia with increasing axial length in this group. Figure 3 illustrates group 3 which consists of 25 eyes and a scattergram does illustrate a weak trend verified by regression analysis of decreasing myopia with increasing axial length. This was explained by a definite decrease in refractive power of the anterior segment. Figure 4 illustrates group 4 consistent with 44 eyes and in this group there was a random distribution of degrees of nearsightedness with increasing axial length. The

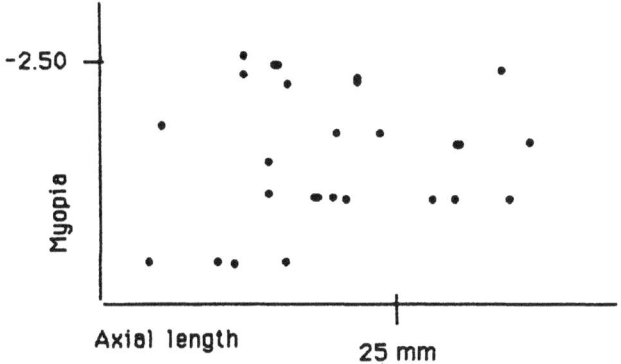

Fig. 2.

highest degrees of myopia are, however, found in the longest axial length in this group. Group 5 is not illustrated but was found to have an increase in myopia with increased axial length.

There is a significant trend in group 1 and 5 towards increasing myopia with increasing axial length. This was also the case for all the myopic sub-group analyzed as a whole. It was interesting that in group 3 there is a weak but significant trend towards decreasing myopia with increasing axial length. This confirms an observation made in a study of 100 cataractous eyes in which there was a slight trend towards decreasing myopia with increasing axial length (Harrie, 1979). Data were also analyzed with respect to the relative contribution of each refractive component towards myopia. This was performed by taking values of each component for the 'model eye', (assumed value of 43.5 for corneal curvature, 13.1 for lens diopter power, and 23.5 for axial length). These are the values required to produce emmetropia in a model eye. To calculate the myopia producing or opposing factor for each component, the

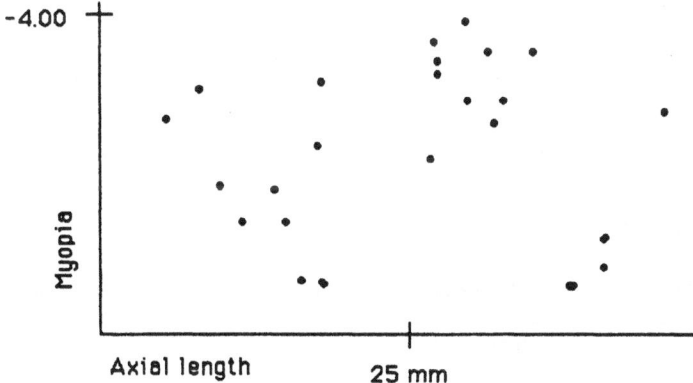

Fig. 3.

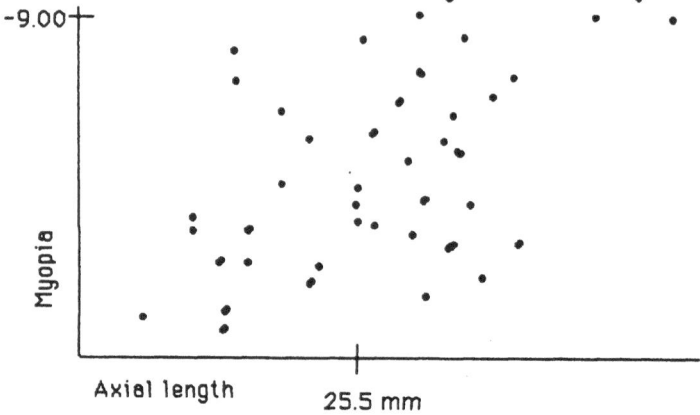

-9.00

Myopia

Axial length   25.5 mm

Fig. 4.

measured value of each component for each eye in my study, was subtracted from the corresponding value in the model eye. This resultant number was assigned a plus or minus value based on either its contribution to the production of myopia or its opposition to the production of myopia.

The analysis of the individual contribution of each component towards or away from myopia is illustrated in the tables. Table 1 illustrates the first group in which it is found that the major factor in the production of myopia in the myopic population below −1.49 diopters is that of the corneal curvature. The axial length has a minimal contribution and the lens power actually has an opposing role in the production of myopia. Table 2 illustrates the group from 1.50 to 2.50 diopters of myopia. Within this group, the major myopia produc-

Table 1. Myopia 0.25 to 1.50.

Refractive component	Myopia producing value	Myopia opposing value
Cornea	1.29	
Axial length	0.11	
Lens		0.3

Table 2. Myopia 1.50 to 2.50.

Refractive component	Myopia producing value	Myopia opposing value
Cornea	0.51	
Axial length	2.01	
Lens		0.88

Table 3. Myopia 2.50 to 4.00.

Refractive component	Myopia producing value	Myopia opposing value
Cornea	0.27	
Axial length	3.21	
Lens		0.61

ing force is that of the axial length with the cornea playing a contributory role. The lens power fairly strongly opposed myopia. Table 3 illustrates group 3 in which the axial length is the strongest force in the production of myopia with a weak contribution from the cornea. Again the lens power opposes myopia. Table 4 illustrates group 4 in which the axial length is the strongest force in the production of myopia with a minor contribution from the cornea and a small opposition by the lens power. Group 5 is illustrated in table 5 and shows a strong trend toward the production of myopia by the axial length and lens power with a small contribution by the corneal curvature. Each of these contributory factors of the refractive components reflect the average value of those calculations for each sub group. The average values for the total group of 118 myopia eyes found that the axial length had a myopia-producing value of 3.15, the cornea had a myopia-producing value of 0.81, and the lens had a myopia-opposing value of 0.05.

The same type of analysis was applied to the smaller group of hyperopic eyes which included 23 eyes in three subgroups. The first subgroup is illustrated in Table 6 in which the cornea has a hyperopia opposing value of 0.04, the axial

Table 4. Myopia 4.00 to 10.00.

Refractive component	Myopia producing value	Myopia opposing value
Cornea	1.13	
Axial length	4.57	
Lens		0.16

Table 5. Myopia 10.00 and up.

Refractive component	Myopia producing value	Myopia opposing value
Cornea	0.23	
Axial length	7.27	
Lens	7.00	

Table 6. Hyperopia 0.25 to 2.00.

Refractive component	Hyperopia producing value	Hyperopia opposing value
Cornea		0.04
Axial length	0.44	
Lens	0.45	

length a hyperopia producing value of 0.44, and the lens a hyperopia producing value of 0.45. The second group is illustrated in table 7 in which the cornea has a hyperopia producing value of 0.7, the axial length a hyperopia producing value of 0.4 and the lens power a hyperopia producing value of 0.82. The third subgroup is illustrated in Table 8 in which only two eyes were studied and the cornea has a hyperopia producing value of 2.5, the axial length a hyperopia producing value of 4.8 and the lens a hyperopia producing value of 5.0. The average values for the entire group of hyperopic eyes were cornea having a hyperopia producing value of 0.14, axial length with a hyperopia producing value of 0.13, and the lens with a hyperopia producing value of 0.27.

Discussion

This study supports the concept that there is a definite process of emmetropization which occurs among the refractive components of the eye. However, it is a complex issue and it is difficult to make generalizations.

Table 7. Hyperopia 2.00 to 4.00.

Refractive component	Hyperopia producing value	Hyperopia opposing value
Cornea	0.70	
Axial length	0.40	
Lens	0.82	

Table 8. Hyperopia 4.00 and up.

Refractive component	Hyperopia producing value	Hyperopia opposing value
Cornea	1.25	
Axial length	2.40	
Lens	2.50	

Several observations did emerge from this study which bear further investigation. It was found in the low myopic group (−0.25 to −1.49) that the cornea curvature seems to be the major determinant in myopia in these patients. Within the group there was a trend towards increased myopia with increased axial length but still overall, the cornea was the major culprit in nearsightedness. One, therefore, might predict that in the low myopic patient he will have a steeper cornea than average and probably an axial length close to a normal value.

As one progressed from group to group within the myopic population, it was found that the axial length became a major determinant of myopia. In a higher myopic population there appears to be a contribution of each component towards myopia but the axial length is the strongest. The one exception to this occurred in the middle myopic group (−2.50 to −3.99). Within this group itself, the shorter axial lengths were found in the lower myopic members of the group, but this was found even more so in the longer axial lengths in this group. There was a large jump to the highest degree of myopia in the mid-axial length eyes within this population. The major force responsible for this decrease in myopia with increase in axial length is a definite trend away from myopia by the lens power.

In his study of myopic eyes, Franceschetti (1966) found the lens to be a major factor toward emmetropization. He also verified this in a population of myopic eyes. This was found to be the case in the present study. The lens was the major factor opposing myopia in each of the subpopulations except for the highest myopic individuals (greater than −10 diopters). This was less true in the hyperopic eyes but the number of eyes in this study is not sufficient for adequate statistical analysis.

The results of this study provide stimulus for further investigation, especially of the lower and middle myopic individual to see if these trends identified in this paper are verifiable with larger numbers.

References

Duke-Elder S. 1969. The Practice of Refraction, St. Louis, Missouri: The C.V. Mosby Company. Pp 60–66.

Franceschetti DA. 1965. Importance of Ultrasonic Echography for Measurements of the Optical Components of the Eye. Tr Am Acad Ophthalmol and Otol, May-June: 465–473.

Franceschetti A, Luyckz J. 1966. Study of Emmetropization Effect of the Crystalline Lens by Ultrasonic Echography. Am J Ophthalmol 61: 1096–1100.

Francois J, Zoes S. 1977. Ultrasonographic Study of 100 Emmetropic Eyes. Ophthalmologica 175: 321–327.

Harrie RP. 1979. Emmetropization Factors. Jules Stein Eye Institute Resident Seminar.

Hartridge H. 1950. The Causes of Errors of Refraction. BR J Physiol Opt 7: 143–149.

Hofstetter HL. 1954. Some Interrelationships of Age, Refraction and Rate of Refractive Change. Am J Optom 31: 161–169.

Michaels DD. 1980. Visual Optics and Refraction. St. Louis, Missouri: The CV Mosby Company. Pp. 499–526.

Ossoinig KC. 1979. Standardized Echography Basic Principles, Clinical Applications and Results in Ophthalmic Ultrasonography: Comparative Techniques. 19 (4): 133–136.

Sorsby A, Benjamin V, Davey JB, Sheridan N, Tanner JN. 1957. Emmetropia and Its Aberrations, a Study in the Correlation of the Optical Components of the Eye. Medical Research Council Report 293, London, Her Majesty's Stationary Office.

Stinstrom S. 1948. Investigation of the Correlation of the Optical Elements of Human Eyes, Translated by Dr. D. Woolf, Am J Optom Monograph No. 58.

A biometric study of aniseikonia

JEFFREY S. HILLMAN and ALAN HAWKSWELL
Leeds, UK

Introduction

The intraocular lens is widely accepted today for the correction of aphakia and there is increasing use of intraocular lenses of power calculated to control the refractive outcome for each individual patient. The surgeon is offered the choice of intraocular lens power for postoperative emmetropia, planned ametropia or iseikonia. Some surgeons have stressed the importance of using iseikonia intraocular lens powers although such calculation requires biometric data from both eyes and may leave the patient with significant postoperative anisometropia. In practice, however, most surgeons largely disregard aniseikonia and use intraocular lenses of powers calculated for near-isometropia.

This ongoing study was undertaken to investigate the amount of postoperative aniseikonia in a series of patients after unilateral cataract extraction with implantation of an intraocular lens and to determine whether it is necessary to calculate iseikonic intraocular lens powers. A biometric study was also made to seek a relationship between aniseikonia and differences of axial length and corneal power in the eye pairs.

Material and method

This study was carried out on a population of 80 patients after unilateral cataract extraction with implantation of an intraocular lens of either calculated or 'standard' power. All of the intraocular lenses were of pupil-supported styles with the optic in the anterior or posterior chamber. 20 patients had either inadequate vision in the fellow eye or suppression indicated by the Wirt Fly test and were excluded from the study as these prevented measurement of image size difference (eikonometry). None of the excluded patients had diplopia problems.

Both eyes of the remaining 60 patients were refracted and with the patient

K.C. Ossoinig (editor), Ophthalmic Echography, ISBN 978-94-010-7988-4

74

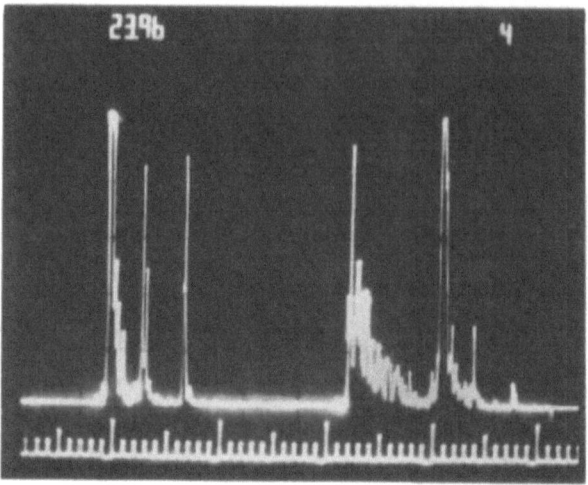

Fig. 1. Axial biometric ultrasound scan of a phakic eye with echoes (Left to Right) from the cornea, lens surfaces and the vitreo-retinal interface.

wearing the current spectacle prescription eikonometry was performed using a home-made portable space eikonometer. This instrument has been described in the literature (Hawkswell, 1975) and gives results which are comparable with eikonometry using size lenses or the American Optical Co space eikonometer. The patient viewed different rod targets with each eye and one rod was moved until it appeared the same distance away as the fixed rod. A black Bjerrum screen background eliminated monocular clues to depth perception and four readings were averaged for each patient.

The axial lengths of both eyes were measured by ultrasound using the Digital Biometric Ruler (D.B.R.) of the Ocuscan DBR-400 with a 12.5 MHz transducer. Accurate axial alignment was indicated by the echo pattern. The phakic eye gave clear high peaks from the cornea, lens surfaces and from the vitreo-retinal interface (Fig. 1). In the pseudophakic eye the intraocular lens behaved as a foreign body with 'ringing' to give a descending cascade of echoes (Fig. 2). Central corneal keratometry was performed using a calibrated Haag-Streit Javal-Schiotz instrument.

Results

The range of postoperative anisometropia is shown as dioptres spherical equivalent in Fig. 3. 45 patients had less than 2 dioptres anisometropia with a mean value (± S.D.) of 1.02 (± 0.59) dioptres and 15 patients had more than 2 dioptres anisometropia with a mean value (± S.D.) of 3.73 (± 1.10) dioptres.

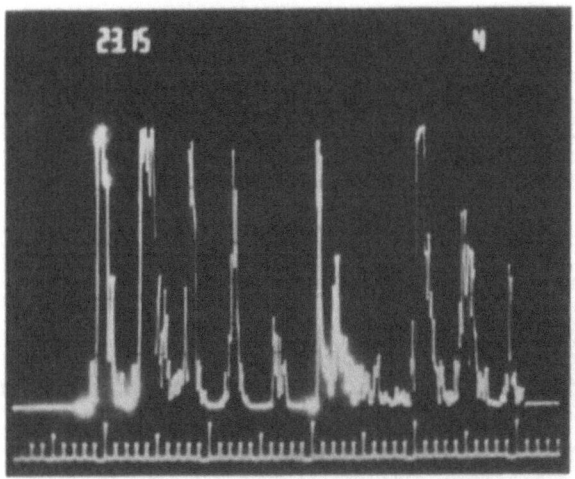

Fig. 2. Axial biometric ultrasound scan of a pseudophakic eye with echoes (Left to Right) from the cornea, 4 echoes 'ringing' from the intraocular lens and the vitreo-retinal interface.

The greatest anisometropia found in this study was 7.1 dioptres.

The range of postoperative aniseikonia is shown in Fig. 4, the mean value (± S.D.) was 1.85 (±1.80)% and the greatest value found was 7.8%.

Table 1 presents the relationship between postoperative anisometropia and aniseikonia. The 45 patients with less than 2 dioptres anisometropia had mean aniseikonia (± S.D.) of 1.30 (±1.19)% and the 15 patients with more than 2 dioptres anisometropia had mean aniseikonia (± S.D.) of 3.52 (±2.23)%.

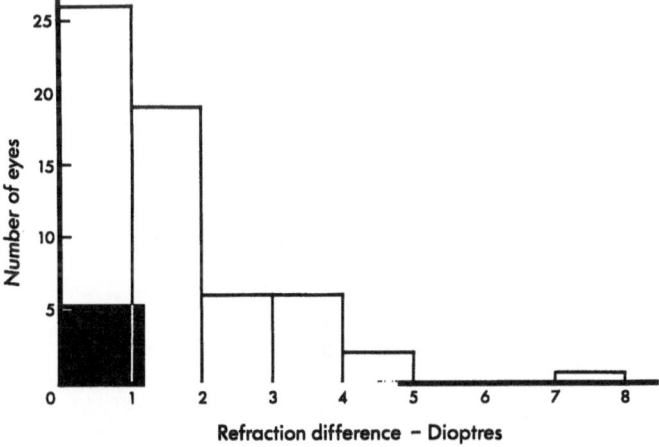

Fig. 3. The range of postoperative anisometropia (dioptres spherical equivalent) in 60 patients after unilateral cataract extraction with implantation of an intraocular lens.

76

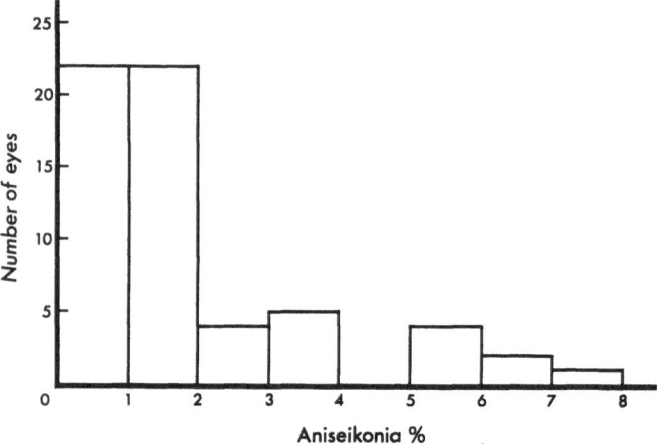

Fig. 4. The range of postoperative aniseikonia (%) in 60 patients after unilateral cataract extraction with implantation of an intraocular lens.

The 21 patients with postoperative isometropia (taken as less than 1 dioptre anisometropia) presented a mean aniseikonia ($\pm$ S.D.) of 1.13 ($\pm$ 0.78)%.

The relationship between postoperative anisometropia and aniseikonia is presented in graphic form in Fig. 5. Statistical analysis shows a statistically significant association with P<0.001.

Statistical analysis of the relationship between postoperative anisometropia and aniseikonia with differences of axial length and differences of keratometry in the eye pairs or with combinations of those differences failed to show an association of statistical significance.

Table 1. The relationship between postoperative anisometropia and aniseikonia.

Refraction difference		Aniseikonia
(Dioptres)	n	Mean ($\pm$ S.D.)
0–1.0	26	1.02 ($\pm$ 0.82)
1.1–2.0	19	1.74 ($\pm$ 1.45)
2.1–3.0	6	3.28
3.1–4.0	6	3.28
4.1–5.0	2	3.30
5.1–6.0	0	
6.1–7.0	0	
7.1–8.0	1	6.80

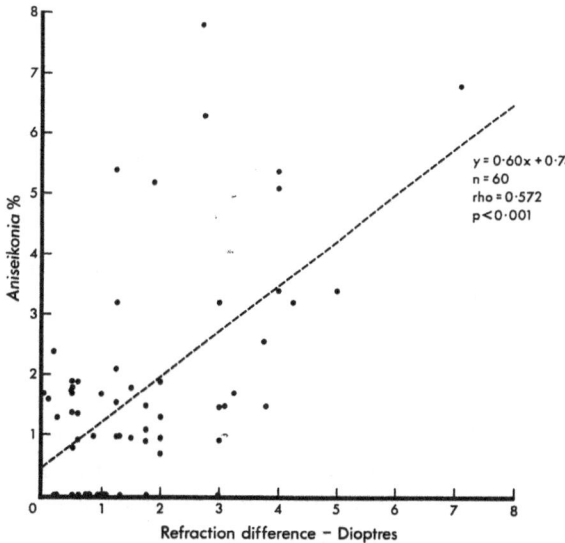

$$y = 0.60x + 0.74$$
$$n = 60$$
$$rho = 0.572$$
$$p < 0.001$$

Fig. 5. Graphic presentation of the relationship between postoperative anisometropia (dioptres spherical equivalent) and aniseikonia (%) in 60 patients after unilateral cataract extraction with implantation of an intraocular lens. There is a statistically significant association with P<0.001.

The refractions and biometric data for the three patients with the greatest aniseikonia is presented in Table 2. It is not possible to explain the high levels of aniseikonia in terms of the biometric differences studied.

Discussion

There is some controversy in the literature regarding the limits of aniseikonia which are compatible with BSV. It appears that the visual system is more tolerant of aniseikonia with intraocular lenses than with contact lenses or with

Table 2. Refractions and biometric data for the three patients with the greatest aniseikonia.

Refraction				Aniseikonia	Ax diff.	K diff.
$\dfrac{-8.0}{\text{D.S.}}$	(6/36)	$\dfrac{-6.50}{+2.50 \text{ ax } 125}$	(6/9+)	7.8%	0	0.025
$\dfrac{-7.50}{+2.0 \text{ ax } 125}$	(6/18)	$\dfrac{-1.0}{+3.25 \text{ ax } 180}$	(6/12+)	6.8%	1.65	0
$\dfrac{-0.75}{+1.50 \text{ ax } 15}$	(6/9)	$\dfrac{+2.50}{+0.50 \text{ ax } 170}$	(6/9)	6.3%	0	0

spectacles – possibly because the optical situation is more physiological. In studies on intraocular lens aniseikonia Nolan & Hawkswell (1974) reported 5%, Crone & Leuridan (1975) suggested 8%, Huber & Binkhorst (1979) suggested 5%, Miyake et al (1981) suggested 9% and Huber et al (1983) suggested 6% as the upper limit of tolerance. In this study aniseikonia of up to 7.8% was found to be compatible with BSV and so we are in agreement with the higher limits suggested by previous studies.

A relationship of statistical significance (P<0.001) was shown between anisometropia and aniseikonia. By the calculation of intraocular lens power for near-isometropia from biometric data it is possible to keep postoperative anisometropia to 2 dioptres or less in almost all cases (Kraff et al (1978), Maloney et al (1979), Hillman (1982, 1983). With this degree of anisometropia the associated aniseikonia is well within the tolerable limits of the visual system. This suggests that the theoretical problems of aniseikonia can be avoided in clinical practice by the calculation of intraocular lens power for isometropia without the more complicated specific calculation of iseikonic intraocular lens powers.

This biometric study failed to show a significant association between post-operative anisometropia and aniseikonia and differences of axial lengths and keratometry in the eye pairs. The mean difference between the keratometry readings for the eye pairs ($\pm$ S.D.) was only 0.10 ($\pm$ 0.10) mm which is equivalent in refraction terms to 0.50 ($\pm$ 0.50) dioptres and one would not expect this to be relevant. Studies by Sorsby et al (1962) on the biometry of phakic anisometropia showed that axial length differences are the major causative factors. The results of this study on pseudophakic anisometropia are not in agreement, possibly because the optical effects of intraocular lens power overshadow the effects of axial length differences. The biometric data of the three patients with the greatest aniseikonia shows that one cannot explain pseudophakic aniseikonia in terms of the factors measured. Two of these patients with 7.8% and 6.3% aniseikonia presented only 2.75 dioptres anisometropia and no differences in axial length or keratometry in the eye pairs.

The establishment of pseudophakic isometropia does not eliminate aniseikonia as one might expect, the 21 isometropic patients still exhibited a mean aniseikonia ($\pm$ S.D.) of 1.13 ($\pm$ 0.78)%. This may be a reflection of the slightly anterior position of the intraocular lenses in this study or the simple optical form of the intraocular lens compared with the complex refractive properties of the natural lens.

In all studies of aniseikonia it must be appreciated that the problem is not a simple optical one. The final image size perceived by the brain may be influenced by variations in retinal photoreceptor density (which may vary with eye size) and the visual signals may be modified during passage through the visual system to the visual cortex.

Summary

This paper reports a study of postoperative refraction, eikonometry and differences of axial length and keratometry of the eye pairs in 60 patients after unilateral cataract extraction with implantation of an intraocular lens. A statistically significant association (P<0.001) was demonstrated between postoperative anisometropia and aniseikonia. The patients studied tolerated aniseikonia of up to 7.8% without problems. 45 Patients with anisometropia of 2 dioptres or less exhibited a mean aniseikonia (± S.D.) of 1.30 (±1.19)% which is well within the limits tolerated by the visual system in pseudophakia. This can be achieved by the calculation of intraocular lens powers for isometropia without the need for specific calculation of iseikonic intraocular lens powers. No statistically significant association was found between anisometropia or aniseikonia and differences of axial length and keratometry. It is suggested that this may be due to the overwhelming effects of intraocular lens power on the optics of the eye.

References

Crone RA, Leuridan OMA. 1975. Unilateral aphakia and tolerance of aniseikonia Ophthalmologica, Basel, 171: 258–263.

Hawkswell A. 1975. The development of a portable space eikonometer. Brit J of Physiol Optics 30: 25–33.

Hillman JS. 1982. Intraocular lens power calculation for emmetropia: – a clinical study Brit J Ophthal 66: 53–56.

Hillman JS. 1983. Intraocular lens power calculation for planned ametropia: – a clinical study Brit J Ophthal 67: 255–258.

Huber C, Binkhorst CD. 1979. Iseikonic lens implantation in anisometropia Am Intra-ocular Implant Soc J 5: 194–202.

Huber C, Meier U, Hess F. 1983. Klinischer Wert der Iseikonie bei der Korrektur des aphaken Auges Klin Mbl Augenheilk 182: 379–382.

Kraff MC, Sanders DR, Lieberman HL. 1978. Determination of intraocular lens power: a comparison with and without ultrasound Ophthal Surg 9: 81–84.

Maloney WF, Kratz RP, Mazzocco TR, Davidson B. 1979. Posterior chamber intraocular lens power calculation in 441 cases Am Intra-ocular Implant Soc J 5: 213–2–6.

Miyake S, Awaya S, Miyake K. 1981. Aniseikonia in patients with a unilateral artificial lens measured with Aulhorn's phase difference haploscope Am Intra-ocular Implant Soc J 7: 36–39.

Nolan J, Hawkswell A. 1974. Clinical aspects of unilateral aphakia Trans Ophthal Soc UK 94: 480–486.

Sorsby A, Leary GA, Richards JM. 1962. The optical components in anisometropia Vision Res 2: 43–51.

Pseudophakodonesis as a major cause of late corneal and retinal complications in IOL surgery

P.E. GALLENGA and G. CENNAMO
Chieti and Naples, Italy

Summary

Pseudophakodonesis is considered the major cause of late corneal and retinal complications in IOL surgery. Three groups of IOL patients were studied with B-scan and M-mode echography – those with anterior chamber lenses, iris fixation lenses and posterior chamber lenses. Only patients with IOLs in the proper position were included in the study. B-scan was used to control the correct position of the IOL, while M-mode echography was used to determine inertial movements of the IOL.

Marked inertial movement was found in the iris fixated lenses; reduced but moderate movement was found in the anterior chamber lenses with flexible loops, and no movements were observed in posterior chamber lenses in the ciliaris sulcus.

Introduction

The echographic examination for intraocular lens implantation (IOL) has become a routine method not only for the calculation of the power of implanted lenses and for the information that we can make decisions regarding the indications or contra-indications for IOL implantation, but also for the possibility for study of the pseudophakia.

In this last case, a post-operative hyphema in the anterior chamber or in the vitreous may also require an echographic examination. In this case we can obtain information on the position of IOL and about the condition of the intraocular structures (Figs. 1, 2, 3 and 4). Moreover, the echographic examination can give us some information on the endophthalmodonesis.

Certain corneal and retinal complications following cataract extraction are not due to surgery, but rather are dependent upon a condition of 'aphakia' (MacInnis et Coll. 1983). These complications usually consist of corneal

K.C. Ossoinig (editor), Ophthalmic Echography, ISBN 978-94-010-7988-4

82

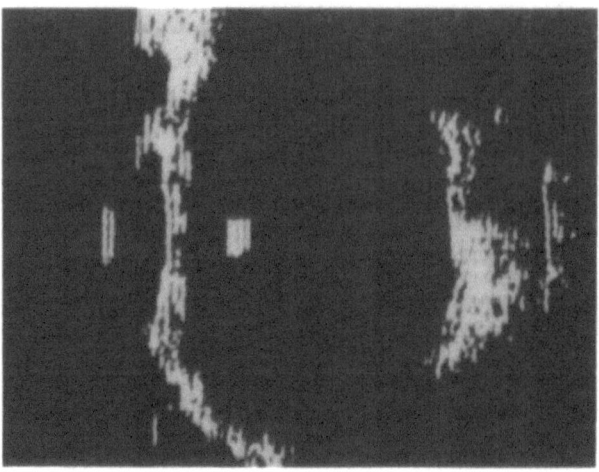

Fig. 1. Inexact position of IOL in the anterior chamber.

edema, edematous maculopatia, papilledema and peripheral retinal degeneration. Many researchers have attributed the appearance of these complications to the loss of the lens-zonule barrier (Ho 1982).

Cataract extraction and the consequent loss of support of the lens to the iris
alters ocular hydrokinetics. Moreover, the saccadic movements of the aphakic
eye generate valid aftermovements of the aqueous humor, the iris and the
vitreous. Furthermore, it has also been noted that these aftermovements of the

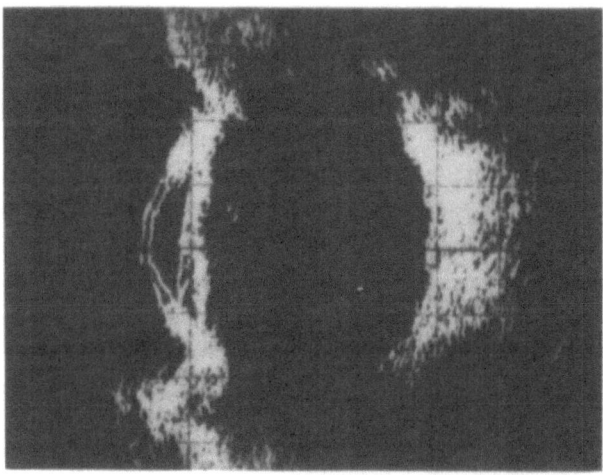

Fig. 2. Exact position of IOL in the posterior chamber.

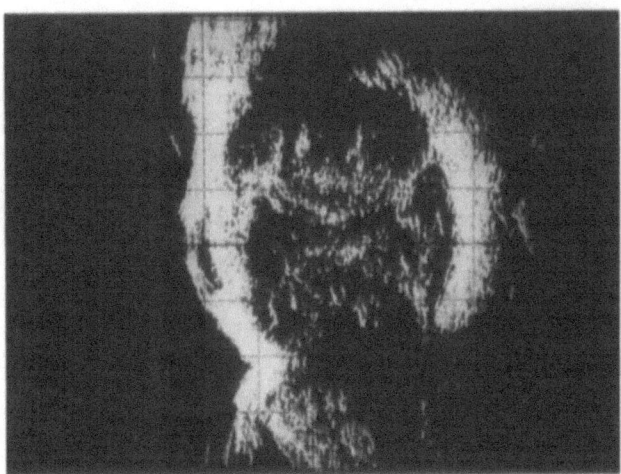

Fig. 3. A case of IOL in the anterior chamber with a postoperative hyphema in the anterior chamber and in the vitreous.

intraocular structures were more pronounced following intraocular extraction (Binkhorst, 1980).

It has been hypothesized that the increased rate of intraocular aftermovements following intracapsular extraction is the primary cause of increased cell loss of the corneal endothelium, and of long-term corneal and retinal complications (Pechereau et coll. 1982).

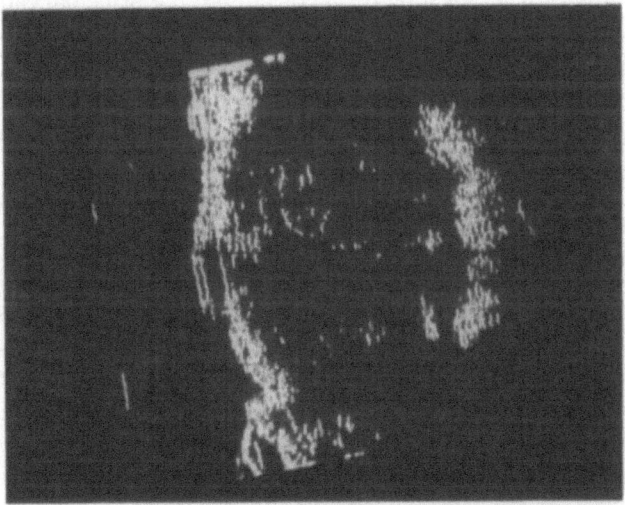

Fig. 4. The same case as in Fig. 3 at increased system sensitivity. The vitreous hemorrhage is better displayed.

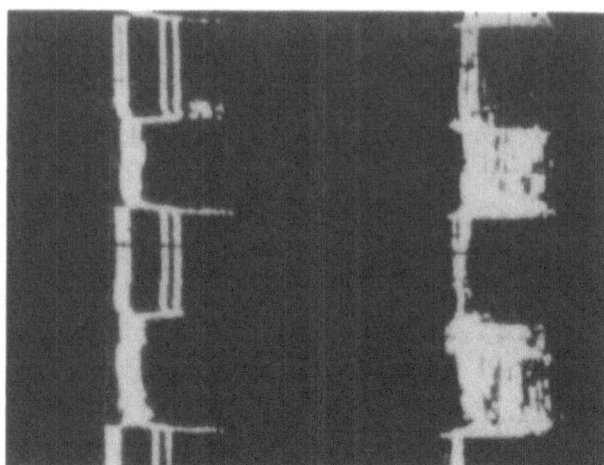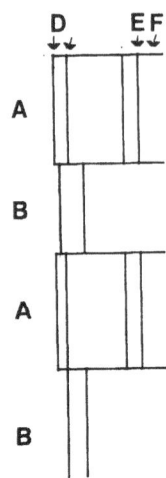

Fig. 5. M-mode echography in patient with IOL in posterior chamber. Absence of aftermovements is shown. A-B: ocular structures after an eye movement. D: anterior and posterior surfaces of the cornea. E: anterior surface of IOL. F: anterior surface of the posterior capsule of the crystalline lens.

Presumably such long-term ocular alterations following cataract extraction are due not only to the continuing trauma of the aqueous and vitreous on the corneal endothelium and retina, but are also due to the subsequently altered distribution of biochemical substances.

The mobility of IOL has long been considered the principal cause of long-term ocular complications. Actually, the rotation of an eye with an IOL induces a series of aftermovements of the aqueous, iris and vitreous movements which may be intensified or diminished by the implant itself; thus, the degree of severity of the endophthalmodonesis will be proportionally related to that of the pseudophakodonesis.

Jacobi and Jagger (1979) analyzed IOL oscillations in patients who had undergone extracapsular or intracapsular cataract extraction. The study was performed by observing the oscillation of luminous reflexes on the anterior surface of the IOL. This study confirmed the presence of more valid aftermovements in patients with IOL following intracapsular cataract extraction.

In our previous study (Bonavolonta' et Coll. 1983) we performed an ultrasonographic study of IOL-induced aftermovements and, subsequently, a study of pseudophakodonesis in a group of 39 patients with various types of implants. An M-mode ultrasonic system (Ophthalmoscan 200, made by Sonometrics) was utilized to examine the aftermovements of IOL.

M-mode systems have been developed to examine temporal variations in

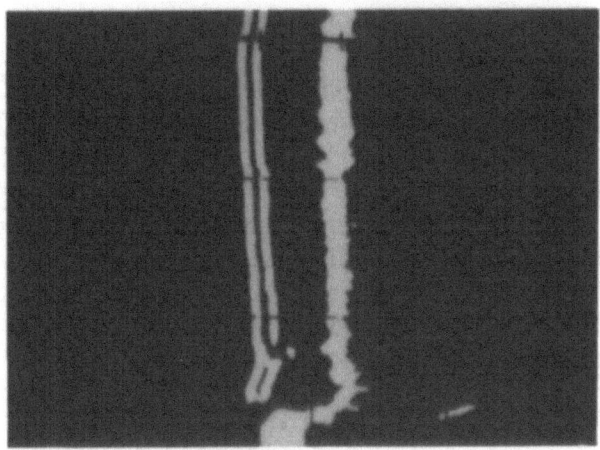

Fig. 6. Absence of aftermovements of the IOL in posterior chamber in a patient with extracapsular extraction.

tissue dimensions. In M-mode operation, a transducer is aligned along a selected axis within the eye. Then the transducer remains fixed while processed echo voltage intensity modulates an oscilloscope beam, delineating the position of each tissue interface. As time progresses, the horizontal display axis is slowly swept down the oscilloscope screen. If all tissue structures remain stationary, a series of parallel lines is displayed. If tissue positions fluctuate over time, corresponding variations occur in the distances between these lines to that a complete time history of tissue position is portrayed (Coleman, Lizzi and Jack 1977), (Fig. 5).

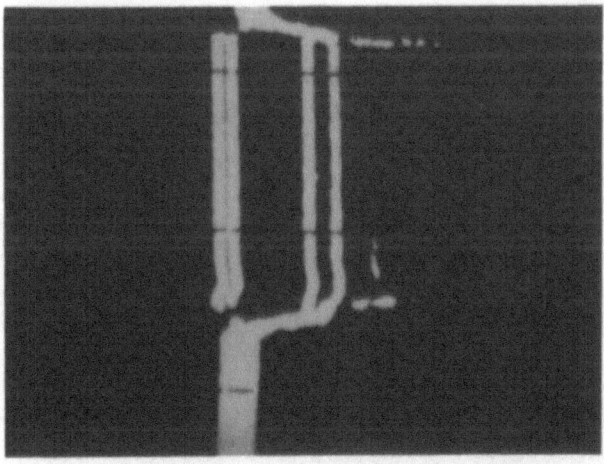

Fig. 7. Aftermovements of the IOL in anterior chamber in a patient with intracapsular extraction.

The aftermovements study of the IOL was obtained by having the patient move his eye to a determinate position, and then immediately returning to the starting position while maintaining the probe in the same direction. Thus, it is possible to pinpoint inertial motions within the global structure after each ocular movement (Bonavolonta' and Cennamo 1984).

Our results showed the presence of significant aftermovements of the IOL in the group of patients who had undergone intracapsular extractions and in the group of patients with an iridocapsular fixation lens (Fig. 6–7). In particular, in the group of patients who had undergone intracapsular extractions the aftermovements of the IOL was found in those cases in which a tri-support point implant was utilized (IOLAB 91 Z lens).

References

Binkhorst CD. 1980. Corneal and retinal complications after cataract extraction. Ophthalmology 87: 609–617.

Bonavolonta' A, Cennamo G. 1983. M-mode echography pattern study in retinal detachment. Hillman JS, Le May MM (eds.), Ophthalmic Ultrasonography, 113–139. Dr W Junk Publishers, The Hague, Boston, Lancaster.

Bonavolonta' A, Cennamo G, D'Avanzo M. 1983. Endoftalmodonesi e cristallino artificiale: studio ecografico. Atti LXIII Congresso della Societa' Italiana di Oftalmologia.

Coleman DJ, Lizzi FL, Jack RL. 1977. Ultrasonography of the Eye and Orbit. Lea & Febiger, Philadelphia, 79–81.

Ho PC, Tolentino FI. 1982. The role of vitreous in aphakic cystoid macular edema: A review, Am Intra-ocular Implant Soc J 8: 257–264.

Jacobi KW, Jagger WS. 1981. Physical forces involved in pseudophakodonesis and iridodonesis. Albrecht von Graefes Arch Klin Exp Ophthalmol 216, I: 49–53.

MacInnis B, Shirley SY, Valberg JD, Gaukrodger WT. 1983. Comparison of iris fixation and anterior chamber intraocular lens implants. Can J Ophthalmol 18, I: 15–17.

Pechereau A, Bordereau X, Baikoff G. 1982. Effets de différentes méthodes d'implantation intra-oculaire sur la population endotheliale cornéenne. Etude en microscopie speculaire. J Fr Ophthalmol 5, 2: 115–120.

Extreme hypermetropia and posterior microphthalmos in three siblings. An oculometric study

H.C. FLEDELIUS and T. ROSENBERG
Hillerød and Hellerup, Denmark

Introduction

Microphthalmos was ultrasonically established in three siblings (all phakic) with hypermetropia close to +20 D. They came to Copenhagen from the Faroe Islands, a North Atlantic community with a population about 40,000, to consult the contact lens section of the National Eye Clinic for the Blind and Partically Sighted. Their expectation was to get more comfortable vision through contact lenses – and to get rid of their thick and unbecoming glasses. Due to the rarity of the condition, and the unique anatomic and optical features, we consider an oculometric report to be of interest.

Material, methods, and results

The siblings were 26 (female), 24, and 15 years old (males) when seen by us. Being No. 1, 2, and 5 out of six children of a non-consanguineous marriage, the family history was reviewed (Fig. 1). Parents, grandparents, and the three remaining siblings had no evidence of significant ametropia, nor was extreme hypermetropia reported in distant relatives. The family revealed no history of mental retardation.

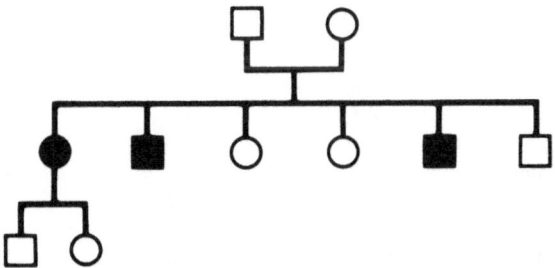

Fig. 1. The family tree of the present report. Filled symbols = extreme hypermetropia.

K.C. Ossoinig (editor), Ophthalmic Echography, ISBN 978-94-010-7988-4

88

General and ophthalmic features are given in Table 1. Glasses were first prescribed around school start. A Zeiss ophthalmometer was used for corneal K-readings, while axial ultrasound measurements were performed by a Kretztechnik 7000 equipment, a 10 Mc Ultrasonolux transducer, and a contact glass technique with a precorneal methocel column (Fledelius 1976). In the anterior chamber depth results given, central corneal thickness is included.

Table 1. Ophthalmic and other parameters in the three siblings with extreme hypermetropia.

	Ena.		Fri.		Bry.	
Sex	f.		m.		m.	
Age at exam. (years)	26		24		15	
Body height (m)	1,66		1,85		1,70	
Head circumference (cm)	56		59		59	
Interpupillary distance (mm)	65		70		67	
Spectacle refraction (D)	+18,75 × 0,75	170	+19,5 × 1,5	20	+19,0 × 1,0	160
	+19,0 × 2,0	0	+18,5 × 1,0	0	+19,5 × 1,5	100
Contact lens power (D)	+21		+21		+27	
	+22		+22		+26	
Corrected visual acuity	0,3		0,5		0,5	
	0,4		0,3		0,5	
Fundus appearence	normal		normal		normal	
Corneal transv. diameter (mm)	11,9		11,0		11,5	
Central corn. curvature rad. (mm)	7,46–7,24		7,32–7,03		7,05–6,78	
	7,44–7,16		7,25–7,0		7,0–6,8	
Ant. chamber depth (mm)	3,5		3,6		2,9	
	3,4		3,5		3,1	
Lens thickness (mm)	4,4		4,0		4,3	
	4,5		4,3		4,3	
Vitreous length (mm)	8,7		9,2		8,2	
	8,7		8,9		8,1	
Axial length (mm)	16,6		16,8		15,4	
	16,6		16,7		15,4	

Discussion

Extreme hypermetropia

Extreme hypermetropia is rare. Phakic refraction of at least +12 D. are to be met only exceptionally by ophthalmologists, most of whom will never encounter the condition. In a recent epidemiological study of refraction in Denmark (Fledelius 1983) only 0.6% had +6 D. or higher (n = 1416, 2832 eyes), the top value being +9.25, and similar experience can be drawn from the classical studies of Table 2.

It is surprising that the present patients had managed so well during early childhood that visual handicap had not been detected. Later, they met the demands of school life with corrected visual acuities of about 0.5. Nystagmus was never present. There was normal colour vision and no hemeralopic complaints. In microphthalmos literature other authors reported on tapetoretinal changes (Franceschetti & Gernet 1965), papillo-macular retinal folds (Boynton & Purnell 1975, Spitznas et al. 1983), or other retinal changes consistent with the low visual acuities acutally found (Fried et al. 1981). Our patients had no such changes, only 'hypermetropic fundus' with some tortuosity of vessels. Optic discs were normal.

A short comment about the power of the contact lens finally to be accepted by the younger brother (cf. Table 1). The high value of +26 D. is consistent with his very short axial length, but in the trial frame he refused spectacle glasses stronger than +19 D.

Oculometric features

Anterior eye segments appeared normal, also in the slit lamp, and microphthalmos would not have been suspected according to classical criteria (microcornea, deep-set eyes). Ultrasound measurement, however, confirmed the diagnosis and helped classifying the microphthalmos. We are dealing with

Table 2. Prevalence of high hypermetropia in some refractive studies.

	Number of eyes	Prevalence of high hyper-metropia	Highest refr. value (D.)
Betch (1929)	12,000	≥+6 D. in 0.4%	+11.0
Kronfeld & Devney (1931)	2,229	≥+6 D. in 0.5%	+8.0
Jackson (1932)	16,092	≥+7 D. in 0.6%	+10.0
Fledelius (1983)	2,832	≥+6 D. in 0.6%	+9.25

neither harmonious nanophthalmos, nor colobomatous or syndrome-like cases, but a posterior microphthalmos with proportions as described by Boynton & Purnell (1975) and Spitznas et al. (1983).

Obviously, posterior eye segment development has been arrested while anterior segments are unremarkable, except the announced corneal curvature. K-readings might be suggestive of keratoconus; astigmatism was however regular and with no bend of axes. – Lenses thicker than expected for age is a feature considered typical of small eyes in general.

In the absence of ocular growth curves from birth, it is not possible to state the critical age period of disproportionate eye growth. Keeping in mind, however, that most published similar cases are hereditary, it is probably prenatal. It is hard to postulate a post-natal influence totally arresting the posterior eye segment, with only a suggested slackening of corneal growth, a component of the anterior segment.

Hereditary transmission

Ophthalmic literature has many families with obvious heredity of (presumed) microphthalmos. Considering only those evaluated and typified by ultrasound, the reports of Franceschetti & Gernet (1965) and of Spitznas et al. (1983) are emphasized due to their similarity to the present family. In spite of lack of known consanguinity, autosomal recessive inheritance is probable, keeping in mind also that the frequencies of specific genes in the population of geographical isolates may deviate from those of larger populations.

Optics of the eye

Practical considerations have been touched upon already, with a hint to the unbecoming glasses of which these patients are dependent. As expected, contact lenses gave a better field of vision, but no significant improvement of visual acuity. A final remark, only, on the unhappy situation if cataract eventually occurs. There will hardly be a contact lens, neither a spectacle solution for the aphakic patient, nor will appropriate intraocular lenses be available. IOL-powers up to 50 D. are thus required to bring about emmetropia.

Summary

Refractive parameters were analysed in three siblings (out of six; age range 15–26 years, one female, two males) from the North Atlantic Faroe Islands. With extreme hypermetropia having been diagnosed around school-start, they now wanted to exchange their unbecoming +18 glasses with contact lenses. Corrected visual acuity was 0.3–0.5.

Microphthalmos was not apparent from anterior eye segment appearance, but vitreous lengths were ultrasonically short (8.1–9.2 mm) and the overall oculometric features consistent with posterior 'microphthalmos'. Axial lengths were 15.4–16.8 mm; hereditary transmission most likely autosomal recessive. There were no associated lesions, ocular or general.

With the present standard of ophthalmic examining techniques, the diagnosis and classification of microphthalmos should not be made without ultrasound measurement.

References

Betch A. 1929. Ueber die menschliche Refraktionskurve. Klin Monatsbl Augenhk 82: 365–379.

Boynton JR, Purnell EW. 1979. Bilateral microphthalmos without microcornea associated with unusual papillomacular retinal folds and high hyperopia. Amer J Ophthalmol 79: 820–826.

Fledelius HC. 1976. Prematurity and the eye. Ophthalmic 10-year follow-up of children of low and normal birth weight. Acta Ophthalmol (Copenh) suppl 128, pp 35–46.

Fledelius HC. 1983. Is myopia getting more frequent? A cross-sectional study of 1416 Danes aged 16 years +. Acta Ophthalmol (Copenh) 61: 545–559.

Fransceschetti A, Gernet H. 1965. Diagnostique ultrasonique d'une microphthalmie sans microcornée . . . nouveau syndrome familial. Arch Ophthalmol (Paris) 25: 105–116.

Fried M, Meyer-Schwickerath G, Koch A. 1981. Excessive hypermetropia, review and case report documented by echography. Ann Ophthalmol 14: 15–19.

Jackson E. 1932. Norms of refraction. J Amer Med Ass 98: 132–137.

Kronfeld PC, Devney C. 1931. Ein Beitrag zur Kentniss der Refraktionskurve. A von Graefes Arch Ophthalmol 126: 487–501.

Spitznas M, Gerke D, Bateman JB. 1983. Hereditary posterior microphthalmos, with papillomacular fold and high hyperopia. Arch Ophthalmol 101: 413–417.

Ultrasonic measurement of fetal eyeball diameter

L. FALCO, M. NARDI, F. PASSANI, M.P. BARTOLOMEI and
V. MAZZEO
Florence and Ferrara, Italy

Abstract

In vivo ultrasonic measurement of fetal eyeball diameter has been performed in 516 women from the 10th to the 40th week of pregnancy. Using the method of the 'best-fit' curve, a logarithmic growth curve of the type y = a + b lnx has been determined.

Th growth curve obtained shows a regular increase of fetal eye diameter; the mean values for each week of pregnancy are slightly higher than those previously reported from anatomical measurements in aborted fetuses. The confidence interval and the measurement interval of this logarithmic curve have been determined in order to formulate a guide for detecting gross abnormalities of fetal eye development during pregnancy.

Introduction

Biometric data regarding the growth of the fetal eye recorded in the literature do not have much clinical significance, as they are derived from anatomical measurements taken from fetuses induced to abort or were spontaneously aborted [4, 5, 6, 11]. The possibility of showing the ocular and orbital structures of the fetus echographically is a recent acquisition [2, 3, 7, 8, 9]. Recently, we have reported a simple and harmless method for the echographic measurement of the transverse diameter of the fetal eye [7, 8].

We have echographically measured the transverse diameter of the fetal eyeball during different gestational periods to determine useful biometric parameters for the evaluation of normal development.

We have subsequently put into practice a statistical analysis of the measurements obtained during the various gestational periods using the 'best-fit' method. The curve obtained best approximates the given data and the relative measurement interval, both of which can be useful in the detection of possible developmental alterations of the fetal eye.

K.C. Ossoinig (editor), Ophthalmic Echography, ISBN 978-94-010-7988-4

Technical note

The ability to detect the fetal ocular structures by ultrasonography during pregnancy is well known [2, 3, 7, 8]. We used an Aloka SSD-250, real time, B-mode ultrasound apparatus with a linear probe of 3.5 MHZ and a lateral resolution of less than 2 mm. By positioning two markers on the video monitor of this apparatus, it is possible to obtain the distance between the two corresponding ocular structures.

We have examined 516 pregnant women with a gestational period ranging between the 10th and 40th week of pregnancy during normal routine tests at the Echographic Diagnostic Laboratory of the Obstetrics-Gynecology Clinic at the University of Florence.

We have not measured women with systemic and/or metabolic diseases, with irregular menstruations and, therefore, doubtful gestation periods. Moreover, we have not measured these fetuses who presented abnormal growth parameters such as head diameter, abdominal circumference or femur length [1].

The eyeball in utero has an almost spherical shape [5]. The transverse eyeball diameter was preferentially measured. The fetal head is usually oriented along an axis which is either oblique or perpendicular to the longitudinal diameter of the mother's abdomen; therefore, we have measured only the eye proximal to the mother's abdomen, either the right or the left eye [7, 8]. With the help of statistical analysis ('best-fit' method), we have obtained the curve which best approximates the given data.

We have also calculated:
a) The correlation coefficient, which conventionally indicates how close the experimental data are to the hypothesis curve;
b) Values of the transverse diameter for the particular week corresponding to the hypothetical curve;
c) The confidence interval: interval of values having a 95% probability of including the real mean value of the measures taken;
d) The measurement interval: interval in which there is a 95% possibility that the measurement of the transverse diameter of the fetal eye is not pathological.

Results

Beginning with the 10th week of pregnancy, it is possible to detect the echoes of the proximal orbital and ocular walls, the transonic area, and the echoes of the distal ocular and orbital walls (Fig. 1).

After the 13th week of pregnancy it is possible to detect, on the front wall of

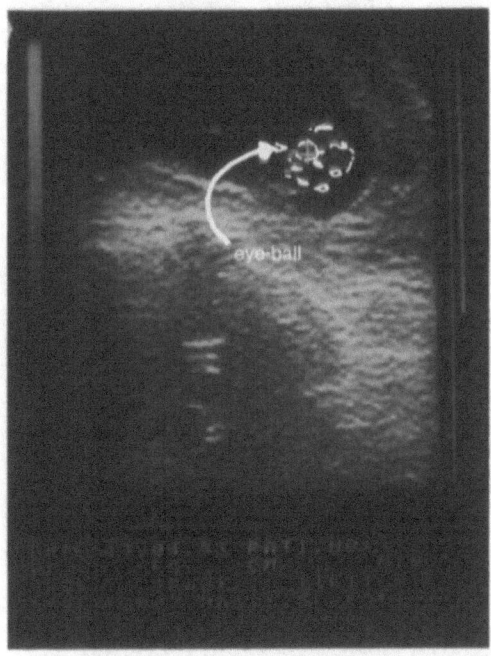

Fig. 1. 10th week of pregnancy. Echoes of the proximal orbital and ocular wall, a transonic area and the echoes of the distal ocular and orbital wall.

the eye, two echo-reflecting interfaces connected with the development of the anterior segment structures (Fig. 2). This facilitates the identification of the major transverse diameter of the eyeball.

After the 22–23rd week of pregnancy, it is possible to detect an area on the anterior part of the globe, showing a higher curvature relating to the cornea (Fig. 3).

Statistically, from the experimental data obtained (Table 1), we have observed that the best curve for the same data is the natural logarithmic function $y = a + b \ln x$. The values given to a and b are: $a = -25.48$; $b = +12.14$. They have been determined in order to minimize variations between values achieved experimentally and those calculated in the hypothetical curve. The correlation coefficient between the hypothetical curve and the experimental data is 0.96.

Figure 4 shows the growth curve obtained from experimental data with the 'best-fit' method; it contains the relative measurement intervals as well as the confidence interval.

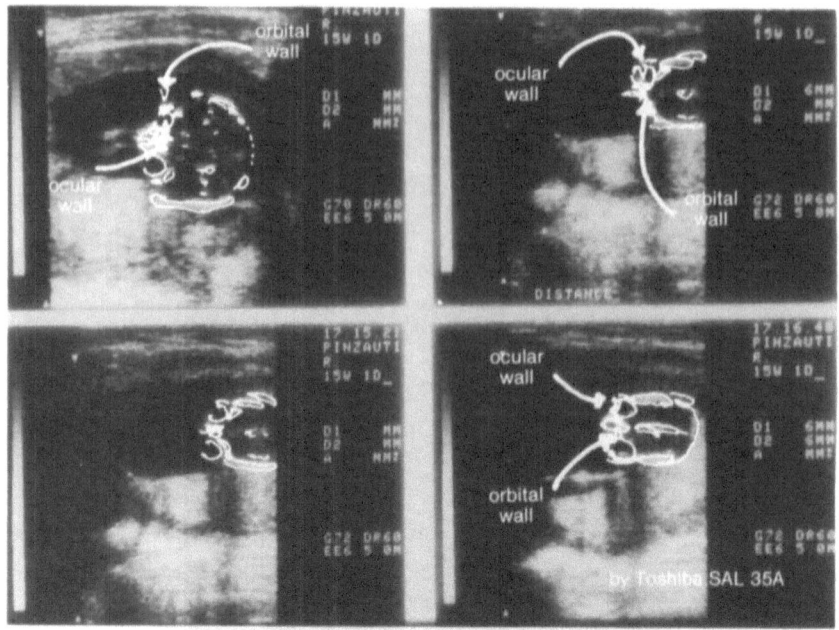

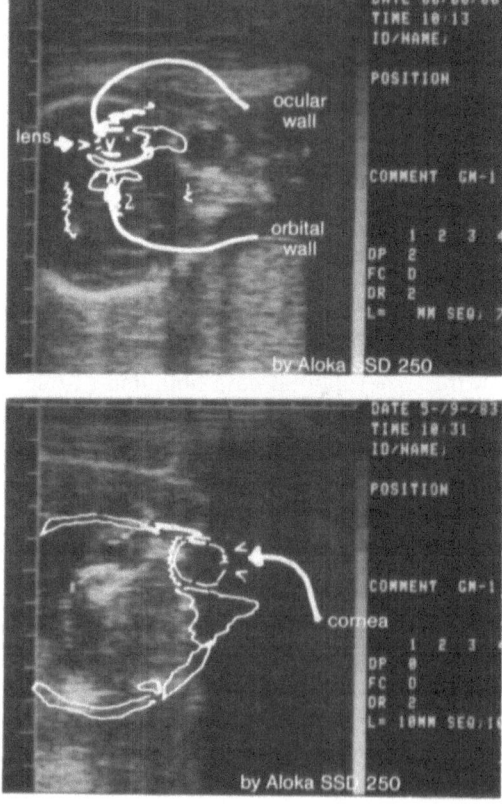

Fig. 2. 15th week of pregnancy. On the front wall of the eyeball are seen two echoreflecting interfaces connected with the development of the anterior segment structures.

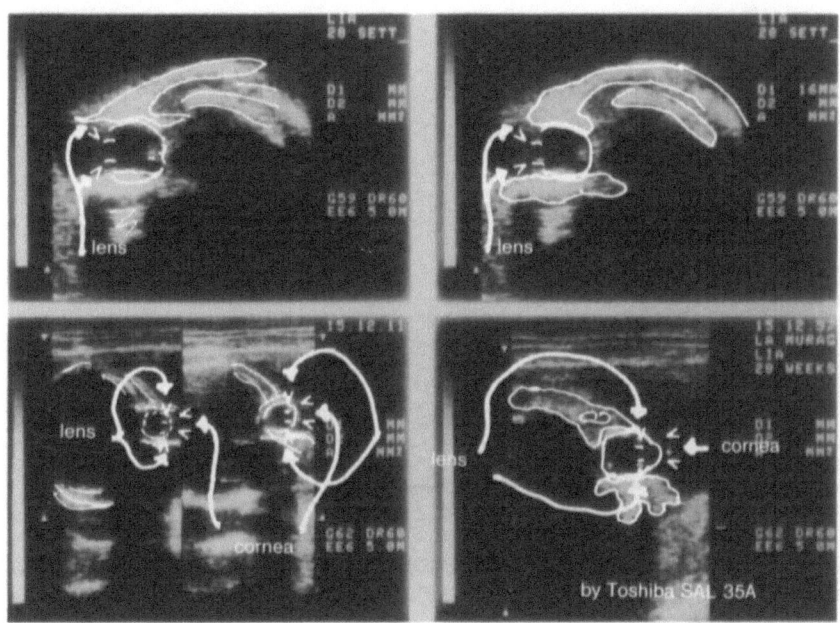

Fig. 3. 28th week of pregnancy. On the anterior part of the eyeball an area is seen showing a higher curvature relating to the cornea (<).

Table 1.

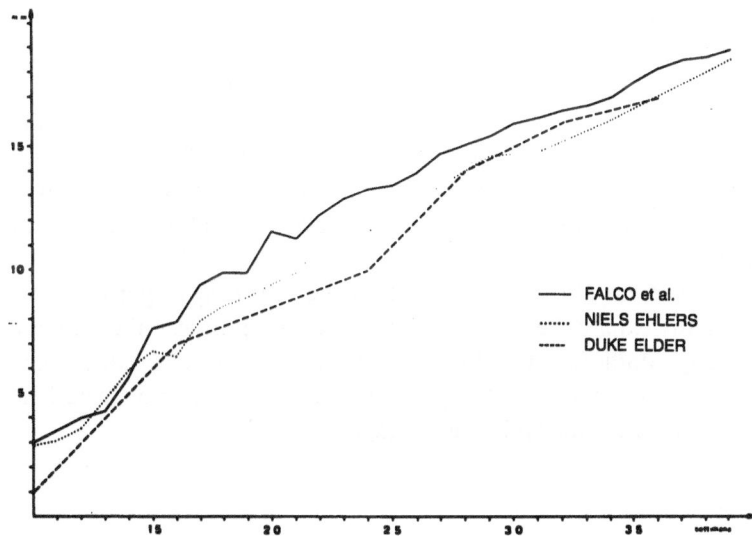

98

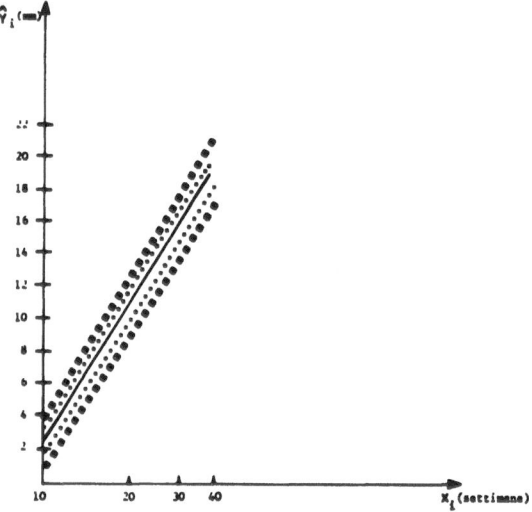

Fig. 4. Growth curve obtained from experimental data (——), measurement intervals (---) and confidence interval (...).

Discussion

A logarithmic curve of the physiological growth of the transverse diameter of the fetal eye in utero was developed from the statistical analysis of the experimental data.

The configuration of this curve is similar to the other growth curves usually utilized for the evaluation of the development of the fetus.

The correlation value of 0.96 demonstrates excellent correlation between the data obtained experimentally and the curve created statistically.

95% of the measurements taken of transverse fetal eyeball diameter during normal pregnancy fall within the measurement interval. This is of particular interest, from a clinical standpoint, because measurements different from those of the measurement interval have only a 5% probability of being taken on normal eyes.

The measurement of the fetal eyeball diameter is easy to perform, it does not significantly extend the time of a routine echographic examination, it does not imply any additional risk [10] and, after assessment of a normal growth curve, will provide the possibility of checking to determine whether the development of the fetal eyeball is normal.

Acknowledgments

The authors wish to thank Ing. C. Tasselli and Ing. L. Terreni for their assistance in statistical elaboration of the experimental data.

References

1. Borrutto F. 1982. Ecobiometria Fetale: Le Misure del Feto con Gli Ultrasuoni. Libr Cortina, Verona, pp. 19–40.
2. Bots R, Nijhuls J, Martin C. 1981. Human Fetal Eye Movements: Detection in Utero by Ultrasound, Early Human Development 5: 87.
3. Catizone FA, Franceschini-Benigni N, Gesmundo G, Carucci A, Pirillo P. 1983. Biometria Orbitaria: Una Integrazione ed Una Alternativa Nella Valutazione Dell'Estremo Encefalico, VIII Congr Naz SISUM: Bologna.
4. De Vlieger M, Strandness DE. 1978. Handbook of Clinical Ultrasound, New York, John Wiley & sons: 848.
5. Duke-Elder SS, Cook C. 1963. Normal and Abnormal Development, in Duke-Elder SS (ed.): System of Ophthalmology, Vol. III, Part 1, Embriology, London, H. Kimpton: 291–304.
6. Ehlers N, Matthiessen ME, Andersen H. 1968. The Prenatal Growth of the Human Eye, Acta Ophthalmol 46: 329–346.
7. Falco L, Pandimiglio A, Bartolomei MP, Nardi M. 1983. Nuovo Parametro di Ecobiometria Fetale: Misurazione del Diametro del Bulbo Oculare, ULTR OST GIN 3–4: 212–216.
8. Falco L, Pandimiglio A, Bartolomei MP, Carelli F, Nardi M. 1984. Curva di Accrescimento del Bulbo Oculare Fetale: Determinazione Ecografica in Gravidanza, Clin Oc 6: 13–15.
9. Anniruberto A, Tajan A. 1981. Lo Studio Ecografico dei Movimenti Oculari del Feto Umano, VI Cong Naz SISUM, Firenze, 273–277.
10. Mazzeo V. 1982. Problemi Relativi Agli Effetti Biologici Degli US, VII Congr Naz SISUM, Palermo.
11. Rivara A, Gemme G. 1965. Misurazione Dell'Asse Oculare Antero-Posteriore e del Potere Diottrico Oculare Dei Prematuri: ANN OFTALMOL 91: 1328–1334.

An ultrasonic comparison of normal eyes and eyes with idiopathic retinal detachment

F.A. YOUNG, T.C. BURTON and K.C. OSSOINIG
Pullman, Milwaukee & Iowa City, USA

Abstract

Sixty patients with idiopathic retinal detachments in one eye were evaluated with A-scan ultrasound using a Kretztechnik 7200 MA unit and Polaroid photography with measurements of the photographs under three-power magnification. This approach provides measures of the depth of the anterior chamber (DAC), lens thickness (LT), depth of the vitreous chamber (DVC) and posterior retinal-scleral thickness (RST) and permits comparison of these measures in the affected/non-affected eyes. While most patients were over 50 years old, there was a group of 12 myopic patients ranging from 13 to 22 years of age. The myopic eyes demonstrated a significantly larger DVC than the non-myopic eyes. The detached eye had a greater depth of the DAC and a greater combined DAC and LT than the non-detached eye. The RST was significantly thinner in the myopic eyes, but there was no significant difference between the detached and the non-detached eyes. The ultrasonic comparisons did not provide definitive evidence as to the possible cause or causes of the retinal detachment.

K.C. Ossoinig (editor), Ophthalmic Echography, ISBN 978-94-010-7988-4

Optical and acoustical measurement of the corneal thickness. A study on phantoms and living human eyes

R.-D. LEPPER and H.G. TRIER
Bonn, FRG

Introduction

The measurement of corneal thickness serves to answer some clinical questions, such as: the early detection of corneal edema; changes in corneal thickness in glaucoma or keratoconus; operative changes in corneal thickness or curvature for refractive improvement. Early experiments for comparative measurements of the corneal thickness by optical and acoustical methods were carried out in the sixties (Lowe, 1967). In clinical routine optical methods (Jaeger, 1952) usually provide a measurement accuracy of about 0.05 mm, while the precision of ultrasonic standard equipment in general is only 0.1 mm. Nowadays specialized pachymeters are on the market which claim to be precise to +/−9 microns. The aim of this study was to determine the limitations and drawbacks of a high resolution ultrasonic counting technique for clinical practice.

Material and methods

We used our RESSOURCE-system with an electronic accuracy of 0.02 mm. Reprogramming the system originally used for implant lens determination, enabled the measurement of thin isolated layers like the cornea (Lepper & Trier, 1984).

Figure 1 demonstrates the screen data display of the computer. The histogram of the values measured easily gives information of measurement quality. The evaluation of the layer thickness is performed on command. A printout to keep with the patient's record is available.

K.C. Ossoinig (editor), Ophthalmic Echography, ISBN 978-94-010-7988-4

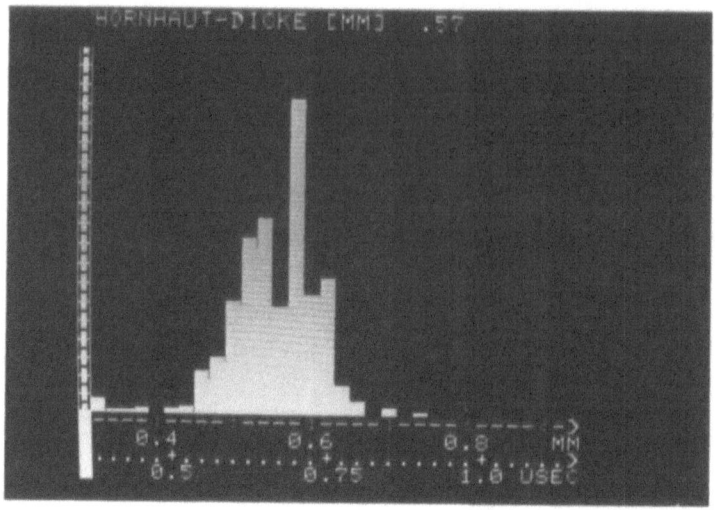

Fig. 1. Screen data display of the measured layer thickness. The indicated thickness value (upper number) is calculated assuming a sound velocity of 1639 m/s.

Results

To confirm absolute accuracy of the system mechanical flat phantoms of fixed and variable thickness were measured. Perspex, glass, metallic plates and two water layer phantoms (Fig. 2 a + b) were examined both mechanically and acoustically. Measurements were consistent. In all cases the two values of the interval 'd' confirmed to 0.02 mm within a thickness range of about 0.32 to 0.75 mm (Table 1).

To determine the system accuracy on shaped structures like cornea we used a perspex phantom. The mechanical thickness of this cornea phantom and the ultrasound measurement were in total agreement (delta = 5 microns). The repeatability of the measurement values in this case is shown in Table 2.

We measured 50 eyes with the ultrasonic system. A contact eye cup was applied which was held in position by the eyelids and then filled with water. The transducer was aligned centrally to the cornea. The values obtained were highly reproducible and in reasonable accordance to the optically measured values (a slit lamp supplement made by Haag-Streit, Bern was used). However both data groups showed a correlation coefficient of 48% only. Figure 3 demonstrates the frequency distribution of the differences between optically and acoustically measured corneal thickness.

When measuring more peripheral corneal thickness the acoustically determined values were far less reproducible then those measured at the center of the cornea. The variability of the values was equal to or less than 0.1 mm.

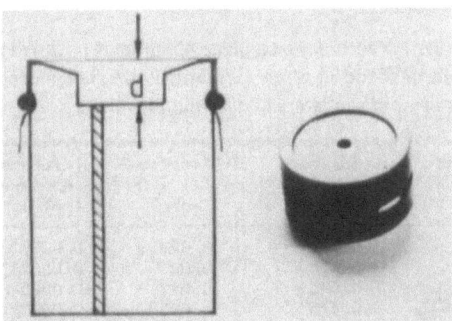

Fig. 2a. Plane phantom with fixed interval 'd' which was determined prior to the acoustical measurement by means of a dial gauge. The membrane's thickness is less than 0.01 mm.

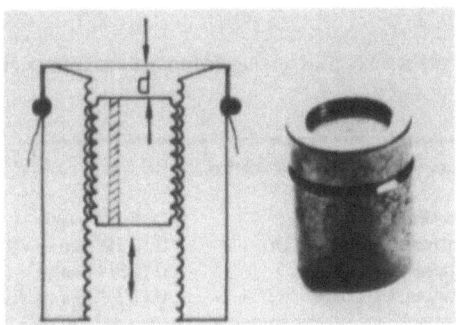

Fig. 2b. Plane phantom with variable interval 'd'.

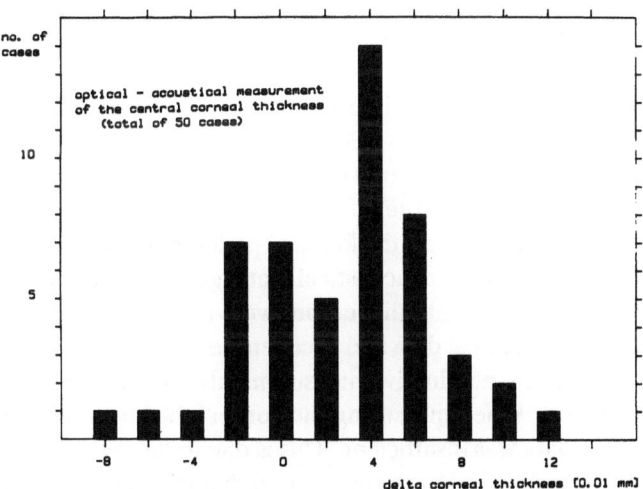

Fig. 3. Histogram of the differences of optical and acoustical corneal thickness measured in vivo (50 cases).

Table 1. Evaluation of the system accuracy on a plane phantom (Fig. 2b). The values of column 2 are converted to the speed of sound in water (Willard, 1967). The mean value of column 3 is interpreted as the zeroing error of the interval 'd' of the phantom.

measurement interval [mm]	ultrasonic measurement [mm]	difference col. 1 - 2 [mm]	difference minus mean [mm]
0.75	0.727	0.023	0.0037
0.656	0.636	0.02	0.0007
0.563	0.545	0.017	-0.0023
0.469	0.445	0.023	0.0037
0.375	0.336	0.039	0.0197
0.313	0.318	-0.006	-0.0133
	mean value:	0.0193 [mm]	

Table 2. Repeatability of the system. The cornea phantom made from perspex was measured 25 times.

number of measurements	25	
arithmetic mean	0.55	mm
standard deviation	0.019	mm
minimum value	0.53	mm
maximum value	0.57	mm

Discussion

The measurements on flat phantom demonstrate a system accuracy in the limits of the electronic resolution. The proof of measurement accuracy at curved surfaces is of considerable importance since the broad sound beam reaches the corneal periphery too (Fig. 4a). The experiments on curved phantoms indicated that the fringe area of the sound beam is of no importance when measuring the central thickness.

The measurement of the corneal thickness of patients and the rather insufficient correlation of optical and acoustical data gave rise to the question whether optical or acoustical or both methods were responsible for this result. Statistical scatter of the optical data and excellent repeatability of the acoustical data on both phantom and in-vivo measurements point to a superiority of the acoustical method. When measuring the corneal thickness off-center the repeatability of the data was insufficient. This is due to the fact that the fringe area of the sound beam now interferes in an undeterminable way (Fig. 4b). The use of a water filled stand-off with a membrane contacting the cornea, instead of the eye cup did not improve accuracy. One reason is that the membrane introduces an additional variable interval. This could be overcome

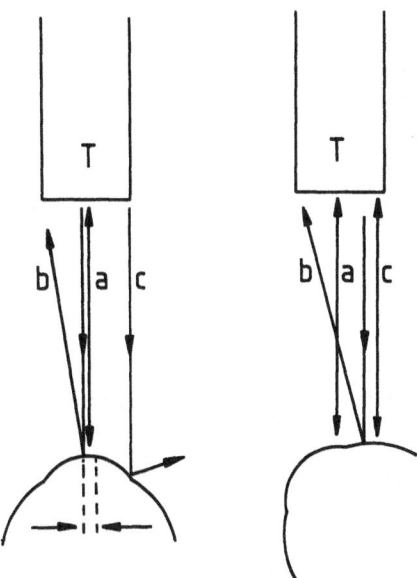

Fig. 4a (left). The sound field of the transducer (T) is symbolized by the three traces a, b, and c. Despite the fact that the transducer and the cornea are comparably thick only a small (indicated) central area of the cornea is 'seen' by the transducer.

Fig. 4b (right). Echotrace 'a' (and its neighbours) only come from the area of interest. The other echoes are reflected from the sclera and therefore interfere heavily. A discrimination of wanted and unwanted echoes is practically impossible.

by using a stand-off technique without membrane. However an accurate topometry of the corneal thickness cannot be achieved with a manually guided transducer.

The cornea gets thinner when pressing a transducer onto it. However, using reasonable assumptions, it can be shown mathematically that this does not contribute significantly to the measurement error.

Conclusions

The central corneal thickness can be determined with an accuracy of 0.02 mm without needing a special transducer. However, non-central measurements can not be performed with this technique. To prevent the outer fringe area of the sound beam from interfering with the central portion, a small transducer only a few millimeters apart from the cornea has to be selected. This improves the definition of the examined corneal area, too. However, a precise topometry of the cornea with this manually guided transducer cannot be performed. Instead, a mechanically steered transducer immersed in water which is very close to the cornea is needed.

Measurement accuracy of the total system is determined by both the electronic and the ultrasonic sub-systems. The inferior resolution of the ultrasonic components in comparison with the superior electronic precision reduces the accuracy of the total system.

References

Jaeger W. 1952. Tiefenmessung der menschlichen Vorderkammer mit planparallelen Platten (Yusatzgeraet zur Spaltlampe). Graefes Arch Ophthal 153: 120–131.

Lepper R-D, Trier HG. 1984. Computer-Aided Ultrasonic Measurements of the Corneal Thickness. Ophthalmic Res 16: 163–167. (S. Karger, Basel).

Lowe RF. 1967. Linear A-scan ultrasonography in the measurement of intra-ocular distances: a stand-off technique. Trans Ophthal Soc Aust 26: 72–77.

Willard GW. 1967. Temperature coefficient of ultrasonic velocity in solutions. J acoust Soc Am 19: 235–242.

Improved ultrasound pachymetry at corneal mid-periphery

M. FREESE
Toronto, Canada

Surgeons performing radial keratotomies currently rely mainly on central and paracentral measurements to set blade depths since the mid-peripheral thickness is normally greater (Martola & Baum, 1968; Tomlinson, 1972). However, the occurrence of corneal irregularities and resultant perforations together with the increasing use of other forms of kerato-refractive surgery suggest that accurate measurements are also required in the mid-peripheral region. A typical example of corneal 'scalloping' is shown in Fig. 1.

Most of the present ultrasonic pachymeters rely on some form of pulse-echo level detection to determine the intervals to be measured. If adequate corrective measures are not taken, this can result in decreased accuracy at the mid-periphery (and periphery) due to the reduced amplitudes and distortion of the corneal echo pulses resulting from the inclination of the anterior and posterior surfaces to each other (typically 2°) at these positions (Fig. 2). Additional error can result from probe misalignment especially if the acceptance angle of the probe is large. The Radionics Medical pachymeter (Corneomap 4500) digi-

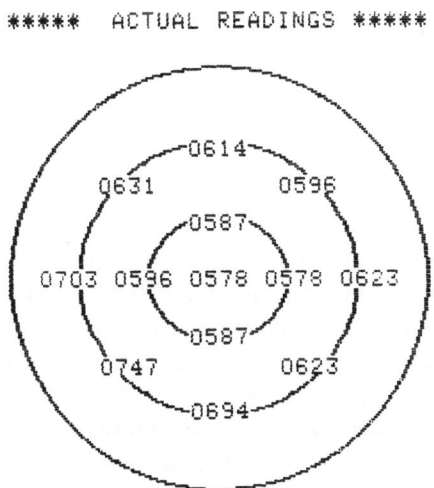

***** ACTUAL READINGS *****

Fig. 1. Corneomap 4500 printout of measurements on a moderately thick cornea indicating the presence of 'scalloping' in the superior temporal quadrant.

K.C. Ossoinig (editor), Ophthalmic Echography, ISBN 978-94-010-7988-4

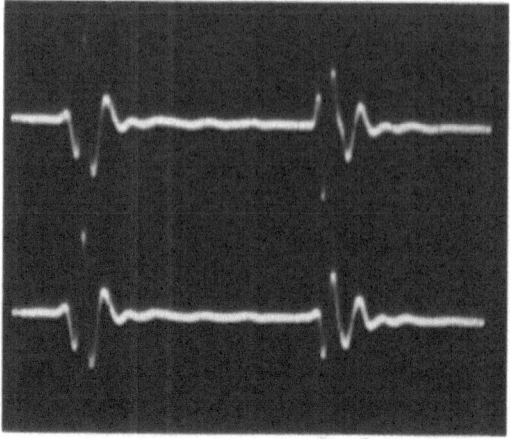

Fig. 2. The upper trace shows echoes from a corneal phantom having parallel anterior and posterior surfaces for the case of perpendicular beam incidence. The lower trace shows the echoes resulting when the posterior surface is inclined at an angle of about 5 deg. to the beam. Note the distortion of the posterior echo. The same phenomenon is observed in the corneal echoes at mid-periphery or periphery for similar beam angles.

tizes the RF A-scans to be measured and employs real time signal processing to overcome these problems (Freese et al., 1983).

This paper describes results of measurements in the central, paracentral and mid-peripheral region using the Corneomap 4500, the Accutome Inc. Corneometer and the Haag-Streit optical pachymeter.

Methods and materials

The Corneomap 4500 employed had a 'liquid' tip (actually a water filled PMMA cone); a more recent model has a solid tip. The liquid tip has a physical diameter of 1.6 mm and a beamwidth at the corneal entrance site of approximately 3/4 mm. The ultrasound frequency is 20 MHz. The two instruments are similar to the extent that both employ liquid probes having approximately the same dimensions, and have a readout resolution of 9 and 10 μm, respectively.

The measurements were performed as part of the normal preoperative workup for RK surgery. Each eye was measured over a three hour interval (usually in the morning) with the optical measurements (employing the catoptric technique – Schachar et al., 1981) being done first. Each measurement was repeated four times.

The order in which the two u.s. pachymeters were used was randomized. However, due to the demands of the clinical practice and the automatic recording nature of the Corneomap, slightly different procedures were employed for recording the measurements. With the Corneomap a single reading was recorded at each measurement site – 8 mid-peripheral, 4 para-central, and the center of the pupil according to the pattern shown in Fig. 1. The first reading obtained at each site was rejected. One or two more readings were then observed before the reading was locked in by the ophthalmologist.

With the Corneometer, the measurements were also made by the ophthalmologist but the numerical readings were recorded silently by an assistant. A deliberate effort was made to determine and map the thinnest part of the central region. Between 10 and 20 separate readings were recorded per eye and averaged.

Results

Although some staircase patterning is evident in the plot of the central thicknesses measured with the two instruments (Fig. 3a) the overall correlation is quite good. The total residual standard deviation of the measurements, s_{tr}, is 11 μm where $s_{tr}^2 = (s_x^2 + s_y^2)(1 - r^2)$ and s_x^2, s_y^2 and r are the variances and the correlation coefficient, respectively. The mean thicknesses listed in Table 1 reflect the experimental bias of the Corneometer measurements towards slightly lower values. Results of an earlier study by Hikishima (1983) on 134 eyes (see Table 1) did not indicate any significant bias in the Corneomap 4500 central zone readings. Also, no significant differences in the mean values are observed at any of the other positions listed in Table 1.

Fig. 3b shows a similar plot of measurements in the paracentral temporal region. The correlation is of the order of 0.9. Similar results were obtained for the other paracentral sectors. It must be emphasized that the data points in Fig. 3b-c correspond to individual readings. In general this does not reflect standard clinical practice where a number of readings are taken, averaged, and compared with adjacent readings, thereby yielding better statistical estimates of the actual thicknesses.

Fig. 3c shows the data obtained at mid-periphery. Even with the two largest thickness values included, the correlation is less than 0.65. Probably the major reason for this poor correlation were errors due to differences in probe positioning on the cornea for the two sets of measurements, as in contrast to measurements taken in the OR, the corneas were unmarked. The other sources of error include instrumental errors, possible variations in corneal thickness during the interval between the measurements, e.g. due to drying

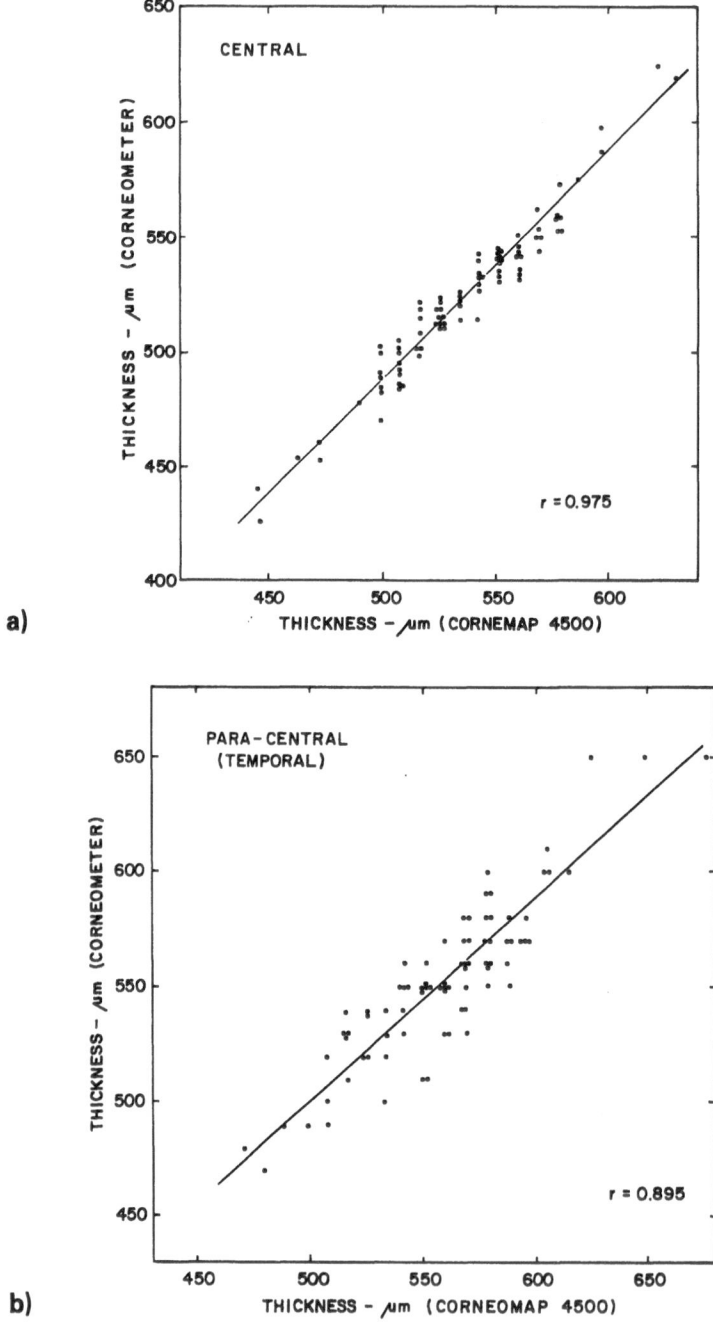

Fig. 3. Correlation of thickness values measured with the Corneometer and the Corneomap 4500. (a) central; (b) paracentral; (c) mid-peripheral (superior or 12:00 o'clock position).

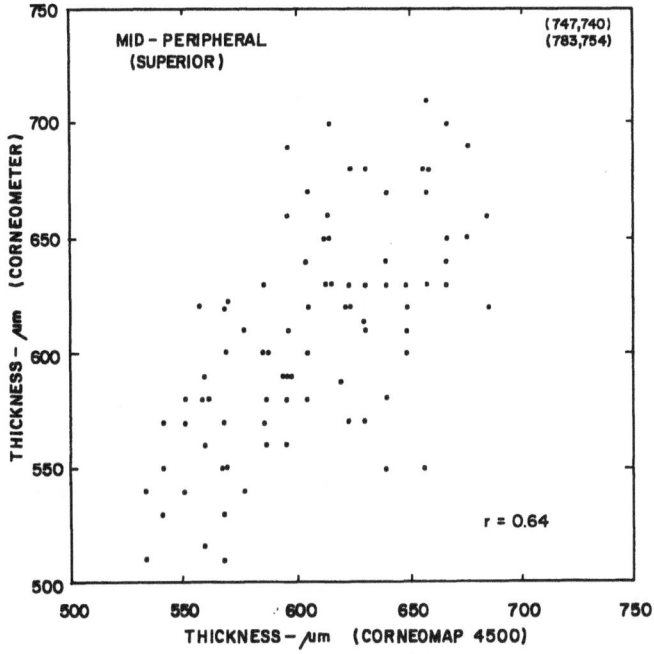

c)

Table 1. Comparisons of corneal thickness.

present study: site	86 eyes no. of eyes	mean age: 32 (18–51) yrs.	
		Corneomap 4500 μm	Corneometer μm
central	84	535 ± 35	523 ± 35
paracentral			
– temporal	79	559 ± 35	552 ± 35
– nasal	83	555 ± 37	537 ± 35
mid-peripheral			
– temporal	81	586 ± 42	588 ± 45
– nasal	83	616 ± 43	607 ± 45
– superior	84	611 ± 47	612 ± 53
Previous studies: Hikishima (1983): Site	134 eyes no.	approx. mean age 51 (22–90) yrs.	
		Corneomap 4500 μm	Haag-streit pach. μm
central	134	526 ± 27 (487–607)	531 ± 25 (462–566)

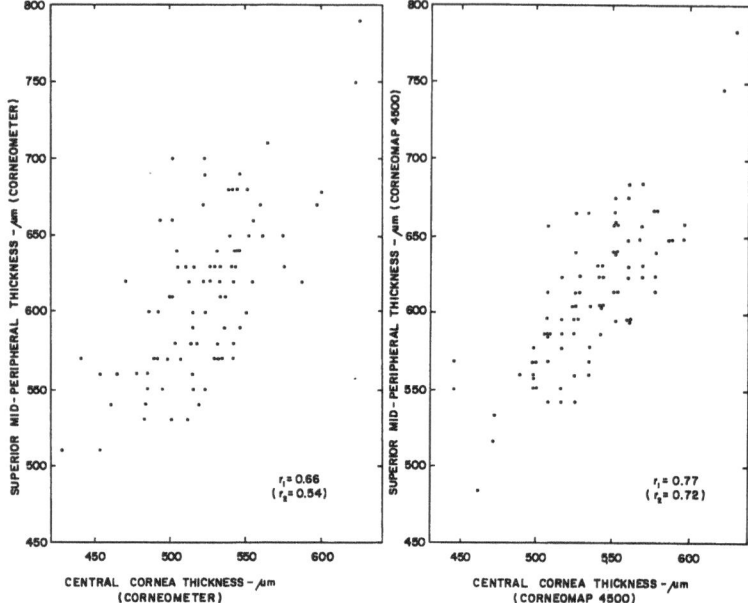

Fig. 4. Correlation of thickness values at the center and mid-periphery for the same eyes using (a) Corneometer; (b) Corneomap 4500. To avoid excessive weighting by the two extreme values at the low and high end of each graph, the correlation coefficient (r_2) has been calculated minus these data points.

(Mishima, 1968) and observer errors. However, despite the poor correlation, the mean mid-peripheral thicknesses differ less than $4 \mu m$, on the average, between the instruments. The s.d. are also comparable (Table 1).

Considerably more insight into the relative performances of the instruments at mid-periphery is obtained by plotting these readings as a function of the corresponding central readings, Fig. 4. Despite the fact that the Corneometer central readings are averaged over 10 to 20 measurements, the correlation of the Corneomap measurements is definitely better. The value of p is roughly in agreement with the results obtained by Tomlinson (1972) using optical pachymetry. To avoid excessive weighting of the regression by the two smallest and the two largest central readings which correspond to the same eyes in both cases, the correlation coefficients were recalculated minus these values. The resultant correlation coefficients of 0.54 and 0.72 indicate a significant difference in performance of the Corneometer and the Corneomap at the mid-periphery. Assuming approximately equal residual variances of $(7.8 \mu m)^2$ for the central thickness measurements (based on the results of the measurements shown in Fig. 3a and Table 1) the residual s.d. calculated from the total residual variances for the Corneometer and Corneomap 4500 mid-peripheral values were $46 \mu m$ and $34 \mu m$, respectively.

Conclusions

The results show that ultrasound pachymeters utilizing the same type of probe and of approximately equal accuracy in the central zone of the cornea may have significantly different accuracies at mid-periphery. The reason for this appears to stem from the differences in response of the detection methods used, to variations in amplitude and distortions in the echo pulse shape resulting from the combined effects of non-parallel corneal interfaces and non-perpendicular beam incidence at mid-periphery.

Acknowledgement

The author would like to thank Dr. M. Deitz (Kansas City, Kan.) for performing the measurements.

References

Freese M, Callway E, Wong P. 1983. Precision thickness gauging using digitized RF waveforms. Ultrasonics Int'l '83, Halifax NS.

Hikishima H, Sasaki K. 1984. Clinical test report. School of Ophthalmology, Kanazawa Medical College, pp. 10.

Martola EL, Baum JL. 1968. Central and peripheral corneal thickness. Arch Ophthal vol 79, pp. 28–30.

Mishima S. 1968. Corneal thickness. Survey Ophthal vol. 13, pp. 57–96.

Schachar RA, Black TD, Huang T. 1981. Understanding radial keratotomy. LAL Publishing, Denison, Texas.

Tomlinson A. 1972. A clinical study of the central and peripheral thickness and curvature of the human cornea. Acta Ophthal vol 50, pp. 73–82.

Ultrasonic measurement of corneal thickness (pachymetry). A comparative study

E. MORAGREGA, E. HERNANDEZ and C. HAYS
Mexico City, Mexico

Summary

This study tries to demonstrate the effectiveness of the ultrasonic pachymeter in the Xenotech 404 high-resolution unit in measuring corneal thickness, and makes a comparison with optical methods.

Introduction

When we have opaque media such as corneal edema, nubeculae or leukoma, it is almost impossible to measure the corneal thickness with optical methods. In these cases, the ultrasonic pachymeter can do such measurement accurately because of the easy recognition of the interfaces of saline-solution / epithelium and endothelium / aqueous humor.

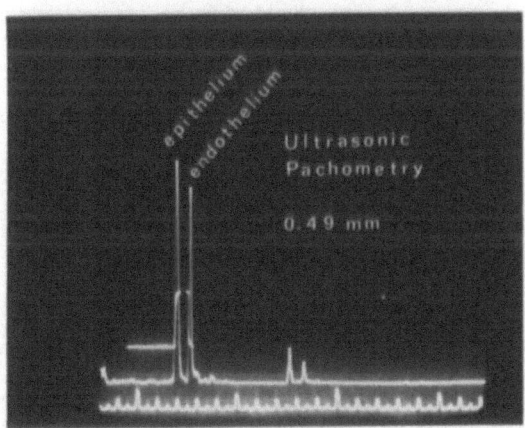

Fig. 1. A-Scan echogram obtained during pachymetry.

K.C. Ossoinig (editor), Ophthalmic Echography, ISBN 978-94-010-7988-4

Material and method

A Xenotech 404 high-resolution unit with a 20-MHz A-scan probe was used for echographic measurements, and the Haag/Streit slit-lamp pachymeter as well as the pachymeter of the specular microscope were employed for optical measurements which then were compared to the results of the acoustic measurements.

300 corneas were studied at the Hospital of the Association to Prevent Blindness in Mexico. 200 corneas were normal and were measured with the three methods; a different examiner performed each type of measurement not knowing the results of the other methods. 100 corneas were pathologic with different degrees of edema, nubeculae and leukoma.

Results

The study of the 200 normal corneas gave us the idea that the three methods provide similar results (Table 1), but in the pathologic corneas we found that the ultrasonic measurements were possible in all of the corneas, whereas measurements were not possile with the optical methods (Table 2).

We believe that the ultrasonic method is very useful in measuring the corneal thickness prior to refractive surgery in order to map the cornea. The possibility of having good perpendicularity of the ultrasonic probe on the corneal surface, in its center as well as in its periphery, is a unique situation that is often very difficult to obtain with the optical methods.

Table 1. 200 normal corneas.

	Ultrasound	Haag-Streit	Specular
Mean	.5034	.5111	.52
Variance	.1204	.1333	.1056
Standard Deviation	.0347	.0365	.0325

Table 2. 100 pathologic corneas.

Utility	Comparative %
Ultrasound	100%
Haag-Streit	62%
Specular	10%

Biometric evaluation of the lens in glaucomatous and normal eyes

G. CENNAMO and N. ROSA
Naples, Italy

Summary

Narrow angle glaucoma produces some biometric variations in the dioptric system of the eye. The purpose of this study is the ultrasonic measurements of lens thickness in a group of patients with narrow angle glaucoma as compared to a group of patients with normal intraocular pressure.

Lens measurements were obtained with the standardized A-scan using the immersion technique. Echograms were measured in microseconds and then converted into millimeters since the ultrasound velocity in the normal lens is 1641 m/sec. Our results show a slight increase in lens thickness in those patients with narrow angle glaucoma. While many factors undoubtedly contribute to the pathogenesis of this disease by involving the closed angle, we conclude that the increased lens thickness represents a high risk condition.

Introduction

Narrow angle glaucoma produces some biometric variations in the dioptric system of the eye. In 1883, Priestley Smith reported measurements of lenses removed from enucleated glaucomatous eyes and eyes from cadavers, and showed that in acute congestive glaucoma the lenses were larger than normal.

The blossoming of ocular biometry for angle closure glaucoma burst forth with the use of time amplitude ultrasonography by Lowe, Delmarcelle and associates, and Toulinson and Leighton. They respectively found lens thickness values of:

K.C. Ossoinig (editor), Ophthalmic Echography, ISBN 978-94-010-7988-4

Normal eyes	Eyes with narrow angle glaucoma
4.50 (0.34)	5.09 (0.34) (Lowe)
4.46 (0.42)	5.43 (0.46) (Delmarcelle et al.)
4.67	5.23 (Toulinson and Leighton)

The purpose of this study is to compare the ultrasonic measurements of lens thickness in a group of patients with narrow angle glaucoma with those obtained from a group of patients with normal intraocular pressure.

Material and methods

Lens measurements were obtained with standardized A-Scan echography using the immersion technique. Since the ultrasound velocity in the normal lens is 1641 m/sec, the echograms were measured in microseconds and then converted in millimeters. In this study we considered 60 patients (105 eyes) affected by narrow angle glaucoma – 29 (50 eyes) in an acute phase and 31 (55 eyes) in a chronic phase varying in age from 42 to 80 years. These patients had never undergone any antiglaucomatous treatment until the biometric evaluation. 35 patients (63 eyes) varying in age from 20 to 80 years with normal intraocular pressure and without pathology were examined. Patients with some opacity of the lens were not included in this study because the ultrasonic velocity is different in the cataractous lens. The results obtained were compared with the normal value averages obtained in the group of non-glaucomatous patients and evaluated in relation to different ages.

During the examination, each patient had to look at a light point situated 3 meters away. This was done to exclude any influence of the accommodation on the lens thickness. We evaluated our results considering the patient's age using a linear regression.

Results

We can summarize our results as follows (Fig. 1–2):
- The increase in lens thickness in normal eyes is 1.2 mm in patients 20 to 80 years of age.
- The increase in lens thickness in normal eyes does not have a linear, but a curvilinear course, reaching a maximum between the ages of 70 and 80.
- Standard deviation from the mean is lower than that found by other authors.

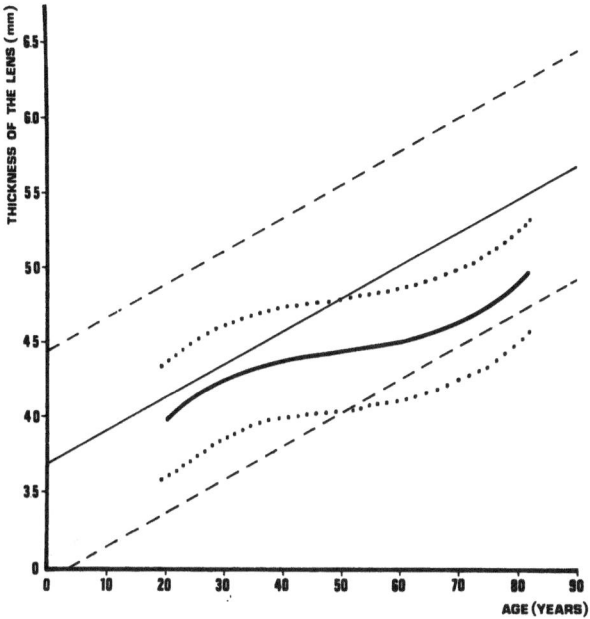

Fig. 1.

------------- Correlation between lens thickness and age in a group of patients with normal intraocular pressure (Delmarcelle et al.)

·:·:·:·:·:·:· Correlation between lens thickness and age in a group of patients with normal intraocular pressure (Cennamo et al.)

– Lens growth in patients with narrow angle glaucoma is higher than normal.
– The kind of growth differs from a normal eye, and has a maximum growth between 55 and 70 years of age.

Discussion

Many factors surely contribute to the pathogenesis of the acute narrow angle glaucoma correlated to biometric alterations regarding different structures of the dioptric system, among which decreased anterior chamber depth is clinically the most relevant. The biometric data correlated with the decreased anterior chamber depth are:
– smaller corneal diameter;
– smaller radius of anterior and posterior corneal curvature;
– thicker lens;
– lens situated in a relatively forward position;
– shorter axial length.

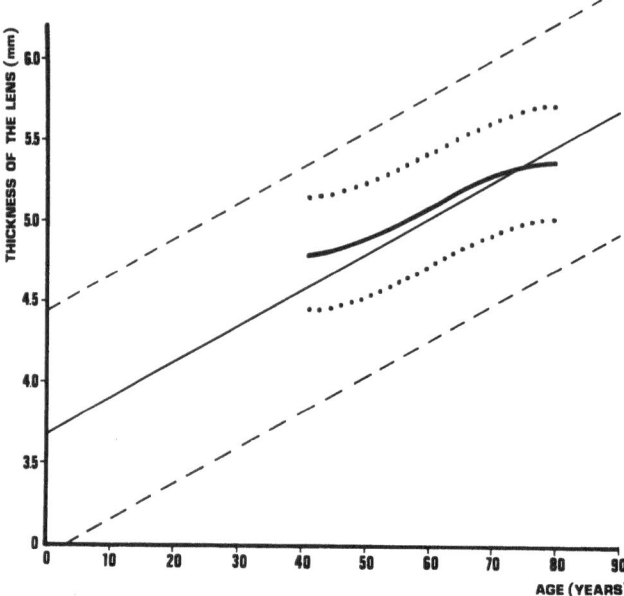

Fig. 2.

---------------- Correlation between lens thickness and age in a group of patients with normal
---------------- intraocular pressure (Demarcelle et al.)

·:·:·:·:·:·:· Correlation between lens thickness and age in a group of patients with narrow
angle glaucoma (Cennamo et al.)

Even if these data play a different role, each of them can contribute to the
pathogenesis of this disease. We think our results confirm the hypothesis that
the thickening of the lens may be one of the most important causes in the
pathogenesis of narrow angle glaucoma.

Moreover, our data indicates that in glaucomatous patients there is an
altered course in the growth of lens thickness. We have pointed out that there
is an increase in the lens thickness in patients varying in age from 40 to 50 years
which is higher in glaucomatous eyes than in normal eyes, but it is between 50
and 70 years of age that we have noticed the biggest difference. In fact, in this
age range the increase of lens thickness in glaucomatous eyes is higher than in
other age groups, while in normal eyes there is a low tendency toward
thickening of the lens. This data could explain the increased incidence of this
pathology in patients varying in age from 55 to 70 years. Finally, we have
pointed out a standard deviation in the 2 groups which was lower than that
found by other authors. Surely this depends on our technique, which is more
accurate with regard to both the lens and the globe.

References

Delmarcelle Y. et al. 1971. Etude biométrique du globe oculaire dans le glaucome a angle fermé. Bull et Mem Soc Franc Opht 84: 449–457.

Franceschetti A, Gernet H. 1965. Importance of ultrasonic ecography measurements of the optical components of the eye. Trans Amer Acad Opht and Otolar 69: 465–473.

Gabai R, Calabrese D, Cennamo G. 1983. Lens Ultrasonographic Biometric Evaluation in Acute Angle Closure Glaucoma. International Symposium on Glaucoma, Jerusalem, Israel.

Gernet H, Franceschetti A. 1967. Ultrasound biometry of the eye, (Review), pp. 175–206, Ultrasonics in Ophthalmology Symposium, Munster, 1966, Basel/N.Y., Karger.

Lowe RF. 1974. Primary angle closure glaucoma. Biometry and the clinician. In Etienne et Paterson, International Glaucoma Symposium, Albi: 247–260.

Lowe RF. 1971. Primary Angle Closure Glaucoma. Ultrasonic investigations. Acta XXI Concil Opht. (Mexico) Part 2 Amsterdam, Excerpta Medica 1082–1084.

Lowe RF. 1968. Time-Amplitude Ultrasonography for Ocular Biometry Amer J Ophth 66: 913–918.

Lowe RF. 1972. Anterior Lens Curvature. Comparison between Normal Eyes and those with Primary Angle Closure Glaucoma. Brit J Ophth 56: 409–413.

Lowe RF. 1969. Causes of Shallow Anterior Chamber in Primary Angle Closure Glaucoma. Ultrasonic Biometry of Normal and Angle Closure Glaucoma Eyes. Amer J Ophth 67: 87–93.

Luyckx-Bacus J. 1971. Contribution de l'Ultrasonographie A à l'étude du Glaucome à angle fermé. In: Bock J et Ossoinig K, Ultrasonographia Medica. Verlag der Wiener Med Akad, 573–577.

Luyckx-Bacus J, Weekers JF. 1967. Contribution a l'étude des glaucomes par ultrasonographie. Ann Oculistique 200: 489–504.

Luyckx-Bacus J, Weekers JF. 1966. Etude biométrique de l'oeil Humain par ultrasonographie. Bull Soc Belge Opht 143: 552–567.

Ossoinig KC. 1979. Ophthalmic Ultrasonography: Comparative Techniques, Winter Vol. 19, N°4.

Rosa N, Cennamo G, Gabai R. Biometric evaluation of the Lens in Glaucoma. VII Congress of the European Society of Ophthalmology, May 84, Helsinki, Finland.

Ultrasonic microbiometry of the eye

E.W. PURNELL, K.E. FRANK, E. HOLASEK and W.D. JENNINGS
Cleveland, USA

A major constraint in measuring the thickness of the ocular coats by acoustic biometry is our lack of knowledge of both the number and identity of the reflecting surfaces. It is probably naive to think that the exact boundaries of the three component layers are appropriately represented on the echogram or that the number of reflecting surfaces are limited to these anatomical boundaries. Yet the potential information obtained from microbiometric ultrasonic analysis could be invaluable in the study of many genetic and acquired chorioretinal diseases *in vivo* during their earliest stages of development.

Our own experience in studying the reflective properties of the retina in the past several years has left us impressed with the dynamic variations in the apparent orientation of these layers during a period of interrogation, and equally impressed with the reproducibility of the data when measurements are repeated on the same individual over a period of time. In addition, while we may conjecture as to the origin of echos from within the retina or choroid we presently believe that the state of the art does not permit us to fully correlate the ultrasonic data with the known histologic features of these tissues.

This paper presents typical results obtained in a study of the effect of the vascular pulse on the reflectivity data, and reflects our understanding of the complexity of the problem we are attempting to solve.

Methods

The posterior coats were interrogated by a 10 MHz broadband focused transducer coupled to the cornea by a degassed water offset. The central portion of the focal zone was placed within the posterior coats of the eye. The transducer assembly was mounted with appropriate counterbalance for corneal applanation on a slitlamp. An electrocardiographic device monitored the patient's heart rate, and the QRS complex triggered a pulse generator. The RF pattern of the posterior coats was monitored on an oscilloscope, and when alignment

K.C. Ossoinig (editor), Ophthalmic Echography, ISBN 978-94-010-7988-4

was deemed statisfactory, RF data was captured by a Biomation transient recorder and dumped to an HP9825 microcomputer for storage. Each interrogation of a specific area of the retina consisted of 16 A-scans taken in succession over a period of approximately 1.2 seconds, beginning with the QRS complex and extending through a period of one and a fraction cardiac cycles, depending on the heart rate. As a rule, 4 or 5 such interrogations were made for each retinal area with the transducer being aligned between each interrogation. Stored data was processed off line by an HP1000 mini computer. The processing rationale has been previously reported (1). It essentially a type of deconvolution which involves creation of an instantaneous power spectrum and reconversion to the time domain by inverse Fourier transformation. Processed data of all sets of 16 scans per interrogation were plotted separately. The location (in time) and power value of each peak represented in the processed data was calculated and printed on the plots in both microseconds and the micron equivalents with '0 time/depth' set at the first echo from the posterior coats. No corrections were made for variations in the speed of sound in the tissues.

Of particular interest in the present report is the data obtained from the first 0.4 microseconds of RF data, representing approximately 300 microns of tissue depth, and includes the entire retina and the inner choroidal vascular layers. Analysis of typical data obtained from the parafoveal area of a normal eye is presented.

Results and discussion

1. Location of the maximum amplitude reflecting surface

The location of that surface which produces the maximum echo amplitude varies during the ultrasonic interrogation, presumably due to changes in tissue plane-transducer orientation with the vascular pulse. Figure 1 shows the location of the maxima in a series of 5 interrogations (80 A-scans) of one individual from data taken between the fovea and the optic nerve of the right eye. In spite of the deliberate attempt to obtain maximum RF amplitudes from the retinal surface, maximum amplitudes were obtained from the vitreo-retinal interface in only 8% of the scans. Most often the maximum reflecting surfaces were contained within the outer layers of the retina or in the anterior choroidal vascular layers.

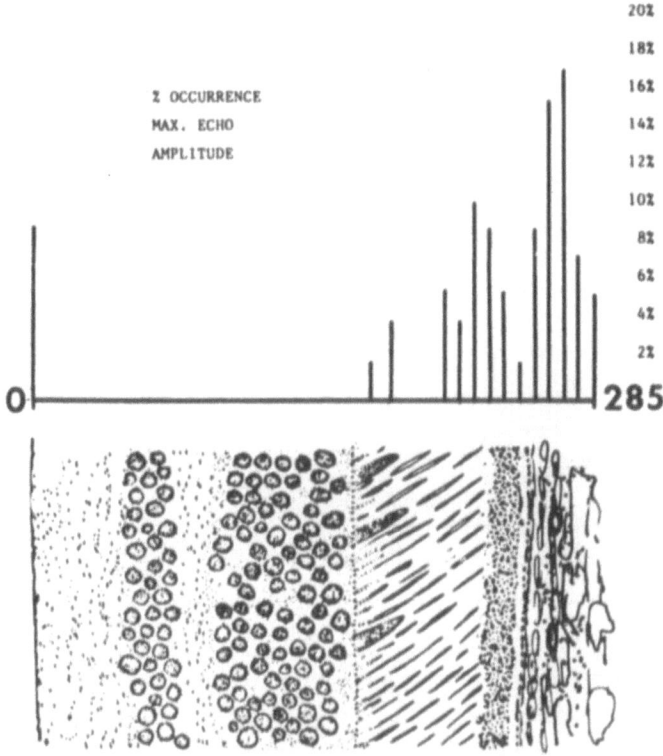

Fig. 1. The location of the maximum reflecting surfaces in a series of 80 A-scans of a single retinal area. Horizontal axis represents depth in tissue in microns. The percentage of occurrences at each location is noted. A drawing of the retina and anterior choroid has been placed below the data.

2. The number and location of all apparent reflecting surfaces to a depth of 300 microns

The number of apparent reflecting surfaces is determined by the resolution bandwidth of the individual A-scans. For any given bandwidth used in the processing algorithm, resolution varies with the cardiac cycle, presumably on the basis of tissue orientation and possibly on the basis of varying distances between the reflecting layers in response to the vascular pulse. When data is analyzed with increasing bandwidths there is greater resolution to the point at which the signal to noise ratio becomes unacceptable. Figure 2 shows plots from four consecutive scans representing the events taking place during approximately the first 1/3 of the cardiac cycle. Variations in apparent resolution of the peaks are noted in this brief period. Figure 3 compares data from one A-scan processed with upper bandwidth limits of 16 and 20 MHz and demonstrates the effect of increasing bandwidth on resolution. At 16 MHz there are 3

126

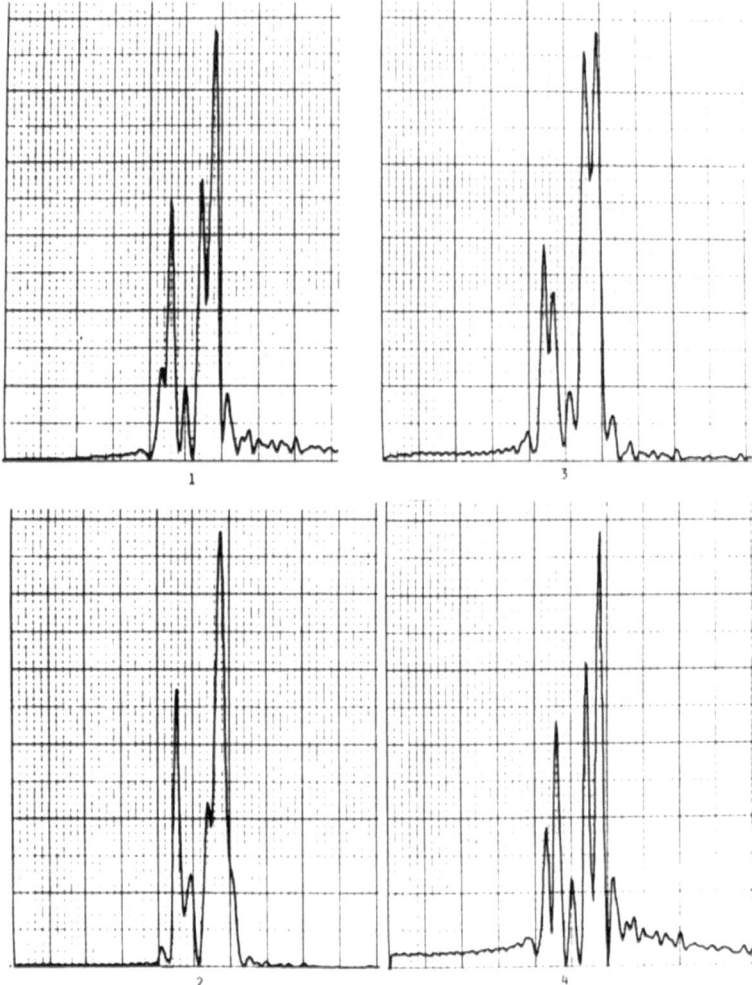

Fig. 2. Four consecutive processed A-scans triggered by the QRS complex demonstrating the apparent resolution of the reflecting surfaces during the first one third of the cardiac cycle. Approximately 600 microns of tissue depth are represented in each A-Scan segment.

significant peaks within the first 300 microns. At 20 MHz the 210 micron peak depicted at 16 MHz is resolved into separate peaks located at 165 and 232 microns.

When a sequence of scans is reviewed it becomes apparent that the shifts in positions of the reflecting surfaces cannot be entirely explained on the basis of varying resolution. Figure 4 shows the 0 to 300 micron data from an entire set of 16 A-scans. Each vertical column represents one A-scan. The location of significant reflective surfaces are indicated for each scan of the series and

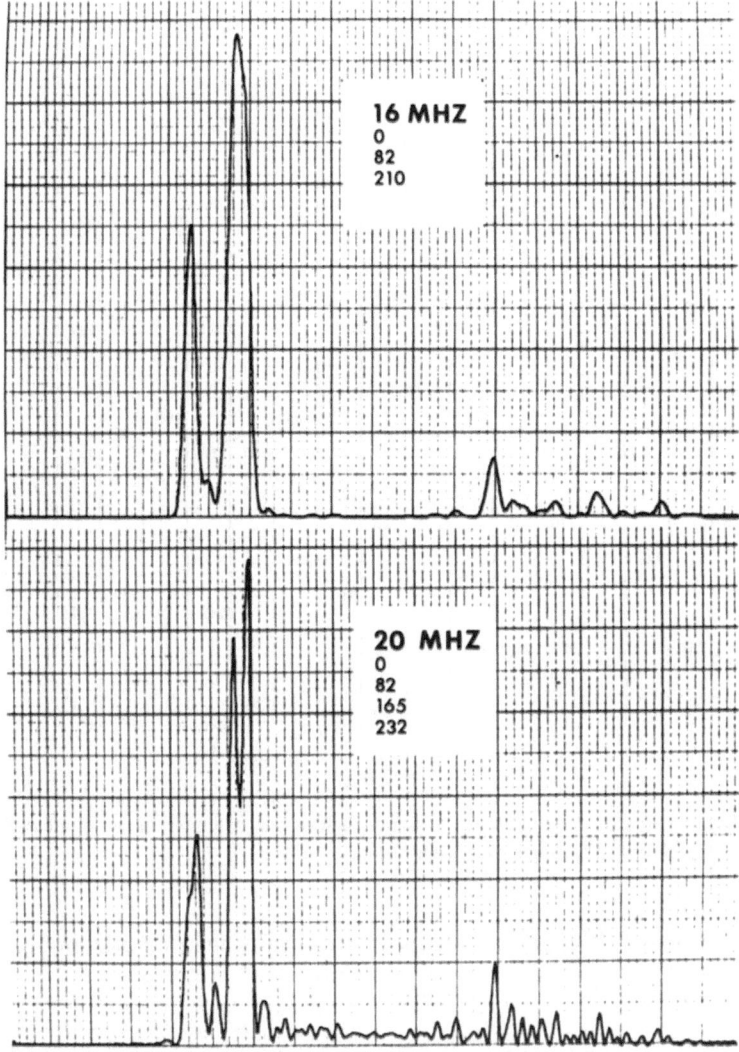

Fig. 3. Comparison of data from one A-Scan processed with upper bandwidth limits of 16 MHz and 20 MHz. Locations of significant reflecting surfaces are noted.

recorded at the appropriate 'depth' from the vitreo-retinal interface (depth 0). On inspection of such tabulated data it is apparent that there is a shifting in depth of the individual reflecting surfaces through the cardiac cycle.

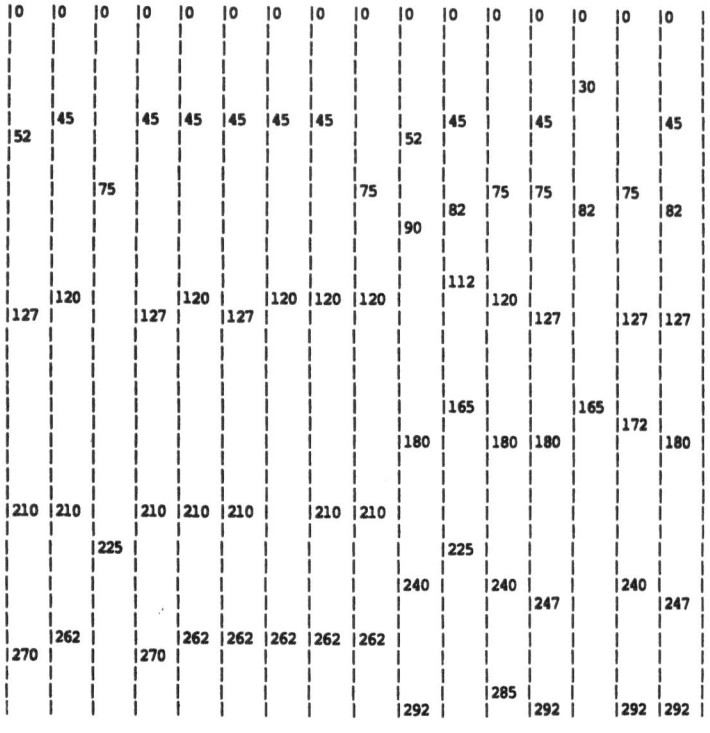

SERIES F29

Fig. 4. Processed data from 16 consecutive A-scans. Each vertical column represents one A-Scan. Locations of significant reflecting surfaces are noted.

3. Establishing 'profiles' of reflecting surfaces within the first 300 microns of tissue depth

It is desirable to compare the reflectivity data of different retinal areas within an individual eye and to compare similiar retinal areas in different eyes while yet taking into account the dynamic changes which are occurring. Visual inspection of the processed A-scans for the purpose of tracking the various reflecting layers is a nearly impossible task. Obviously some method of averaging the data must be devised which will profile each interrogated area over many cardiac cycles. The possible sources of error resulting from tissue transducer orientation can be taken into account by averaging the results of multiple interrogations of the same area. One such 'profile' can be constructed by formulating an incidence plot of all reflective surfaces resolved in a standard interrogation protocol (Fig. 5). The location of any resolved peak is plotted and the incidence of peaks at that location is noted. Figure 6 shows an

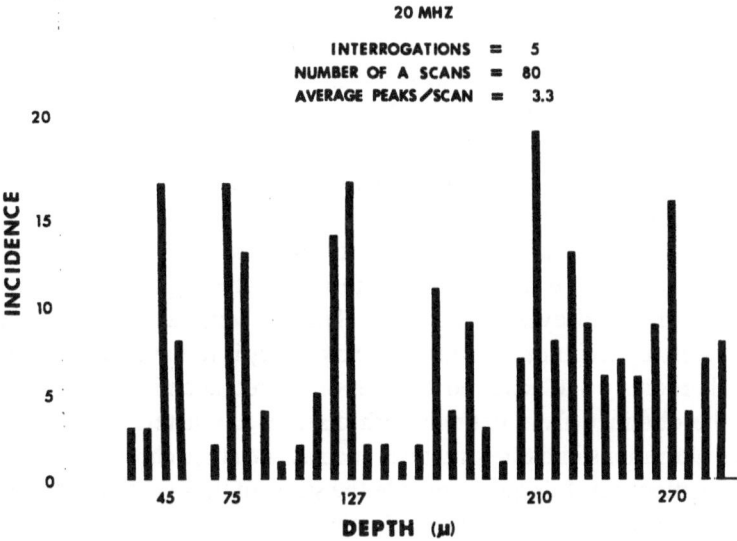

Fig. 5. The locations in depth of all significant reflecting surfaces in a total of 80 A-scans of a single retinal area by 5 interrogations are plotted against the incidence of occurrence at each location.

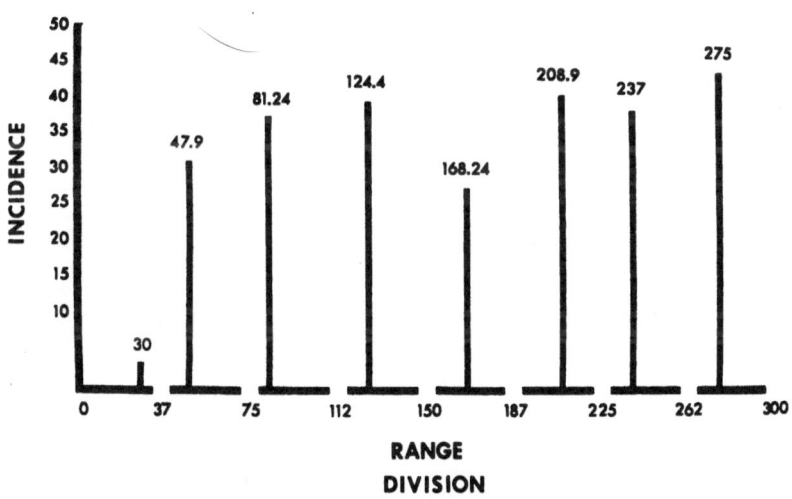

Fig. 6. The average location of significant reflecting surfaces contained within sequential 37.5 micron increments is plotted against the incidence of reflecting surfaces within each increment.

alternative profile, one we are currently employing because of its simplicity. The 300 micron segment of interest is divided into 37.5 micron intervals. The locations of all depicted surfaces within each interval is averaged and weighted according to the number of surfaces within the interval. In the example shown, a reflective surface will be depicted in a 37.5 depth segment between 225 and 362 microns 40 times during 5 interrogations of 16 A-scans each and will have an average position of 237.5 microns.

We are as yet unable to judge which profile of these data will be most useful. For this reason we are maintaining a library of the digitalized RF data of normal and diseased eyes for future analysis by some as yet unformulated signal processing technique. If ultrasonic biometry is to have some role in the study of hereditary and acquired diseases of the retina and choroid, data will have to be obtained from patients with diseases characterized by generally accepted alterations in tissue structure, such as end stage chronic glaucoma or retinitis pigmentosa. It is quite possible the study of these patients will permit us insight as to the location of the reflecting surfaces in the normal retina.

Reference

Purnell EW. 1981. Ultrasonic biometry of the posterior ocular coats. Transactions of the American Ophthalmological Society, LXXCVIII, 1027–1078.

The microscopic biometry of the thickness of human retina, choroid and sclera by ultrasound

S. TANE, J. KOHNO, K. OHASHI, A. KOMATSU and J. SUZUKI
Kawasaki, Japan

Summary

We developed a system that permits exceptionally accurate measurements of human retinal, choroidal and scleral thickness *in vivo* by means of ultrasound and Fourier analysis.

Introduction

With minicomputer techniques, the complementary functions of the time and spectral domains of the reflected sound can be used to permit measurements accurate to less than $20\,\mu m$ at 10 MHz center frequency.

The average thickness of the retina, choroid and sclera in all age groups was $151.2 \pm 28.03\,\mu m$, $370.0 \pm 92.08\,\mu m$, and $708.0 \pm 11.34\,\mu m$ respectively. The average retinal thickness in individuals older than 51 years was significantly greater than that in younger groups, i.e., those less than 30 years old.

Determination of the exact thickness of the retina, choroid and sclera in living eyes provides quantitative information for the diagnosis of various eye diseases, and is very useful for the classification and the diagnosis of stage of diseases.

Determination of the exact thickness of thin tissue membranes of less than 1 mm by usual A- and B-mode ultrasonic measurements has conventionally been difficult. We identified accurate echowaves of the retina, choroid and sclera by the active application of computer wave form analyzer DATA-6000 and by microscopic pulsation of the choroid and performed a Fourier analysis of the wave forms. The exact thickness of the living eye wall was first measured microscopically in normal human eyes.

The subjects were 46 healthy persons (81 normal eyes) consisting of 20 men and 26 women between the ages of 14 and 80. In these eyes, eye-wall thickness was measured microscopically.

K.C. Ossoinig (editor), Ophthalmic Echography, ISBN 978-94-010-7988-4

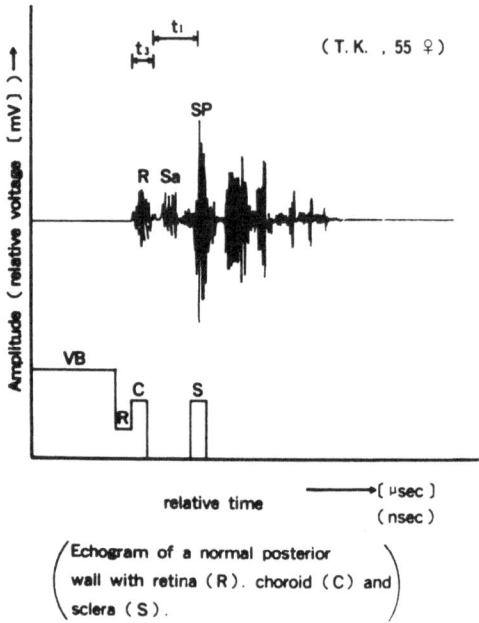

Fig. 1. Echogram pattern of a normal human posterior wall with retina, choroid and sclera.

Microscopic measurement was undertaken with a focused PZT transducer (10 MHz) by means of St. Marianna's high resolution ophthalmic diagnostic ultrasonic equipment, according to the supine immersion method or the direct contact method. Measurement through the lens, which can cause strong absorption and refraction of the echo-beam, was avoided. While echo-beam was directed through the sclera, with the subjects in a state of lateral fixation, probes were placed under the careful observation of A-mode and B-mode so that the beam would be directed at a right angle to the eye wall (on the nasal or aural side) to an area slightly posterolateral from the equator of the eyeball. In addition, the A-mode waves reflected from the probes were ascertained on monitor Braun tube, introduced to Hitachi's 610 oscilloscope, and input to the computer wave form analyzer (DATA-6000). The data were immediately displayed in real-time on a synchroscope. The data which were estimated to have precise wave forms were semi-automatically processed by microcomputer via the interface of a built-in GPIB, and the wave form and the obtained values were stored in the memory.

As Fig. 1 shows, the obtained wave forms definitely showed three types of patterns: the echo-spike (R), with which the echoes from the anterior and posterior surfaces of the retina interfaced; the echo (Sa) from a boundary surface between the choroid and the sclera; and the echo (Sp) from the posterior surface of the sclera.

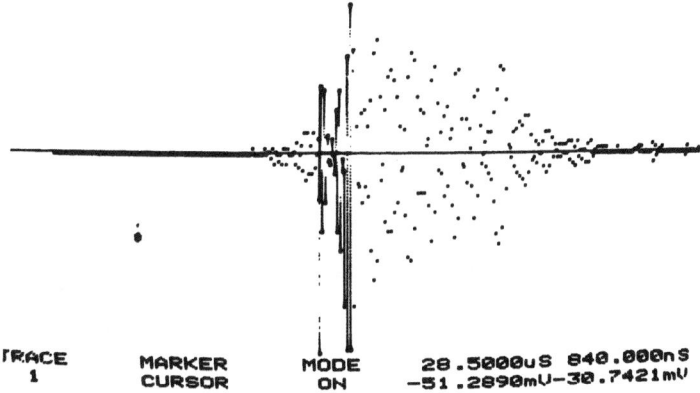

```
TRACE          MARKER     MODE    20.5000uS 840.000nS
  1            CURSOR      ON     -51.2890mV-30.7421mV
```

Fig. 2. The actual three echo spikes patterns-R, Sa. and Sp. (Particularly, the echo spike shown by a thick line exhibits thickness of the sclera, from anterior surface to the posterior surface).

Figure 2 shows the actual three echo-spike patterns – R, Sa and Sp. The echo-spike shown by a thick line, in particular, exhibits thickness of the sclera from the anterior surface to the posterior surface.

When these echo-spikes were vague, regular movements of Sa and Sp due to venous congestion of the choroid were determined by jugular compression (50 mm Hg, 5 minutes) to identify the wave forms. The sound speeds for the retina, choroid and sclera were 1.54, 1.57 and 1.65 mm/μsec, respectively. The thickness of the sclera was calculated according to the formula $t_1 \times 1.65 \times 10 \times 1/2$ μm after the interval (t_1 μsec) between the echo from a boundary surface between the choroid and the sclera, and the echo from the posterior surface of the sclera was determined from the data stored in the memory.

Since the retina is very thin, measurement of the interval between wave forms was impossible because of the interference of echoes from the anterior and posterior surfaces of the retina. Therefore, radio-frequency (RF) signal waves from the retina were treated by FFT processing by means of DATA-6000.

Power spectra of these waves were then determined by Fourier analysis by DATA-6000, and the cycle width was measured. This sign curve of a scalloped shape is an interfering wave which occurred at the frequency of the transducer. The cycle width corresponds reciprocally to the distance between the anterior and posterior surfaces of the retina (Fig. 3). The longitudinal axis was displayed with db. The interval between the echo from the anterior surface and the echo from the posterior surface of the retina was determined from a reciprocal of the cycle width ($\triangle$fMHz) between the troughs of the spectral peaks, and the thickness of the retina was calculated according to the formula t_2 $1.54 \times 10^3 \times 1/2$ m. The thickness of the choroid was calculated in a way

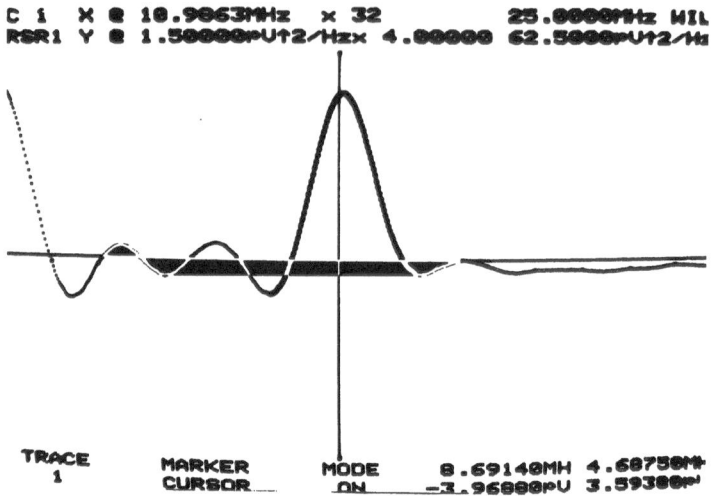

Fig. 3. Computer-treated interfered wave-form of retina.

similar to that shown in the previous formula; that is, the interval ($t_3 \mu$sec) between the echo from the anterior surface of the retina and the echo from a boundary surface between the choroid and the sclera was determined from the data stored digitally, and the thickness of the choroid was calculated according to the formula $(t_3-t_2) \times 1.57 \times 10^3 \times 1/2 \ \mu$m.

The mean thickness of the living eye wall for 81 eyes of 46 normal subjects was $151.2 \pm 29.03 \ \mu$m for the retina, $370.0 \pm 92.08 \ \mu$m for the choroid and $708.0 + 11.34 \ \mu$m for the sclera. These values involved the eye wall at a polar site posterior from the equator (Table 1).

There were significant differences ($P<0.05$) in the thickness of the retina between a group of subjects aged 30 years or less and a group of subjects aged 51 years or older. There were no significant differences in eye-wall thickness between other age groups.

Next, the thickness of the eye wall was determined in morbid eyes. Twenty-two non-operated eyes of 11 patients with primary open angle glaucoma (POAG) consisting of 5 men and 6 women between the ages of 38 and 73 were examined. The intraocular tension was controlled within a range of 12 mm Hg to 25 mm Hg. These patients had early or middle stage disease. No patients in the late stage of disease were involved. If possible, any use of eye lotion or eye drops or internal medication was withdrawn for three days before measurement. As shown in Table 2, the mean thickness was $144.4 \pm 29.32 \ \mu$m for the retina, $414.21 \pm 114.94 \ \mu$m for the choroid and $755.25 \pm 102.23 \ \mu$m for the sclera. There was no significant difference in the mean thickness of the retina or sclera between the normal subjects and the patients, but the thickness of the choroid increased significantly in patients with glaucoma ($P<0.05$).

Table 1. The thickness of the retina, choroid and sclera in living normal human eyes by means of ultrasonic RF signal analysis.

age groups (cases)	Sclera		Retina		Retina + Choroid	Choroid	
	t_1	μm	t_2	μm	t_3	t_3-t_2	μm
30 y $\geqslant$	848.6	700.1	175.4	135.5	670.8	500.0	392.5
(6 cases, 9 eyes)	± 11.53	± 95.23	± 34.26	± 26.56	± 118.09	± 97.82	± 76.80
31–50 y	854.3	704.9	194.2	149.9	714.0	460.5	361.5
(14 cases, 23 eyes)	± 14.19	± 11.70	± 34.68	± 26.94	± 202.11	± 16.56	± 13.01
51–70 y	850.3	701.5	201.2	155.0	708.1	469.3	368.5
(21 cases, 39 eyes)	± 13.53	± 11.16	± 40.06	± 30.98	± 14.12	± 97.56	± 76.57
71 y $\leqslant$	904.0	745.8	201.8	155.4	677.1	478.9	376.0
(5 cases, 10 eyes)	± 16.05	± 13.25	± 22.98	± 17.93	± 78.67	± 84.16	± 65.91
Average	858.1	708.0	196.1	151.2	702.8	471.3	370.0
(46 cases, 81 eyes)	± 13.75	± 11.34	± 36.23	± 28.03	± 15.49	± 11.73	± 92.08

There was no significant difference in the thickness of the retina between the normal eyes and operated eyes with POAG, although the number of operated eyes was small. The thickness of the choroid and sclera increased significantly ($P<0.05$) in the operated eyes (Table 3).

Conclusion

The thickness of the retina, choroid and sclera at a polar site slightly posterior

Table 2. The mean wall thickness of the non-operated eyes with primary open angle glaucoma.

Case No.	Name	age sex	Retina (μm)		Choroid (μm)		Sclera (μm)	
			R	L	R	L	R	L
1	T.Y.	69♂	123.2	134.8	471.0	302.2	792	660
2	F.M.	73♀	160.9	207.5	338.3	511.0	726	759
3	M.M.	68♀	98.6	123.2	527.5	471.0	759	990
4	M.T.	47♀	164.2	185.5	303.8	282.6	858	825
5	T.A.	62♀	123.2	123.2	471.0	471.0	660	660
6	Y.M.	68♀	123.2	123.2	408.2	282.6	825	858
7	T.H.	42♂	123.2		596.6		891	858
8	K.K.	38♂	164.2	123.2	492.2	282.6	693	660
9	K.M.	51♀	159.3	164.2	339.9	303.8	693	660
10	T.T.	38♀	164.2	197.1	680.6	489.8	792	759
11	M.S.	40♂	123.2	123.2	361.1	314.0	693	544
	mean		144.4		414.3		755.3	
	+S.D.		± 29.32		± 114.94		± 102.34	

Table 3. The thickness of the retina, choroid and sclera of the eyeball operated on for primary open angle glaucoma.

Case	Name	age sex	Retina (μm)		Choroid (μm)		Sclera (μm)	
			R	L	R	L	R	L
1	H.K.	57♂	157.7	197.1	404.3	646.8	891	858
2	Y.T.	59♀	254.4	164.2	530.0	366.6	825	660
3	A.K.	57♂	123.2	133.6	565.2	585.6	759	627
4	K.T.	59♀	140.8	164.2	578.5	335.2	825	792
	mean		166.9		501.5		779.6	
	± S.D.			± 42.03		± 116.06		± 93.23

to the equator was microscopically determined in 81 living eyes of normal persons between the ages of 14 and 80 years by means of digital wave form analyzer DATA-6000 on the basis of RF signals obtained by A-mode ultrasonic measurement using probes at 10 MHz.

The mean thickness of the eye wall in normal eyes was 151.1 μm for the retina, 370.0 μm for the choroid and 708.0 μm for the sclera. The thickness of the retina, particularly, in groups of subjects more than 50 years of age was significantly thicker than in groups of subjects aged 30 years or less. In contrast, the choroid and sclera showed no variation in thickness with age.

The examination of morbid eyes revealed a significant difference in the thickness of the choroid between the normal eyes and non-operated eyes with primary open angle glaucoma, and significant differences in the thickness of the choroid and sclera between the normal eyes and operated eyes with this condition. As for the retina, however, no variation in eye-wall thickness was observed in non-operated or operated eyes, as compared with normal eyes.

References

1. Coleman DJ, Lizzi FL. 1979. In vivo choroidal thickness measurement. Am J Ophthalmol 88: 369–376.
2. Thijssen JM, Cloostermans MJTM, Verhof WM. 1982. Ultrasonic tissue differentiation in Ophthalmology, Ultrasonic Tissue Characterization, (Martinus Nijhoff Publishers, the Hague), 146–158.
3. Trier HG, Decker P, Lepper RD, Irion KM, Reuter R, Kottow M, Müller-Breitenkamp R, Otto KJ. 1984. Ocular tissue characterization by RF-signal analysis, Ophthalmic ultrasonography, (Proceeding of the 9th SIDUO Congress Edited by J.S. Hillman) Dr W Junk Publishers, The Hague, 455–466.
4. Tane S, Kohno J, Horikoshi J. 1984. The study on the microscopic biometry of the thickness of the human retina, choroid and sclera by ultrasound: Acta Societatis Ophthalmologicae Japonicae; 1412–1417.

Standardized A-scan and B-scan in vivo evaluation and measurement of the retino-choroidal layer

K.C. OSSOINIG and K. CODY
Iowa City, USA

Abstract

Ever since standardized A-scan was introduced as a method for echographic screening of the posterior eye segment in the mid 1960's, it has been used regularly for evaluation and measurement of the retinal and choroidal layers throughout the entire fundus. Over the years the normal thickness range of these layers and the critical measuring values that help distinguish between normal and abnormally thick layers were established for different portions of the eye. In the macular region, retinochoroidal thickness of more than 1.7 mm, or a thickness that is at least 0.2 mm greater than the thickness of the reti-nochoroidal layer in the macula of the normal fellow eye, should be considered abnormal. The same values hold true for the regions of the vortex veins. In other fundus areas a thickness of more than 1.2 mm is abnormal unless a similar thickness (within 0.2 mm) is found in the corresponding fundus region of a normal fellow eye. Naturally, even values well within the normal range must be considered abnormal if the same area in a normal fellow eye is more than 0.2 mm thinner.

Today such A-scan evaluation is routine for every intraocular clinical examination. It not only helps to detect thin fundus lesions such as choroidal nevi, macular edema or retinal hemorrhages, but also helps distinguish between different flat or shallow lesions on the basis of different reflectivities and distribution. Choroidal hyperemia, for instance, causes diffuse regular thickening of the choroidal layer with sustained high reflectivity. Inflammatory infiltration of the choroid in endophthalmitis, by contrast, produces irregular (nodular) thickening of the retina and choroid with decreased reflectivity. Accuracy in measuring retino-choroidal layers by the standardized A-scan method ranges from ± 0.05 to ± 0.1 mm depending on how extensive and how regular the thickening happens to be. The use of low measuring sensitivities and peak-to-peak measurements is essential for achieving this high measuring accuracy.

K.C. Ossoinig (editor), Ophthalmic Echography, ISBN 978-94-010-7988-4
© 1987, Martinus Nijhoff/Dr W. Junk Publishers, Dordrecht.

138

References

1. Ossoinig KC. 1979. Standardized Echography: Basic Principles, Clinical Applications and Results. In: Ophthalmic Ultrasonography: Comparative Techniques (Dallow R.L., ed.) Int. Ophthal. Clin., 19/4 (1979), 127–210. Little, Brown & Co., Boston.
2. Ossoinig KC. 1983. How to Obtain Maximum Measuring Accuracies with Standardized A-Scan. Ophthalmic Ultrasonography. J.S. Hillman and M.M. LeMay (eds.), The Hague: Dr W. Junk Publishers, pp. 197–216.
3. Ossoinig KC. 1985. Standardized Ophthalmic Echography of the Eye, Orbit and Periorbital Region. A comprehensive Slide Set (774 slides) and Study Guide, Third Edition. Iowa City, Iowa: Goodfellow Company, Inc.

In vivo study of the human retino-choroidal layers by RF signal analysis. I. Visual echogram interpretation. Part 1: Techniques

R.-D. LEPPER, H.G. TRIER, S. REINERT and R. REUTER
Bonn, FRG

Introduction

With conventional diagnostic ultrasound devices it is very difficult or perhaps even impossible to obtain information on the internal structure of retina and choroid. In vitreoretinal diseases, a retinal detachment sometimes cannot be excluded, when the echo of a suspicious membrane is analyzed. In such cases the indirect examination approach could be helpful. By this approach the presence or absence of the retina at the wall of the eye is detected. The measurement of choroidal pulsations serves (a) as a means for identification of acoustical landmarks in the indirect examination approach, and (b) it gives information on circulatory disorders of the choroid or of drug effects. Therefore, measurement of the backwall structure is of interest to several fields of ophthalmology.

Material and methods

The anatomical structure discussed is less then 1 mm thick. Therefore, only 10 to 20 ultrasonic waves fall into that interval depending on the ultrasonic frequency used. The analysis of A-mode signals is of no use in this case, as these RF signals are rectified and smoothed by a low pass filter. The best resolution can be achieved when the original RF signal is analyzed.

Mathematically speaking the echo of the posterior pole of the eye is a convolute of the distribution of the reflectors and the transmitted ultrasonic signal. In terms of physics there is enhancing and destructive interference within the echoes. Consequently a large echo corresponds not necessarily to a single strong reflector but might result from enhancing interference of several adjacent small reflectors. Visual interpretation of an RF echogram therefore need not give the real geometrical distance of anatomical structures but nevertheless gives reproducible parameters describing the tissue layers. When

K.C. Ossoinig (editor), Ophthalmic Echography, ISBN 978-94-010-7988-4

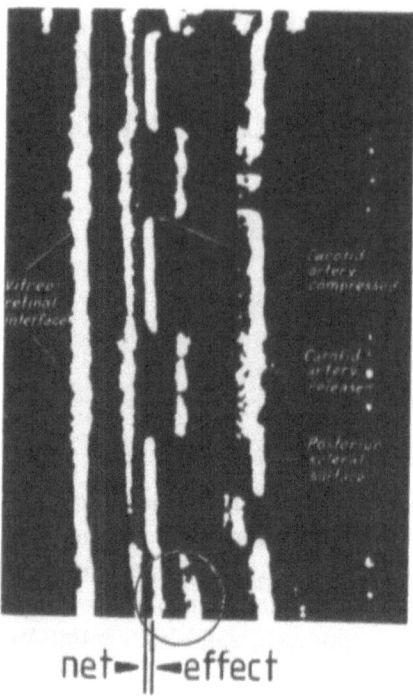

net→‖←effect

Fig. 1. Bistable M-mode picture of the posterior wall of a dog's eye during cyclic carotid occlusion. The alternative appearance of two different layers can be misinterpreted as a layer shift. The small net effect as indicated has to be assumed (from Coleman, 1969).

measuring dynamical changes due to blood pressure variations within the posterior layers the physical restrictions are less severe than in the case of absolute static measurements. If major parts of the layers are displaced then we have a good chance of measuring the displacement of these layers correctly with the resolution and precision of the system used.

A number of authors have performed measurements of backwall structures and their dynamic variations, probably first described by Coleman & Weiniger (1969). Figure 1 is taken from this paper and demonstrates the variations of the posterior pole of a dog's eye caused by cyclic carotid compression. The authors probably believed that the layers were displaced in the indicated way. The data displayed had been measured with a trigger level unit and therefore only the two levels black (below level) and white (above level) are visible. What really happens is shown on the right hand side of this picture: There are two different reflectors which are above and below the trigger level alternatively. The true net effect of the carotid occlusion seems to be very small and is indicated by a pair of arrows.

In 1978 we demonstrated that thickness variations of the backwall layers of

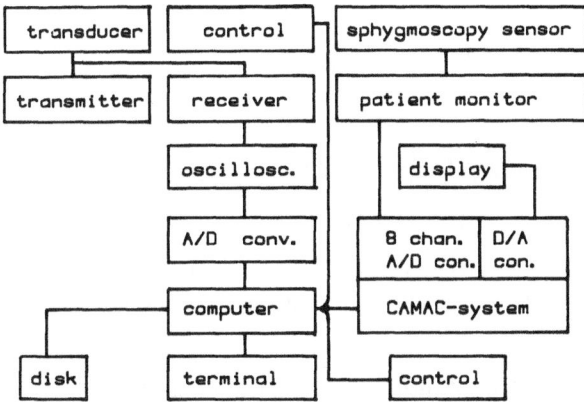

Fig. 2. Block diagram of the measuring system in use. Measurement, data storage, and off line visual analysis are performed with this setup.

the human eye are likely to be less than 30 microns (Lepper, 1978; Lepper et al., 1981). At that time we could not measure in synchronism to the blood pulsation. Therefore, we had to improve our system. Figure 2 shows the functional block diagram of the system used. A hand held transducer (center frequency 15 MHz) with a water filled stand off was placed onto the patients eye globe. The transducer was focused onto the posterior wall (Fig. 3). The individual sound field of the transducer was evaluated by means of an automatic measurement system which steered a special reflector in three planes (Lepper, 1982). The ultrasonic echoes are band limited to 30 MHz and then digitized with a sampling frequency of 200 MHz. The timebase error of the transient recorder (AD 7612, Tektronix) is (according to the specifications)

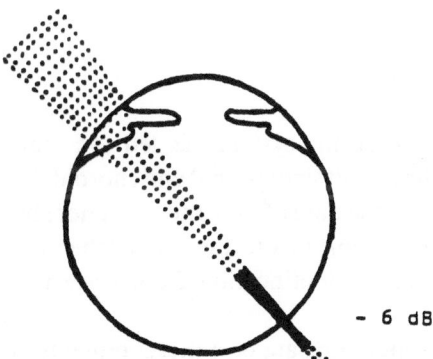

Fig. 3. The transducer focus is positioned onto the posterior wall. The scaled image indicates the −6 dB zone of the focus area.

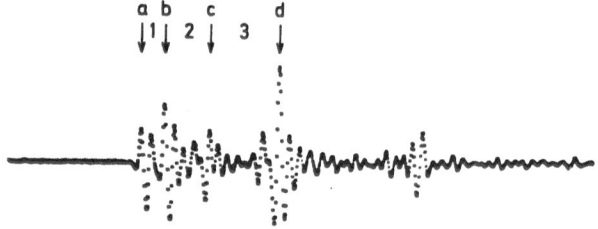

Fig. 4. Digitized RF signal of a typical back wall echo. The markers indicate echo layers which can be found in nearly all echo data of different patients and corresponding areas of interest.

negligible. The signal amplitude within the frequency band used is resolved to effectively 64 levels which proved to be sufficient. Up to ten microseconds of RF signal can be recorded in one trace which corresponds to a length of 7.5 mm. Signal acquisition is monitored on an A-mode oscilloscope screen and the digitized signal interval is displayed on a computer monitor.

The echo data together with the sphygmoscopy data are stored on a magnetic disk with a rate of 4 measurements per second for an off-line analysis. The off-line data display is programmed so that the echoes are zoomed to see the single data points. As the resolution in time is 5 ns the echo traces are easily adjustable to that resolution in time. By setting and moving a cursor to selected parts of the stored echoes, all traces can be shifted to an equivalent position of the time axis. After aligning all data a non overlapping data display of all traces can be chosen to get visual information about similarity of the total set of signals. By setting a cursor to selected points of the echotraces the mutual distances of these points within all traces are evaluated and printed. Figure 4 demonstrates a typical backwall echo after digitization with superimposed markers for the different layer parts.

Experimental experience

Improvement of our measuring system has led to a device with which the measurement and off line analysis of retinal and choroidal pulsations can easily be done. When analyzing the data off line the examiner always knows whether a single trace sufficiently conforms to the rest of the data block. Ambiguity problems concerning peak identification from trace to trace is practically excluded.

The relatively low repetition rate of 4 measurements per second however does not allow a synchronous detection of pulsations with the aid of the sphygmoscopy data. With a heart rate of approximately 1 Hz the theoretical minimum repetition rate would be 2 Hz to avoid aliasing. Increasing the repetition rate of 4 Hz by a factor of 2 could improve detectability of pulsatory components within the back wall echo.

References

Coleman DJ, Weiniger R. 1969. Ultrasonic M-mode technique in ophthalmology. Arch Ophthal, Chicago 82: 475–479.

Lepper R-D. 1978. Ultraschallmessungen an der Rueckwand des lebenden menschlichen Auges. Thesis Univ Bonn, Bonn-IR-78-5.

Lepper R-D, Trier HG, Reuter R. 1981. Ultrasonic measurements at the posterior wall of living human eyes. Ophthalmic Res 13: 1–11 (S. Karger, Basel).

Lepper R-D. 1982. Computer-aided quality assurance of ultrasonic transducers for use in medical diagnostics. Biomedizinische Technik, 27, 1–2, pp. 2–6 (Schiele & Schoen, Berlin).

In vivo study of the human retino-choroidal layers by RF-Signal analysis. I. Visual echogram interpretation. Part 2: Results on choroidal thickness and pulsation under physiological conditions and under tonometry

H.G. TRIER and S. REINERT
Bonn, FRG

Abstract

Using off-line visual interpretation of the stored RF-signal trace and finge: pulse recordings, the retino-choroidal layers were studied in 20- to 30-year olc volunteers. It is shown that portions of the RF-echogram demonstrate heart cycle correlated pulsations of usually $10-30\,\mu$ under physiological conditions The pulsating layer may further be subdivided in two parts with differen phases of pulse. The pulsating layers show considerable thickness variation. during and after increase of the intraocular pressure provoked by means of ε Schiøtz's tonometer test. The ultrasonic findings are correlated to anatom and function of the choroidal layer.

K.C. Ossoinig (editor), Ophthalmic Echography, ISBN 978-94-010-7988-4
© 1987, Martinus Nijhoff/Dr W. Junk Publishers, Dordrecht.

In vivo study of the human retino-choroidal layers by RF-Signal analysis. II. Automated digital image analysis on the M-scan

K.M. IRION, H.G. TRIER and R.-D. LEPPER
Bonn, FRG

Abstract

A computer-assisted interactive method has been developed for the quantitative determination of small tissue movements in the posterior ocular wall. An ultrasonic M-scan has been reconstructed from a sequence of digitized RF-signals obtained from a region in the fundus of the eye. The repetition rate is four signals/sec. The RF-representation of the M-scan is transformed into an image with 256 grey levels and is displayed on a color screen. Axial shifts of each signal caused by relative movements of the transducer and patient are corrected by digital phase-correction, thus preserving axial changes in the layers. After phase-correction, layers of interest may be defined interactively in one RF-line. Dynamic changes and tissue movement caused by the pulsation of internal blood vessels are determined by changes of layer distances as a function of time. The detection and registration of the dynamics in all RF-lines is performed by an adapted image processing software. To prove the dependence of tissue movements on the heart rate, the correlation between changes of distances and the finger-pulse is calculated. The finger-pulse signal is digitized and stored synchronously with each RF-signal.

A special high resolution RF-data acquisition system is necessary for these measurements since detected changes in distances of the layers are usually smaller than 15 μ. The signal processing procedure and results of the analysis of M-scans taken from the normal posterior ocular wall will be presented.

K.C. Ossoinig (editor), Ophthalmic Echography, ISBN 978-94-010-7988-4
© 1987, Martinus Nijhoff/Dr W. Junk Publishers, Dordrecht.

Ultrasonic measurement of transverse lens diameter during accommodation in emmetropic and myopic eyes

J.K. STOREY and E.P. RABIE
Manchester, UK

Abstract

A new method is introduced which makes possible *in vivo* measurement of transverse lens diameter (T.L.D.) with ultrasound for the first time. This method was found to be reliable when ultrasonic and optical measurements of T.L.D. were compared in both eyes of an aniridic subject. Horizontal T.L.D. was measured for 7 emmetropic and 7 myopic subjects at 0, 2, 4, 6 and 8 dioptres of stimulus to accommodation. Unaccommodated T.L.D. was directly proportional to the refractive error, axial length, anterior chamber depth and sagittal lens thickness. T.L.D. changed more per dioptre of stimulus in myopic than in emmetropic eyes. The mean unaccommodated T.L.D. was found to be larger than in-vitro measurements reported in the literature.

Introduction

During accommodation lens fibres are rearranged so that the thickness of the lens increases whilst its transverse or equatorial diameter (T.L.D.) becomes smaller. This change is directly observable in aniridic eyes only.

Grossman (1903) was the first investigator to measure unaccommodated and accommodated T.L.D. in a 26 year old aniridic hypermetrope. Without drugs he found the T.L.D. to be 11.50 mm, with homatropine 12.25 mm and with eserine 10.25 mm. Story (1924) reported an apparent decrease of 1.5 mm in the T.L.D. of an 18 year old aniridic subject with eserine. Fincham (1935) photographed the lens of a 22 year old emmetrope with traumatic aniridia and reported a T.L.D. of 10.20 mm unaccommodated and 9.75 mm accommodated. His photographic measurements did not correct for any corneal magnification. A method for *in vivo* measurement of T.L.D. is introduced in this paper which avoids unwanted magnification effects and can be used on subjects with normal irides.

K.C. Ossoinig (editor), Ophthalmic Echography, ISBN 978-94-010-7988-4

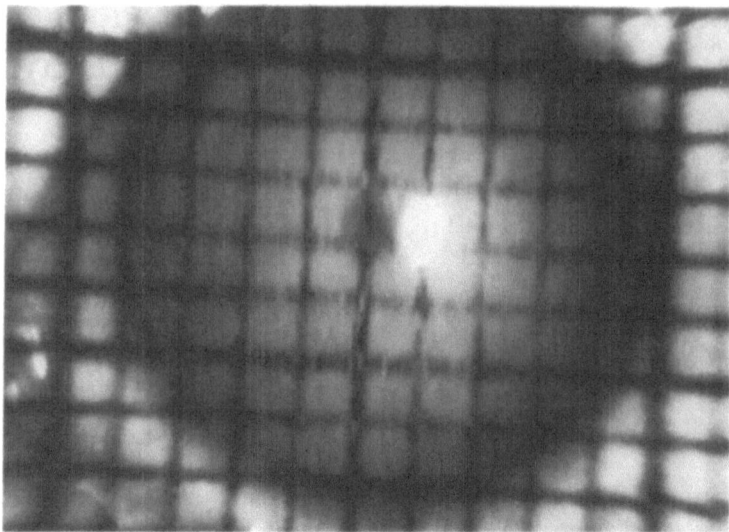

Fig. 1. Transverse lens diameter of an aniridic subject photographed through a fundus camera is overlaid on a photograph of graph paper divided in 1 mm squares, placed at the focal plane of the same camera and photographed without alteration of the camera settings.

Methods

In order to test the reliability of the ultrasonic method, T.L.D.'s of both eyes of a 15 year old aniridic subject were measured ultrasonically with accommodation paralyzed by instillation of 1% cylopentolate. The T.L.D.'s were also photographed using a Zeiss fundus camera with the astigmatic setting at −9.00 D so that a clear focus could be obtained at the periphery of the crystalline lens. Subsequently graph paper graduated in 1 mm squares was positioned at the focal plane of the fundus camera and photographed separately without alteration of the focus or the astigmatic setting of the fundus camera. The two films were then overlaid (Fig. 1) and measured on a travelling microscope. An attempt was made to photograph the crystalline lens through a fundus examination lens as this would have neutralized corneal magnification; however, this proved unsuccessful as there was too much eye movement under the fundus examination lens.

T.L.D. was measured at 5 accommodative stimulus steps for each of 7 nearly emmetropic and 7 myopic subjects ranging from 21 to 27 years in age. All subjects had at least 8.00 dioptres amplitude of accommodation with no accommodative difficulties at near. Subjective and objective refraction was performed at 6 meters. The amplitude of accommodation was measured with minus lenses before one eye as a 20/20 line of letters was viewed on a transilluminated chart with a luminance of 90 cd/m.

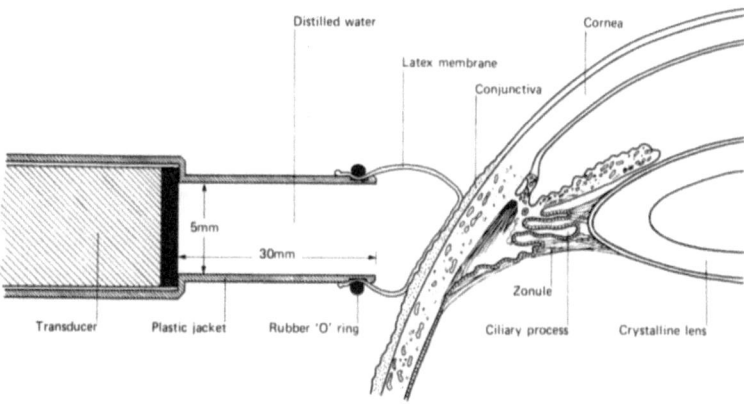

Fig. 2. The position of the transducer for T.L.D. measurement.

Anterior corneal curvature was measured with a Zeiss keratometer and axial biometry done with the Storz Alpha 20/20 instrument. A head-band trial frame adapted for monocular use was adjusted before the left eye and the refractive error placed in the back cell at a vertex distance of 14 mm. The subject was seated erect and instructed to keep a 20/20 line of letters on the chart clear as minus lenses of 2, 4, 6 and 8 dioptres were introduced before the left eye. T.L.D. was measured in the occluded right eye whilst the consensual left eye actively accommodated. As the eyes accommodated, the chair was rotated so that convergence was about equal in both eyes.

The Kretz 7200 MA A-scan ultrasonoscope was calibrated as suggested by Ossoinig (1984)and the amplification set at 60 db. A Kretz 10 MHz plane wave transducer was eased into a plastic jacket and a thin latex membrane mounted at the front of the jacket leaving about 3 mm of slack membrane at the tip. Distilled water was injected though a hole into the jacket until it was full and after elimination of air bubbles, the hole was sealed with tape. Benoxinate 0.5% was instilled in the right eye, normal saline applied to the membrane and the transducer positioned at the temporal limbus as shown in Fig. 2 to obtain the traces shown in Fig. 3.

Often other echoes appeared from the ciliary processes and within the lens, but an attempt was made to avoid them by repositioning the transducer as this made the results more repeatable. The initial complex includes the membrane, temporal sclera and ciliary body, and the two peaks following it represent the temporal and nasal lens equators respectively. No other peaks follow these because the nasal ciliary body and sclera reflect sound at an oblique angle to the transducer. Only surfaces normal to the transducer are acoustically detectable, so the transducer had to be pointed normal to both equators of the lens for a suitable trace. This very precise position considerably reduced errors due

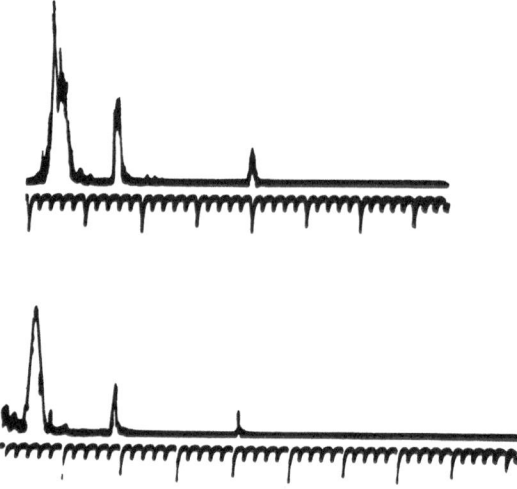

Fig. 3. Unaccommodated (above) and fully accommodated (below) T.L.D. for subject 7 of the emmetropic group. The initial complex (left) includes the membrane and the temporal sclera and ciliary body. The two following peaks represent the temporal and nasal lens equators respectively. Each small division on the scales below the traces is one micro-second.

to obliquity of the beam. The distance from the initial complex to the lens equator has been studied and will be the subject of a later paper.

At least 5 traces were photographed for each accommodative step using a Nikon camera equipped with a macro lens and motor drive. The negatives were measured peak to peak on a travelling microscope to 0.01 mm. A velocity of 1640 m/s was used as suggested by Jansson and Kock (1962) to convert the time scale to lenticular distances.

Results

The results for the aniridic subject are shown in Table 1. If it is assumed that the cornea is spherical and that the distance of the lens equator from the cornea is equal to the anterior chamber depth, the photographed T.L.D. would be about 9% larger than the true T.L.D. in both eyes. This figure subtracted from the photographic dimensions is 7.57 and 7.60 mm for the right and left eyes respectively, suggesting that the ultrasonic method is reliable to about 0.3% for this subject.

The axial dimensions of the 7 emmetropic subjects are shown in Table 2 and the change in T.L.D. during accommodation appears in Table 3. Tables 4 and 5 present similar data on 7 myopic subjects. The emmetropic T.L.D. data can be approximated with a straight line of slope −0.08 mm/D (Fig. 4) and the myopic data with a line of slope −0.15 mm/D (Fig. 5). The standard deviation

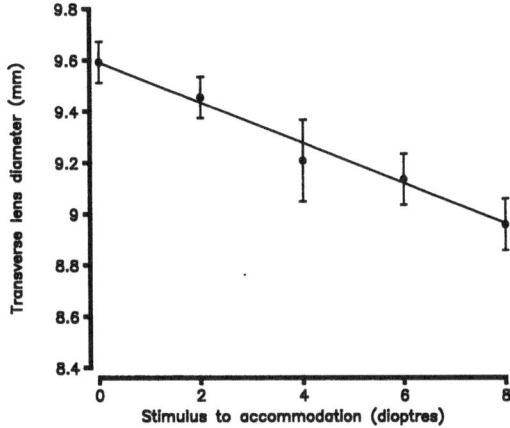

Fig. 4. The mean transverse lens diameters (mm) for 7 nearly emmetropic subjects plotted against the stimulus to accommodation (D) at the spectacle plane. The slope of the regression line is −0.08 and the correlation coefficient is −0.99.

of the slopes of the regression lines between subjects was 0.02 for the emmetropic group and 0.03 for the myopic group. Significant linear correlations were found between the unaccommodated T.L.D. dimensions for each subject and slope of the regression line, refractive error, axial length, anterior chamber depth and sagittal lens thickness, but not with corneal radius (Table 6).

Discussion

Horizontal T.L.D.'s were measured for 7 nearly emmetropic and 7 myopic

Table 1. Results for an aniridic subject.

	R.E.	L.E.
Photographic T.L.D. (mm)	8.32 ± 0.03	8.35 ± 0.06
Ultrasonic T.L.D. (mm)	7.59 ± 0.13	7.63 ± 0.11
Axial length (mm)	22.06	22.00
A.C. depth (mm)	2.84	2.75
Lens thickness (mm)	2.86	2.94
Mean corneal radius (mm)	8.58	8.57
Equivalent sphere refraction (D)	+5.50	+5.50
Visual acuity	6/24	6/12

152

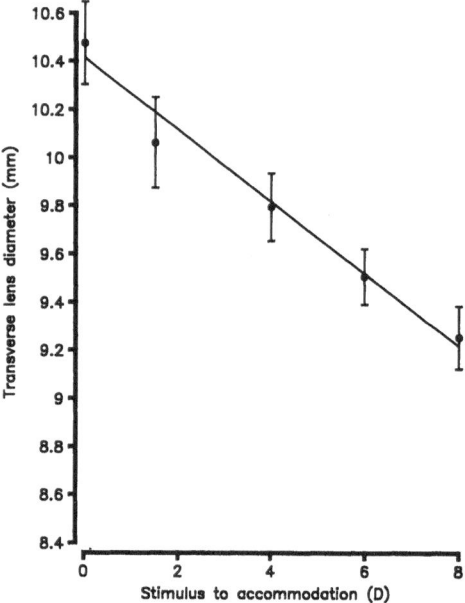

MYOPIC SUBJECTS

Fig. 5. The mean transverse lens diameters (mm) for 7 myopic subjects plotted against the stimulus to accommodation (D) at the spectacle plane. The slope of the regression line is −0.15 and the correlation coefficient is −0.99.

Table 2. Axial dimensions for seven emmetropic subjects.

Subjects	1	2	3	4	5	6	7	Mean
Axial length (mm)	22.14	22.87	23.40	23.23	23.22	23.38	23.27	23.07
Anterior chamber depth (mm)	3.70	3.53	3.08	3.25	3.39	3.34	3.35	3.38
Lens thickness (mm)	3.71	3.72	4.04	3.56	3.65	3.73	3.77	3.74
Mean corneal radius of curvature (mm)	7.33	7.53	8.25	7.70	7.75	7.87	7.90	7.76
Equivalent sphere refraction at the cornea (D)	+0.50	−1.00	+0.50	+0.50	+0.25	−0.25	+0.50	+0.14

Table 3. Transverse lens diameters for seven emmetropic subjects.

Stimulus to accommodation (D)	Transverse lens diameter (mm)							
	Subjects							
	1	2	3	4	5	6	7	Mean
0	9.22	9.37	9.37	9.43	9.74	9.92	10.08	9.59
2	9.15	9.24	9.24	9.30	9.64	9.71	9.90	9.45
4	8.87	9.04	8.90	9.02	9.44	9.63	9.86	9.25
6	8.65	8.96	8.84	8.86	9.42	9.51	9.75	9.14
8	8.52	8.84	8.50	8.66	9.28	9.43	9.48	8.96
Slope of regression line	−0.10	−0.70	−0.10	−0.10	−0.06	−0.06	−0.07	−0.08

subjects during accommodation. The mean changes in this dimension were 0.08 mm/D for emmetropic subjects and 0.15 mm/D for myopic subjects. In a previous paper (Storey and Rabie 1981) we reported that sagittal lens thickness changes 0.05 mm/D in emmetropic subjects and 0.08 mm/D in myopic subjects. We therefore conclude that the crystalline lens moves more per dioptre of accommodation both sagitally and transversally in myopic subjects than in emmetropic subjects.

The accommodative stimulus levels quoted are from the spectacle plane. There is a practical convenience in making measurements from the spectacle

Table 4. Axial dimensions for seven myopic subjects.

Subjects	1	2	3	4	5	6	7	Mean
Axial length (mm)	25.84	25.38	26.01	25.81	24.89	25.77	25.75	25.64
Anterior chamber depth (mm)	3.81	3.94	3.83	4.03	4.29	4.12	3.84	3.98
Unaccommodated sagittal lens thickness (mm)	3.81	3.52	3.77	3.55	3.50	3.63	3.58	3.62
Mean corneal radius of curvature (mm)	7.81	7.63	8.11	7.79	7.30	7.70	7.63	7.71
Equivalent sphere refraction at the cornea (D)	−4.00	−6.50	−4.00	−5.25	−5.00	−5.25	−5.50	−5.07

Table 5. Transverse lens diameters for seven myopic subjects.

Stimulus to accommodation (D)	Transverse lens diameter (mm)							
	Subjects							
	1	2	3	4	5	6	7	Mean
0	9.65	10.36	10.50	10.55	10.57	10.70	11.01	10.48
2	9.52	9.61	10.22	10.28	9.92	10.47	10.49	10.07
4	9.19	9.48	9.88	10.05	9.56	10.22	10.20	9.80
6	8.99	9.31	9.61	9.60	9.25	9.92	9.92	9.51
8	8.66	9.13	9.31	9.38	8.91	9.76	9.64	9.26
Slope of regression line	−0.12	−0.14	−0.15	−0.15	−0.20	−0.12	−0.16	−0.15

plane since most ametropic subjects in fact accommodate with their spectacles on in daily life. However it is necessary to be clear as to the relationship between the quantity thus measured and the accommodative stimulus at the eye. Vertex distance effects and the finite chart distance must be taken into consideration. When the eye is ametropic, the power of the distance correcting lens also enters the relationship between ocular and spectacle accommodation. When the stimulus to ocular accommodation is plotted against T.L.D. the slopes of the regression lines become 0.09 and 0.19 mm/D for the emmetropic and the myopic groups respectively.

Unaccommodated T.L.D. dimensions found in this study are larger than in-vitro dimensions reported in the literature. T.L.D. of the cadaver lens

Table 6. Statistical analysis of data.

Unaccommodated Transverse Lens Diameter (mm) versus	Correlation Coefficient (n = 14)	t-statistic (d.f. = 12)	Probability (p) that the null hypothesis is true
Slope of accommodative stimulus – T.L.D. line (mm/D)	0.67	3.14	p<0.005
Axial length (mm)	0.80	4.54	p<0.001
Anterior chamber depth (mm)	0.70	3.37	p<0.005
Sagittal lens thickness (mm)	0.52	2.09	p<0.05
Mean corneal radius (mm)	0.02	0.07	p = 0.47
Equivalent sphere refraction (mm)	0.81	4.72	p<0.001

measured in-vitro has been given as between 8.7 and 9.0 mm between the ages of 20 and 30 years (Francois 1959 and Duke Elder 1961). The mean unaccommodated T.L.D. in-vivo was found to be 9.59 mm and with 8 dioptres of stimulus to accommodation, it was 8.96 mm in this age group. The crystalline lens in the cadaver eye is in the fully accommodated state due to a fall in intraocular pressure and loss of tonus of the ciliary muscle.

In conclusion, a new method is introduced which makes possible *in vivo* measurement of transverse lens diameter with ultrasound. This method was found to be reliable when ultrasonic and optical measurements of T.L.D. were compared in both eyes of an aniridic subject. Unaccommodated T.L.D. was directly proportional to the refractive error, axial length, anterior chamber depth and sagittal lens thickness, T.L.D. changed more per dioptre of accommodation in myopic than in emmetropic eyes. To our knowledge, T.L.D. has not been measured before with any ultrasonic technique.

References

1. Duke Elder S. 1961. System of Ophthalmology Vol 2, Henry Kimpton: London; 312.
2. Fincham EF. 1935. A study of accommodation by photography of the living lens and ciliary body in a case of aniridia. Trans Ophthalmol Soc UK; Vol 50: 145–158.
3. Francois J. 1959. In: Cataract and Abnormalities of the Lens, ed. JG Bellows, Grune & Stratton Inc: New York, 1975: 139.
4. Grossman K. 1903. The mechanism of accommodation in man. British Medical Journal; Vol 2: 726–731.
5. Jansson F, Kock E. 1962. Determination of the velocity of ultrasound in the human lens and vitreous. Acta Ophthalmologica; 40: 420–433.
6. Ossoinig KC. 1984. How to obtain maximum measuring accuracies with standardized A-scan, Proceedings of the 9th SIDUO Congress, Documenta Ophthalmologica Proceedings Series 38. Dr W Junk Publishers, The Hague; 197–216.
7. Storey JK, Rabie EP. 1981. Biometry of the Eye During Accommodation, Proceedings of the 9th S.I.D.U.O. Congress, Documenta Ophthalmologica Proc. Series 38, Dr W Junk Publishers, the Hague, 295–301.
8. Story J.B. 1924. Aniridia: notes on accommodation changes under eserine. Trans Ophthalmol Soc UK, Vol 44: 413–417.

Measurement of accommodative changes in human eyes by means of a high-resolution ultrasonic system

R.-D. LEPPER and H.G. TRIER
Bonn, FRG

Introduction

The measurement of accommodative changes by means of ultrasound has been described in the literature by different authors (Storey & Rabie, 1984). Due to the older technique of the ultrasonic devices most often these examinations are performed in a stationary manner: The intraocular distances are measured with and without accommodation (Coleman et al., 1969). In cases of photographic documentation and off line evaluation the measurements evaluated only give information on the steady state conditions of the eye, and are deteriorated by a relatively high degree of systematic error.

Obviously, only the differences of the intraocular intervals due to accommodation are of interest. If we measure the change of these intervals over a period of time steady state conditions of the eye as well as additional dynamic information such as accommodative slew rate will be given. In 1980 we published a paper demonstrating M-mode images of accommodation (Lepper et al., 1980). The clock frequency of the time base used was 10 MHz only. Therefore, small changes of lens thickness were resolved insufficiently. The instrumentation used at that time was impracticable.

Experimentally, the influence of drugs onto accommodation could be of interest. This question could be solved optically; however to measure the dynamic phenomena a recording optical device has to be used. Clinically it could be of interest whether the accommodative mechanism of an eye is affected traumatically. If there is a severe intraocular bleeding, there is no way to solve this question optically. It was our aim to develop a simple measurement technique for accommodative changes of the intraocular distances which can be used in clinical routine.

K.C. Ossoinig (editor), Ophthalmic Echography, ISBN 978-94-010-7988-4

Material and methods

Obviously a maximum of resolution is achieved with the RF signal. Therefore, the use of our RF signal acquisition and evaluating system would give a maximum of flexibility in evaluating the accommodation dynamics. However the costs and complexity of such a system do not coincide to our aim to develop a routine method. The resolution of 0.02 mm of our RESSOURCE-system BMS 811 Echocomp (now GBS, Grieshaber) appeared to be be sufficient for measuring accommodative changes. Also, programming of this system promised to be much easier than that of the RF-system because the intraocular distances need not be evaluated by additional software but are mainly determined by hardware. For these reasons we decided to work with the RESSOURCE-system.

Attaching the transducer to the eye is a problem: We did not want the measuring technique to influence the accommodative mechanism. Therefore, a contact coupling of the transducer to the cornea with the consequence of impressing it did not seem feasible. The use of aiming devices appeared not to be fruitful due to two facts: (1) The individual corneal curvature has to be taken into consideration for a reproducible refractive change of the target's position. (2) If the accommodation is impaired due to trauma, the eye examined might have a very low visual acuity. We decided, therefore, to use the fellow eye for the accommodative stimulus. However, when accommodating the globe normally rotates to converge. To keep the eye to be measured in line with a stationary transducer we arranged the targets according to Fig. 1. The accommodation stimulus was nearly 5 dptr.

The measurement values derived from our RESSOURCE-system are just numbers. To get a clear information on the accommodative process monitored, we programmed a pseudo M-mode display. The display scale is non-linearly compressed. No absolute distances can be extracted but the dynamical change is clearly shown with a resolution better than 0.1 mm.

Results

Only a limited number of volunteers could be measured until now. Thirteen examinations derived from 6 volunteers appeared to be useful. Table 1 shows the result of the examinations. Figure 2a shows a typical M-mode. As can be seen in this case the major part of the accommodation is performed by a thickening of the lens by shifting the posterior surface back towards the posterior wall of the eye. The small oscillatory components of the eye length data are presumably due to oscillations of the convergence of both eyes. This phenomenon is clearly visible in Fig. 2b. A remarkable increase in eye length is

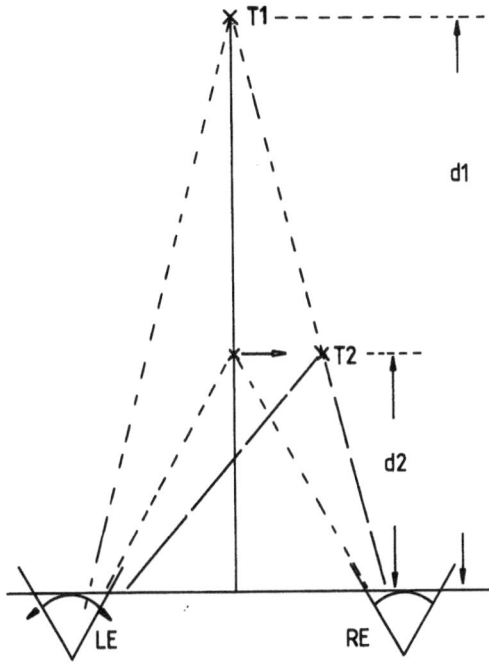

Fig. 1. The patient's right eye is to be measured. Two fixation targets (T1 & T2) 20 cm (d2) and more than 2 m (d1) apart from the eyes give an accommodation stimulus of nearly 5 dptr. The two targets are arranged in line for the right eye to avoid rotation of that eye due to convergence. Minimization of the rotation is achieved by a fine adjustment of the lower target.

Table 1. Compilation of the results of the examinations. The minus indicates a decrease of a distance.

Name	Age	Refr. Dptr.	Shift [0.01 mm] AC	LE	EL
ad	21	− 2.75	− 11	16	21
			− 16	16	19
pb	21	0.0	− 11	16	0
			− 13	16	− 5
			− 14	21	− 8
sch	21	0.0	− 16	19	0
			− 8	11	0
			− 5	13	0
rb	24	0.0	− 21	21	13
			− 8	16	0
li	36	− 0.25	0	11	0
			0	11	0
bu	37	0.0	− 11	21	5

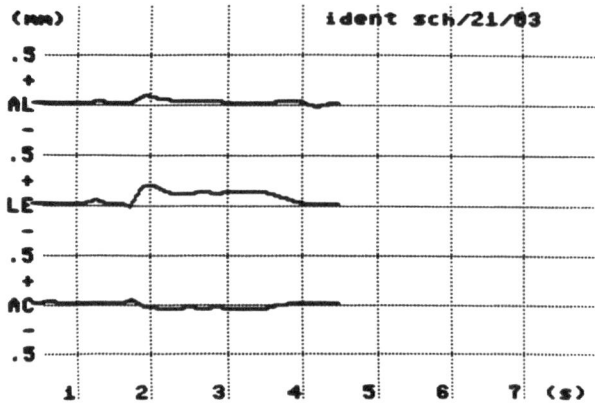

Fig. 2a. Pseudo lengthening of the eye due to small rotations of the globe.

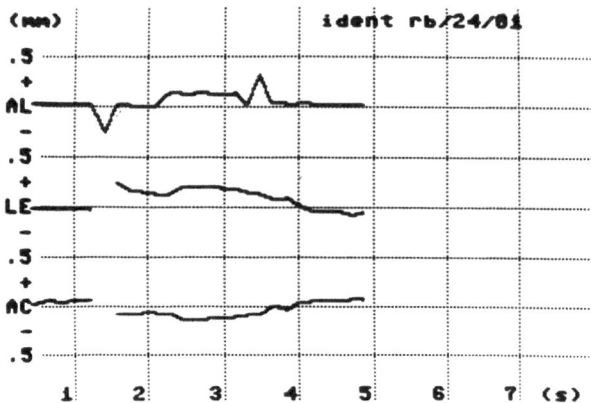

Fig. 2b. Example of a back and forth rotation before and after accommodation.

demonstrated in Fig. 3a, whereas a decrease is to be seen in Fig. 3b. Figure 4 demonstrates a practically constant eye length and anterior chamber length.

Discussion

The small number of examinations does not allow for a conclusive answer to all questions. We believe that measurements of the change of eye length were not based on artefacts. In some cases, we found a change of eye length. Naturally, we would expect only a lengthening, but shortening also happens. In most cases, however, we find no remarkable change of the length of eye during accommodation. These results are consistent with the results published by other authors.

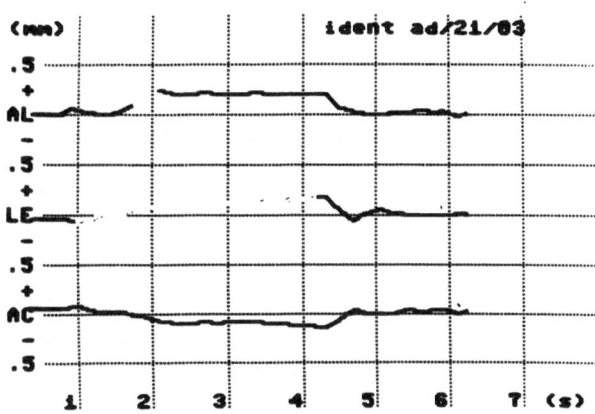

Fig. 3a. Example of an increasing eye length.

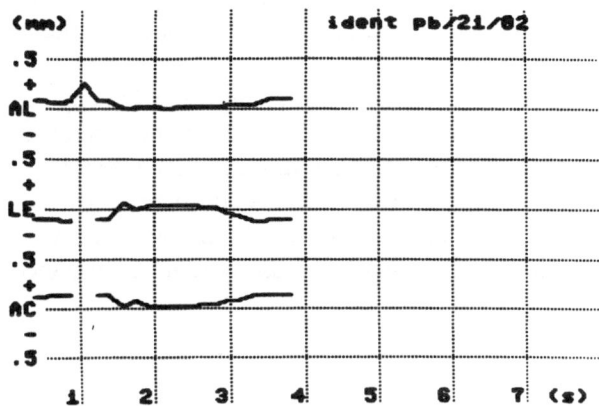

Fig. 3b. Example of a decreasing eye length.

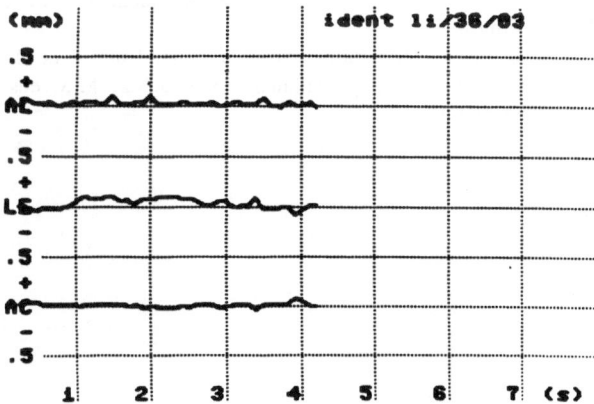

Fig. 4. Example of an accommodation with a shift of the posterior lens surface only.

Often, the lens accommodation is achieved by mainly shifting the anterior lens surface towards the cornea, thus reducing anterior chamber length. Sometimes, there is a more symmetric movement of the two lens surfaces; and in rare occasions we find a shift of the posterior lens surface only.

Conclusions

The number of patients or volunteers examined is not sufficient enough to obtain statistically significant results. However, the small number of examinations shows that there is a variety of physiological techniques to accommodate.

The biggest problem in performing these measurements is to couple the transducer to the eye. The rotational movement of the eye had to be excluded subjectively by the examiner. This was performed very carefully in these cases. However in clinical routine a fixation of the transducer to the eye would be necessary to obtain accurate results.

Two fixation methods could be used: either a sucking cup technique or a pressing of the transducer onto the eye. The first method increases intraocular pressure and could influence accommodation. The second method changes the shape of the globe and therefore also seems not to be very useful.

As the electronic accuracy is no longer the limiting factor we have to solve the transducer coupling problem to increase system performance.

References

Coleman DJ, Wuchinich D, Carlin B. 1969. Accommodative changes in the axial dimension of the human eye. In Gitter: Ophthalmic Ultrasound (Mosby, St Louis).

Lepper R-D, Trier HG, Reuter R. 1980. Neuartige Ultraschallbiometrie. Klin Mbl Augenheilk 177/101–106 (F. Enke, Stuttgart).

Storey JK, Rabie EP. 1984. Biometry of the eye during accommodation. Proc SIDUO IX, Leeds, U.K. 1982, in Ophthalm. Ultrasonography Hillman, J.S. & Le May, M.M. eds. pp. 295–301 (W Junk Publishers, The Hague).

Echographic findings in accommodation

HORACIO M. SORIANO
Buenos Aires, Argentine

The existence of accommodation has been established by different experiments. Sheiner, in 1619, elaborated an elegant demonstration of accommodation and established that the young eye has a mechanism for changing focus. Thomas Young (1801) demonstrated that this change does not occur in the cornea or in the length of the eyeball. All evidence indicated that the dioptric change in accommodation results from a change in the form of the lens. Young also demonstrated that accommodation could be exerted despite the neutralization of the cornea.

The change in the form of the lens during accommodation has been proved by optical methods and with echography in a study of accommodative spasm induced by pilocarpine [3]. Our aim was to observe the changes in the eye during physiological accommodation in young, healthy people and with different pathologies. We were particularly interested in the degree of thickening of the lens and in movement of the posterior lens surface.

Material and methods

We measured the ocular components of 25 persons, five emmetropic, five myopic ranging from −1.5 to −4 diopters, five hyperopic ranging from +2 to +4 D., five anisometropic, two with one myopic eye and three with one hyperopic eye, three patients with retinal detachment in one eye and two patients with choroidal melanoma in one eye. The ages ranged from eight to 32 years old with a mean of 17.4 years. The sex distribution was seven women (28%) and 18 men (72%).

Measurements were performed with the Kretz 7200 apparatus with a 10 MHz transducer. The equipment was calibrated before each examination. The patients, in a supine position, fixate a point at three meters distance with one eye. The other eye is examined using local anesthesia and a methocel-filled contactring. During accommodation the other eye fixates a number

K.C. Ossoinig (editor), Ophthalmic Echography, ISBN 978-94-010-7988-4

corresponding to Jaeger 1 at a distance of 15 cm. The best zones of the oscilloscope screen were utilized for the measurements by applying a (10–12 mm) precorneal methocel column.

The amplification of the equipment was 50 db. The ultrasonographic measurements were made between the peaks of the echospikes. In all cases we were able to separate the echo of the anterior and posterior surface of the cornea and the echo of the iris from the anterior lens surface signal. In our calculation we did not take into account the corneal thickness. The conversion to eye distances was based on the tables published by Poujol, J. [5].

Results

Emmetropic eyes

Five emmetropic persons (10 eyes) were examined and the main values for the anterior segment, lens thickness and vitreous length, with and without accommodation, were calculated (Table 1). The average narrowing of the anterior chamber with accommodation was 0.56 mm. The average thickening of the lens with accommodation was 0.6 mm. The average narrowing of the vitreous space was 0.04 mm. The accommodation produces a thickening and a forward bulging of the lens, causing the narrowing of the anterior chamber. The vitreous length remains practically unchanged. The axial length remains unchanged with and without accommodation.

Myopic eyes

Five myopic persons (10 eyes) were examined (Table 2). The average narrowing of the anterior chamber with accommodation was 0.17 mm. The average thickening of the lens with accommodation was 0.32 mm. The average narrow-

Table 1. Mean value for the anterior segment, lens thickness and vitreous length of the emmetropic eyes without and with accommodation.

	Without accommodation	With accommodation	
Number of emmetropic eyes examined	10	10	
Anterior segment	3.40 mm	2.84 mm	−0.56 mm
Lens	3.43 mm	4.03 mm	+0.6 mm
Vitreous	15.40 mm	15.36 mm	−0.04 mm
Axial length	22.23 mm	22.23 mm	−

Table 2. Mean value for the anterior chamber, lens thickness and vitreous length of the myopic eyes without and with accommodation.

	Without accommodation	With accommodation	
Number of myopic eyes examined	10	10	
Anterior chamber	3.45 mm	3.28 mm	−0.17 mm
Lens	3.75 mm	4.07 mm	+0.32 mm
Vitreous	16.87 mm	16.72 mm	−0.15 mm
Axial length	24.07 mm	24.07 mm	−

ing of the vitreous was 0.15 mm. The accommodation produces a less important thickening of the lens than in emmetropia and the narrowing of the anterior chamber and the vitreous space was almost the same. The axial length remained unchanged.

Hyperopic eyes

Five hyperopic persons (10 eyes) were examined (Table 3). The average narrowing of the anterior chamber with accommodation was 0.49 mm. The average thickening of the lens with accommodation was 0.51 mm. The average narrowing of the vitreous space was 0.02 mm. Accommodation produced more thickening of the lens than in myopia but less than in emmetropia. The vitreous length remained practically unchanged. There were no changes of the eye length.

Anisometropic eyes

Three patients with one hyperopic eye were examined (Table 4). The shallow-

Table 3. Mean value for the anterior chamber, lens thickness and vitreous length of the hyperopic eyes without and with accommodation.

	Without accommodation	With accommodation	
Number of hyperopic eyes examined	10	10	
Anterior chamber	3.36 mm	2.87 mm	−0.49 mm
Lens	3.39 mm	3.90 mm	+0.51 mm
Vitreous	15 mm	14.98 mm	−0.02 mm
Axial length	21.75 mm	21.75 mm	

Table 4. Mean value of the anterior chamber, lens, vitreous and axial length in anisometropic patients.

		Ant. chamber	Lens	Vitreous	Axial length
3 Hyperopic eyes	Without acc.	3.7 mm	3.1 mm	15.7 mm	22.5 mm
	With acc.	3.1 mm	3.7 mm	15.7 mm	22.5 mm
3 Emmetropic eyes	Without acc.	3.7 mm	3.2 mm	16.45 mm	23.35 mm
	With acc.	3.6 mm	3.3 mm	16.45 mm	23.35 mm

ing of the anterior chamber in the emmetropic eye was less than in the emmetropic group (range 3.7 mm to 3.6 mm). There was practically no change in the thickening of the lens. The unilaterally hyperopic eyes showed comparable changes to those of the hyperopic group. The average thickening of the lens was 0.6 mm (range 3.1 to 3.7 mm). The average narrowing of the anterior chamber with accommodation was 0.6 mm (range 3.7 to 3.1 mm).

Two patients with one myopic eye were examined (Table 5). The average narrowing of the anterior segment in the emmetropic eye with accommodation was 0.8 mm (range 3.8–3.0 mm). The average thickening of the lens was 0.7 mm – there was an increase 0.1 mm in vitreous length with accommodation. The unilaterally myopic eyes showed comparable changes to those of the myopic group. The average narrowing of the anterior segment with accommodation was 0.1 mm (range 3.95 to 3.85 mm). The average thickening of the lens was 0.3 mm (ranging from 3.9 to 4.2). The average thickening of the vitreous space was 0.2 mm (ranging from 16.2 to 16 mm).

Table 5. Mean value of the anterior chamber, lens, vitreous and axial length in anisometropic patients.

		Ant. chamber	Lens	Vitreous	Axial Length
2 Myopic eyes	Without acc.	3.95 mm	3.9 mm	16.20 mm	24.05 mm
	With acc.	3.85 mm	4.2 mm	16 mm	24.05 mm
2 Emmetropic eyes	Without acc.	3.8 mm	3.3 mm	14.6 mm	21.7 mm
	With acc.	3.0 mm	4.0 mm	14.7 mm	21.7 mm

Table 6. Retinal detachment in one eye.

		Ant. chamber	Lens	Vitreous	Axial length
3 Eyes with detachment	Without acc.	2.7 mm	4.1 mm	16.8 mm	23.6 mm
	With acc.	2.7 mm	4.2 mm	16.7 mm	23.6 mm

Retinal detachment eyes

Three patients with retinal detachment in one eye were examined (Table 6). The anterior segment and the axial length remained unchanged with accommodation. The thickening of the lens was 0.1 mm (range 4.1 to 4.2 mm). The shortening of the vitreous space was 0.1 mm (range 16.8 to 16.7 mm). The normal eye was not examined.

Choroidal melanoma eyes

Two patients with a peripheral choroidal melanoma with normal visual acuity were examined (Table 7). In the normal eye the narrowing of the anterior chamber was 0.6 mm (range 3.6 to 3.0 mm). The thickening of the lens was 0.4 mm (range 3.2 to 3.6 mm). The vitreous space enlarged 0.2 mm (range 16.8 to 17.0 mm). The axial length remained unchanged. The melanoma eye showed a narrowing of the anterior chamber of 0.5 mm. The thickening of the lens was 0.5 mm. The vitreal space and the axial length remained unchanged.

Discussion

The shape of the lens depends upon the elasticity of its capsule, a relatively

Table 7. Peripheral choroidal melanoma in one eye.

		Anterior chamber	Lens	Vitreous	Axial length
2 Melanoma eyes	Without acc.	3.2 mm	3.7 mm	16.1 mm	23.0 mm
	With acc.	2.7 mm	4.2 mm	16.1 mm	23.0 mm
2 Normal eyes	Without acc.	3.6 mm	3.2 mm	16.8 mm	23.6 mm
	With acc.	3.0 mm	3.6 mm	17.0 mm	23.6 mm

Table 8. Values of the increase of thickness of the lens compared with the decrease of length in the anterior chamber and vitreous.

	Emmetropic	Myopic	Hyperopic
Anterior chamber	−0.56 mm	−0.17 mm	−0.49 mm
Lens	+0.6 mm	+0.32 mm	+0.51 mm
Vitreous	−0.04 mm	−0.15 mm	−0.02 mm

thick basement membrane of the lens cells, and on the traction on the zonulae. Fincham [1] says that in extreme accommodation the ciliary ring has contracted to such an extreme that the zonulae are relaxed and the lens becomes displaced in the direction of gravity.

In our study only in myopic eyes did we find a shortening of the vitreous space. In those cases the thickening of the lens was less important than in emmetropic or hyperopic eyes, but it became displaced in the direction of gravity (Table 8).

This is a paradoxical situation because we expected to find this in hyperopic eyes where we have an extreme accommodation. Maybe the vitreous condition could be the explanation of this finding.

The mean lens thickness in myopic eyes without accommodation was 3.75 mm, very close to that finding by Francois and Goes [2] of 3.54 mm. The most important changes with accommodation were found in the emmetropic eyes with a mean shortening of the anterior chamber of 0.56 mm and a lens thickening of 0.6 mm (Table 7). In the hyperopic eyes the main shortening of the anterior chamber was 0.49 mm and the lens thickening of 0.51 mm (Table 8).

In cases of anisometropic patients with one hyperopic eye, we don't find an explanation for the results in the emmetropic eyes, with almost no variation with accommodation. We need a larger series of patients to make a conclusion. In cases of anisometropic patients with one myopic eye the results were the same as those for each type of the refractive groups.

Summary

Accommodation of 25 persons with different refractive and pathologic conditions were examined with ultrasound. The mean changes were given in the anterior chamber, lens, vitreous and axial length in emmetropic, hyperopic, myopic, anisometropic, retinal detachment and choroidal melanoma eyes, with and without accommodation. In myopia the thickening of the lens was less pronounced than in emmetropic or hyperopic eyes, and we also observed a displacement of the lens in the direction of gravity.

References

1. Fincham E. 1937. The mechanism of accommodation, Br J Ophthalmology 8: 1–9.
2. Francois J, Goes F. 1975. Oculometry of progressive myopia. Ultrasonography in Ophthalmology Bibl Ophthal 83: 277–282 (Karger, Basel).
3. Francois J, Goes F. 1975. Ultrasonographic comparative study of the effect of pilocarpine and aceclidine on the eye components. Ultrasonography in Ophthalmology. Bibl Ophthal 83: 320–327 (Karger, Basel).
4. Helmholtz H. 1924. Treatise on physiologic optics, Vol. 1, New York, Dover Publications, Inc.
5. Poujol J. 1973. Tables de transformation des micro-secondes de temps d'echo en millimètres de longueur oculaire. In Echographie de l'oeil et de l'orbite, par Hammard H, Massin M, Poujol J. Bull Soc Ophthal France, numéro spécial, p. 183–184.

Ultrasonic measurements of accommodation in phakic and pseudophakic eyes

G.L. VAN DER HEIJDE and W.A.E.J. DE VRIES-KNOPPERT
Amsterdam, the Netherlands

Abstract

A method is presented to continuously registrate intraocular distances by accurately transforming the time-period between successive echoes of reflecting surfaces into a voltage.

In such a way it is possible to recognize alterations in the measured distances, for instance due to eye blinks or small eye movements. Another application is the continuous registration of the position of the lens in the (pseudo-)phakic eye during accommodation.

Results are shown of static and dynamic accommodation experiments. An interesting phenomenon was found in some unilateral pseudophakic patients with their IOL fixed in the capsular bag: by presenting an accommodation stimulus to the normal fellow eye, the IOL in the pseudophakic eye moved slightly in a forward direction.

Introduction

During accommodation the lens in the eye changes its refractive power in order to sharply focus an object onto the retina. In man the change in refractive power can be accomplished by altering the shape of the lens: when fixating a nearby object the lens will become more convex consequently increasing its axial thickness.

Many investigators have studied the changes in the refractive state of the lens during accommodation using IR optometers.

The use of high-resolution echography in ophthalmology extended our knowledge of the properties of the accommodation system. For instance, results of static echography of the position of the lens during accommodation forced Coleman (1970) to revise the classical theory of Helmholtz on accommodation.

K.C. Ossoinig (editor), Ophthalmic Echography, ISBN 978-94-010-7988-4

During accommodation the maximal displacements of the lens in the eye generally do not exceed 0.6 mm (Coleman, 1970). Therefore, to measure small changes of intraocular distances, standard clinical methods will not meet the necessary high accuracy. Another disadvantage of commercially available echographic instruments is their lack to give an impression of the variability of the measured values. In clinical circumstances, usual single measurements of intraocular distances are performed by photographing the echogram in combination with an electronic ruler. Due to instabilities of the electronic circuit and, what is more important, significant errors in reading the scale, inaccuracies may be about 0.5 mm.

A better accuracy can be achieved by using quartz controlled electronic counters (Van der Heijde et al., 1977). In that case, accuracy is limited by the clock frequency of the counter. Instruments based on this principle, such as the one described by Lepper and Trier (1981), are therefore powerful to calculate IOL power, but are not simply suitable to measure variations in ocular distances smaller than about 0.1 mm.

Its our purpose to present a method to register also these small fluctuations in order to study accommodation.

Methods

In the method presented here, the time between echoes was linearly transformed into a voltage, that could be plotted continuously, or processed by a computer to enable off-line inspection of the registered data (Fig. 1).

Subjects were in a supine position. The echo probe was mounted in a contact ring filled with water to allow for easy centering of the probe with respect to the optical axis of the eye.

Accommodation stimuli were presented to the fellow eye. For that purpose the subject fixated a checkerboard pattern mounted in an optical stimulator according to the principle of Badal.

Results

Figure 2 shows a simultaneous registration during 30 seconds, of the depth of the anterior chamber (A.C.), the lens, the vitreous and axial length of the eye of a normal phakic patient. The effect of voluntary blinking is demonstrated in the first part of the registration. The eyelid may have pressed the contact glass with echoprobe downwards resulting in a measurement of the echo of the iris instead of the front surface of the lens.

Combining the measurements of the depth of the A.C. and the thickness of

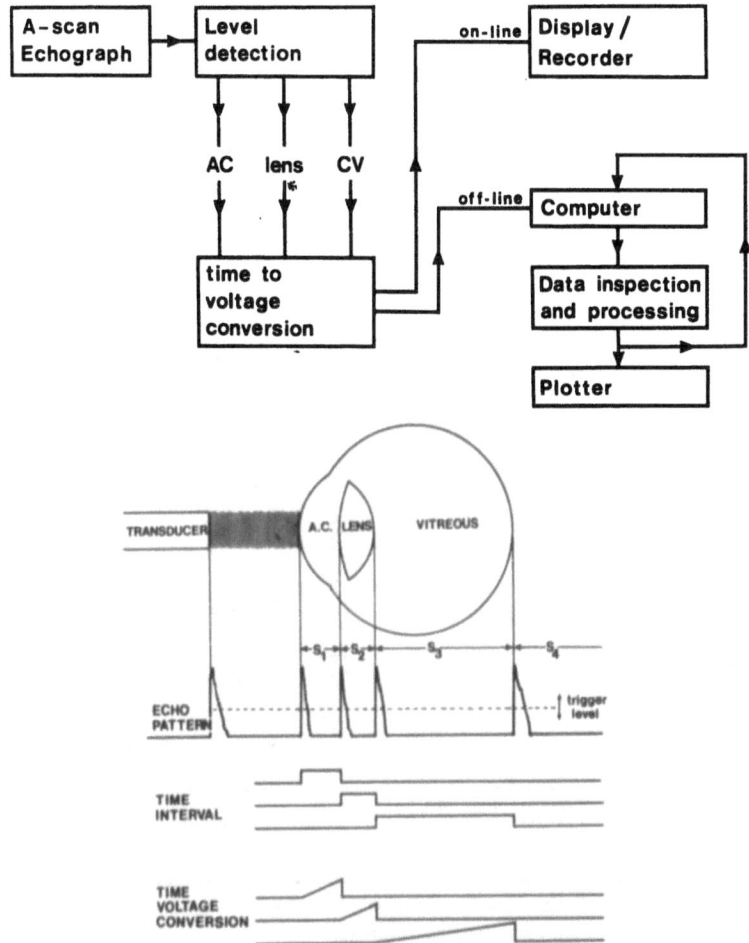

Fig. 1. Principle of the transformation of the time interval between echoes to voltage.

the lens, results in the smooth registrations of the position of the posterior surface of the lens during blinking. Clearly, blinking deteriorates the proper determination of the front surface of the lens.

Large eye movements also can seriously influence the accuracy of the measurement. Figure 3 shows the effect of a 10 degrees lateral movement of the eye on the measured intraocular distances. The absolute magnitude of the deviation depends, of course, on the way the ultrasound probe is fixated with respect to the eye. During accommodation the front surface of the lens moves anteriorly as was shown by Coleman (1970). We found on average a decrease in A.C. depth of 0.08 mm/diopter (Fig. 4). The thickness of the lens increases in the same rate, so the posterior surface of the lens will stay on its place.

174

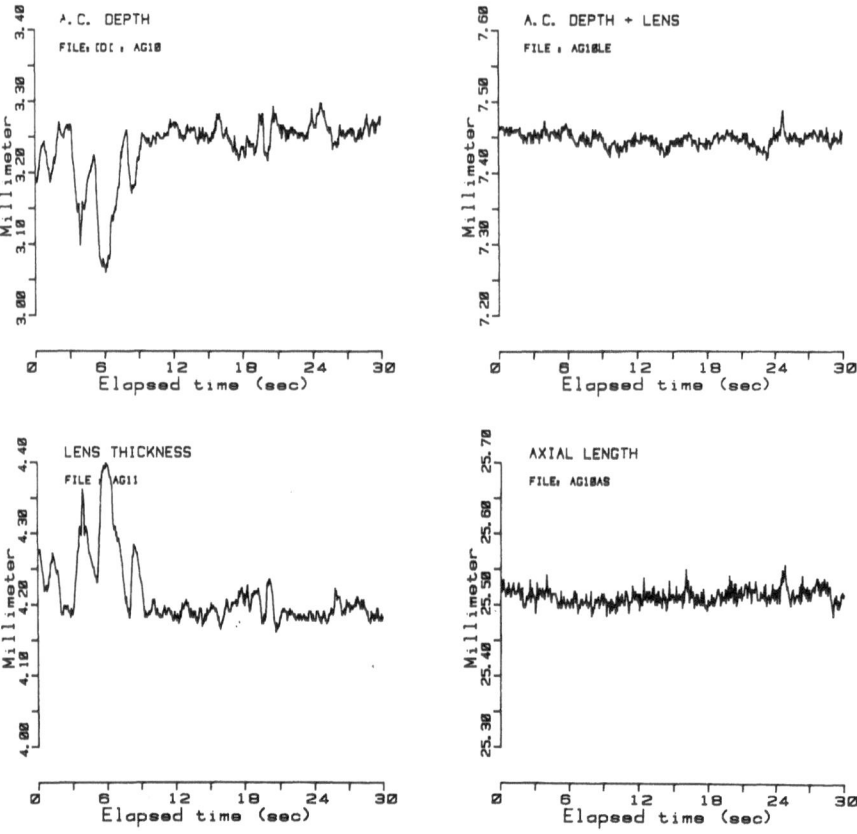

Fig. 2. Continuous registration during 30 seconds of intraocular distances in a normal phakic patient. The effect of voluntary blinking can only be demonstrated in the first part of the registrations of the A.C. depth and the lens thickness.

The ciliary muscle moves during accommodation to a forward position. To test the hypothesis that also in the pseudophakic eye with an intact ciliar muscle, the IOL moves anteriorly, we measured young pseudophakic patients with an IOL fixed in the capsular bag. When stimulating the normal fellow eye, we were able to show that the pseudophakic eye indeed showed a very small, but detectable, (pseudo-)accommodation.

Figure 5 shows results of biometric measurements on a 12 year old boy, who underwent extracapsular lens extraction followed by implantation of a J-loop IOL in oct 1983 after a trauma due to a staple in the right eye in march 1983. Both haptics of the IOL were placed in the capsular bag.

The fellow eye was emmetropic and was able to accommodate 12 diopters. The depth of the anterior chamber of the pseudophakic eye decreases about 0.05 mm/diopter accommodation.

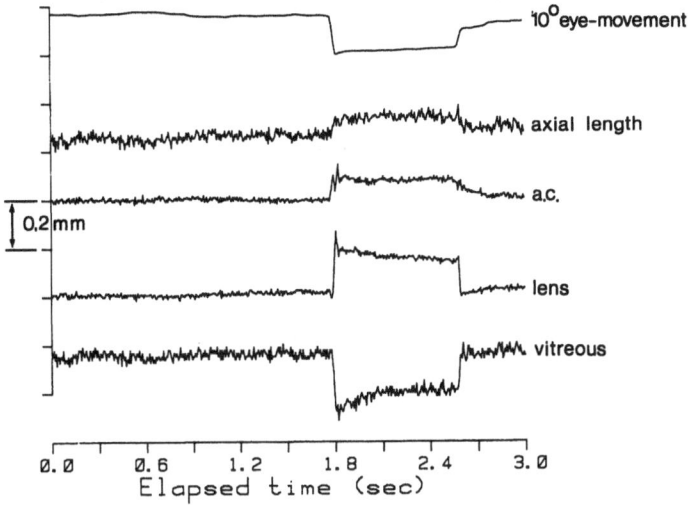

Fig. 3. Effect of a saccadic eye movement of 10 degrees on the measurement of A.C. depth, lens thickness, length of vitreous and axial length.

Conclusions

Our method to registrate intraocular distances continuously, enables:
- determination of the variation within the measurement.
- off-line inspection of the raw material.

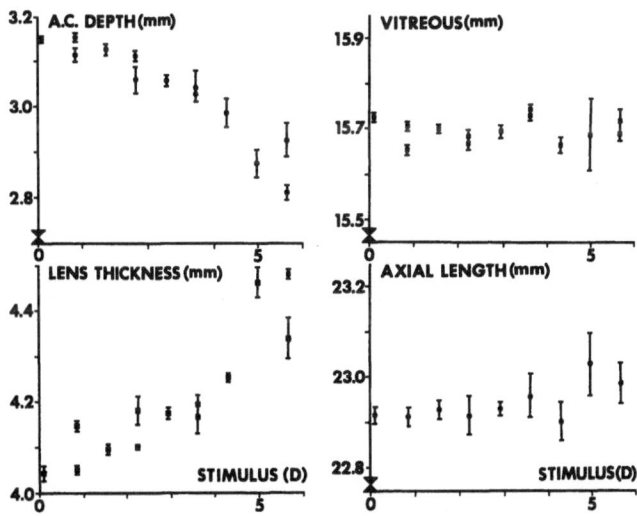

Fig. 4. Alterations of intraocular distances during accommodation in a normal phakic subject.

176

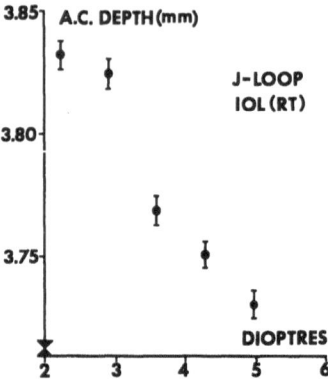

Fig. 5. Decrease of anterior chamber depth in a pseudophakic patient during static accommodation of the fellow eye.

– detection of small displacements of the healthy lens and of an IOL in the capsular bag, during accommodation.

References

Coleman DJ. 1970. Unified model for accommodative mechanism; Am J Ophthal 69 (6): 1063–1078.
Lepper RD, Trier HG. 1981. A new device for ocular biometry; Docum Ophthal Proc Series 29: 473–477.
Van der Heijde GL, Meinema AJ, Vlaming MSMG. 1977. Digital A-scan ultrasonography used to measure ocular distances; Am J Ophthal 83 (2): 276–277.

Electronic linear scanning ultrasonic diagnostic equipment in ophthalmology

A. SAWADA, Y. BABA, H. TORII, A. YAMAMOTO and Y. KODAMA
Miyazaki, Japan

Abstract

Electronic linear-scanning ultraonic diagnostic equipment, the ECHO Camera 210 DX (Aloka, Japan), was used. It has many advantages, particularly in regard to the mobility of intraocular disorders.

Introduction

Electronic linear-scanning ultrasonic diagnostic equipment for ophthalmic practice has recently been developed and its clinical value in the detection, characterization and differentiation of ocular disorders has been recognized (Susal et al., 1983). Recently, the ECHO Camera 210 DX (Aloka, Japan) appeared on the market as the first electronic scanner for ophthalmic use in Japan. Several trial experiences with this electronic scanner have been reported (Tane et al., 1983; Yamamoto et al., 1984). It has been used in the diagnosis of many, ocular disorders at Miyazaki Medical College Hospital.

Materials and methods

The ECHO Camera 210 DX is equipped with a 5.0 MHz transducer with an effective sweeping range of 34 mm in width and 65 mm in depth. If desired a 7.5 MHz transducer is available. A resolution power for both directions to within 1 mm. The frame rate is 30 per second. The dimensions are 25 cm in width, 20 cm in height, and 36.5 cm in depth, and it weighs 8.0 kg. Figure 1 shows the frontal view of the equipment. The probe can be placed directly on the patient's closed eyelids for the contact method, and it can be used with a water bath for the immersion method.

More than 100 eyes with various kinds of intraocular and orbital disorders

K.C. Ossoinig (editor), Ophthalmic Echography, ISBN 978-94-010-7988-4

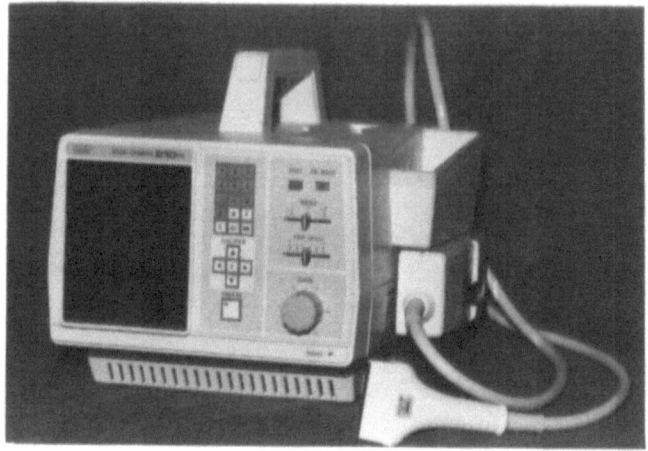

Fig. 1. Electronic linear scanning ultrasonic diagnostic equipment, ECHO Camera 210 DX (Aloka, Japan).

were examined with the ECHO Camera 210 DX. At the same time other kinds of mechanical and electronic B-mode ultrasonic diagnostic equipment were used. The results were compared with those from different types of equipment.

Results

The representative cases will be illustrated.

Lid Lesions. A 60-year-old woman with a left lower lid abscess was examined. A-scanning was done directly on the skin of the lid. Mechanical and electronic B-scanning was done by the immersion method using a surgical drape and wooden frame in which a sharply outlined lesion was displayed in the subcutaneous tissue. The inner reflectivity using the Kretztechnik 7200 MA was weak. In an electronic scanning echogram (Fig. 2) using a 5.0 MHz probe, the lesion was displayed beneath the echolucent eyeball and was found to be relatively unchanged by compression. The strong reflective portion in the lesion was suspected to contain a small foreign body. Upon incision, a quantity of pus was drained away but the foreign body was not found. By using the immersion method with a waterbath a lid lesion, as well as a lesion in the superficial layer of the orbital tissue may be easily evaluated as a whole. The relationship to the tissue surrounding the lesion was also clearly displayed. Fig. 3 shows electronic-scanning echograms of a dermoid cyst located in the left upper lid of a 21-year-old man; the sharply outlined posterior wall was

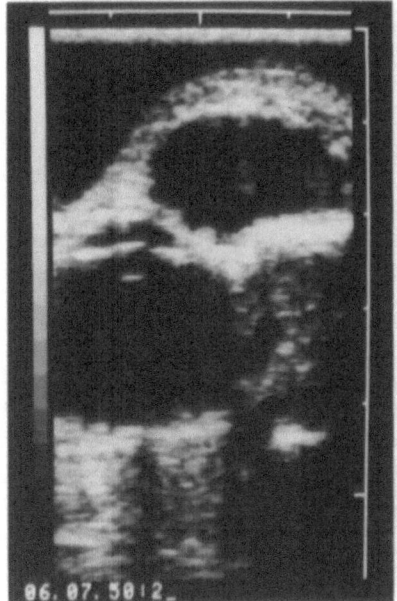

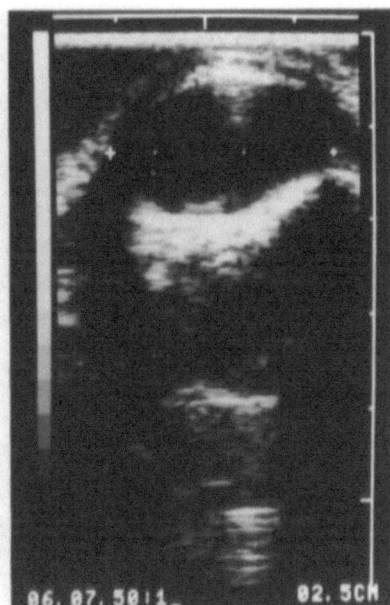

Fig. 2. Vertical scanning section with water-bath of the eyeball and lid abscess.

Fig. 4. A foreign body in the vitreous.

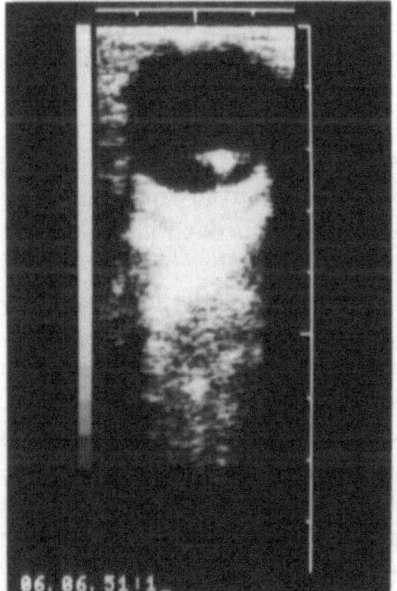

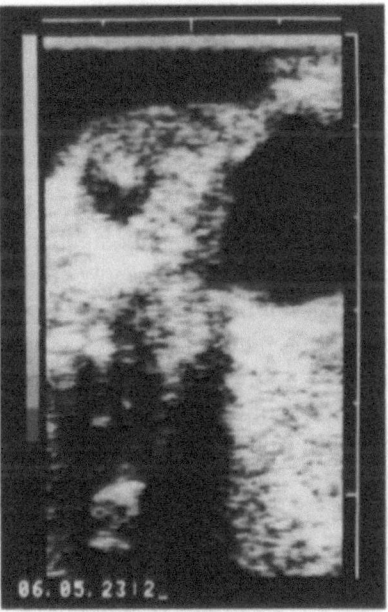

Fig. 3. Dermoid cyst. Left: vertical scanning section with waterbath of the eyeball and an echolucent tumor above it. Right: horizontal scanning section of the tumor. The horizontal size measured with built-in calipers as 2.5 cm.

180

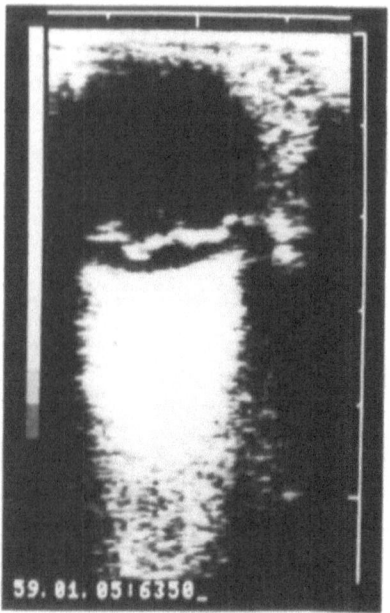

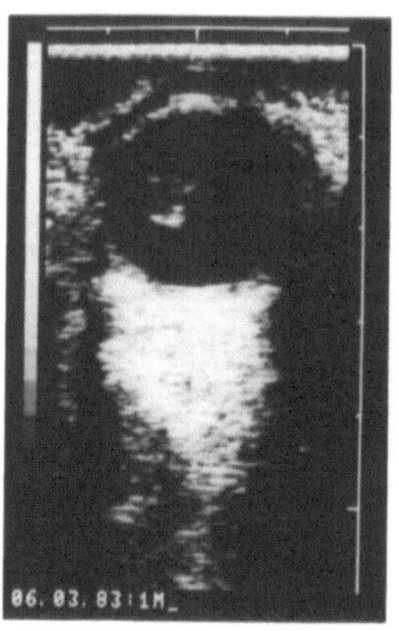

Fig. 5. Subluxated lens in the vitreous space.

Fig. 6. Vitreous hemorrhage in Terson's syndrome.

clearly displayed. As shown in the picture on the right, the horizontal size of the tumor was measured with the use of built in calipers, and the value was digitally displayed as 2.5 cm.

Intraocular foreign body and luxated Lens. Figure 4 is an electronic scanning echogram of a 29-year-old man who had been exposed to an explosion fifteen years before and had many small pieces of glass embedded in the bullous cornea of the left eye. A sharply outlined, strongly reflective point-like lesion with distinct multiple signals was displayed in the center of the vitreous, which is pathognomonic for a foreign body.

Figure 5 is an electronic scanning echogram of a lens subluxated into the vitreous space of the eye of a 28-year-old woman with neovascular glaucoma. An oval, sharply outlined mass in the vitreous was displayed, which also contained low inner reflectivity with some granule-like echogenic materials. The lesion moved, rapidly in a pendulum-like fashion as the eyeball moved. It was strongly suggested that the oval mass adhered partly to the surrounding tissue. With electronic B-scanning, change in the position of the lesion is very easily detected and very accurately evaluated.

Vitreous disorders. Figure 6 is an electronic scanning echogram of a vitreous hemorrhage in the right eye of a 60-year-old man with Terson's syndrome. A

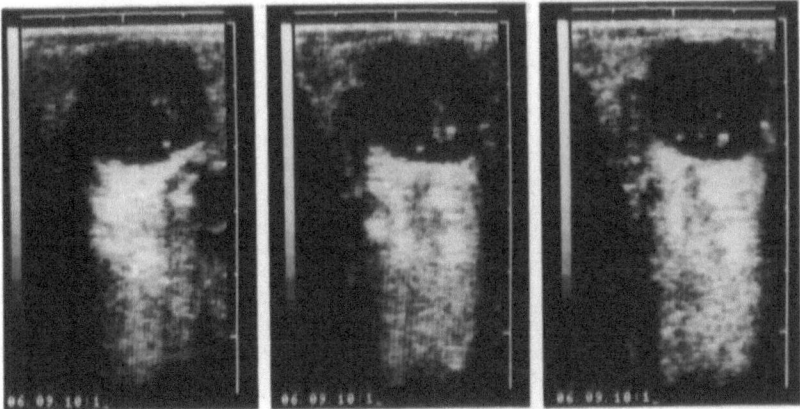

Fig. 7. Horizontal scanning echograms of asteroid hyalitis in kinetic echography. Left: in the temporal gaze position. Center: in primary position. Right: in the nasal gaze position.

membrane with a somewhat irregular thickness, parallel to the posterior wall of the eye at a certain distance, was displayed. The clearness of the image using Aloka's electronic B-scanner was almost identical in comparison to Bronson-Turner's scanner. Kinetic characteristics of the lesion were more easily visualized with the electronic B-scanner. The reflectivity to the ultrasonic wave was very strong. The value of $\triangle$ dB in quantitative echography using Kretztechnik 7200 MA was 16.

Figure 7 shows echograms of asteroid hyalitis in the right eye of a 53-year-old-man. Multiple small point-like lesions of high reflectivity were displayed. These lesions, located in the mid vitreous and separated from the fundus structure by a clear zone, were dense and remained on the screen at a decreased amplification setting. With kinetic echography high mobility was presented.

Retinal detachment. In several cases of retinal detachment the results with Aloka's equipment was compared with those using other types of B-scanners, either mechanical or electronic. A rhegmatogenous retinal detachment in the left eye of a 48-year-old woman was examined. In an A-scan with Kretztechnik 7200 MA a steeply rising, extremely high single spike was displayed in the vitreous space (the value of $\triangle$ dB in quantitative echography was 13). In a B-scan using mechanical Bronson-Turner equipment, a somewhat thick membrane-like lesion parallel to the fundus structure was displayed. When using electronic Aloka's equipment a thick membrane-like lesion was displayed, as it was also using the mechanical equipment. Mobility of the lesion was definitely demonstrated with a change in the gaze position (Fig. 8). In this particular case, the lesion responded slowly and minimally to eye movements.

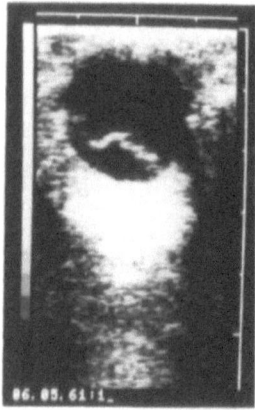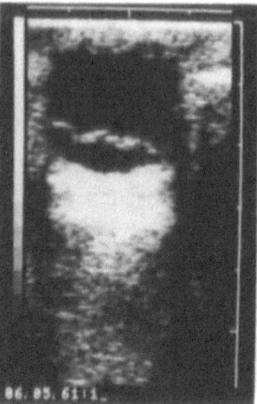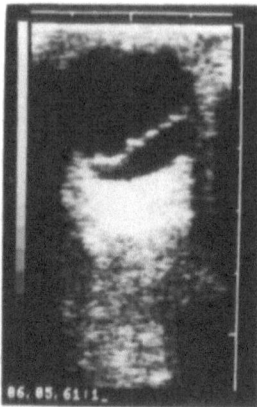

Fig. 8. Horizontal scanning echograms of retinal detachment of the left eye in kinetic echography. Left: in the nasal gaze postion. Center: in primary position. Right: in the temporal gaze position.

Aftermovement was of short duration, and was limited to a small range.

By watching the TV monitor during the examination or by checking the videotapes following the examination, precise information on the mobility of the membrane-like lesions in question were obtained.

Diabetic vitreoretinopathy. Figure 9 is an electronic scanning echogram showing diabetic retinopathy with vitreous hemorrhage and posterior hyphema in a 66-year-old man. Several point-like and massive lesions were scattered throughout the center of the vitreous. Just in front of the fundus structure a flat membrane-like lesion was seen stretching across the fundus like a bridge. The membrane-like lesion shifted easily following a change in gaze direction.

Figure 10 is an electronic scanning echogram of the left eye of a 26-year-old woman with tractional retinal detachment caused by diabetic vitreous hemorrhage. An irregular, membrane-like lesion in the vitreous with unequal thickness was seen on the echogram; the lesion was densely connected to the posterior wall of the eye at the point near the optic disc. Bronson-Turner's equipment was superior to Aloka's in determining the location of adherence – this was probably due to the proper size and shape of the probe. However, in those cases where movements of the lesion are diagnostic, electronic B-scanning is superior to mechanical scanning.

Intraocular tumors. Figure 11 is electronic scanning echograms showing retinoblastoma in a 6-month-old boy. An extremely highly reflective lesion of an irregular shape, protruding from the fundus into the vitreous space, was displayed. In the left eye (left side of the figure) more than two-thirds of the vitreous space was obstructed by the tumor. In the right eye, the tumor

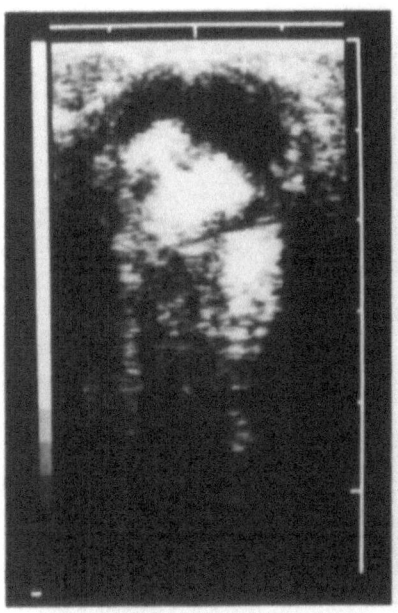

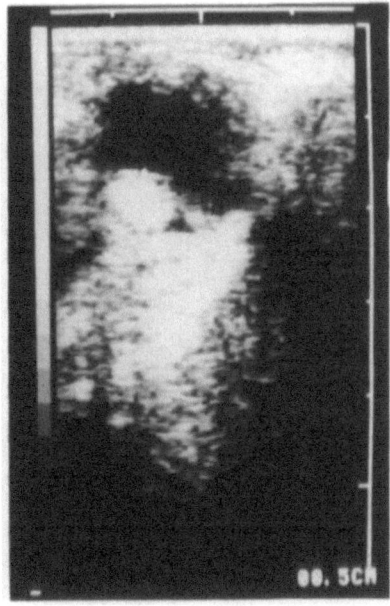

Fig. 9. Diabetic vitreous hemorrhage and posterior hyphema, whch resembles retinal detachment.

Fig. 10. Retinal detachment in proliferative diabetic retinopathy, connecting densely and firmly to the optic disc.

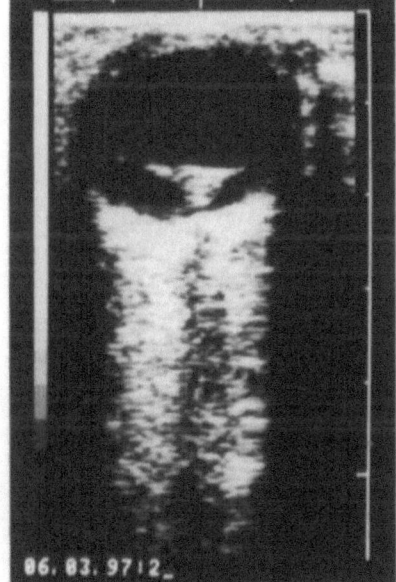

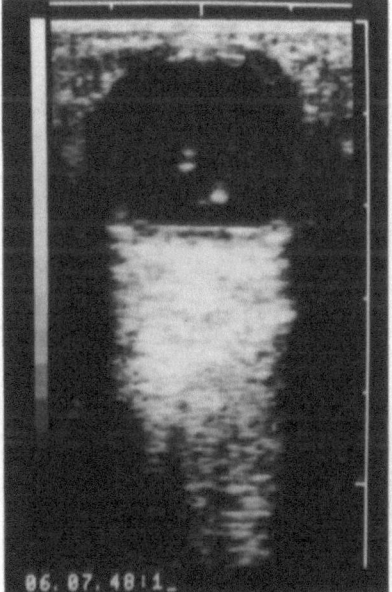

Fig. 11. Retinoblastoma in both eyes. Left: in the left eye more than two-thirds of the vitreous space was occupied by the tumor. Right: in the right eye the protrusion of the tumor measured with built-in calipers as 0.5 cm.

184

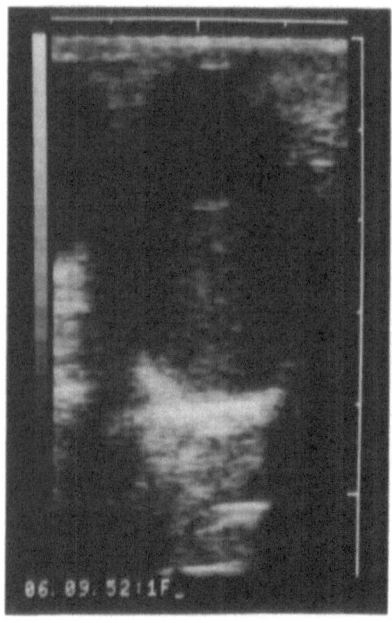

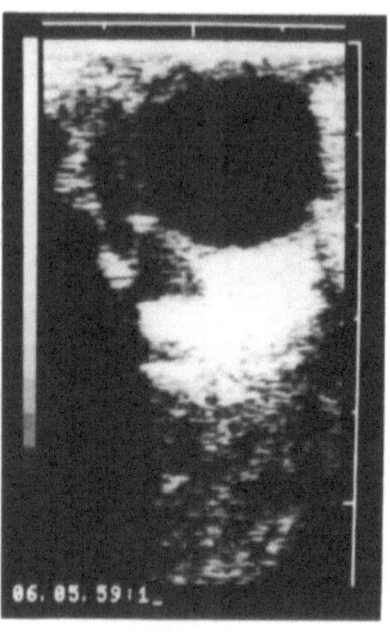

Fig. 12. A vertical scanning echogram of externally extended retinoblastoma, displayed as an echolucent area beneath the upper lid.

Fig. 13. Orbital pseudotumor localized posteriorly and laterally to the right eyeball.

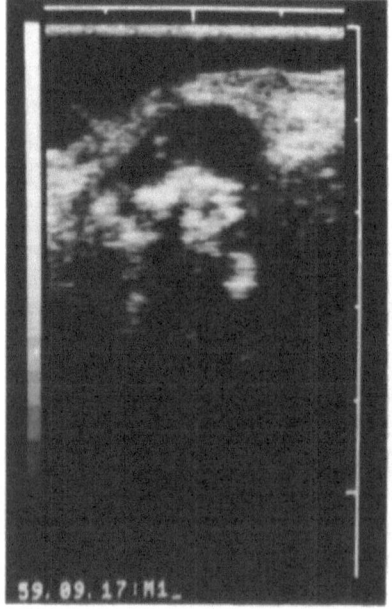

Fig. 14. Recurrent ethmofrontal pyocele. A huge, extremely low reflective area displayed on the right side of the eyeball, in which a quantity of weak echogenic material was accumulated.

protruding into the vitreous space was measured with built-in calipers, and the value was shown digitally in the lower right corner of the screen.

Figure 12 is an electronic scanning echogram of an externally extended retinoblastoma in the right eye of a two-year-old boy. His left eye had been enucleated due to the presence of retinoblastoma two years before. Cryotherapy and radiation therapy could not stop the development of the tumor in the right eye. In the echogram the echolucent area behind the upper lid was displayed. After enucleation it was seen that the echolucent area contained undifferentiated cells without calcium deposits extending from the inside of the eye through the sclera.

Orbital disorders. Figure 13 is an electronic scanning echogram of an orbital tumor in a 53-year-old woman. Computerized tomography (CT) revealed that the lesion stretched backward along the lateral wall of the orbit. A part of the lesion was excised, and histopathologically proved to be chronic nongranulomatous inflammatory pseudotumor. A low reflective mass stretching from the anterior to the posterior temporal side of the eyeball was displayed on the electronic linear scanner.

Figure 14 is an electronic scanning echogram of a recurrent ethmofrontal pyocele in a 66-year-old woman. A huge, clearly outlined, extremely low reflective area was displayed in the center of the screen. It was located on the nasal side of the right eyeball. In the lower part of the echolucent area, weak echogenic materials were accumulated. At surgery it was confirmed to be pus.

Discussion

Electronic-scanning ultrasonic diagnostic equipment has been widely used in medical fields other than ophthalmology. Nevertheless, the development of this kind of equipment is lacking because the ocular and orbital tissues, which do not move so well spontaneously, are not well visualized. However, when the prescribed movement is given in kinetic echography different kinds of information, which are not given by the usual method using mechanical scanners, are provided. The image provided by the new scanning type of equipment is clear and is in real time. The new equipment is, in particular, highly sensitive to movements of point- and membrane-like lesions in the vitreous. A study to ascertain the correct movements necessary for a precise evaluation is now being undertaken.

After almost one year of clinical study at the Miyazaki Medical College Hospital, the following can be concluded: First of all, kinetic echography can be done easily and precisely using electronic-scanning equipment. Other equipment advantages include, for example, the fact that lesions in the lid or in the anterior part of the eye can be displayed using either the contact method or the immersion method; foreign bodies or luxated lenses can be easily and precisely located; adhesions of the surrounding tissues and their precise locations can be found using kinetic echography; and point-like or membrane-like structures in the vitreous are clearly displayed. The site and extent of connection of these structures to the eyeball can be discerned. Mobility of these strucures can be evaluated. Also, the elevation of the detached retina and the size of the intraocular tumor can be digitally measured with electronic calipers; the connection of the tumor to the surroundings can be exactly displayed; the change with eye movement can show the real character of the tumor; and, the tumor image can be frozen at any time, making it easy to take pictures at the optimal time and to discuss the findings during the examination. The displayed image can also be recorded on videotape, which can be reproduced at any time.

On the other hand, disadvantages have also been found: the size of the probe is too large to always apply the ultrasonic wave to the site in a perpendicular fashion; effective vertical scanning is impossible; and the posterior boundary of the eyeball is not as sharply delineated.

Conclusion

With the newly-developed electronic scanner, clearer real time images may be produced than those by the mechanical scanner. Using the electronic scanner, rapid progress in kinetic echography would be expected.

References

1. Baba Y, Sawada A, Yokomatsu M, Torii H, Yamamoto A. 1984. Clinical usefulness of a diagnostic ultrasonic unit with electronic scanner (Renaissance A/B scan). Rinsho Ganka 38: 782–783.
2. Susal AL, Gaynon MW, Walker JT. 1983. Linear array multiple transducer ultrasonic examination of the eye. Ophthalmology 90: 266–271.
3. Tane S, Komatsu A, Kondo K, Suzuki J, Kogakura H, Yamamoto Y, Hirano S, Sugata Y. 1983. Studies on ultrasonic diagnosis in ophthalmology Report 18. The clinical application of handy high-frequency electronic high-speed scanning ultrasonic diagnostic equipment (Echo Camera XA-55) for ophthalmological imaging diagnosis. Folia Ophthalmol Jpn 34: 2478–2482.
4. Yamamoto Y, Hirano S, Sugata Y, Tane S, Komatsu A, Suzuki J. 1984. Image treatment in the eye in ultrasound diagnosis: Its clinical significance XV. Clinical application of new electronic scanning ultrasonograph. Folia Ophthalmol Jpn 35: 114–117.

Computer-assisted clinical A-mode analysis in ophthalmic ultrasonography

W. HAIGIS
Würzburg, FRG

Summary

It was shown how different statistical parameters may be extracted from ophthalmic echograms using commercial instruments and a low-cost personal computer system. Attenuation estimates for normal orbital fat consistent with literature data were obtained with two different ultrasonic instruments after allowance had been made for their individual performance characteristics. Finally, the possible value of an autocorrelation analysis for tissue characterization was illustrated in the case of a normal orbit and a tumour of the ciliary body.

Introduction

Quantitative tissue characterization may be described as the attempt to find a set of numbers which are related to physical properties of a specific tissue in question. These parameters have to be extracted from appropriate measurements making use of methods from the theory of signal analysis. Consequently, the most promising way is to digitize the radio frequency (rf) signals coming from the transducer and let a computer perform the data processing (see e.g. references in: Thijssen, 1980).

However, applying commercial diagnostic instruments presently available, two problems arise: first, these instruments are not designed to perform measurements in a strict sense, second, digitizing rf signals calls for analogue-to-digital converters with very high sampling rates (up to 100 MHz) which are still very expensive.

A solution to the first problem lies in performance measurements characterizing the ultrasonic equipment (Haigis and Buschmann, 1984); the second one may be tackled by exploiting the demodulated (video) signals rather than the rf signals (e.g. Thijssen et al., 1981).

K.C. Ossoinig (editor), Ophthalmic Echography, ISBN 978-94-010-7988-4

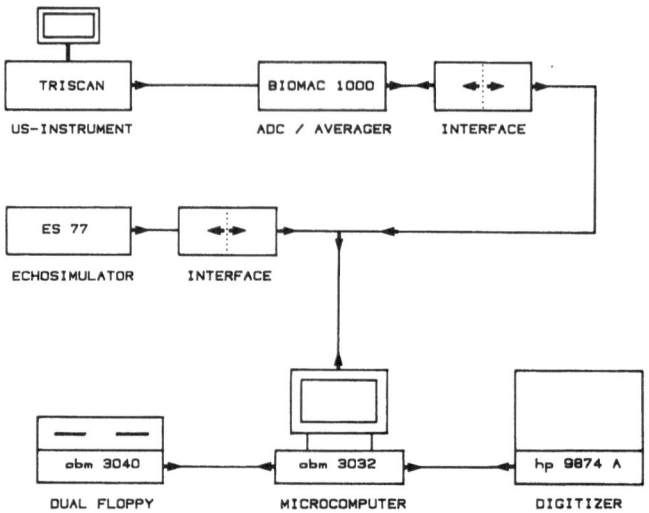

Fig. 1. Block diagram of clinical data acquisition system.

In the following results of clinical A-mode (video) analysis obtained on the basis of performance data shall be reported.

Materials and methods

Equipment

The system for clinical measurements is depicted in the block diagram of Fig. 1. An ECHOSIMULATOR (references in: Haigis and Buschmann, 1984) is interfaced to a personal computer system (COMMODORE) to be used in performance measurements. Clinical ultrasonic data are acquired by a TRISCAN working in the S-gain mode (A-display dynamic range: 34 dB). Different A-transducers nominally ranging from 8 to 10 MHz were applied. Further experimental details are listed in Table 2.

Every 20 msec the TRISCAN video signal was digitized by a BIOMAC 1000 AVERAGER. An interface developed in our laboratory served as a link to the computer (presently a COMMODORE C64 is adapted to the system).

1024 samples with an amplitude resolution of 7 bit represented a period of 80 μsec after the transmitter pulse, thus yielding a temporal resolution of 80 nsec. Sampling was performed over a time of 640–1280 msec. The resulting averaged echogram, therefore, includes the effect of 'spatial averaging' (Thijssen et al., 1981) during this time due to slight movements of the transducer and the sonified tissue.

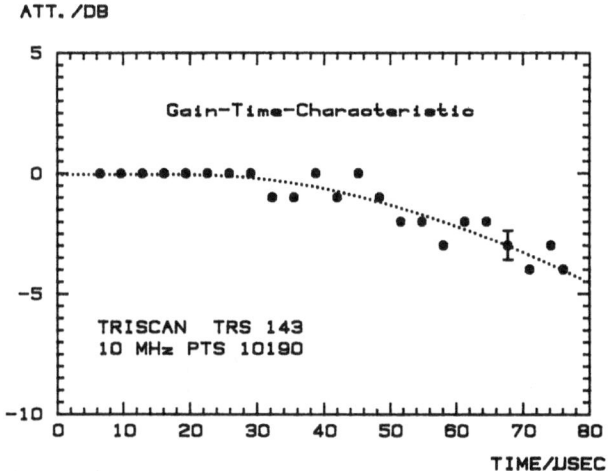

Fig. 2. Gain-Time characteristic for TRISCAN (S-gain mode) and 10 MHz transducer.

After averaging the digitized A-trace was transferred to floppy disk (5.25 '') for further off-line processing. With a record length of 1 kbyte a total of 167 traces may be stored on a single mini disk.

Presently, processing of the stored data consists of the following steps:
– display of data (256 × 220 pixels).
– cursor-controlled definition of region of interest.
– recalibration of signal amplitudes.
– regression line analysis under the assumption of an exponential decay of amplitudes from the region of interest.
– calculation of statistical signal parameters.

Data analysis

An important part of the processing program is the recalibration of the echo amplitudes in units of dB relative to the W38 (test reflector) reflectivity. This method has been described elsewhere (Haigis and Buschmann, 1984). The resulting amplitudes may then readily be related to the perfect reflector's reflectivity in an absolute manner. The recalibrated echo train, however, is still disturbed by the gain-time characteristic of the ultrasonic equipment. This characteristic reflects the influences of diffraction effects associated with the sound field as well as possible gain-time variations of the ultrasonic instrument itself. Fig. 2 shows a typical example of the resulting curve which was obtained by measuring the increase in system gain necessary to maintain constant signal amplitudes as a flat (W38) reflector is moved away from the transducer. The

190

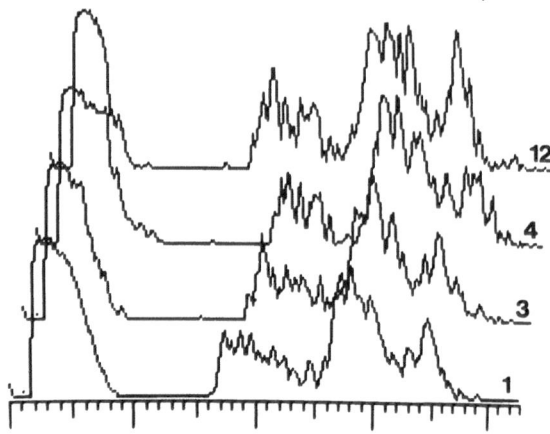

Fig. 3. Computer display of 4 digitized echograms from a tumour of the ciliary body. The echograms were taken from adjacent positions, each one representing the time-domain average of 64 single sweeps.

scatter in the data of Fig. 2 is mainly due to the resolution of the TRISCAN's gain control. After correction for this gain-time effect using curves like that of Fig. 2 the resulting echogram is then – to a certain degree of approximation – free from equipment characteristics. The recalibration procedure is illustrated in Figs. 3 and 4. Whereas Fig. 3 shows the computer display of four echograms

Table 1. Statistical tissue parameters.

Measure-ment No.	Tissue	Amplitudes/dB			Correl. Coeff./%	Att.Coeff. dB/μsec	Measured at Work. Frequ./MHz
		mean	min	max			
1 *)	orbital fat	-40 ± 1	-54	-19	70–91	-0.9 ± 0.2	8.2
2	orbital fat	-43	-50	-31	67	-1.3	8.2
3	orbital fat	-47	-58	-35	67	-0.9	9.8
4	orbital	-54	-65	-42	70	-1.2	9.6
	fat						
5	MM of ciliary body	-48 ± 2	-61	-33	44–81	-1.0 ± 0.3	8.2
6	intraocular MM	-58 ± 2	-75	-42	68–87	-2.1 ± 0.4	8.3

*) = aphakic eye.

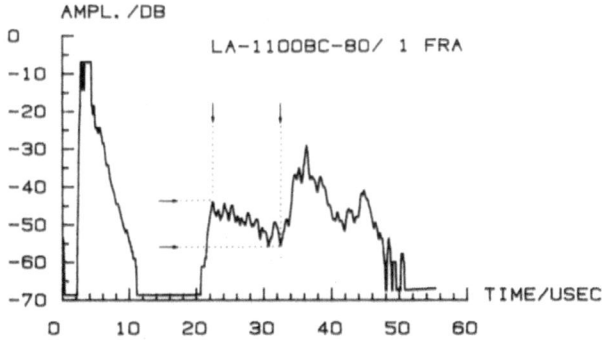

Fig. 4. Recalibrated tumour echogram (bottom trace of Fig. 3), arrows indicating region of interest and amplitude range for signal analysis.

with no processing other than averaging, Fig. 4 exhibits the bottom trace of Fig. 3 now calibrated in dB (relative W38) versus μsec and corrected for the gain-time dependence. So far, with the system described, we have examined three cases of normal orbital fat and one case of a malignant melanoma (MM) of the ciliary body.

Statistical results are compiled in Table 1 with experimental details given in Table 2.

For measurements nos. 3 and 6 digitizing was performed manually via a HEWLETT PACKARD hp 9874 A DIGITIZER (cf. Fig. 1). Furthermore, in these cases a SONOMETRICS OCUSCAN 400 and a KRETZTECHNIK 7200 MA served as diagnostic instruments.

The mean amplitude for measurement no. 1 is higher than for the other cases

Table 2. Experimental details for Table 1.

Measure-ment No.	No. of averaged echograms	US-Instrument type	frequency response	Transducer working frequency	data/MHz bandwidth	Digitized via
1	5 × 64	Triscan	broad	8.2	1.2	Interface
2	1 × 64	Triscan	broad	8.2	1.2	Interface
3	1 × 1	Ocuscan	broad	9.8	1.9	Digitizer
4	1 × 128	Triscan	broad	9.6	0.9	Interface
5	5 × 64	Triscan	broad	8.2	1.2	Interface
6	4 × 1	Kretz 7200 MA	narrow	8.3	3.0	Digitizer

192

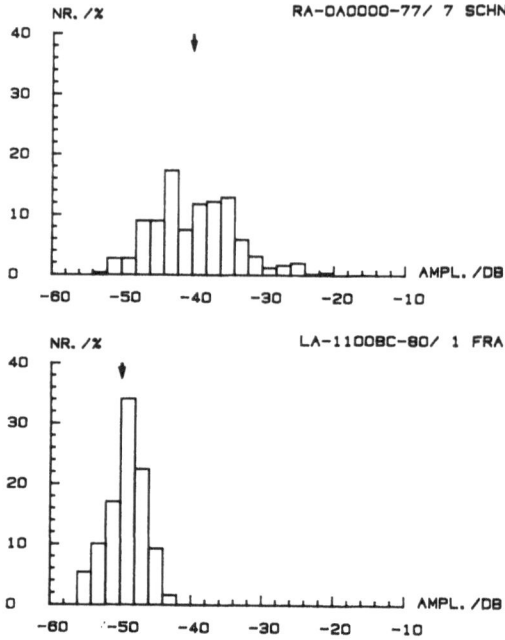

Fig. 5. Amplitude histograms of a normal orbit (top) and a malignant melanoma (MM) of the ciliary body (bottom). Arrows indicate mean amplitudes. Horizontal axes are scaled in dB relative to the W 38 reflectivity (Haigis and Buschmann, 1984).

of orbital fat. Since this eye has been the only aphakic one, there are no reflection losses due to the lens. For the attenuation in normal orbital fat, Thijssen et al. (1981) have measured a value of $\alpha = 1.47$ dB/mm, whereas Lizzi and Coleman (1977) report $\alpha = 1.5$ dB/(MHz · mm). With a velocity of sound of $v = 1.5$ mm/μsec and making allowance for the double time of flight as well as for the working frequencies of our transducers, these values become 1.10 dB/μsec (Thijssen et al.) and 0.92–1.10 dB/μsec (Lizzi and Coleman) for our cases.

It may be seen from Table 1 that there is a surprisingly good agreement between our results and these data, especially in the case of measurement no. 1, where averaging was performed over a total of 320 single echograms. With regard to measurement no. 3 it may be stressed that these results were obtained using a different digitizing technique as well as a different ultrasonic instrument (cf. Table 2).

Figure 5 shows amplitude histograms for a normal orbit (top, measurement no. 1) and a tumour (bottom, measurement no. 5). These histograms are not corrected for the attenuation as e.g. was done by Thijssen et al. (1981). At present, we are using the absolute position on the abscissa (means, indicated

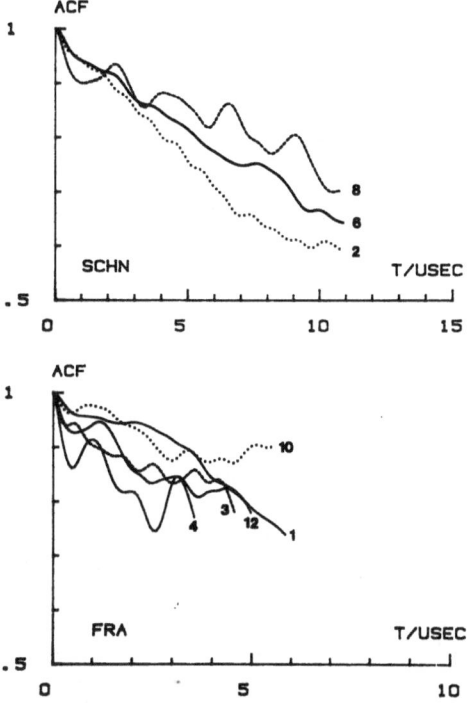

Fig. 6. Autocorrelation functions (ACF) of a normal orbit (top) and the tumour of Figs. 3 and 4 (bottom). Only the first half of the ACF coefficients are plotted, since the ACF becomes more and more unreliable as fewer points are included in the computation.

by arrows) and the spreading of the amplitude distributions as an estimate for the homogenity and isotropy of a tissue when comparing echgrams from different positions.

Just recently we started to study the use of the autocorrelation function (ACF) for tissue differentiation. The ACF is given by its coefficients (Joynt et al., 1980).

$$ACF(j) = \frac{A}{N-j} \sum_{i=1}^{N-j} f(i) \cdot f(i+j); \# j = 1 \ldots N-1$$

with N = number of samples f(i) of the digitized video signal f = f(t) (t: time).

Being the Fourier transform of the power spectrum of f(t), the ACF may be calculated either by a FFT- (Fast Fourier Transform) algorithm or – as was done here – rather straightforward by the above formula. Structure information like periodicities in the tissue is detected and enhanced in the autocorrelation function. In addition, as was pointed out by Gore et al. (1979), the ACF may prove useful to monitor temporal changes of echo patterns (e.g. response

194

to tumour treatment) with each tissue acting as its own reference.

Figure 6 shows calculated ACFs for a normal orbit (top) and the tumour of measurement no. 5 (bottom). Each curve represents an echogram from a slightly differing position. Since our database as well as our experience with this sort of analysis is yet too limited, we dare not draw quantitative conclusions out of Fig. 6. Attempting to interpret these results in terms of characteristic distances within the tissues, it seems that these are smaller in the tumour than in the orbital fat.

It should be worthwhile to continue studies on the possible value of the autocorrelation function for tissue characterization.

References

Gore JC, Leeman S, Metrewelli C, Plessner NJ, Willson K. 1979. Dynamic Autocorrelation Analysis of A-Scans in vivo. In: Ultrasonic Tissue Characterization II, M. Linzer, ed., NBS Spec. Publ. 525 (U.S. Government Printing Office, Washington, D.C.) p. 275.

Haigis W, Buschmann W. 1984. Performance Measurements and Quantitative Echography. In: Ophthalmic Ultrasonography, Proc of the 9th SIDUO Congress, Leeds, 1982. J.S. Hillman and M.M. Le May, eds., Doc Ophthal Proc Series, Vol. 38, Junk, Den Haag, p. 433.

Joynt L, Martin R, Macovski A. 1980. Techniques for in vivo Tissue Characterization. In: Acoustical Imaging, Vol. 8, A.F. Metherell, ed., Plenum Press, N.Y., p. 527.

Lizzi F, Coleman DJ. 1977. Ultrasonic Spectrum Analysis in Ophthalmology. In: Recent Advances in Ultrasound in Biomedicine, D.N. White, ed., Research Studies Press, Forest Grove, p. 117.

Thijssen JM (ed.). 1980. Ultrasonic Tissue Characterization, Stafleu's Scientific Publishing Company, Alphen aan den Rijn/Brussels.

Thijssen JM, Bayer AL, Cloosterman M. 1981. Computer-assisted Echography: Statistical Analysis of A-Mode Video Echograms obtained by Tissue Sampling. In: Med Biol Engng & Comp 19, p. 437.

The clinical application of the new versatile high-powered ophthalmic contact A-, B-Scan equipment

S. TANE, N. TAKAHASHI, J. SUZUKI and Y. KIMURA
Kawasaki, Japan

Summary

A versatile ultrasonic device has been developed for investigation of the structure of the human eye. The equipment consists of a hand-held probe head with a mechanical 40 degree sector scan of 10 MHz focused transducer, and an electronic display unit. In addition to the conventional A- and B-mode pictures, a three-dimensional D-mode can also be displayed in real time. The unit includes an interval caliper for accurate measurements of axial distances in all three modes. The ultrasound examination is carried out by means of the focused transducer with a 40 degree mechanical sector scan which is pressed either against the eyelid or directly against the sclera. The real-time display is obtained by either A-mode, B-mode or D-mode scanning. In clinical applications, both the resolution and the sensitivity of the device are good. A-mode scanning gives the greatest accuracy in amplitude measurement, while the B-mode and D-mode yield the most concrete topographic picture of the target.

In recent daily clinical practice, ophthalmic ultrasonic examination using the contact method instead of the immersion method has become more common, except in cases of detailed examination. This trend is based on the following advantages of the ophthalmic contact ultrasonic diagnostic apparatus: First, it allows simple and rapid manipulation; second, it is minimally influenced by the skill of the operator; third, it provides images of good reproducibility; fourth, it allows the real-time dynamic diagnostic display of intraocular tissue. However, it is still true that the contact method is inferior to the immersion method in terms of resolution and quality of fine images.

The probe is placed directly on the palpebra, to which Scopisol has been applied: B-mode, A-mode, vector A-mode, and D-mode images can be obtained by the contact method (Fig. 1). Polaroid photography is also possible using the foot-switch. The probe has a built-in, non-focused PZT-transducer (or zircon titanic lead-transducer) measuring 4 mm in diameter with a fre-

K.C. Ossoinig (editor), Ophthalmic Echography, ISBN 978-94-010-7988-4

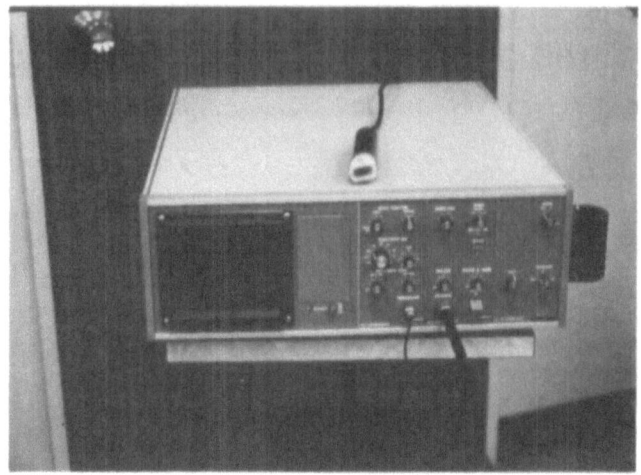

Fig. 1. The versatile new high-powered ophthalmic contact A- and B-scan equipment (Topscan).

quency of 10 MHz which allows sector scanning at 30 sweeps per second *(Table 1)*.

Vector A-mode imaging in particular is possible, as well as A-mode and B-mode imaging. The nickname of this equipment is 'Topscan'. This apparatus is very convenient in that the attached measuring instrument allows simple determination of the degree of artificial intraocular lenses (which have recently been used widely), and provides a digital display of the value. Of course, the anterior chamber depth, the anteroposterior diameter of the lens (or lens thickness), and total axial length can also be determined. Several dozen patients with intraocular and orbital diseases were actually diagnosed using this apparatus.

Presented first are the B-mode, vector A-mode, and D-mode images of the

Table 1. Specifications of the equipment.

Specifications
1) A-scan, B-scan, Vector A-scan, D-scan
2) Contact method
3) 10 MHz, 4 mmØ, non-focused transducer
4) Mechanical sector scan (40°), 30 frames/sec, Scanning lines → 110 lines/scan
5) Attenuator: +6~−60 dB
6) I.O.L. power calculation
7) Weight: 23 kg

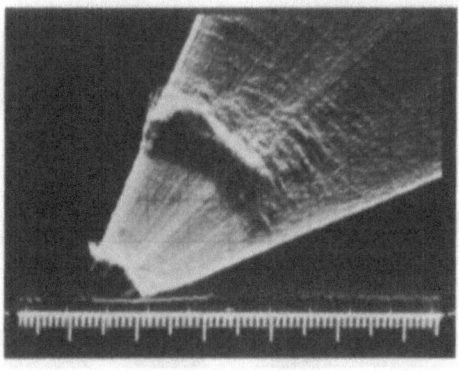

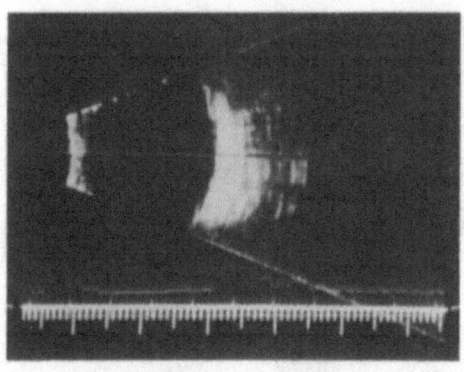

Fig. 2. B- and D-scan ultrasonogram of normal eye.

normal eyes of a 20-year-old man. Because the vitreous is normal, there are no abnormal intraocular echoes. D-mode imaging illustrates a wall-like rise that represents the posterior wall (Fig. 2). The range and angle of D-mode imaging are freely adjustable.

Figure 3 shows a display of retinal detachment in a 46-year-old woman. The upper left part shows detachment echoes imaged by B-mode; the lower left is a B-mode image of the same eyes obtained for comparison by a Bronson-Turner Ophthalmic B-scan system. The upper right is a D-mode image obtained by Topscan, and the lower right is a B-mode ultrasonogram obtained by the immersion method using a St. Marianna high-resolution ophthalmic ultrasonic diagnostic apparatus.

Figure 4 shows the presence of a retinal detachment in a mass vitreous hemorrhage of an 81-year-old man. A D-mode image of retinal detachment echoes is expressed as an A-mode image overlapped with a B-mode image.

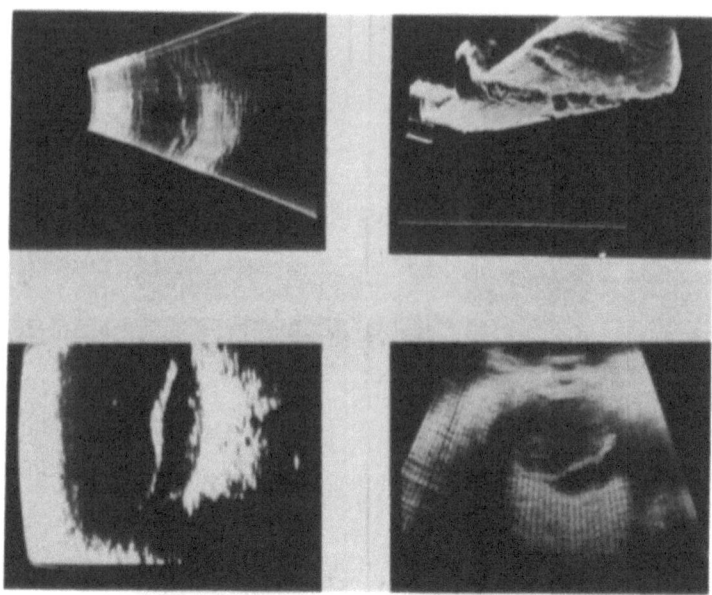

Fig. 3. B-scan and D-scan ultrasonogram of a case of retinal detachment.

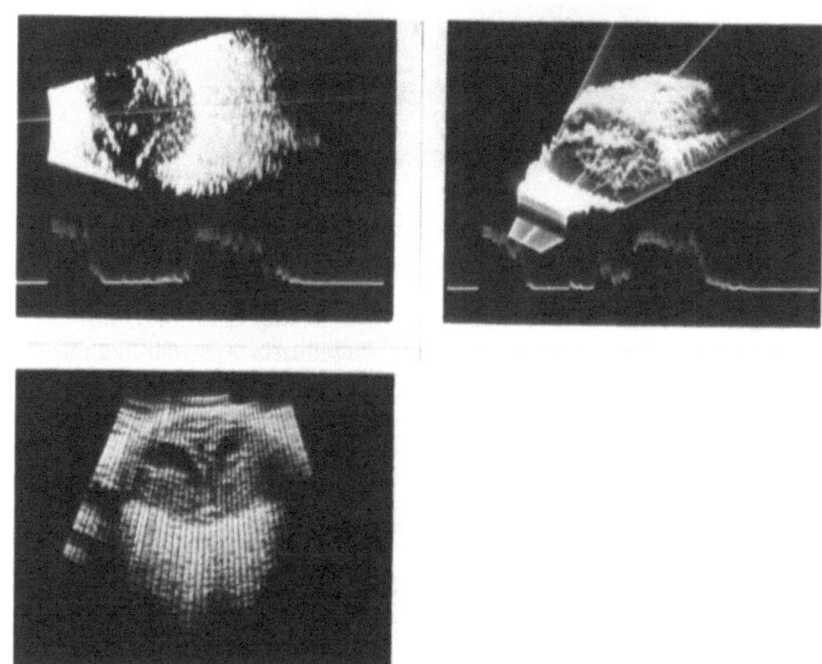

Fig. 4. B-scan and D-scan ultrasonogram of a retinal detachment with massive vitreous hemorrhage (upper left: contact B-scan, upper right: contact D-scan, lower left: immersion B-scan).

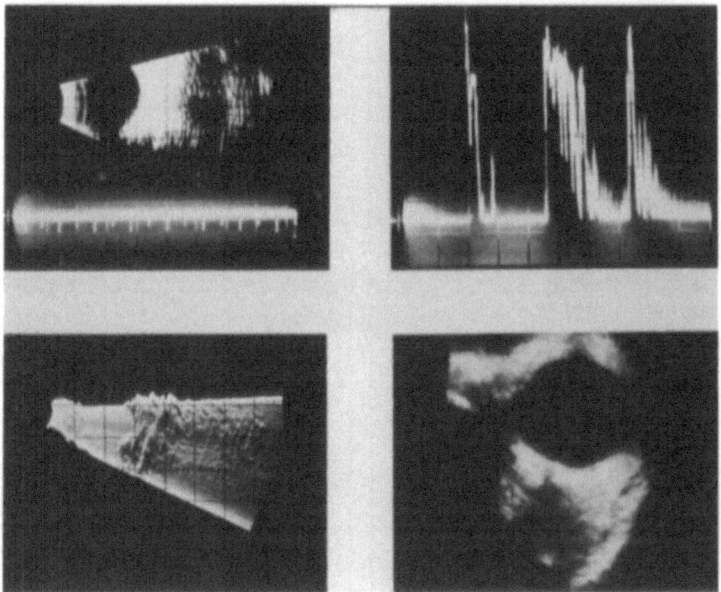

Fig. 5. A-scan, B-scan and D-scan ultrasonogram of a case of orbital meningioma.

Ascertaining the presence of retinal detachment is easy because a pattern markedly higher than the rising of vitreous hemorrhage echoes is shown.

Figure 5 shows an image obtained from a 72-year-old woman with orbital disease. B-mode, A-mode and D-mode images of intraorbital meningioma obtained by Topscan, and an immersion-method B-mode image obtained by the St. Marianna apparatus are shown.

Thus, it can be said that Topscan is a high quality clinical apparatus, and we think that it is effective and reliable for use in daily ophthalmologic practice.

Possibility of ocular tissue differentiation by means of false-color assisted echography

A. REIBALDI, T. AVITABILE, S. GUERRIERO and M.G. UVA
Bari, Italy

Introduction

The Eye Clinic of the Bari University and the Signal and Image Processing Institute (I.E.S.I.) of C.N.R. in the framework of the 'Progetto Finalizzato Tecnologie Biomediche' of C.N.R. are carrying out research on diagnostic methodologies of eye echography through the introduction of digital image processing. This is being done in order to develop techniques capable of extracting the maximum amount of information possible from echo patterns.

Preliminary results obtained in this effort are reported in this paper. The images have been analyzed using false color techniques on a B-scan whose normal output can be visualized in gray levels.

Materials and methods

In preliminary tests on the applicability of false color digital techniques in the diagnostic echography of eye pathology it was decided to use the equipment available both at the Eye Clinic and at the I.E.S.I. in order to find out new instrumental solutions through specific clinical experiments.

The device used was the Storz Echograph Renaissance A/B scan together with an ultrasonic electronic scanning probe characterized by the capacity to memorize single digital mode images in the internal memory of the Z-80 microprocessor. The image is stored in a 256×560 pixels format, and codified at 64 gray levels. This equipment can also store image sequences by means of a videorecorder.

A certain number of interesting clinical cases were selected, and for each of them an adequate number of image sequences containing the maximum information for a B-scan diagnosis were recorded. The most interesting images were first stored in the Tesak VDC-501 graphic/pictorial bi-dimensional memory in digital form, and then transferred to a Vax 11/780-PDP11/45 pro-

K.C. Ossoinig (editor), Ophthalmic Echography, ISBN 978-94-010-7988-4

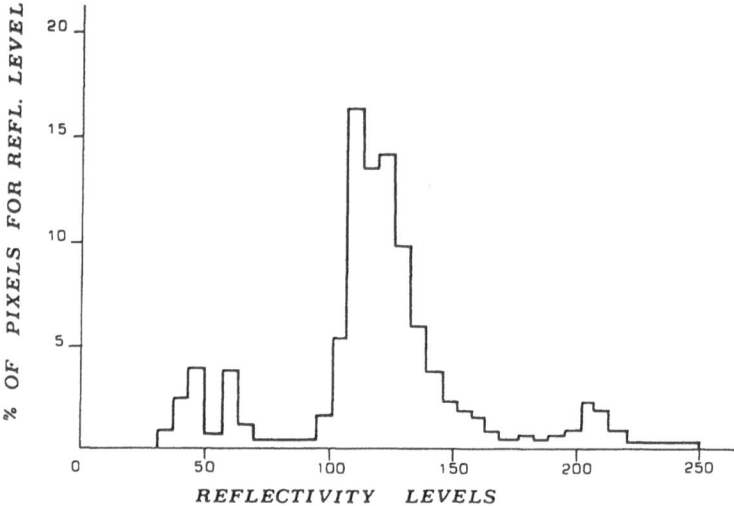

Fig. 1. Histogram presentation of gray level frequency distribution.

cessing system disc specializing in the treatment of images and signals.

Thanks to the videocassette recordings the acquisition took place at the Eye Clinic, while the analysis was carried out on the digital images processing system at the I.E.S.I. using the following interactive procedures:

1. Display of the recorded sequences on the TV screen, both in gray levels and in false color, applying standard transposition scales.
2. Selection of particular images of the sequence and storage in digital form. This is achieved by sending the analog signals from the videorecorder to a fast converter which samples and translates the analog levels into numbers from 0 to 255. Each number corresponds to the gray level of a picture element (pixel).
3. Histogram presentation of gray level frequency distribution. Individuation of maximum and minimum reflectivity of the tissues under analysis can be achieved by selecting the corresponding values on the frequency distribution. Moreover, the subdivisions of the histogram in steps of properly chosen amplitudes allows the determination of equally spaced subintervals related either to the tissue reflectivity or to the pixels number. The operator can assign the limits of each interval using an interactive procedure.
4. Attribution to the pixels of a definite color belonging to a specific reflectivity range. The system allows the subdivision of the interval between the minimum and the maximum reflectivity values into a 256 color scale, and also represents each pixel with the color corresponding to its interval reflectivity. Each color is selected through the interactive specification of its chromatic coordinates (red, green, blue) with values ranging from 0 to 255.

5. As an alternative, it is possible to attribute a color interval to each reflectivity interval, specifying first the extreme values of reflectivity and then the two extreme colors by means of the respective chromatic coordinates. A linear interpolation procedure translates the reflectivity values into different colors; in this way shaded scales of false colors are obtained.
6. Storage of the selected color scales. Additional color scales can be used alternatively on the same image to improve and facilitate the echographic interpretation.
7. Display on a color screen of the complete videorecorded sequences in order to verify a) the validity of the conversion scale chosen; b) the stability of reflectivity values of the internal eye structures, both for images of the same eye in various echograms and for corresponding eye structures of different patients.

Results

The distribution of the gray levels in digital echographic images is shown in Fig. 1. By presenting the points corresponding to each chosen interval of the reflectivity values (density slicing), the following connections can be detected (average results):
1. From level 0 to level 26: artifacts due to the external image contours.
2. From level 27 to level 110: normal vitreous and image background.
3. From level 111 to level 180: vitreous disorganization.
4. From level 181 to level 200: vitreous membranes.
5. From level 201 to level 210: retina and retrobulbar structures.
6. From level 211 to level 255: artifacts due to the external image contours.
The color scales were singled out according to their efficiency in discriminating the reflectivity levels relevant to the diagnosis of the eyes' pathological situation; when a definitive diagnosis could not be made on the basis of the echogram it was shown in black and white (Figs. 2, 3, 4 and 5).

In order to produce shaded scales for each interval, the extreme colors have been specified together with their chromatic coordinates. Following this procedure the video recordings of 1,211 patients were analyzed (Table 1). For these cases the intra-vitreal structures could not be easily classified as retina, membrane or vitreous disorganization using the standard gray level technique.

The visualization in false color helped us to establish the presence of a real difference in reflectivity among the parts because they appeared in different colors; in particular it was possible to determine the presence of the retina detachment by virtue of a higher reflectivity. Such attributes were confirmed during the surgical operation which followed the echographic examination.

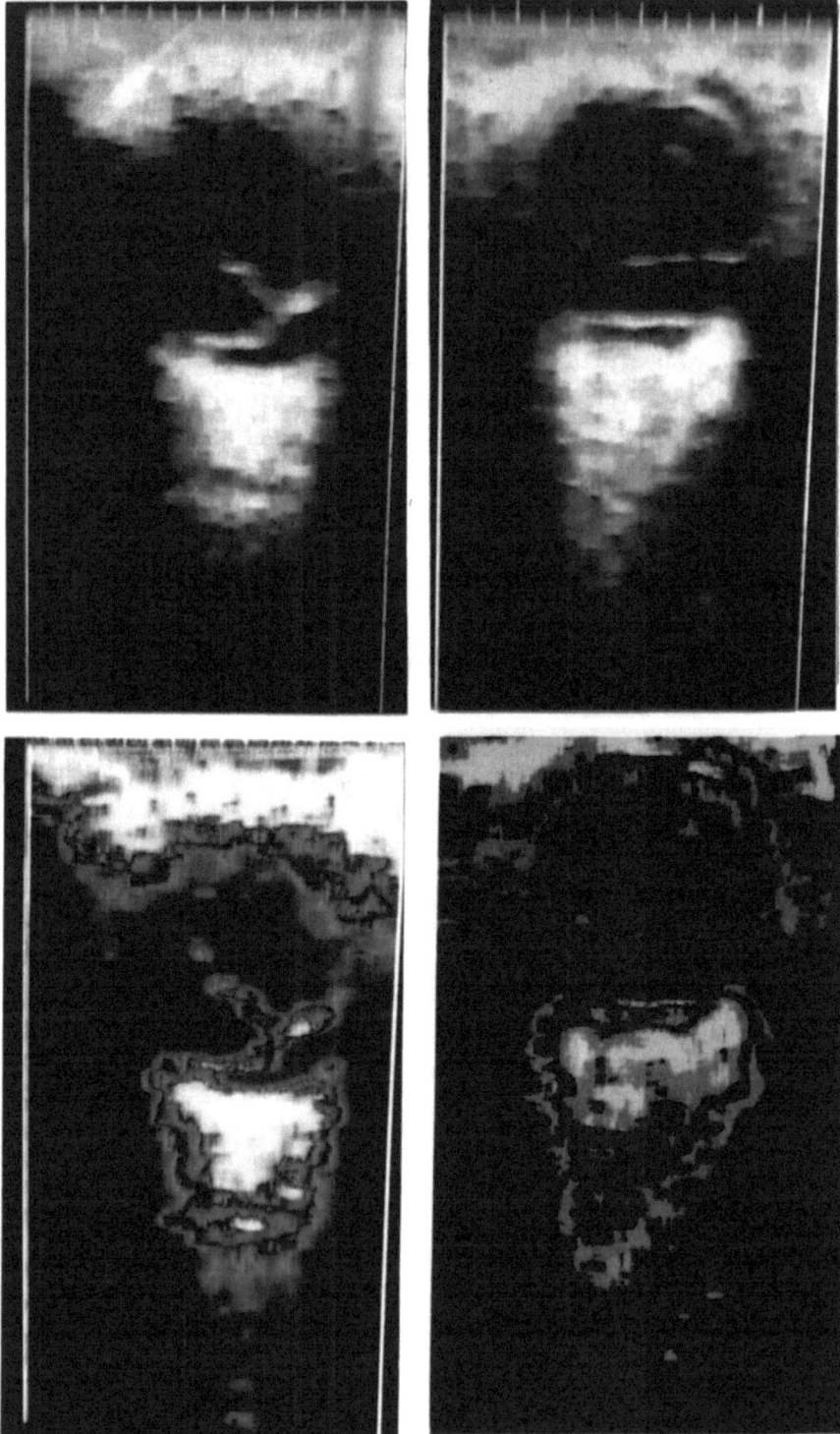

Fig. 2. (Reibaldi and associates). A typical case of two membranes that, in the gray level image, are apparently indistinguishable from each other.

Fig. 3. (Reibaldi and associates). The same image of Fig. 2 processed in false colors allows the differentiation of the two structures which appear in different colors, allowing immediate perception of the different reflectivity levels existing between them: a vitreous membrane (the first one), a retinal detachment (the second one).

Fig. 4. (Reibaldi and associates). An analogous case in which the gray scale is not discriminating between the structures present in the vitreous.

Fig. 5. (Reibaldi and associates). The same case of Fig. 4 shown in false colors where the difference in reflectivity between the retinal detachment and the vitreous membrane (which exerts a traction on the retina itself) is visible.

Conclusions

The results obtained in this first phase of the research program seem to confirm the remarkable diagnostic potential of eye echography if integrated with digital techniques. In fact, combinations of the two technologies favor the extraction of the maximum amount of information from normal and pathological tissue echography.

The simple technique of density slicing also seems to be promising in regard to current diagnostic tools. Moreover, the flexibility and interactive capacity of the digital system allows a dynamic choice of color scales for the presenta-

Table 1. Case report.

– normal eyes	n.	430
– vitreous floaters	n.	210
– vitreous membranes	n.	124
– vitreous hemorrhage	n.	71
– posterior vitreous detachment	n.	112
– persistent hyaloid system	n.	5
– persistent primary vitreous	n.	2
– retinal detachment	n.	156
– choroidal detachment	n.	9
– choroidal hematoma	n.	2
– choroidal malignant melanoma	n.	12
– metastatic carcinoma	n.	3
– luxation of lens	n.	5
– endobulbar foreign bodies	n.	60
– orbital tumors	n.	10
Total	n.	1211

tion of the reflectivity levels. This fully utilizes the amazing capacity of the human eye.

This is only the beginning of the information we are striving to obtain from computer-assisted echography. In fact at present, after having singled out the point of study, we have applied various mathematical operations (Standard deviation, variable analysis, etc.) to increase the information about the tissue texture analysis, represented in false colors, so that these results are easily intelligible. With these methods of texture analysis we are already getting the first results; these are not, however, definitive, and we will therefore be further expanding upon them in the future.

Summary

According to our evaluations, the A-scan ophthalmic echography gives information about tissue reflectivity, while the B-scan relays information regarding topography. Even in a bi-dimensional image (especially obtained by new equipment with many gray levels), all the information is contained regarding the reflectivity of the tissue even if it cannot be easily visualized by the human eye. The authors, using bi-dimensional images obtained by equipment with a good gray scale, sent the images to a computer where they were changed first to digital form, and then into colors. Different colors corresponded to different gray levels not easily differentiated by the human eye.

References

Baum G, Greenwood I. 1958. The application of ultrasonic locating techniques to ophthalmology: II Ultrasonic slit lamp in the ultrasonic visualization of soft tissues. Arch Ophthalmol 60: 263–279.

Baum G. 1972. Quantized ultrasonography. Ultrasonics 10: 14–15.

Cardia L, Reibaldi A, Avitabile T, Guerriero S, Veneziani N, Distante A. 1984. First results about echographical ocular tissue characterization by false colors. Poster VII Cong. European Society of Ophthal Helsinki, May.

Coleman DJ, Katz L. 1974. Color coding of B-scan ultrasonograms. Arch Ophthalmol 91: 429–431.

Coleman DJ, Lizzi FL, Jack RL. 1977. Ultrasonography of the eye and orbit. Lea & Febiger, Philadelphia.

Purnell E. 1966. Ultrasound in ophthalmological diagnosis, in Grossman C, et al. (eds): Diagnostic Ultrasound. pp. 95–109, Plenum Press, New York.

Reibaldi A, Avitabile T, Guerriero S, Distante A, Veneziani N. 1983. Primi risultati sulla possibilita'di differenziazione ecografica tissutale mediante falso colore. Comun. 8, Cong. S.I.S.U.M., Bologna, 13–15 Nov.

Three-dimensional display of the ocular region. Improvement of scanning method

Y. YAMAMOTO, Y. SUGATA, M. TOMITA and M. ITOH
Tokyo, Japan

Abstract

A new system was developed to display in three-dimensional fashion the interior of the eyeball and to calculate the volume of an intraocular mass. In this system, sampling of echowaves is performed by a spirally scanning transducer covering the area from the central axis to the periphery of the eyeball. Using this system, scanning of the entire eye can be completed within four minutes compared with the former method of piling up cross-sectional layers. Echo waves were digitized to 256 grades and were stored on a floppy disk with the space positions noted. This rapid sampling is advantageous since it minimizes spacial displacement, which is the major cause of decreased sharpness of three-dimensional displays on CRT and of errors in measuring volumes of intraocular space or mass. To display a three-dimensional view of the desired intraocular surface from a given direction on CRT, brighter color is given to the layers closer to the surface and each layer is intensity-graded using a black and white system. To measure volume, an image-processing method of smoothing and a Laplacian process were applied to the surface with the aid of a microcomputer, and the inner pixels of the closed space were counted. This three-dimensional mode of display provides an overview of the shape and the extent to which the tissues of interest are involved. It is also especially helpful in cases with opacification of the ocular media.

Introduction

The shape and the extension of the tissues of an eye with opaque mdia are mentally reconstructed by the echographer during the examination. The three-dimensional (3-D) display is intended to directly visualize the ocular structure of interest [1, 5]. The image-processing method enables us to provide the view from the direction which is inaccessible by an ophthalmoscope, as

K.C. Ossoinig (editor), Ophthalmic Echography, ISBN 978-94-010-7988-4

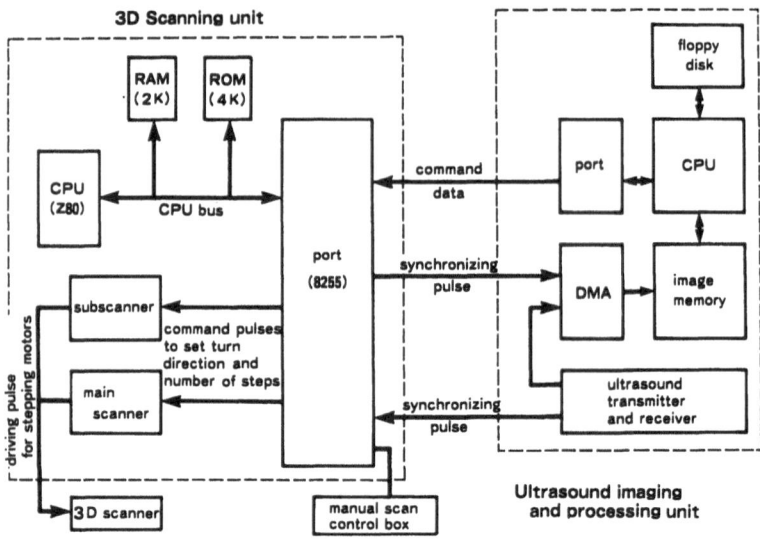

Fig. 1. Block diagram of the scanning unit, and the imaging and processing unit.

well as to determine the volume measurement of a closed surface of interest [4]. Rapid and homogeneous sampling is the key to the practical use of this method. A major improvement for the 3-D mode of display is the scanning method which is performed spirally in contrast to repeated sector scanning.

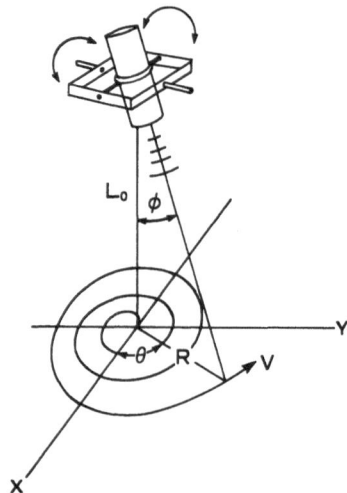

Fig. 2. Scheme for the spiral scanning.

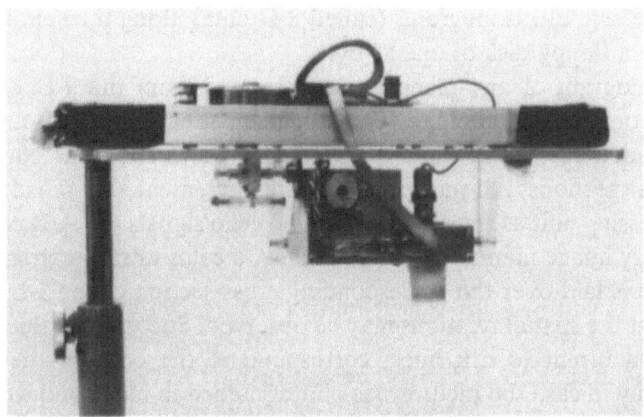

Fig. 3. Scanning unit.

System

An apparatus used for sampling is the ultrasonograph ZD-252 made by General Co. [3] with a concave polyvinylidene fluoride transducer (10 MHz, 10 mm in diameter and focused to 44 mm). For the purpose of the present study, the image-processing unit and 3-D scanning unit are connected to the ultrasonograph. In order to obtain 3-D information of tissues from the ultrasound echo signals, the spacial distribution of echo data should be as uniformly dense as possible. We developed a programmable 3-D scanning unit which drives a probe in several modes; among them is a spiral scan method suitable for the construction of 3-D images and ultrasonograms of any sectional plane. It also provides a volume scan consisting of successive plane sector scans, which can be used for the fast display of 3-D images. The block diagram of the unit is shown in Fig. 1. Two stepping motors are controlled by CPU. The principle of spiral scanning is shown in Fig. 2. The angular velocity is inversely proportional to diameter R, so that the revolution velocity V stays at a constant level. Figure 3 shows the profile of the scanning unit.

The spiral scanning method has the following advantages:
1. The distance between the adjacent lines of a spiral locus can be set at any distance. This distance varies according to the depth. The minimum angle is 50/128 = 0.2 degrees/step.
2. Since the velocity V is constant, the interval of ultrasound beams can be adjusted, and because of this:
3. We can vary the spacial sampling density of scanning lines.
4. The uniformity of scanning density yields uniform 3-D tissue information, preventing the loss of data by not scanning all areas.

5. The successive ultrasonograms (called 3-D data) along the spiral line are stored on a floppy disk of one M-byte.

The ultrasonogram of any plane is reconstructed from the 3-D data by a coordinate conversion technique. The 3-D image is constructed from a set of intensity-graded black and white plane images which show the contours of specific tissue sections. All such processes are implemented in the ultrasound image-processing unit as shown in Fig. 1. The echo signals are A/D converted for temporary image memory storage. Finally, a color ultrasonogram using a special scale is laid over the corresponding cross-section of the 3-D contour image so that the spatial relations may be observed. Successive value changes ranging from bright to drk hues, correspond to the color-gradient scale, including gray in case the picture was photographed in black and white [2].

Results

The posterior half of the 3-D display of a dislocated lens was compared with a usual B-mode image (Fig. 4). To give a 3-D view, 128 layers of spiral echo waves were collected sectorially and reconstructed (Fig. 5). Five layers of reconstruction gives a rough image of a lens (Fig. 6), and the whole eye region done by using 12 layers gives an image of an eyelid and eyelashes (Fig. 7). A case of choroidal detachment following glaucoma surgery was displayed by the usual B-mode using the new color grading scale (Fig. 8). A 3-D display of 128 layers of the posterior half gives a picture of a concave detached choroid (Fig. 9). Sector scans are also reconstructed by the image-processing unit (Fig. 10).

The most promising characteristic of the present method is that the desired section profile can be displayed in combination with a 3-D view of the desired structure. The section profile was drawn by the same color gradient scale as that used in the B-mode image (Fig. 11). A one-minute drive of the transducer near the central axis of the eye creates an image the approximate size of a lens (Figs. 12 and 13). To cover an area 0.9 cm in diameter at a depth of 5 cm, a 72-second drive is actually required that is corresponds to 8 out of 29 frames per disk. The transducer is intermittently driven every 9 seconds because of the limitation of the frame memory. The closed area surrounded by an extracted contour line (Fig. 14) was piled up to create a mass (Fig. 15). Trial calculations of the volume of a lens gave similar values of 0.328, 0.357 and 0.333 cm^3 by using three different section profiles: vertical, horizontal and coronal, respectively.

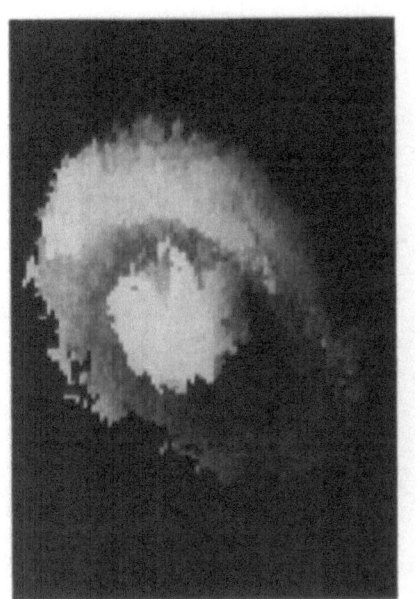

Fig. 5. Three-dimensional display of the dislocated lens.

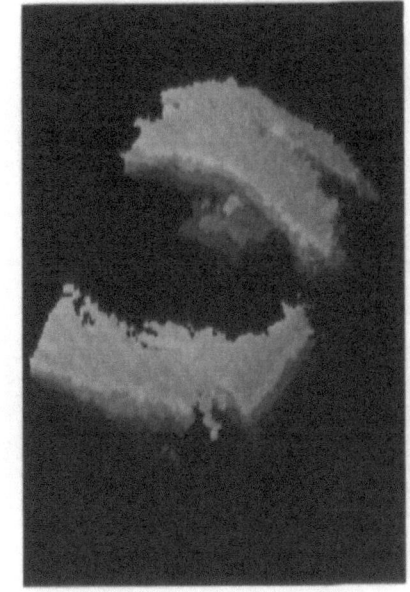

Fig. 7. Reconstruction of the image of the dislocated lens in 12 layers.

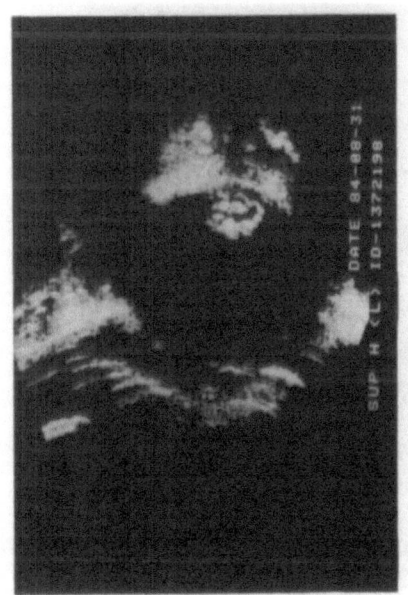

Fig. 4. B-mode image of a dislocated lens.

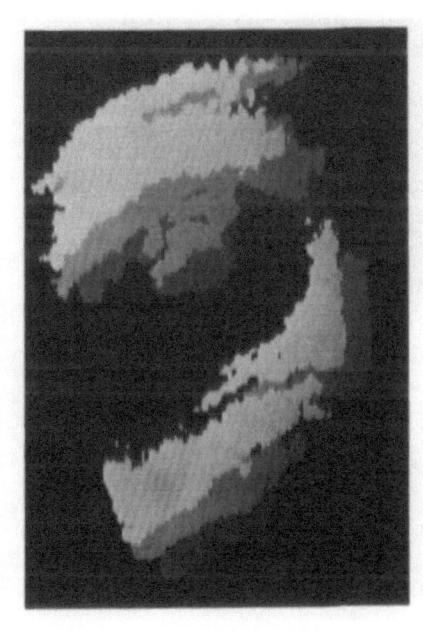

Fig. 6. Reconstruction of the image of the dislocated lens in 5 layers.

212

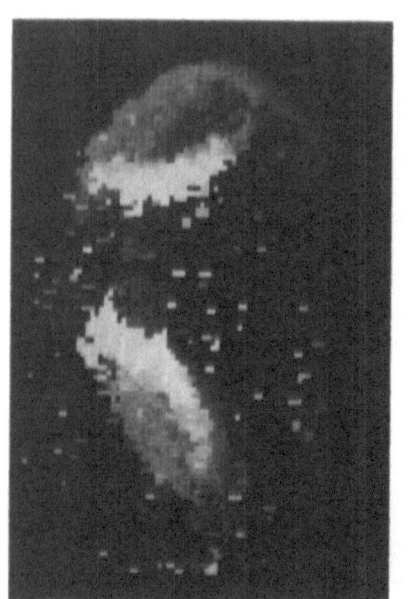

Fig. 9. Three-dimensional display of the detached choroid.

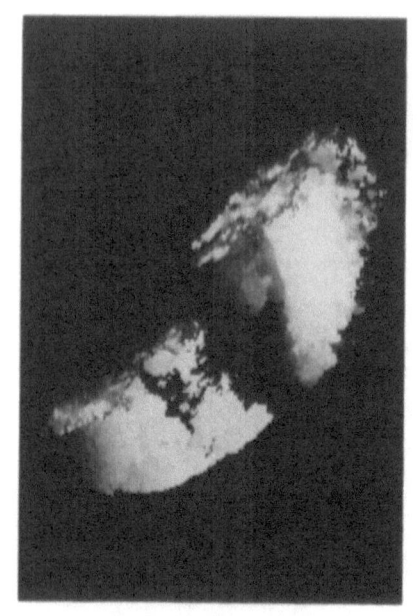

Fig. 11. Three-dimensional display of the dislocated lens with a cross section.

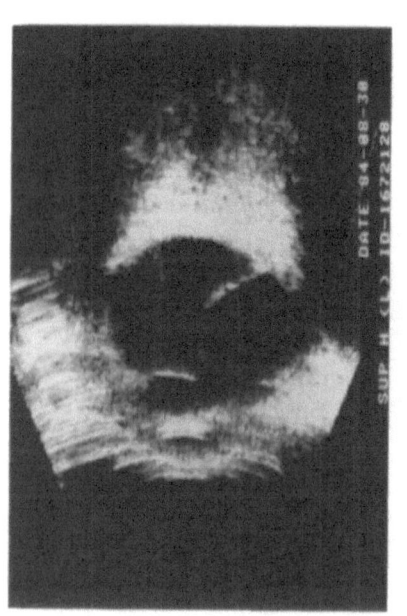

Fig. 8. B-mode image of the detached choroid.

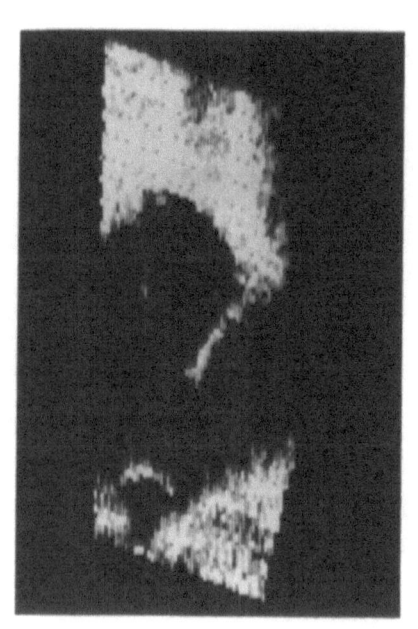

Fig. 10. Sector-sector display of detached choroid.

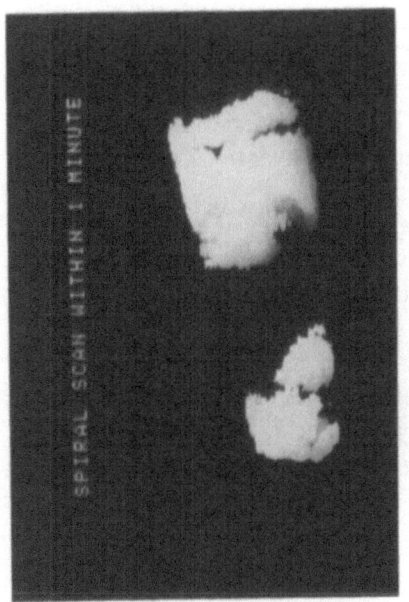

Fig. 13. A side view of the three-dimensional display of first 8 frames.

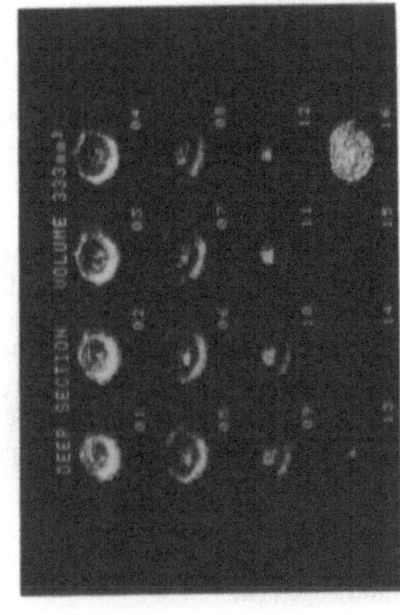

Fig. 15. Cross sections before applying contour line extraction for calculating the volume of a lens.

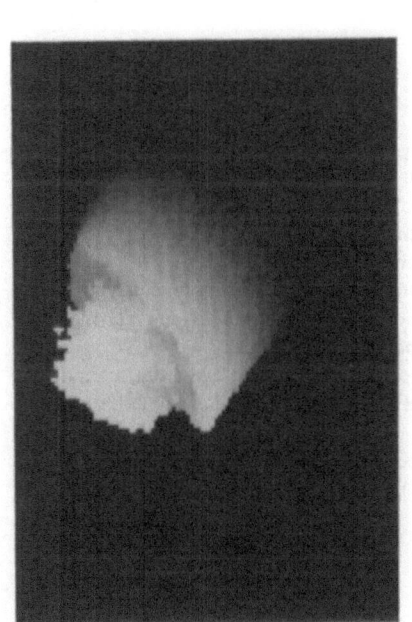

Fig. 12. Three-dimensional display of a lens using first 8 frames out of 29 frames.

Fig. 14. A closed area surrounded by an extracted contour line.

214

Discussion

Sampling of echo waves is performed by a spirally scanning transducer from the central axis to the periphery of the globe. This was formerly done by piling up cross-sectional layers, a time-consuming method which often took over 30 minutes to store information from one eye on the magnetic tape. Ocular movements during sampling cause displacements from layer to layer, and this increased the chance for error when measuring volumes.

It takes only 4 minutes to complete one eye using the new method. This is tolerable for the patient and the shorter time will be sufficient to memorize a major part of the ocular region, if the desired structure is restricted to a smaller area (Fig. 12). Another characteristic of the system is taking view from the desired direction and combining it with a cross-section of a mass with the color grade corresponding to the strength of the echo waves (Fig. 11). It will be possible to minimize the examination time by introducing a hard disk or an image memory with a large capacity. This may lead to an almost real-time 3-D display of intraocular structures.

Acknowledgement

The authors express greatly their thanks to Mr. Satoshi Miki for his fine technical assistance.

References

1. Hirano S, Yamamoto Y, Sugata Y, et al. 1982. Image treatment in the eye in ultrasound diagnosis and clinical significance. X. Contour line extraction and three-dimensional display. Jpn J Clin Ophthalmol 36: 475–480.
2. Hirano S, Sugata Y, Tomita M, et al. 1983. Image treatment in the eye in ultrasound diagnosis and clinical significance. XIII. Color gradient scale. Jpn J Clin Ophthalmol 37: 830–831.
3. Sugata Y, Hirano S, Tomita M, et al. 1982. Image treatment in the eye in ultrasound diagnosis and cliical significance. XI. Improvements of images on cathode ray tube by new polymer transducer and new color grading. Acta Soc Ophthalmol Jpn 86: 1004–1011.
4. Yamamoto Y, Hirano S, Sugata Y, et al. 1983. Image treatment in the eye in ultrasound diagnosis and clinical significance. XIV. Measurements of vitreous volume. Folia Ophthalmol Jpn 34: 2473–2477.
5. Yamamoto Y, Hirano S, Sugata Y, et al. 1983. Microcomputer aided imaging techniques in ophthalmic B-mode. In Ophthalmic Ultrasonography pp. 467–477 (eds Hillman JS and May MM, Dr W Junk Publishers, The Hague).

Clinical artifacts in real-time examinations

A.L. SUSAL
Stanford, USA

Introduction

Ultrasonic evaluation of the eye gives an accurate representation of the tissues and structures under observation. There are several artifacts which can occur in ultrasonic examinations, however, which tend to confuse the clinical picture and may lead to an erroneous diagnosis. Real-time ultrasonic studies may produce a disturbing number of image artifacts which confound the clinical picture. Multiple-element transducers can produce their own artifacts which add to the confusion. By recognizing these artifacts and understanding the mechanism of their production, the sonographer can avoid mistakes and use ultrasonic equipment more effectively at its higher sensitivity levels. This paper will discuss those artifacts frequently encountered in real-time clinical ultrasonic examinations, particularly artifacts which may be related to multiple array transducers and higher ultrasonic sensitivity. An exhaustive discussion of all ophthalmic ultrasonic artifacts is beyond the scope of this communication.

Physics and clinical examples of artifacts

The major ultrasonic artifacts encountered in real-time clinical examinations are due to:

I   Reduplication artifacts
II Transducer artifacts
    1. Grating lobe source
    2. Side lobe source
III Equipment noise artifacts
IV Standard artifacts
    1. Shadowing

K.C. Ossoinig (editor), Ophthalmic Echography, ISBN 978-94-010-7988-4

216

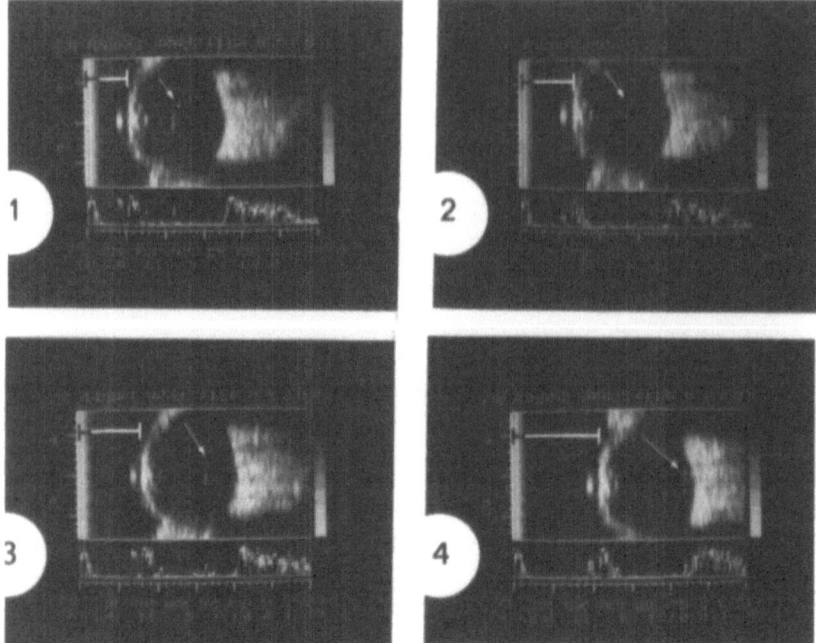

Fig. 1. Reduplication Echoes. The distance between the transducer and the highly reflecting iris surface is marked by a measure in these photos. As this distance progressively increases, the reduplicated iris echo (arrow) is progressively shifted deeper in the eye region.

2. Reflection, refraction
3. Ringdown

Reduplication artifacts

The reduplication artifact is an erroneous echo complex which can appear either within the eye or the orbit [1, 2, 3]. Reduplication artifacts are caused by double reflection of the ultrasonic tissue echoes with the second reflection usually occurring at the transducer surface. (Echo reflection between tissues rarely cause such artifacts).

The reduplication artifact usually involves a secondary corneal/iris/anterior lens complex of echoes that are erroneously displaced on the display behind their normal orientation (Fig. 1). They are produced when large echo signals (from these tissues) returning to the transducer are reflected at the transducer face (acting as a mirror) and return to the eye as a secondary ultrasonic wave. This secondary wave is again partially reflected at the highly reflecting tissue interface and returns to the detecting transducer to produce a second set of ultrasonic echoes on the display tube. Due to the reflection of the original pulse wave from tissue to transducer surface, back to the tissue interface and finally back to the transduer (acting as a detector) a double acoustic path length is created which causes the reduplication echo to appear on the screen at twice its normal distance from the transducer.

Reduplication echoes can appear with either contact or immersion scanning. With immersion scanning the transducer to tissue distances are usually more easily recognized and the reduplication artifact is displaced deeper in the eye image.

Reduplication echoes are easily recognized in real-time ultrasonic studies by observing the display as the transducer is pressed closer to the highly reflecting tissue interfaces. By shortening the distance between transducer and tissue reflector by a factor of one (IX) the reduplication echoes are shifted forward by a factor of two (2×) due to the double path length with these artifacts. Thus the artifacts are recognized on the display to move twice as fast toward the transducer as the regular ultrasonic image moves. Real-time examinations enable the sonographer to eliminate most reduplication echoes by tilting the transducer face to the side, tilting the reduplication echoes off to a position outside the field of the detecting transducer.

Transducer artifacts

Muliple element ultrasonic transducers produce artifacts which are unique to real-time electronically scanned imaging systems [4, 5, 6, 7]. These artifacts are mainly due to grating lobe and side lobe ultrasonic signals which are generated at the transducer at the same time the main ultrasonic pulse is produced.

Grating lobes

Ultrasonic transducers deform while producing ultrasonic waves – mainly oscillating in an axial direction to produce the main ultrasonic wave, but also becoming fatter and thinner (Fig. 2) to produce secondary ultrasonic waves that tend to travel out along the face of the transducer [8, 9]. In a multiple element transducer having a spacing pattern of approximately one wavelength between ultrasonic elements, the secondary ultrasonic waves tend to add to one another to produce a side oriented wave (a grating lobe) which almost parallels the face of the transducer (Fig. 3).

Grating lobes produce ultrasonic pulses which are strongest in the direction of the multiple element array. When these grating lobes are echoed from a strong reflecting surface (such as a wire speculum), they return to their originating transducer elements with a time delay that is equivalent to the linear distance between the element and the reflector. This produces a grating

218

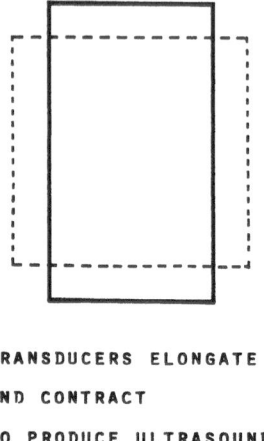

TRANSDUCERS ELONGATE

AND CONTRACT

TO PRODUCE ULTRASOUND

Fig. 2. Grating lobe production. The elongation and contraction of ultrasonic transducers in a direction perpendicular to the main axial movement of the transducer will produce side oriented ultrasonic waves.

lobe artifact (Fig. 4) which is a low amplitude line which extends approximately 45 degrees from the transducer surface and seems to emanate from the high reflector (Figs. 5 and 6).

A secondary ultrasonic echo produced perpendicular to the long axis of a transducer array will travel in a plane almost parallel to the transducer surface. This secondary ultrasonic wave can be reflected from a strong acoustic inter-

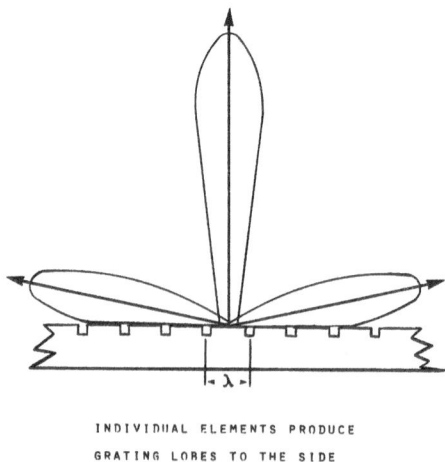

INDIVIDUAL ELEMENTS PRODUCE
GRATING LOBES TO THE SIDE

Fig. 3. Grating lobe artifacts. Ultrasonic energy generated from an oscillating transducer produces side traveling waves which tend to be additive with one wavelength spacing between transducer elements.

219

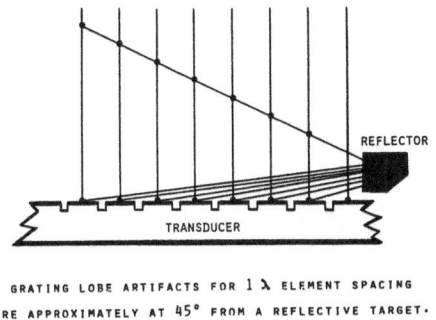

GRATING LOBE ARTIFACTS FOR 1 λ ELEMENT SPACING
ARE APPROXIMATELY AT 45° FROM A REFLECTIVE TARGET·

Fig. 4. Schematic diagram – Grating lobe artifacts. Grating lobe echoes from a strongly reflecting target produce artifactual linear echoes approximately 45 degrees from the transducer orientation.

face (as produced by a wire speculum) and be reflected back to each element of the transducer array at approximately the same distance (Fig. 7). This produces a straight line artifact which parallels the axis of the transducer. A double line artifact produced from both sides of the wire in a speculum is seen in Figs. 8 and 9.

Side lobes

Side lobe signals are also produced when the main ultrasonic wave is gener-

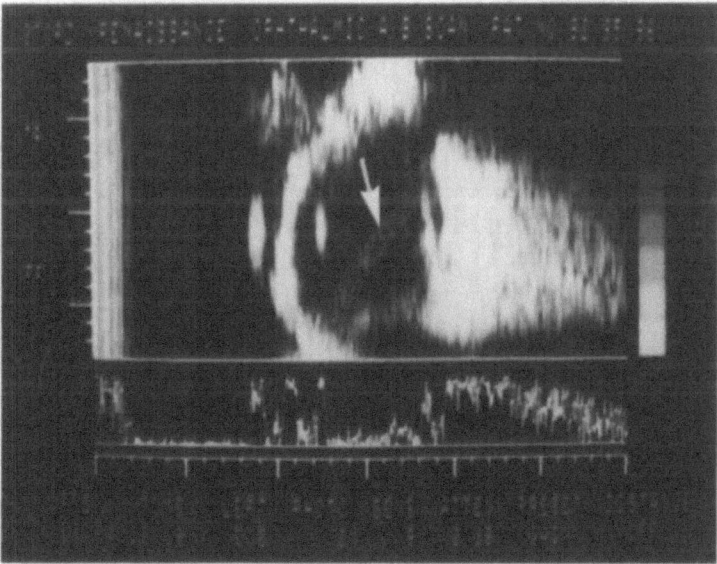

Fig. 5. Grating lobe artifact. This artifactual line (arrow) produced at 45 degrees to the transducer axis is caused by a high reflection from a wire speculum.

220

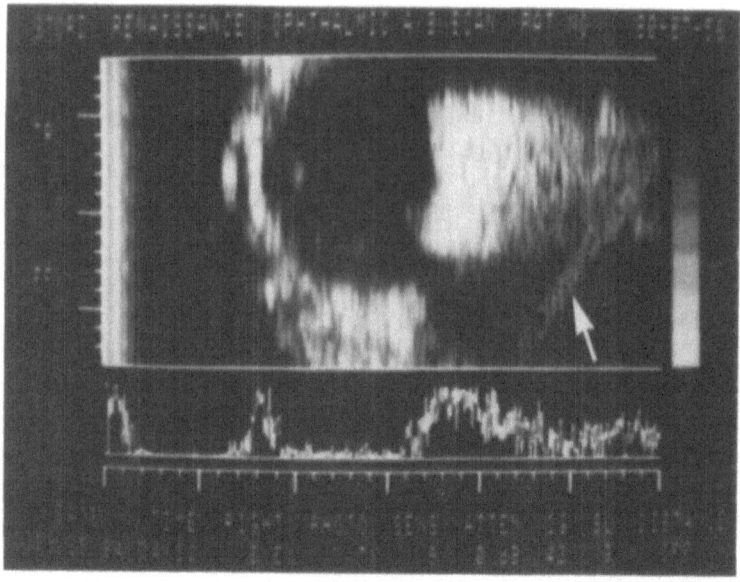

Fig. 6. Grating lobe artifact. This 45 degree artifactual line is produced by a grating lobe reflecting from the air/water interface of the immersion bag.

ated. These side lobe signals will spread out the effective sound field emanating from a transducer to produce a broader wave pattern [10]. When the side lobes are echoed from a strong reflector they produce a hyperbolically curved artifactual echo which extends in a convex manner away from the highly reflecting surface (Fig. 10).

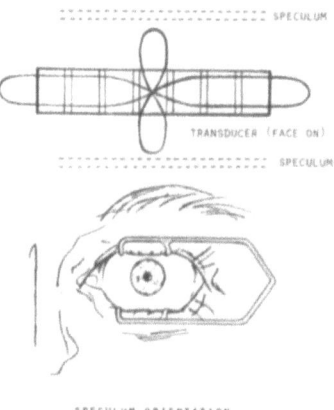

Fig. 7. Grating lobe signals traveling perpendicular to the long transducer axis are reflected from a wire speculum to produce linear artifactual echoes on the display screen. (Speculum orientation shown below).

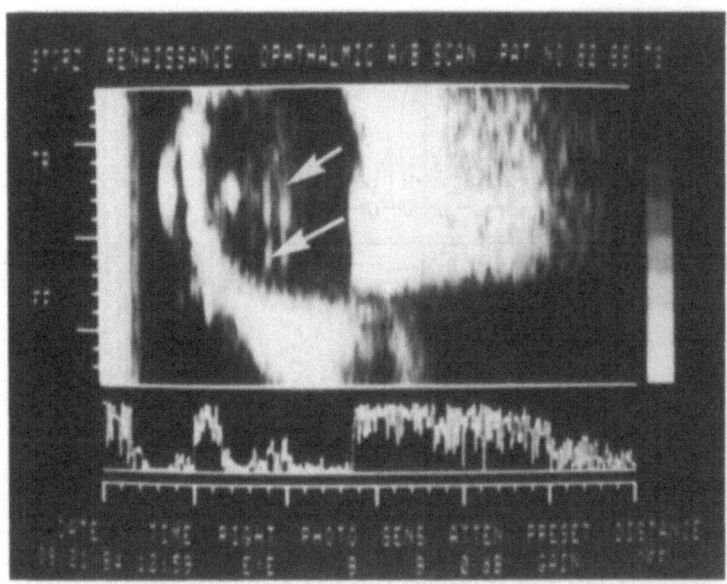

Fig. 8. Secondary grating lobe artifacts. These parallel lines are produced by side generated grating lobes which reflect from the wire speculum used to separate the patient's lids.

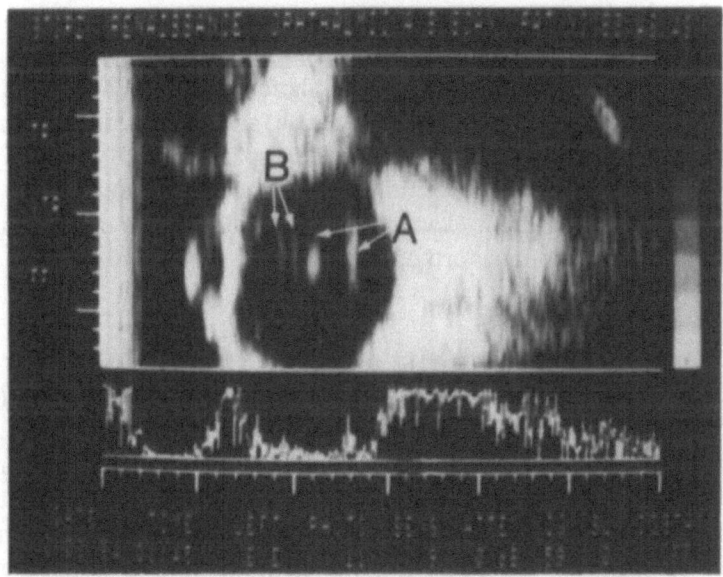

Fig. 9. Reduplication and secondary grating lobe artifacts. Reduplication echoes of the cornea and iris surface (A) and secondary grating lobe artifacts due to speculum reflections (B) are imaged in the vitreous cavity.

222

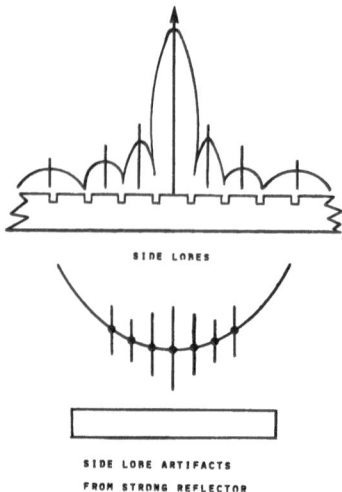

SIDE LOBES

SIDE LOBE ARTIFACTS
FROM STRONG REFLECTOR

Fig. 10. Side lobe artifacts. A curved artifact is produced by side lobes because the echo from progressive order side lobes travel successively longer distances to the generating transducer.

Transducer artifacts can be effectively decreased by proper design of the transducer array. (Most small organ scanning systems cannot be used in ophthalmic applications due to the higher levels of their transducer artifacts). The weak artifactual echoes which are clinically observed on highly sensitive real-time ophthalmic apparatus can geneally be eliminated by either reorientation of the transducer (with tilting and angulation), adjustment or elimination of high reflective targets (such as wire speculae) and decrease in the gain of the receiver. Real-time examinations where the display screen is constantly visualized while the transducer is positioned in front of the patient and the gain is actively varied for different examination procedures helps in detecting and minimizing these transducer artifacts.

Equipment noise artifacts

Equipment noise artifacts will produce radiating lines or speckle (snow) artifacts on the display screen [13]. They are due to extraneous signals that are introduced to the receiver section of the ultrasonic apparatus. These artifacts can often be produced by noise generating equipment (such as motors or defective fluorescent ballasts). They can be recognized by their intermittent and random nature. Separating the noise generating source from the ultrasonic equipment, eliminating the source altogether or turning down the receiver gain will help to eliminate these artifacts [14].

Standard artifacts

Standard artifacts are those artifacts which are associated with the interaction of sound with tissues and foreign matter [15]. These artifacts occur in both static and real-time examinations.

Shadowing

Shadowing artifacts occur when a strong reflecting or absorbing media attenuates the penetrating ultrasonic pulse and decreases its energy. This causes the attenuated pulse to display tissue echoes at lower amplitudes. In addition, the pulse cannot penetrate as deeply into tissues to produce imaging signals – thus less deeper tissue is displayed. Shadowing often occurs in the imaging of deeper structures behind dense tumors such as orbital 'drop-out' from a melanoma or a lack of posterior bulbar details behind a particularly dense cataract. (Choroidal excavation may also be a simple shadowing effect beneath some melanomas).

Reflection and refraction

Reflection and refraction artifacts cause tissues to appear displaced in their orientation or to not be imaged at all. A common refraction artifact is due to the higher velocity of sound in the lens as compared to other ocular tissues. This can cause a scalloped posterior bulbar wall echo due to refraction of the sound wave at the periphery of the lens. A common reflection artifact makes it difficult to image the sides of the globe with ultrasound. Sound waves at the sides of the globe are reflected slightly at the global periphery but are not reflected sufficiently in an axial orientation to return the echo to the detecting transducer. Thus the sides of the eye are poorly imaged.

Shadowing, reflection and refraction artifacts are especially easy to recognize on real-time displays when a part of the image appears to fill in or disappears as the transducer orientation is changed. By judicious choice of the transducer scanning orientation these artifacts can be effectively minimized.

Ringdown

Ringdown artifacts usually occur as sound waves bounce within a highly reflective structure (such as a wire speculum or metallic foreign body). Part of the reverberating wave returns to the detecting transducer to produce a continuous line of echoes deep to the generating structure. The ringdown appears to extend from this structure and to diminish in amplitude as it gets deeper. Ringdown echoes can regularly occur from metallic foreign bodies

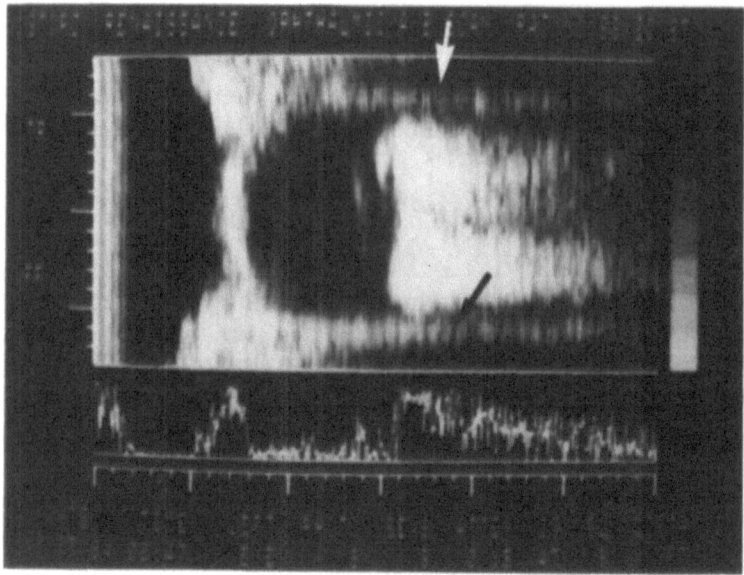

Fig. 11. Ringdown artifact. Ringdown from the upper and lower wires of the lid speculum are seen in most of the display.

around the eye (Figs. 11 and 12) but may also be seem from highly reflective tissues (such as the calcified lens in Fig. 13). Ringdown artifacts aid in clinical examinations by calling attention to highly reflecting objects in the sound field.

Conclusion

Real-time ophthalmic ultrasound is capable of producing clear clinical images with a minimum of extraneous echoes. However there are some artifacts which are especially unique when conducting a real-time examination.

The use of sensitive real-time ultrasonic receivers increases the prevalence of reduplication echoes, particularly of the cornea, iris and anterior lens surfaces. Real-time examinations clearly demonstrate the twice-as-fast motion of these artifactual images on the display screen as the transducer is pressed closer to the eye region.

Multiple arrays can produce grating lobe and side lobe artifacts which introduce linear and curved false echo patterns. Proper gain adjustment of the receiver and re-orientation of the transducer will help to clarify the image in these cases. By scanning the eye from different directions and tilting the transducer probe during real-time studies, it is possible to overcome refraction

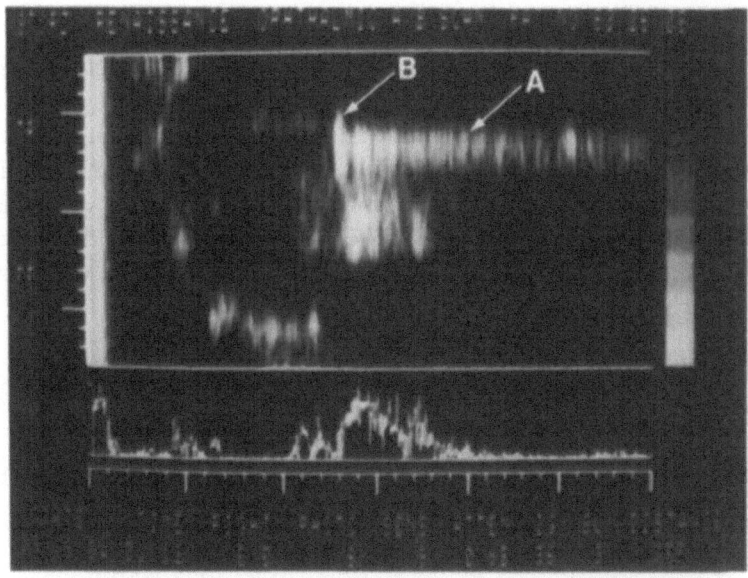

Fig. 12. Ringdown artifact. Ringdown from a BB foreign body (A). The BB (B) is located in the posterior bulbar wall.

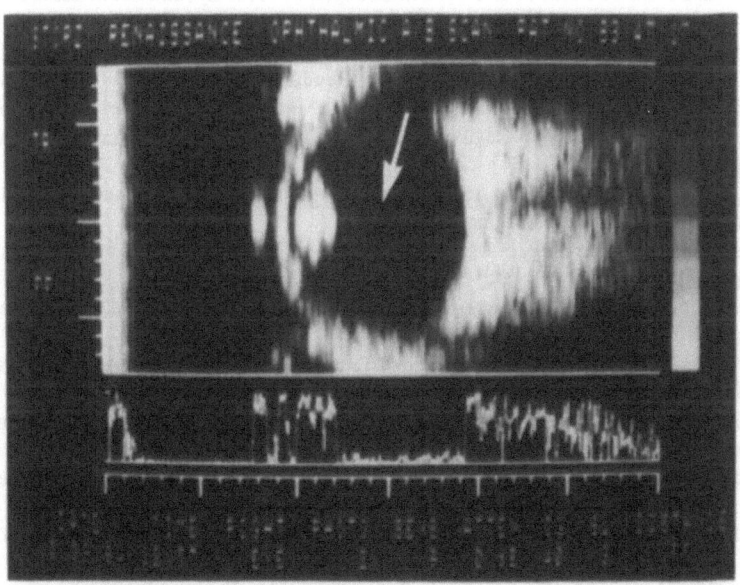

Fig. 13. Ringdown artifact from a cataractous lens. At high gain a cataract can also produce a subtle ringdown artifactual image.

and reflection artifacts which degrade or obscure the clinical picture.

Ringdown artifacts can be seen from highly reflecting foreign bodies or calcific degenerative changes. Once these artifactual echoes are recognized they can help to localize the strong reflector in the ultrasonic image.

The direct feedback the clinician enjoys between observing the real-time image while simultaneously moving the transducer in front of the eye helps to detect and eliminate most false ultrasonic echoes. In this manner the clinician can effectively eliminate artifacts which confuse and degrade the clinical picture.

Acknowledgement

This work was supported, in part, by an unrestricted grant from Research to Prevent Blindness, Inc.

References

1. Baum G. 1969. Ultrasonics in Orbital Diagnosis: B-Mode; in International Ophthalmology Clinics – Ultrasonography in Ophthalmology. Ed. A. Wainstock, Little, Brown & Co., Vol. 9, No. 33, pp. 589–594.

2. Coleman DJ, Lizzi FL, Jack RL. 1977. Ultrasonography of the Eye and Orbit. Lea & Febiger, pp. 72–75, 166–171, and 297–301.

3. Thijssen JM, Bakker JH. 1975. Intensity modulation in B-Scan systems: Correction of non-scanning speed and a devise for suppression of Reduplication Artifacts. In Kazner E, et al., Ed. Ultrasonics in Mecicine, Amsterdam. Excerpta Medica. W3, Ex 89, No. 363, pp. 115–120.

4. Bom N. 1979. Technology of Real-Time Ultrasound. Part II. Contrib-Gynecol-Obstet, Vol. 6, pp. 11–18.

5. Hanafy A. 1980. Characterization of Multielement Acoustic Arrays by Acousto-optic Diffraction Methods. Ultrasonic Imaging 2, pp. 122–134.

6. Kossoff G. 1979. Technology of Real-Time Ultrasound, Part 1. Contrib-Gynecol-Obstet, Vol. 6, pp. 2–10.

7. Lizzi FL, Feleppa EJ. 1979. Practical physics and electronics of ultrasound. Int-Ophthalmol-Clin, Vol. 19, No. 4, Winter, pp. 35–63.

8. Powis RL, Jones TB. 1984. Second Wave of Technology Sweeps Phased Arrays. Diagnostic Imaging, Vol. 6, No. 10, Oct., pp. 80–83.

9. Borburgh J, Feigt I, Hini P, Zurinski V. 1980. Bildqualitat bei Ultraschallgruppenantennen fur die medizinische Realzeitdiagnostik, Teil 1. Artefakte (Image Quality with Ultrasonic Arrays for Medical Real-time Diagnostics, I. Artifacts)., Siemens forsch entwicklungsber Res Dev Rep Vol. 9, No. 2, pp. 116–119 (Springer-Verlag).

10. Laing FC, Kurtz AB. 1982. The importance of Ultrasonic Side-Lobe Artifacts. Radiology, Vol. 145, No. 3, pp. 763–768.

11. Kino GS, DeSilets CS. 1979. Design of Slotted Transducer Arrays with Matched Backings. Ultrasonic-Imaging, Vol. 1, No. 3, July, pp. 189–209.

12. Kossoff G. 1979. Analysis of Focusing Action of Spherically Curved Transducers. Ultra-sound-Med-Biol, Vol. 5, No. 4, pp. 359–365.

13. Hassani SN, Bard RC. 1978. Real Time Ophthalmic Ultrasound. Springer-Verlag, pp. 180–186.

14. Baum G. 1983. A comparison of the performance of Commercial Ultrasound Breast Scanners vs. A Laboratory Instrument. J Clinical Ultra, Vol. 11, No. 8, Oct, pp. 405–413.

15. Farrell EJ. Backscatter and Attenuation Imaging from Ultrasonic Scanning in Medicine, IBM J Res and Dev, Vol. 26, No. 6, pp. 746–758.

Differential diagnosis of intraocular tumors with the echomemory of ophthason A 11

V. TANEV and N. MUDROV
Sofia, Bulgaria

In the routine practice of ophthalmic echography, the problem of confirming or ruling out the presence of an intraocular tumor occurs rather often. Ophthason A 11 is an instrument for A-scan examination. With its memorizing possibilities, it helps the accurate diagnosis of intraocular tumors.

The equipment is standardized according to W. Buschmann to achieve maximal sensitivity, so that it secures an ultrasound conductivity of a 43 mm standard paraffin solution (corresponding to a 730% levulose solution) at 20° C for a 7 MHz probe. For the more thorough echogram analysis and for the acoustic characterization of the established lesion, a decibel dial is used. Clinically, such a sensitivity may be checked with K.C. Ossoinig's 'Tissue phantom', J. Poujol's 'scleral echo', etc.

The examination begins with topographic echography, which helps to define the shape, the size and the localization of the suspected tumorous lesion. The surrounding tissue is explored too. For this purpose, one may also apply indirect kinetic echography with a probe placed opposite the globe. By quantitative echography of various points, the area which is suspicious of a tumor is disclosed.

Echograms needing a more detailed analysis may be memorized on the oscilloscope display with the aid of storage facilities. This allows the analysis of echograms from small lesions, observed only at a defined position of the probe.

The amplitude of the echoes which are not 'cut off' from the display along the 'Y' axis e.g., the internal echoes of the tumor tissues may be measured in decibels; the prominence of the lesion can also be measured.

As the echo amplitudes are often higher than the capacity of the screen, it becomes often necessary to reduce them by decreasing their amplification (db dial). After that the desired image can be memorized.

In accordance with other authors (J. Poujol, etc.) we found that the internal tumor echoes are lost between 80 and 50 decibels of attenuation as this occurs in ordinary selective echography and in other lesions of the vitreous body such

K.C. Ossoinig (editor), Ophthalmic Echography, ISBN 978-94-010-7988-4

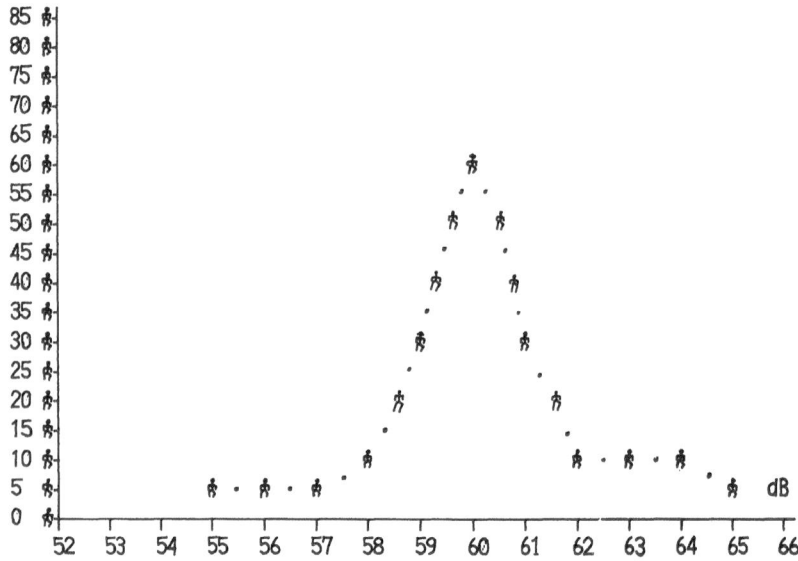

Fig. 1.

as blood, opacities and membranes (Fig. 1).

In the differential diagnosis of intraocular tumors and subretinal hemor-rhages, 'soft tissues', etc., the fading of the ultrasonic signals from the investig-ated lesion is of great importance. With the echo-memory Ophthason A 11, we proceed as follows: during a normal working setting, the position of the lesion's maximal prominence is displayed. The internal echoes are erased from the screen and the echogram is memorized by pushing a foot switch or manual knob, called 'memory'. The first marker is put on the echo signal of the lesion's anterior surface. The second one – upon the scleral signal. After the lesion's prominence is measured, the echogram is erased.

The probe is again in the same position and the amplitude is reduced to 5 mm. The dotted line is drawn in this position of the oscilloscope screen. After that the probe is applied symmetrically to the other eye under the same angle and with the same pressure. The obtained echo is observed on the display and memorized. Here the instrument's memory is especially useful as even the most skilled echographer may retain the probe in a symmetrical position only for a short time. The memorized scleral echo is measured in decibels with the decibel 'memory' dial. The decibels are graded along the prominence, defined in microseconds. Thus we find the attenuating of the echo intensities within the lesion in terms of decibels per microsecond (db/ms).

An analysis of variance procedure revealed highly significant differences ($p < 0.001$) between the average amounts of ultrasonic energy received from

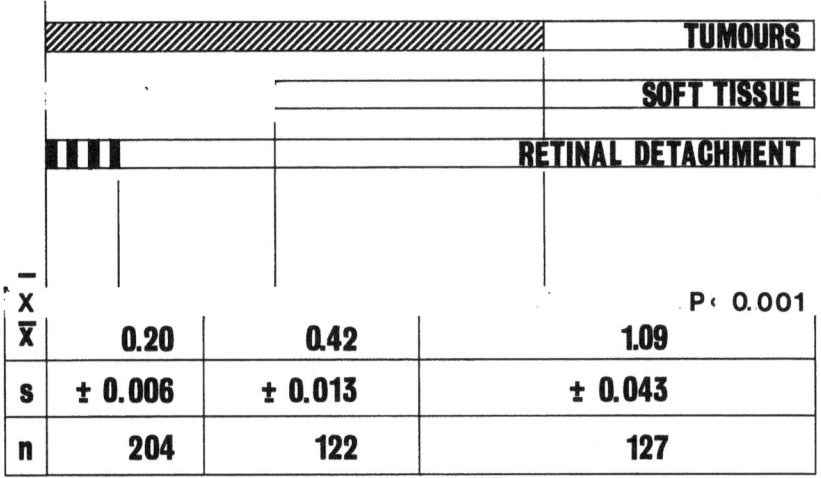

X̄	0.20	0.42	1.09
s	± 0.006	± 0.013	± 0.043
n	204	122	127

Fig. 2.

choroidal melanoma, from 'soft tissues' (retroretinal hemorrhage, localized vitreal hemorrhage, vitreal membrane conglomerate), and from retinal detachment (Fig. 2).

The correlation between tumor prominence in microseconds and the reduction of echo intensity in decibels is presented. There is a moderate negative correlation (r = −0,46) between the prominence and the degree of echo intensity reduction (Fig. 3).

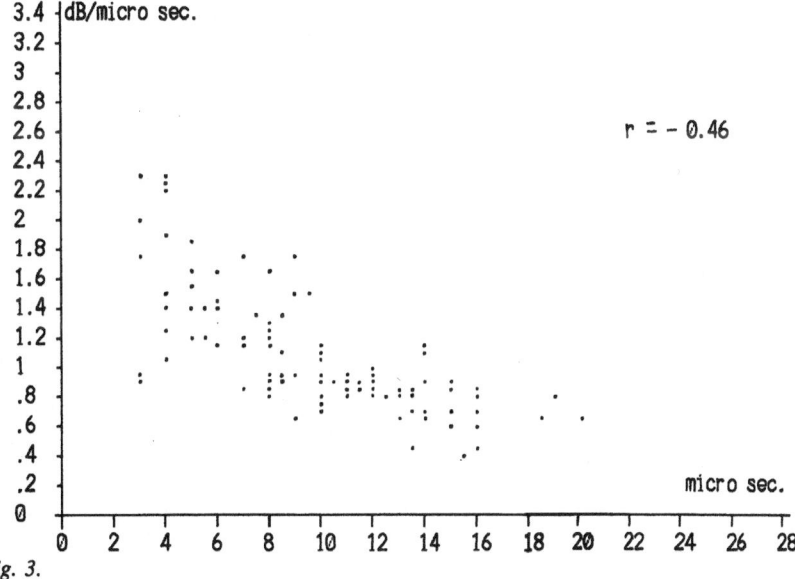

Fig. 3.

The ophthason A 11 echo memory aids in the differential diagnosis of intraocular tumors.

References

1. Buschmann W. 1984. Ausgewalte Falle aus der Arbeit der Ultraschalldiagnostischen Abteilung der Charite Augenklinik. Klin Mbl Augenheilk 144: 147–148.
2. Ossoinig KC. 1966. Standardization problems in ultrasonic diagnostics of the eye. Graefe Arch Klin exp Ophthal 169: 241–249.
3. Poujol J. 1981. Echographie en ophthalmologie Masson.

The echographic evaluation of spontaneous vitreous hemorrhage

R.L. GREEN
Los Angeles, USA

Introduction

The causes of spontaneous vitreous hemorrhage are well known. The frequency of the various etiologies of these hemorrhages has been reported by several authors (Winslow, '80, Butner, '82, Morse, '74). Diabetes has been shown to be the most common cause of spontaneous vitreous hemorrhage, with the second and third most common causes retinal tears and rhegmatogenous retinal detachments. The density of the hemorrhages in these cases varied from microscopic blood to very dense hemorrhage. Echographic examination of these latter cases is usually performed to evaluate the posterior segment.

We studied the causes of the clinically dense spontaneous vitreous hemorrhage in those patients referred to our echography laboratory. We compared the frequency of these causes to clinical studies reported previously.

Subjects and methods

Eighty patients with clinically dense spontaneous vitreous hemorrhage were studied in the echography laboratory over a three year period. These patients had no history of diabetes, previous intraocular surgery or trauma. All patients were evaluated with standardized echography utilizing the Kretz 7200 MA standardized A scan and a contact B scan. In each case the density and location of the vitreous hemorrhage was determined. In addition, the presence or absence of a posterior vitreous detachment was documented with specific reference to localized areas of vitreoretinal adherence. In every case the presence or absence of a tumor, retina or choroidal detachment, and/or retinal tear were evaluated.

K.C. Ossoinig (editor), Ophthalmic Echography, ISBN 978-94-010-7988-4

234

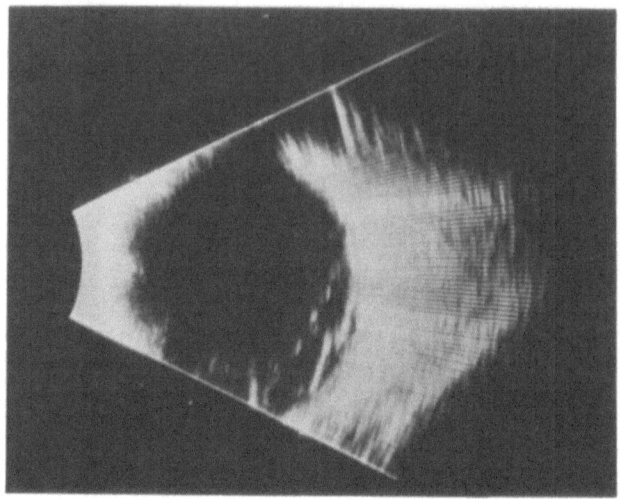

Fig. 1. B-scan echogram showing posterior vitreous detachment with adherence to a retinal tear.

Results

Of the eighty patients, 8 were found to have retinal tears (Table 1). These were found by echography to usually be mild vitreous hemorrhages with at least a partial posterior vitreous detachment. Very seldom was there blood in the sub-vitreal space.

Rhegmatogenous retinal detachment accounted for 8 of the cases. In several of these, we were able to identify the location of the retinal tear (Fig. 1). 20 of the cases were caused by either a central or a branch vein occlusion. The

Table 1. Causes of spontaneous vitreous hemorrhage.

Cause	No. of patients	%
Vein occlusion	20	25
Disciform degeneration	19	23.5
Retinal detachment	11	14
Retinal tear	8	10
Retinal vasculitis	6	7.5
Posterior vitreous detachment	3	4
Pars planitis	1	1
Leukemia	1	1
Unknown	8	10
TOTAL	77	96%

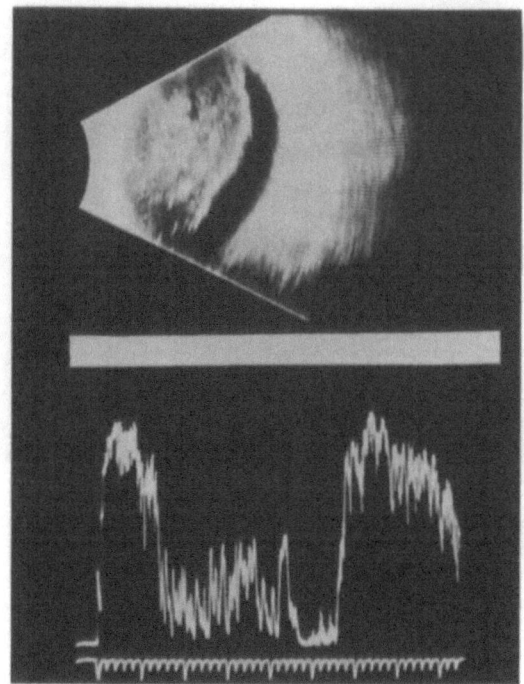

Fig. 2. B scan and A scan echogram showing dense vitreous hemorrhage secondary to a vein occlusion.

density of the hemorrhages in the eyes ranged from mild to quite severe (Fig. 2). These patients often presented initially with dense sub-vitreal hemorrhage (Fig. 3), which on follow-up would be seen to infiltrate the vitreous gel.

The second most common cause of spontaneous vitreous hemorrhage in our series was disciform degeneration, accounting for 19 of the cases. Most of these lesions were located in the macula; however, 5 were eccentric, located in the periphery. Disciform degeneration was usually seen in elderly patients, the average age being 68.

Three of the spontaneous vitreous hemorrhages were choroidal melanomas. We did not see any case of spontaneous vitreous hemorrhage related to a metastatic lesion to the choroid. Six of the cases were secondary to a retinal vasculitis.

Discussion

In previous clinical studies analyzing the frequency of spontaneous vitreous hemorrhage, after diabetes, the most common causes were retinal tears and

236

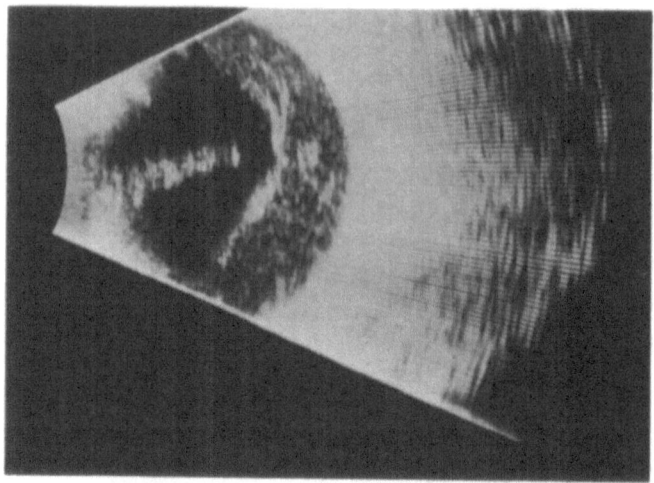

Fig. 3. B scan echogram showing dense sub-vitreal hemorrhage secondary to a vein occlusion. Note blood in Cloquet's canal.

rhegmatogenous retinal detachments. These hemorrhages are very often mild, allowing the fundus tó be visualized with the ophthalmoscope. Other common causes in the series included vein occlusion and posterior vitreous detachments. The cases in our study differ somewhat from those in other series in that ours are skewed toward more clinically dense hemorrhages. At our institution only those patients in whom the fundus cannot be visualized are referred for an ultrasound examination. Therefore, our patients usually present with clinically dense spontaneous vitreous hemorrhage.

Retinal tears, without detachments, represented 10% of the vitreous hemorrhages in our series, and these hemorrhages were usually mild by echographic standards. This compares to 20 and 25% frequency in some of the other series. This is due primarly to the fact that these, clinically, are very often not dense hemorrhages and therefore, the posterior segment can be visualized with an ophthalmoscope. The same applies to rhegmatogenous retinal detachments, which represented 14% of our cases and which, in the clinical series were significantly greater.

The most common cause of vitreous hemorrhage in our series was either central or branch vein occlusion, accounting for 25% of the cases. As previously mentioned, these often present initially with dense sub-vitreal hemorrhages that later may break into the vitreous gel. The second most common cause of spontaneous vitreous hemorrhage in our series was disciform degeneration, both macular and eccentric disciform lesions. This etiology is either not mentioned or noted as a rare cause of spontaneous vitreous hemorrhage in the previously mentioned series. The reason for this is that these are usually very dense hemorrhages in elderly patients. These hemorrhages often do not

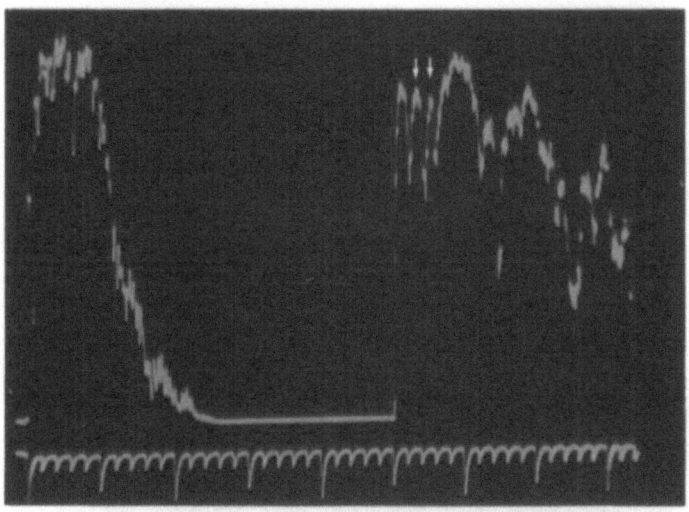

Fig. 4. A scan echogram of a disciform lesion showing typical high reflective internal spikes (arrows).

clear on their own and, due to the advanced age of the patient, a vitrectomy is not often performed. Therefore, the etiology may be difficult to establish clinically.

Nevertheless, these disciform lesions can very often be easily detected by echography. The echographic characteristics of disciform degeneration (Fig. 4) have been described by various authors using standardized echography (Ossoinig, '74, Byrne, '82). It is not unusual to see a shallow hemorrhagic retinal detachment associated with the disciform lesion (Fig. 5).

A few of the cases of spontaneous vitreous hemorrhage were found to be caused by intraocular tumors. In each of these instances the tumor was a large choroidal melanoma. It is therefore very important to look carefully by echography for choroidal melanomas in the presence of a dense vitreous hemorrhage, as the tumor signals very often can be confused with those of the hemorrhage. Specifically, with the standardized A scan it is important to look for the lack of after movement of the signals, thus confirming the presence of a solid lesion.

Conclusions

Eighty patients with dense spontaneous vitreous hemorrhage were evaluated by standardized echography. The frequency of the causes of the hemorrhages in this series differed somewhat from a previously published series of spontaneous vitreous hemorrhage. Our results indicate that the causes of clinically

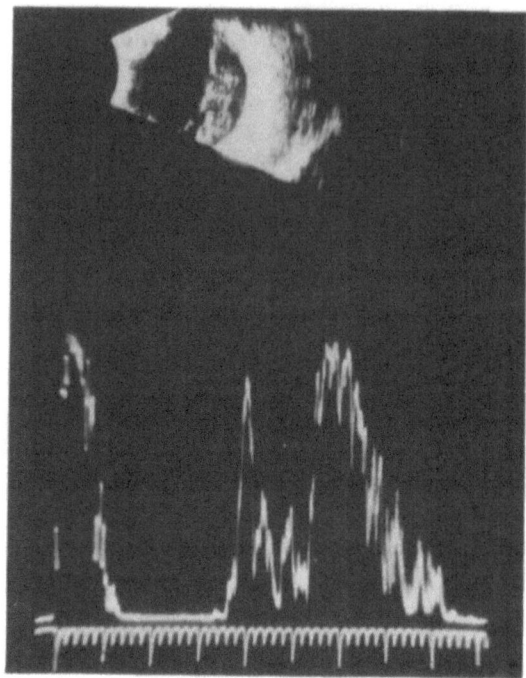

Fig. 5. B scan and A scan echogram showing a hemorrhagic retinal detachment.

dense vitreous hemorrhages are somewhat different from those of vitreous hemorrhages in general.

References

1. Butner RW, McPherson AR. 1982. Spontaneous Vitreous Hemorrhage. Ann Ophthalmol 14: 268–270.
2. Byrne SF. 1982. Differential Diagnosis of Disciform Lesions Using Standardized Echography. Ophthalmic Ultrasonography. Proceedings of the 9th SIDUO Congress. Edited by J.S. Hillman and M.M. LeMay. pp. 149–162.
3. Morse PH, Aminlari A, Scheie HG. 1974. Spontaneous Vitreous Hemorrhage. Arch Ophthalmol 92: 297–298.
4. Ossoinig KC, Blodi FC. 1974. Preoperative Differential Diagnosis of Tumors with Echography: III. Diagnosis of Intraocular Tumors, in. Blodi, F.C. (ed): Current Concepts in Ophthalmology, St. Louis. C.V. Mosby Co, Vol 4, pp. 296–313.
5. Winslow RL, Taylor BC. 1980. Spontaneous Vitreous Hemorrhage: Etiology and Management. Southern Medical Journal. 73: 1450–1452.

Combined echography and fluorophotometry in the detection of vitreous disorders

A. SAWADA, Y. MASUYAMA, Y. KODAMA and T. HAYASHIDA
Miyazaki, Japan

Abstract

In 7 eyes with posterior vitreous detachment and 4 eyes of familial exudative vitreoretinopathy, echography and vitreous fluorophotometry were done. In the former group, no correlation between echographic findings and the mid-vitreous values was found. In the latter group, the midvitreous values in the advanced eyes containing more distinct abnormal echographic findings were higher than those in the less affected eyes showing minimal echographic changes.

Introduction

Various changes in the vitreous space have been the object of ultrasonic examination. It is especially important to characterize and differentiate membrane-like lesions in the vitreous. On the other hand, vitreous fluorophotometry (VFP), which was developed as a new technique to evaluate the breakdown of the blood-retina barrier, is influenced by the various states of the vitreous (Yoshida et al., 1984). The purpose of this study is to investigate the possibility of differences in VFP values in a variety of vitreous disorders which frequently show similar patterns on ultrasonic imaging. In the short time of this study, the conclusion for most types of vitreous disorders cannot be drawn. However, the relation of echography and VFP with the different stages of familial exudative vitreoretinopathy is very interesting.

Materials and methods

In many cases with changes in the vitreous, echography and vitreous fluorophotometry were done in Miyazaki Medical College Hospital. Echography was done using Kretztechnik 7200 MA for A-scan, and mechanical scanning

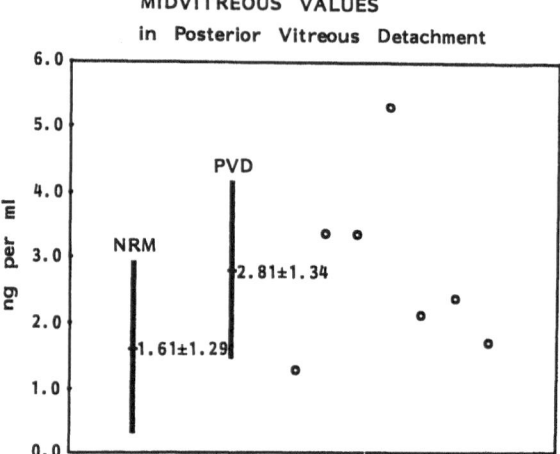

MIDVITREOUS VALUES
in Posterior Vitreous Detachment

Fig. 1. Mean midvitreous value in VFP of the normal eyes and eyes with posterior vitreous detachment. Open circles represent midvitreous detachment. They ranged between 1.40 ng/ml and 5.30 ng/ml.

equipment (Bronson-Turner ophthalmic B-scan and Santesonic, Japan) and electronic linear scanning equipment (Aloka 210 DX, Japan) for B-scan.

Vitreous fluorophotometry was done with Metricon Model 120 Fluoro-photometer. Measurements were taken before (for baseline) and 60 minutes after an antecubital venous injection of 7 mg/kg bodyweight of 10% fluorescein sodium. Baseline-corrected fluorescein values (60 minutes – baseline) at midvitreous were adopted for the study.

In the present study, the results in 7 eyes of posterior vitreous detachment and 4 eyes of familial exudative vitreoretinopathy will be shown.

Results

In all 7 eyes with posterior vitreous detachment abnormal echoes in the vitreous space were more or less displayed with some of the equipment used. The baseline-corrected midvitreous values in these eyes ranged between 1.40 ng/ml and 5.30 ng/ml, which fell into the normal range as shown in Fig. 1. There is no significant difference between the midvitreous values in the normal eyes and those in eyes with posterior vitreous detachment.

In echography of the eye, in which the midvitreous value was the lowest (1.4 ng/ml), a very few point-like lesions were displayed in the center of the vitreous. In the echograms of the eye, in which the value was the next lowest (1.7 ng/ml), a distinct echogenic membrane parallel to the fundus structures

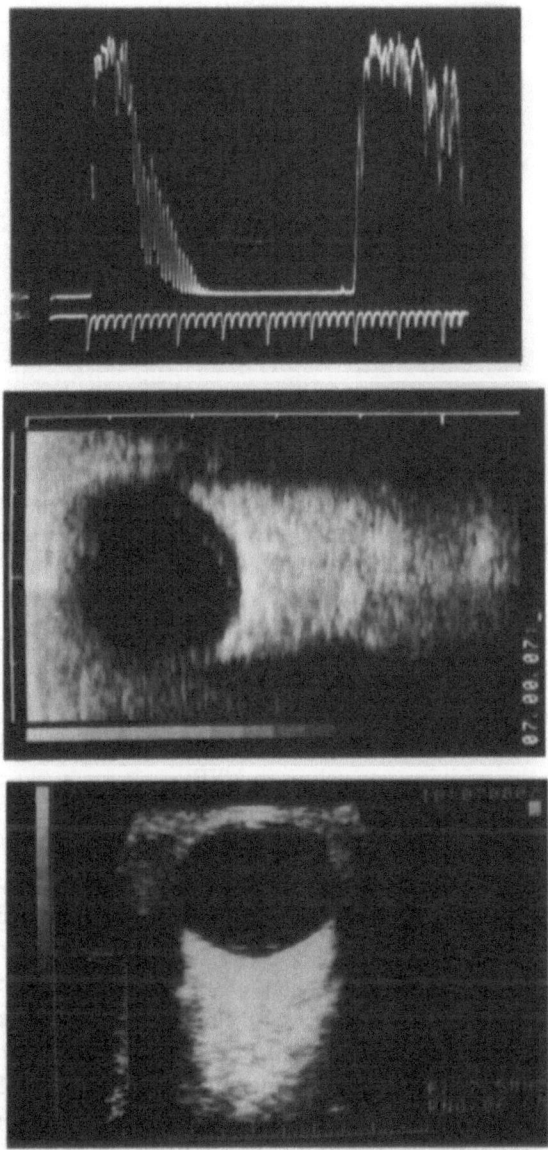

Fig. 2. Posterior vitreous detachment is displayed as a distinct echogenic membrane with an electronic (middle) and a mechanical (bottom) scanner. The midvitreous value in VFP is 1.7 ng/ml.

was noted in the posterior part of the vitreous (fig. 2). The membrane was concave anteriorly. Mobility with prompt response and limited range was clearly shown in kinetic echography. On the other hand, in those echograms showing the highest value (5.3 ng/ml), a very similar membrane-like lesion was displayed (Fig. 3). The visibility of the displayed images was inferior to those

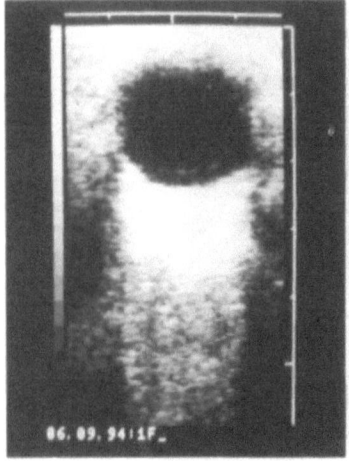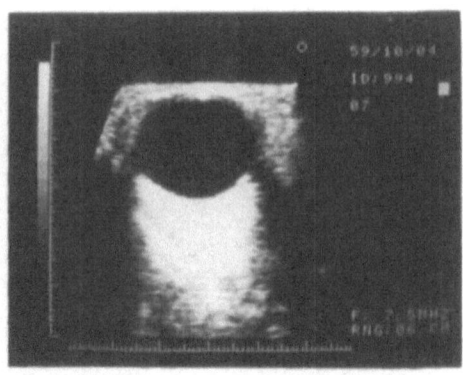

Fig. 3. Posterior vitreous detachment is displayed as an interrupted membrane when using an electronic scanner (left), and as a very thin echogenic membrane when using a mechanical scanner (right). The midvitreous value in VFP is 5.3 ng/ml.

in the eye with the value of 1.7 ng/ml in Fig. 2. A specific relationship between the midvitreous values and the degree of abnormality in vitreous echography was not found.

Two cases of familial exudative vitreoretinopathy will be illustrated with echograms and the midvitreous values in VFP:

Case. 1. A 35-year-old woman, in whose right eye the central vision was good. Posterior vitreous detachment was observed in the whole fundus. In the temporal periphery an avascular zone was observed and the retina was found to be degenerated. In the left eye the central vision was moderately deteriorated. The vitreous was totally detached and a thick vitreous membrane was formed. In the temporal periphery abnormalities of the retinal vessels with fibrovascular proliferation as well as localized areas of tractional retinal detachment were observed. Clinical findings in the right and the left eye corresponded to Stage 1 and 2 of Gow and Oliver's classification for familial exudative vitreoretinopathy (Gow and Oliver, 1971). The midvitreous value in VFP was 24.9 ng/ml in the right eye and 68.2 ng/ml in the left eye.

Figure 4 shows echograms of the right eye, in which only a few point-like lesions were displayed. Fig. 5 shows echograms of the left eye. Two layers were displayed in the posterior portion of the vitreous. The inner, thin and interrupted layer was mobile, the outer, thick and uninterrupted layer was less mobile. Part of the outer layer was taut and showed high reflectivity to ultrasound.

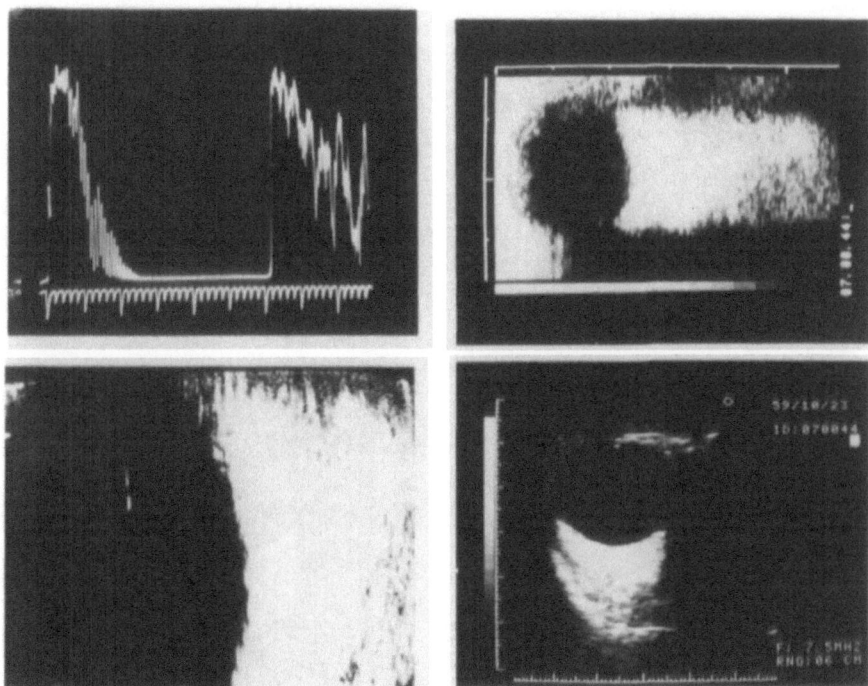

Fig. 4. Familial exudative vitreoretinopathy in the right eye of a 35-year-old woman. Only a few point-like lesions are displayed with an electronic scanner (top right) and a mechanical scanner (bottom left and right). The midvitreous value in VFP is 24.9 ng/ml.

Case 2. A 7-year-old boy with good central vision in both eyes. In the right eye posterior vitreous detachment, dragged disc and ectopic macula were observed. In the temporal periphery, fibrovascular proliferation with resultant tractional retinal detachment was clearly seen. In the left eye, vitreous changes including posterior vitreous detachment was mild and weaker than those in the right eye. In the posterior pole the retina was not affected. In the temporal periphery, mild retinal degeneration with exudation was observed. Clinical findings in the right and the left eye fell into the classification of Stage 2 and Stage 1. The midvitreous value in VFP was 5.6 ng/ml in the right eye and 0.6 ng/ml in the left eye. Figure 6 shows echograms of the right eye. Only a few point-like lesions were displayed in the posterior part of the vitreous. In the left eye, few point-like lesions were displayed, even with high sensitivity setting.

Discussion

With echography, it is relatively easy to detect and differentiate vitreous

244

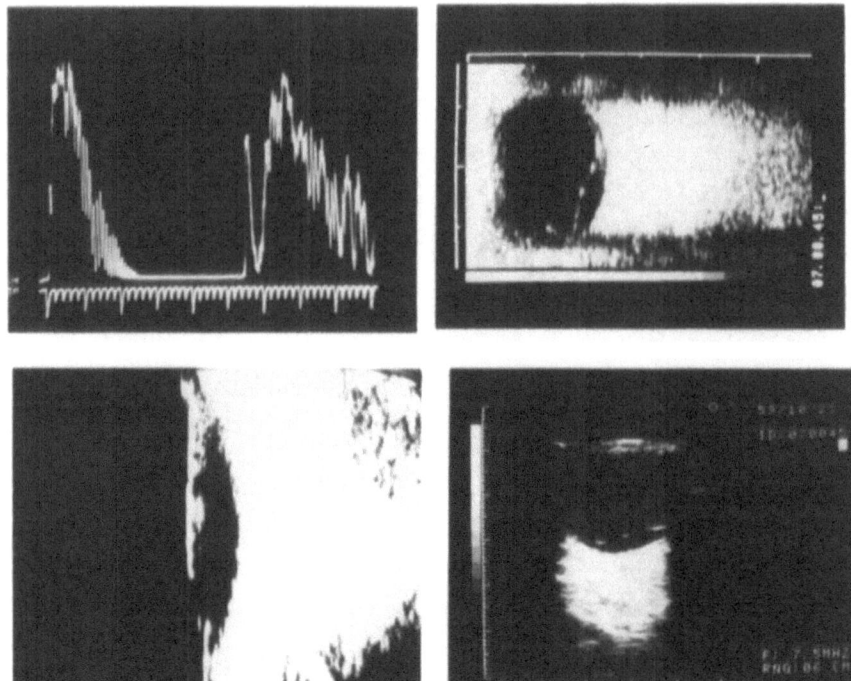

Fig. 5. Familial exudative vitreoretinopathy in the left eye of a 35-year-old woman. Two layers are displayed in the posterior vitreous. The inner layer is thin, interrupted and less mobile. The outer layer is thick, uninterrupted and less mobile; part of this outer layer is highly reflective to ultrasound. The midvitreous value in VFP is 68.2 ng/ml.

disorders in eyes with retinal detachment, vitreous membrane formation, and proliferative diabetic retinopathy (Sawada et al., 1984). However, it is sometimes difficult to delineate a posterior vitreous detachment when hemorrhage or inflammatory processes are not present. On the other hand, the significance of posterior vitreous detachment on the mechanism of vitreous hemorrhage and retinal detachment as well as the effect of posterior vitreous detachment on the prognosis of these diseases, have previously been stressed.

To locate minute changes in the posterior part of the vitreous, the combined use of echography and VFP was challenged.

In the present study on 7 eyes with posterior vitreous detachment, no distinct echographical differences among them were found, irregardless of the VFP midvitreous values. Further studies on other vitreoretinal disorders displaying point- or membrane-like patterns are going on. Of these disorders, two cases of familial exudative vitreoretinopathy were reported. In both cases, the unilateral eye was highly affected. The midvitreous values in VFP in more highly affected eyes were greater than those in less strongly affected eyes. The

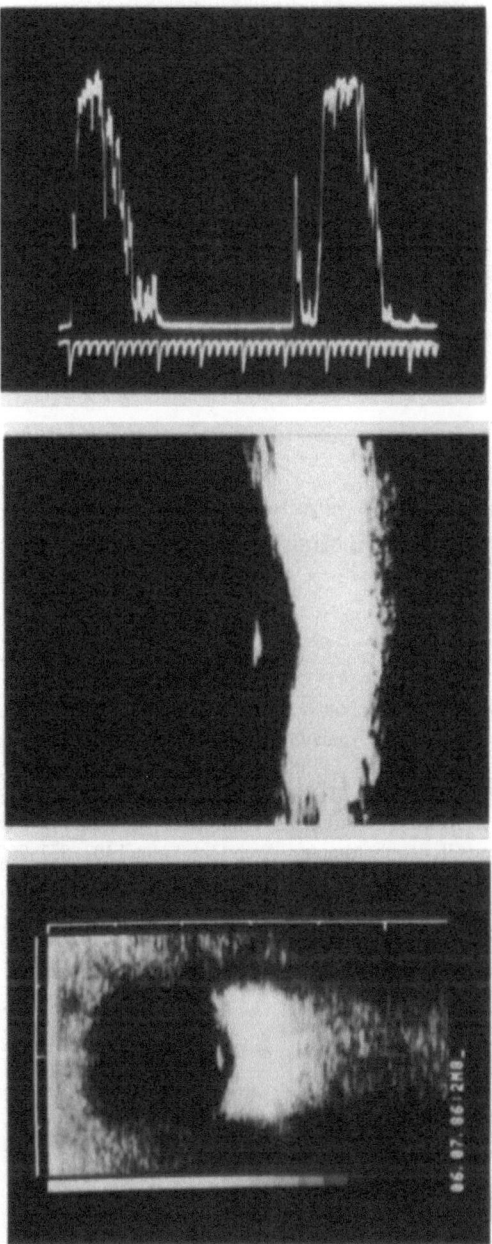

Fig. 6. Familial exudative vitreoretinopathy in the right eye of a 7-year-old boy. An A-scan echogram shows weak to medium reflectivity. B-scan echograms show a few point-like lesions in the posterior part of the vitreous. The midvitreous value in VFP is 5.6 ng/ml.

question as to where the value differences in Case 1 and Case 2 originate will be answered in further investigations. The patient's age, progression of disorders, and other unknown factors should be considered.

Conclusion

To define essential qualities of point- and membrane-like lesions in the vitreous more precisely, it is useful to combine echography with other techniques of investigation. VFP may be one of these techniques.

Acknowledgment

This study was supported in part by a grant-in-aid for scientific research (59480349) from the Japanese Ministry of Education.

References

Gow J, Oliver GL. 1971. Familial exudative vitreoretinopathy. Arch Ophthalmol 86: 150–155.

Sawada A, Masuyama Y, Baba Y, Oyamada Y. 1983. Evaluation of quantitative echography for intraocular membrane-like lesions. Hillman JS and Le May MM (eds) Ophthalmic Ultrasonography, Dr W Junk Publishers, The Hague, p. 95–105.

Yoshida A, Furukawa H, Delori FC, Busell SE, Trempe CL, McMeel JW. 1984. Effect of vitreous detachment on vitreous fluorophotometry. Arch Ophthalmol 102: 857–860.

Echographic findings in Terson's syndrome

K.C. OSSOINIG, D.S. RESHEF, T.A. WEINGEIST, J.C. FOLK and
A.J. PACKER
Iowa City, U.S.A.

Abstract

Standardized Echography studies were performed on 11 eyes of 6 patients with
Terson's syndrome prior to pars-plana vitrectomy. In each case either a total
or subtotal posterior vitreous detachment was observed in association with a
dense vitreous hemorrhage. In addition, a very thin and smooth, minimally
mobile, preretinal membrane extended over the posterior pole. All vitreous
structures were extremely mobile. The preretinal membrane, though suggestive of retinal detachment in B-scans, was clearly less reflective and thinner
than detached retina when evaluated with Standardized A-scan. This membrane appeared to be dome-shaped in some cases, but was less elevated in
others.

The combination of a very mobile vitreous hemorrhage and (sub)total
posterior vitreous detachment, along with a thin, smooth preretinal membrane overlying the posterior pole of the eye, appears to be specific for
Terson's syndrome. Thus, Standardized Echography is a useful diagnostic tool
which helps to confirm Terson's syndrome in addition to ruling out retinal
detachment or other posterior segment lesions that might reduce the otherwise excellent prognosis of vitrectomy in these cases. This report describes and
explains the echographic findings specific for Terson's syndrome.

Introduction

At the beginning of this century, Terson [1] first reported upon the association
of vitreous hemorrhage and intracranial hemorrhage. Subsequent reviews of
this phenomenon by Timberlake and Kubik [2], by Manschot [3], by Walsh
and Hoyt [4], and by Shaw, Landers, and Sydnor [5] indicate that between
10% and 40% of adults and about 70% of children with subarachnoidal or
subdural hemorrhage develop bilateral, or at least unilateral, intraocular

K.C. Ossoinig (editor), *Ophthalmic Echography*, ISBN 0-89838-873-2.

248

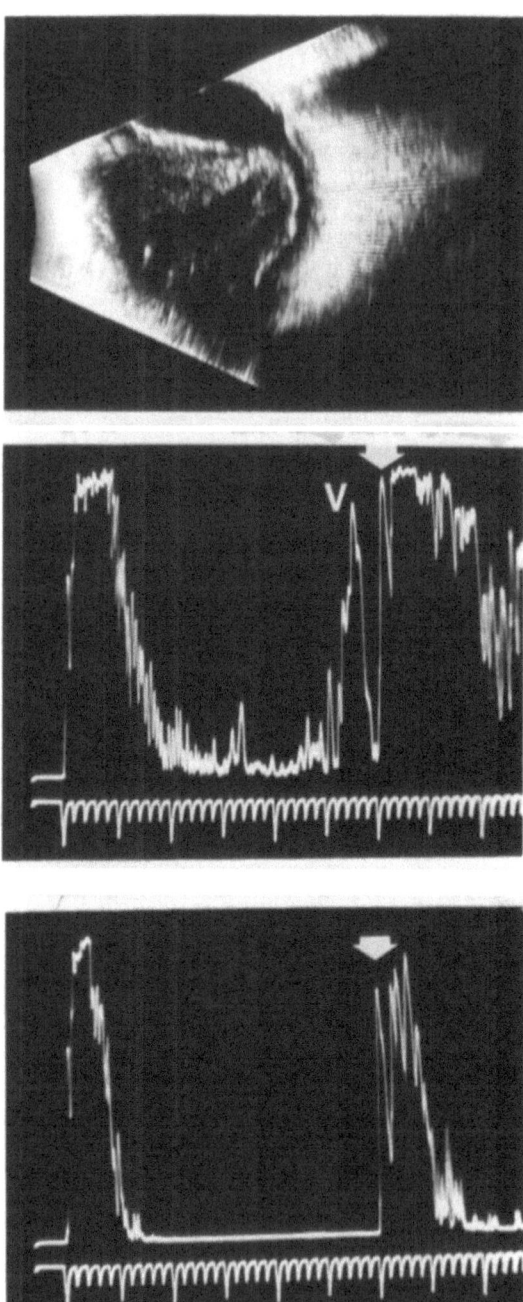

Fig. 1. Echograms from the right eye of a patient with Terson's syndrome. Horizontal B-scan shows total posterior vitreous detachment and vitreous hemorrhage. A dome-shaped membranous structure extends from the disc toward the macula. A-scan echogram at T + 6 (center) shows a complete chain of low spikes from dense vitreous hemorrhage. V = 95% high spike from detached posterior vitreous surface; arrow = signal from thin and smooth preretinal membrane. Bottom A-scan echogram, obtained at T-9, shows better separation of the maximal membrane spike from the fundus signals.

hemorrhages. Most of these hemorrhages remain limited to the retina or the subhyaloid space and rarely penetrate into the vitreous cavity. Shaw and Landers [6] reviewed 320 patients with subarachnoidal hemorrhage and found that only 7 had documented vitreous hemorrhage. It is in those rare cases in which dense vitreous hemorrhage is present, that echography is indicated, particularly prior to pars-plana vitrectomy (which is recommended when the vitreous hemorrhage persists) [7].

Echographic results

Since 1974, eleven eyes in six patients with Terson's syndrome have been studied with Standardized Echography [8] prior to vitrectomy. The following echographic findings were observed in all of these eyes and, in combination with each other, appear to be specific for Terson's syndrome.

Dense, very mobile vitreous hemorrhage with total, or at least subtotal (funnel-shaped), posterior vitreous detachment

With both Standardized A-scan and contact B-scan dense, dispersed vitreous opacities were detected (Figs. 1–6). These vitreous opacities were clearly visible in the B-scans when maximum or only slightly reduced system sensitivities were applied. Sometimes the opacities appeared to be denser and to contain larger interfaces at and near the detached posterior vitreous surface. The posterior vitreous detachment was usually complete (Fig. 1). Occasionally the detachment was incomplete, with the posterior vitreous surface forming a funnel that inserted into the optic disc (Fig. 6). In B-scans, the posterior vitreous surface appeared as an enhanced signal whenever the sound-beam incidence was not too oblique. This phenomenon is typical of a large and rather coarse surface. The vitreous opacities produced low echo spikes in the A-scans at Tissue Sensitivity, forming a complete (Fig. 2) or incomplete (Fig. 6) chain. This is due to the dispersed character of the long-standing hemorrhage. At six decibels higher system sensitivity (T + 6), however, the chain of opacity spikes was always complete (Figs. 1 and 4), indicating very dense hemorrhage. Occasionally, the opacity spikes were high near the posterior vitreous surface signal when the hemorrhage was layered (Fig. 4). As is typical of vitreous and subvitreal hemorrhages, the posterior vitreous surface was acoustically enhanced, producing a very high surface spike when reached by a perpendicular sound beam (Fig. 4). This posterior vitreous surface spike is not visible in A-scan echograms when the surface is lying on the fundus or on another membranous structure (Fig. 2), or when it is reached by an oblique sound beam (Fig. 6). Even when maximized, the posterior vitreous surface

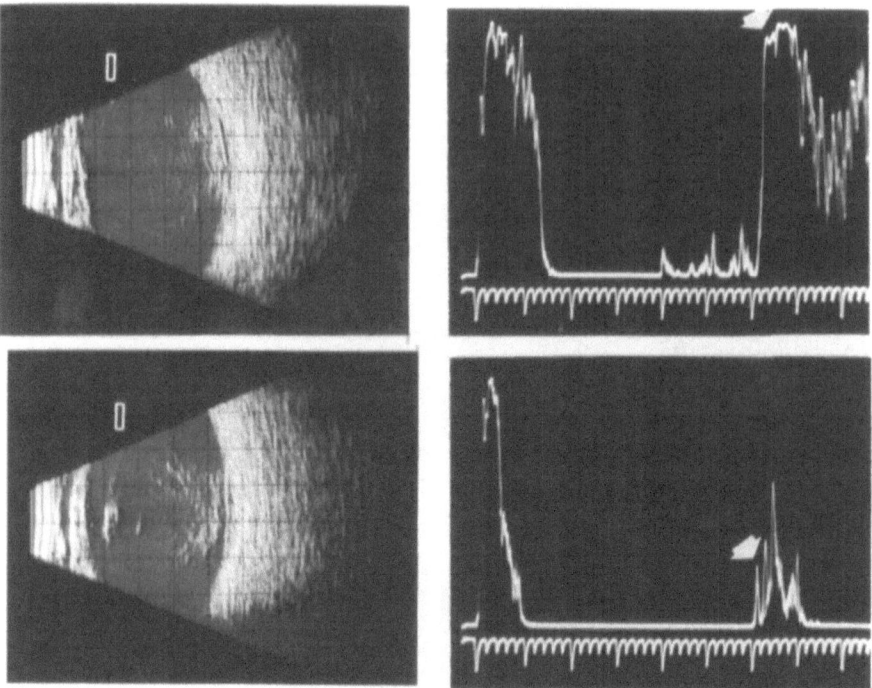

Fig. 2. Echograms from the right eye of a patient with Terson's syndrome displaying shallow elevation of the preretinal membrane. Top B-scan was obtained in a horizontal cut angled 30 degrees superiorly (above macula where maximally elevated). Bottom B-scan represents vertical cut through macula. Hemorrhagic vitreous is lying on top of membrane. Top A-scan displayed at Tissue Sensitivity: the preretinal membrane signal does not appear separate from the retinal spike (but membrane signal appeared mobile and therefore was recognized even at Tissue Sensitivity). Again, hemorrhagic vitreous appears attached to membrane, but promptly lifted off the membrane during kinetic echography. The membrane spike appears separate from the retinal signal at low Measuring Sensitivity (bottom A-scan). Arrow = membrane spike.

spike does not show a sharp rise (left ascending limb appears rugged and rises with several peaks interrupting its course as illustrated in Fig. 1). This is explained by the coarseness of the posterior vitreous surface in the presence of vitreal or subvitreal hemorrhage, and clearly sets it apart from smooth surfaces such as the surface of the retina or the preretinal membrane in Terson's syndrome.

The echographic findings of a dense vitreous hemorrhage and a (sub)total posterior vitreous detachment are not, in themselves, pathognomonic of Terson's syndrome. They are, after all, frequently associated with dense vitreous hemorrhage from ocular trauma and from proliferative diabetic retinopathy. What makes the echographic findings in Terson's syndrome so special is the pronounced mobility of all vitreous structures during and follow-

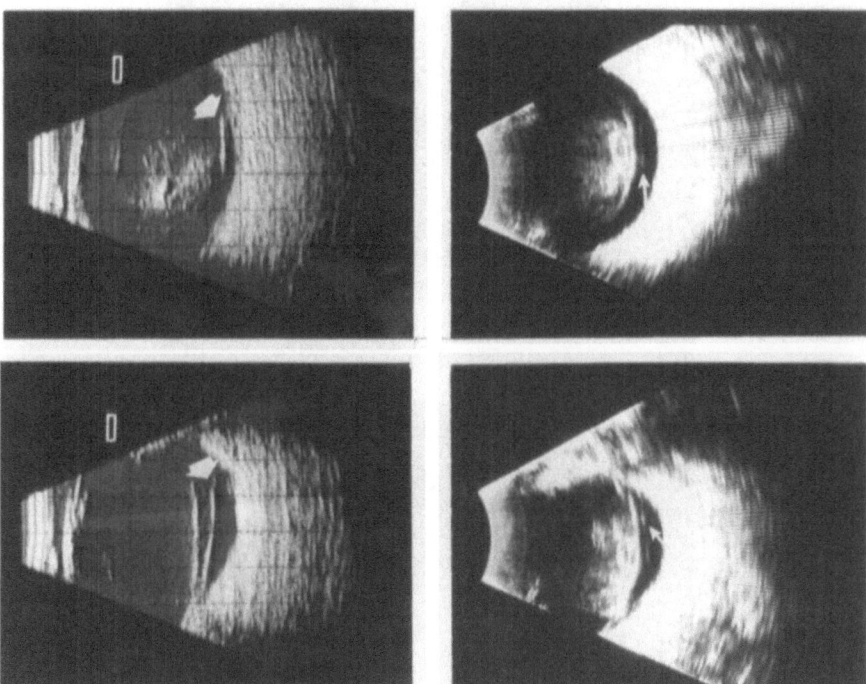

Fig. 3. B-scan echograms from the left eye of a patient with Terson's syndrome (same patient as in Fig. 2) demonstrating vitreous hemorrhage, posterior vitreous detachment, and extensive and highly elevated preretinal membrane. The left echograms wer obtained with the Ocuscan 400 model by Cilco/Sonometrics, whereas the right patterns were displayed with the Ultrascan by Cooper Vision. Note the distinct difference in the performance of these two B-scan units: the vitreous hemorrhage is better displayed with the Ultrascan, whereas the smooth preretinal membrane (arrow) is better documented with the Ocuscan.

ing extensive eye movements. This pronounced mobility and the obvious lack of proliferative changes within the vitreous cavity are well documented with kinetic A-scan and B-scan echography.

Thin, smooth, preretinal membrane overlying the posterior pole

In all eleven eyes examined with Standardized Echography, a very thin and smooth, minimally mobile membrane was documented rising from the optic disc and extending over the posterior pole. This membrane was sometimes dome-shaped (Fig. 1), or occasionally flatter and more widespread (Fig. 3). In other eyes the membrane was only slightly elevated above the retina (Figs. 2 and 5), and in one case it was separated so minimally from the retina that it was not recognizeable in the B-scan, but was visible only in the A-scan (Fig. 6).

252

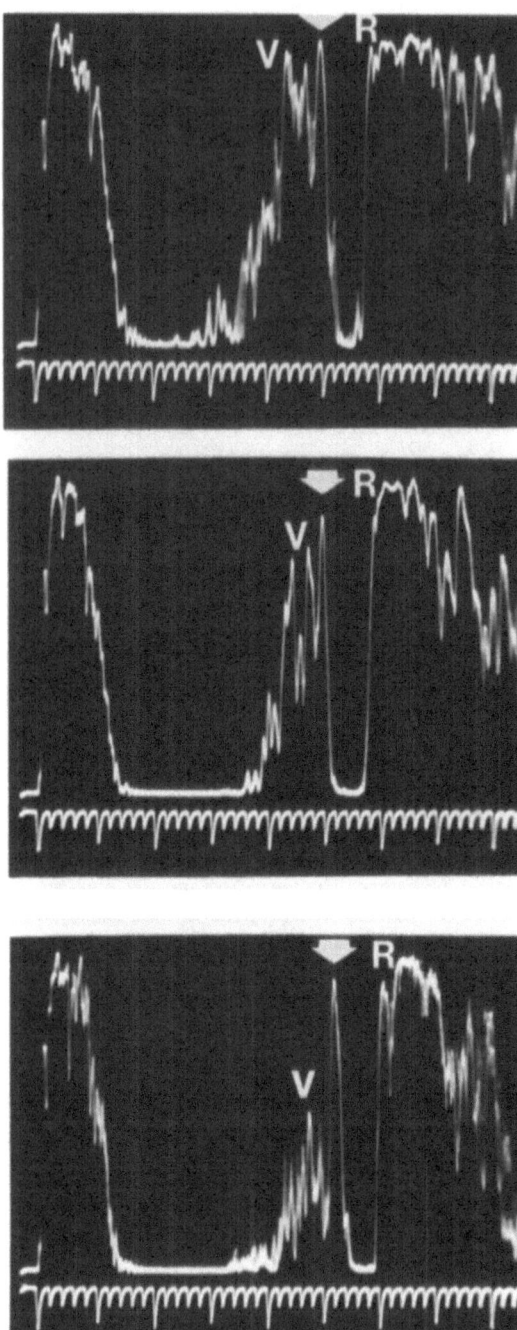

Fig. 4. A-scan echograms from the left eye (same eye as in Fig. 3) of a patient with Terson's syndrome. The vitreous hemorrhage in this eye is particularly dense (increasing spike height) near the detached posterior vitreous face (V). The top A-scan echogram, obtained at T + 6, indicates mild hemorrhage even in the most anterior portion of the vitreous (lack of anterior hemorrhage spikes at T as shown in center and bottom echograms). The preretinal membrane (arrow) is clearly separated from the retina (R); the hemorrhagic vitreous seems to be attached to the membrane, but lifts off promptly from the membrane during kinetic evaluation. The vitreous hemorrhage spikes are lower and appear blurred in a late phase of this movement as captured in the bottom echogram.

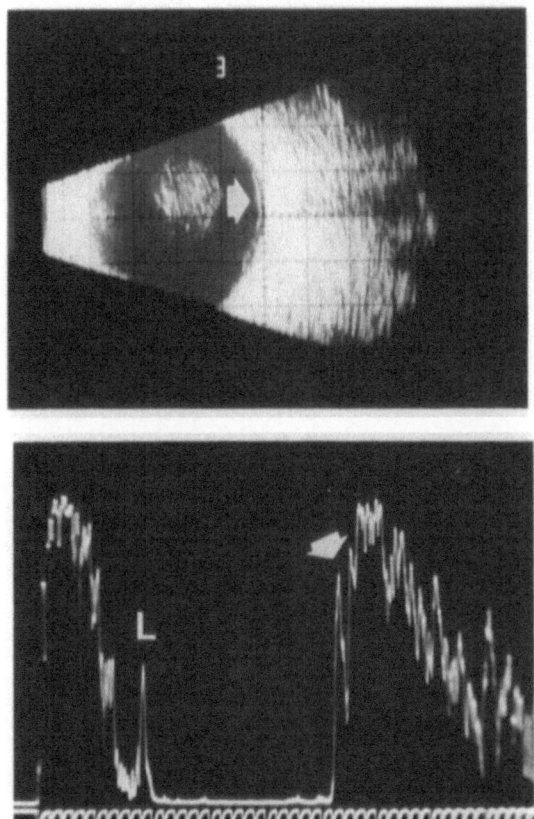

Fig. 5. Echograms from the right eye of a patient with Terson's syndrome. A dense hemorrhage in detached vitreous and shallowly elevated preretinal membrane (arrow) are demonstrated. The hemorrhage spikes are very low and do not form a complete chain of spikes at Tissue Sensitivity in the A-scan echogram, despite dense hemorrhage, because the sound beam is aimed almost axially through the lens which attenuates the beam (L = posterior lens spike).

In our first case observed in 1974 the preretinal membrane was dome-shaped and overlying the macula. Following the pars-plana vitrectomy a transparent, cellophane-like membrane was visible in front of the macula by ophthalmoscopy and slit-lamp biomicroscopy. Echographically, this membrane was less elevated postoperatively than prior to vitrectomy. Over the following years the membrane could not be detected and presumably flattened out over the fundus. Based on this observation in our first case, we assumed that the preretinal membrane occurring in Terson's syndrome was a detached internal limiting membrane. Recently Weingeist [9] demonstrated with light and electron microscope studies that the preretinal membrane observed in chronic

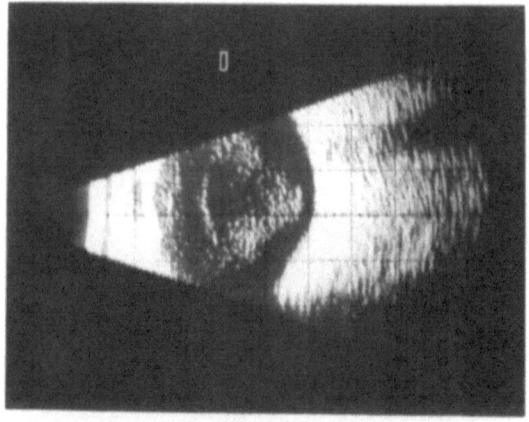

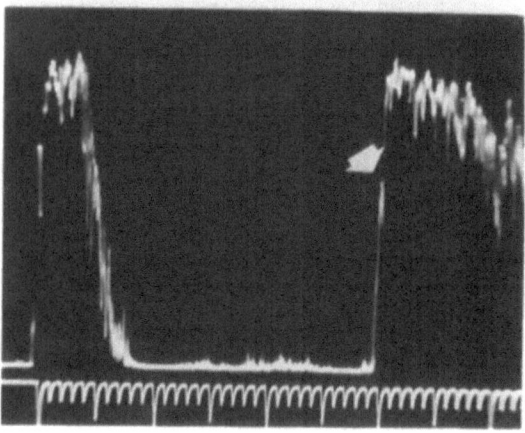

Fig. 6. Echograms from left eye of patient with Terson's syndrome. The B-scan shows the funnel-shaped posterior vitreous detachment barely missing the insertion into the disc. It does not reveal the minimally separated preretinal membrane (arrow) which, in the A-scan, can barely be seen, but can be demonstrated more clearly by showing its after-movement during kinetic echography.

Terson's syndrome consisted of glial cells and basement membrane material, and that in acute cases the membrane was derived from the posterior hyaloid face.

There are two echographic pitfalls that should, and may easily, be avoided: confusion of the peculiar preretinal membrane with either (1) a detached retina, or (2) the horizontal surface of a posterior hyphema. The B-scan appearance of the membrane may closely resemble a detached retina (Figs. 1 and 2). When Standardized A-scan is performed, the membrane is readily shown to be thinner and much less reflective than a detached retina. With quantitative echography [10], the delta db values found in the eleven eyes examined ranged from 18 to 30, whereas the delta db values characteristic of retinal detachment are 15 or less. At first glance, the surface signal of the preretinal membrane in some cases of Terson's syndrome may resemble the signal from the horizontal surface of a posterior hyphema (Figs. 2, 3 and 5). With both the A-scan and the B-scan procedures of Standardized Echography the fixed position of the preretinal membrane in Terson's syndrome can easily be documented and contrasted to the shifting character of a posterior hyphema [11].

The maximal A-scan spikes from preretinal membranes in Terson's syndrome are very slim compared to most maximal signals from detached retinas, indicating the extremely thin dimension of these membranes. Sharply rising and slim maximal spikes may be found in retinoschisis and in some tractional retinal detachments; however, the location of the preretinal membrane in Terson's syndrome is different from the typical site of retinoschisis. The insertion of proliferative bands or membranes can clearly be demonstrated in tractional retinal detachments, whereas the preretinal membranes found in Terson's syndrome were always completely separated from the vitreous structures. While the appearance of the B-scans in Figs. 2 and 3 may suggest insertion of vitreous structures into the preretinal membrane, it was always easy to prove that these structures were lying loosely on the preretinal membrane and they promptly lifted off the membrane during kinetic echography. By contrast, vitreous structures remain adherent to a tractional retinal detachment throughout a kinetic procedure.

As in retinoschisis, the extremely smooth surface of the preretinal membrane in Terson's syndrome becomes obvious echographically from the sudden onset of maximal height when, during angling of the sound beam, the perpendicular sound-beam incidence is achieved. Upon perpendicular sound-beam exposure the left ascending limb of the membrane spike rises sharply, clearly contrasting the membrane signal from the maximal echo spike of the posterior vitreous surface (Fig. 1).

In our series of eleven eyes in patients with Terson's syndrome, other echographic findings have been seen occasionally, including mild to moderately dense subvitreal opacities and a coarseness of the fundus surface behind the preretinal membrane. Retinal detachment or posterior hyphema was not detected in any of these eyes.

Conclusions

The following combination of Standardized Echography findings is specific for Terson's syndrome: a dense vitreous hemorrhage with a total or subtotal posterior vitreous detachment, and a pronounced mobility of all vitreous structures; a very thin and smooth preretinal membrane extending over the posterior pole including the optic disc and the macula, which is clearly less reflective than retina and which is completely separated from the vitreous; and the absence of retinal detachment or other posterior segment lesions. Standardized Echography, therefore, is very helpful in confirming or ruling out the diagnosis of Terson's syndrome.

From the Echographic Service of the Department of Ophthalmology, University of Iowa Hospitals and Clinics. This research was supported in part by an unrestricted grant from Research to Prevent Blindness.
Reprint requests to Karl C. Ossoinig, M.D., C.S. O'Brien Library, Department of Ophthalmology, University of Iowa Hospitals, Iowa City, Iowa 52242, U.S.A.

References

1. Terson A. 1900. De l'hemorrhagie dans le corps vitre au cours de l'hemorrhagie cerebrale. Clin Ophthalmol 6: 309.
2. Timberlake WH, Kubik CS. 1952. Follow-up report with clinical and anatomical notes on 280 patients with subarachnoid hemorrhage. Trans Am Neurol Assoc 77: 26.
3. Manschot WA. 1954. Subarachnoid hemorrhage. Intraocular symptoms and their pathogenesis. Am J Ophthalmol 38: 501.
4. Walsh FB, Hoyt WF. 1969. Clinical Neuro-ophthalmology, 3rd ed. Baltimore, Williams and Wilkins Co., p. 1786.
5. Shaw HE, Landers MB, Sydnor CF. 1977. The significance of intraocular hemorrhages due to subarachnoid hemorrhage. Ann Ophthalmol 9: 1403.
6. Shaw HE, Landers MB. 1975. Vitreous hemorrhage after intracranial hemorrhage. Am J Ophthalmol 80: 207.
7. Clarkson JG, Flynn HW, Daily MJ. 1980. Vitrectomy in Terson's syndrome. Am J Ophthalmol 90: 549.
8. Ossoinig KC. 1979. Standardized Echography: Basic principles, clinical applications, and results. Int Ophthalmol Clin 19 (4): 127.
9. Weingeist TA, Goldman EJ, Folk JC, Packer AJ, Ossoinig KC. 1986. Terson's Syndrome: Clinicopathologic Correlations. Ophthalmology 93/11, pp. 1435–1442.
10. Ossoinig KC. 1974. Quantitative Echography – The Basis of Tissue Differentiation. J Clin Ultrasound 2(1): 33.
11. Ossoinig KC. 1984. Echographic Detection and Classification of Posterior hyphemas. Ophthalmologica 189: 2.

Echographic findings after intravitreal silicone injection

S. CLEMENS and P. KROLL
Münster, FRG

Summary

In 105 patients treated by silicone injection combined with pars plana vitrectomy in severe retinal detachment various positions of the retina were sonographically examined in the state of clear media. Reproducible phenomenons could be found that revealed the situation of the retina in eyes with opacification of the lens or cornea.

Introduction

By Cibis [1] in the early sixties silicone oil was introduced in the treatment of retinal detachment. The first results reported were not encouraging because of severe secondary complications. Scott [10], Leaver et al. [6] and Zivojnović [14, 15] combined the procedure of silicone injection with pars plana vitrectomy since 1975 and reported much better results. Poujol and Massin [7] and Verbeek, Bayer and Thijssen [12] have described general problems in echographic diagnosis in eyes treated with silicone oil. Detection of position of the retina was assumed to be impossible after instillation of silicone oil. Reibaldi, Pilato and Tritto [9] found a characteristic foreign body like echo that is quantitatively distinguishible from eye structures.

We echographically examined 105 patients who had undergone pars plana vitrectomy and silicone oil instillation in severe retinal detachment in the state of clear media.

Methods

We used a standardized Kretz-Technik 7200 A-scan with a slightly focussed 10-MHz/5F probe, A Bronson-Turner B-scan with a 10-MHz probe and a

K.C. Ossoinig (editor), Ophthalmic Echography, ISBN 0-89838-873-2.

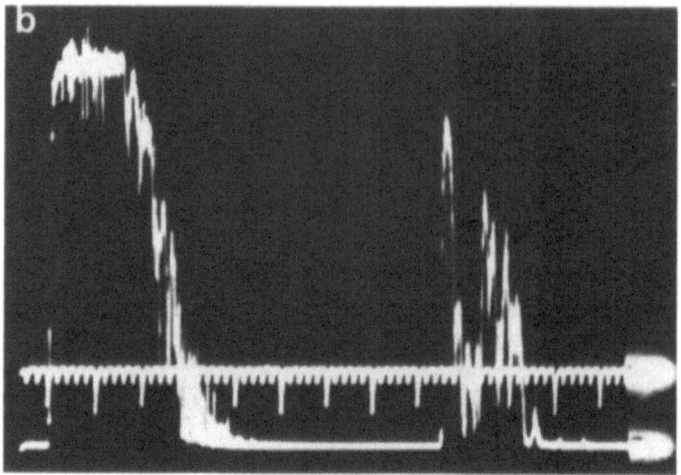

Fig. 1. End of intravitreal silicone bubble at 6 o'clock without contact to the retina.

Biophysic medical Triscan A and B scan, both with 10-MHz probe. The standardisation employed the criteria of Ossoinig [7], the tissue phantoms of Till [11] and test reflectors of Haigis and Buschmann [5].

Results

Some typical situations of the retina after silicone oil instillation are echographically demonstrated as follows:
  Figure 1 demonstrates with the highest peak the end of the silicone bubble without contact to the retina. The peak is symmetrical and narrow (1.5 μsec).
  Figure 2 shows a reattached retina at 12 o'clock in contact with the silicone oil by A-mode.
a) by Krets μsec scale
b) by Triscan mm-scale for normal eye.
The vitreous cavity measures more than 35 μsec after silicone oil instillation. The highest peak represents the end of the silicone bubble. In cases of contact to the retina it is asymmetric in shape with steps. Especially with Kretz A-scan there is an enlargemnt of the peak to 2.5 μsec at tissue sensitivity. This could not be found so constantly in Triscan A-mode. The scleral and orbital echos are rarefied.
  In *Figure 3* the same situation as before is examined with B-mode
a) by Bronson-Turner
b) by Triscan with vector scan.

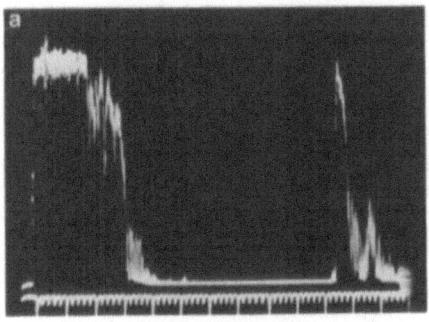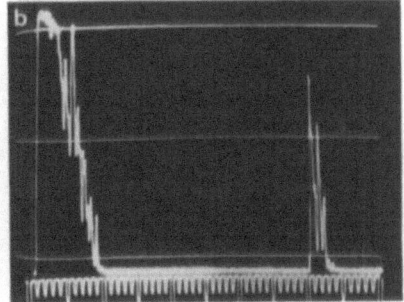

Fig. 2. End of silicone bubble in contact with the reattached retina at 12 o'clock; a) Kretz A-mode, b) Tri-Scan A-Mode.

The brightest echo again represents the end of the silicone bubble in contact to the retina. The demonstrated sector is smaller than in normal eyes, especially in Bronson-Turner. The orbital echos are rarefied.

Figure 4 shows a retinal detachment with preretinal silicone oil (A-mode). The highest peak represents the end of silicone bubble in contact to the retina.
a) Kretz
b) Triscan.
In Kretz examination the peak is widened to 2 μsec at 70 dB, enlarged at the top and asymmetric.

Figure 5 shows the same situation with B-mode.
a) Bronson-Turner
b) Tri-Scan with vector scan.
The first bright membrane-like echo (a in Bronson) represents the detached retina with preretinal silicone oil. In the vector scan there is an enlargement of the silicone peak to about 2 μsec.

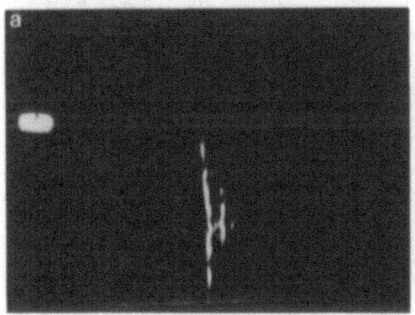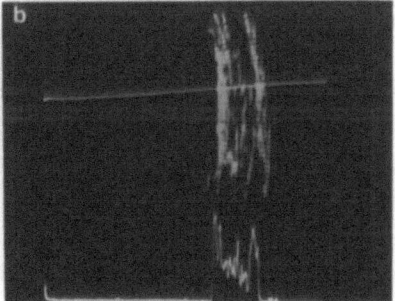

Fig. 3. Same situation as in Fig. 2; a) Bronson-Turner B-mode, b) Tri-Scan B-mode.

260

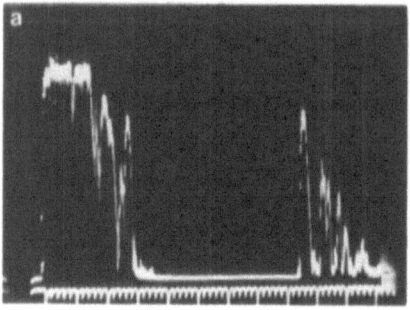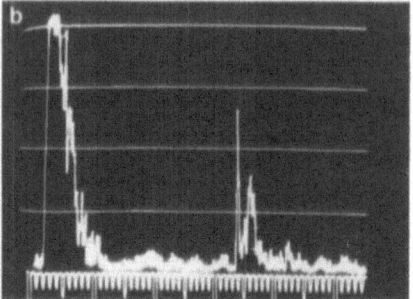

Fig. 4. Intravitreal silicone bubble in contact with detached retina; a) Kretz A-mode, b) Tri-Scan A-mode.

If the silicone does not completely fill the vitreous body and has less density than salt solution it rises leaving only a small unfilled area at the bottom. To avoid having the sound wave strike the 6 o'clock meridian diagonally, the patient should bend over so that the silicone bubble is in direct contact with the retina.

Figure 6 demonstrates the echographical result of diagonally striking the 6 o'clock meridian.

a) scetch

b) Kretz A-scan.

a = end of silicone bubble in contact with the detached retina, only weak echo.

Figure 7 shows the improved representation by causing the patient bend over so that the silicone bubble is in enlarged contact with the retina and the striking of sound wave is in right angle.

a) scetch

b) Kretz A-scan.

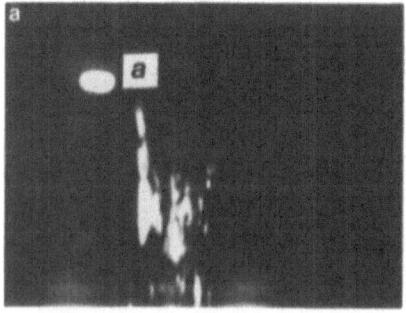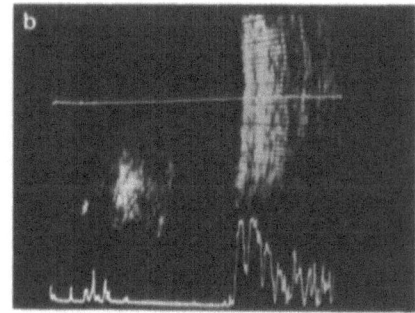

Fig. 5. Same situation as in Fig. 4; a) Bronson-Turner B-mode, b) Tri-Scan B-mode with vector scan.

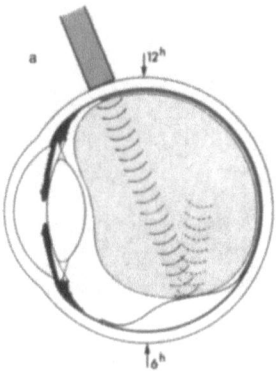
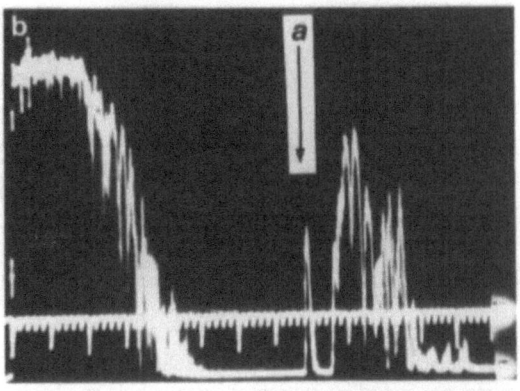

Fig. 6. Diagonally striking of sound bundle at 6 o'clock in cases of uncomplete filling of the vitreous cavity by silicone oil. a) scetch, b) Kretz A-mode. a = end of silicone bubble in contact to the retina.

a = end of silicone bubble in contact with the detached retina, high peak, enlargement to 2.5 μsec.

Figure 8 shows a detached retina with pre- and subretinal silicone.

a) Kretz A-mode
b) Bronson-Turner.

The peak a has a double top and is enlarged to 2.5 μsec, it shows the end of the preretinal and the beginning of the subretinal silicone bubble, a positive kinetic phenomenon is visible at the first top. Peak b is the end of the subretinal silicone bubble, c is the sclera. On the B-mode a lateral shifting of the 2 parts of the peak a is visible.

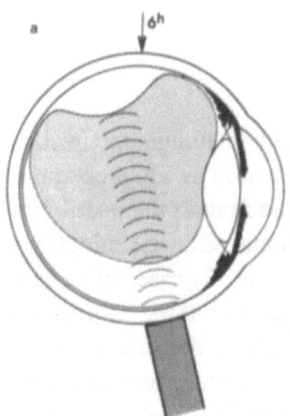
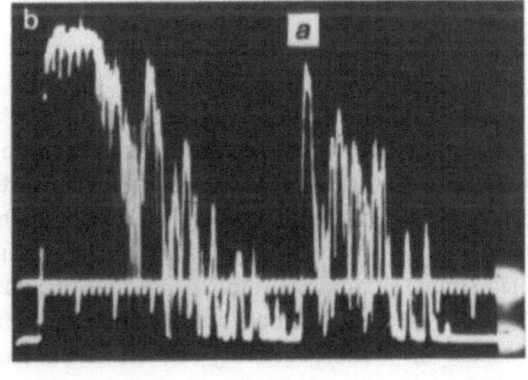

Fig. 7. Improved examination when patient bends over; a) scetch, b) Kretz A-mode. a = end of silicone bubble in contact with detached retina.

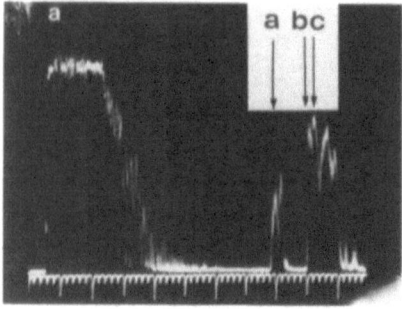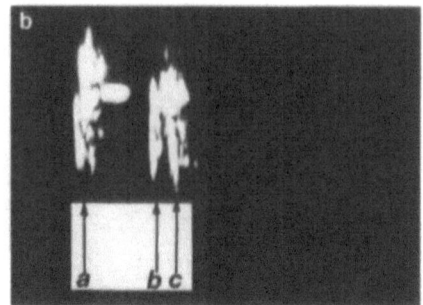

Fig. 8. Detached retina with pre- and subretinal silicone. a) Kretz A-mode, b) Bronson-Turner B-mode. a = end of intravitreal silicone bubble and beginning of subretinal bubble, b = end of subretinal bubble, c = sclera.

The better quantitative differentiation of a retinal detachment in contact with silicone oil by Kretz A-mode than by Tri-Scan A-mode was evident.

The 10 MHz 5F probe of Kretz was focussed in salt solution on 3 to 4 cm distance. The diameter of the probe is 5 mm and the diameter of the focussed bundle is 5 mm. By focussing of the silicone bubble a further concentration of the bundles' diameter at the retina of 3 to 4 mm is expected. The 10 MHz Tri-Scan probe had a diameter of 3,5 mm and was slightly focussed on 3 cm. The diameter of bundle was 2 mm in salt solution. The axial resolution measured by 6 dB-criterion was 0.4 mm for the Kretz probe and 0.1 mm for the Tri-Scan probe. The scanned area at the retina is larger in Kretz device, it is more sensitive to small deviations from the ideal round surface of the bubble in contact to the retina. The scanned area is dependent on the radius of the silicone bubble at the entrance of the sound bundle.

Discussion

In accordance with Poujol and Massin [8] we observed an elongated vitreous distance by a slower sound conduction in silicone oil as well as a higher sound absorption. Verbeek, Bayer and Thijssen [12] reported first on the possibility of echographic reproducibility of retinal detachments. Our examinations showed that an exact diagnosis of the retina is possible. In cases of retinal detachment treated with silicone besides the increased wave at the choroid we found in the retinal area further criterions as for example the double-peak. Because of possible mobility of silicone bubble our method offers new possibilities in the diagnosis of the retina after silicone instillation. Inclusions of air or vitreous in the silicone bubble as described by Verbeek, Bayer and Thijssen [12] could not be found in our examinations.

Summary

1. Prolongation of the vitreous length of 50% because of the delayed sound velocity in silicone oil. We measured a speed of 1010 m/sec in silicone oil at 20 centigrade.

2. Increased absorption of ultrasound in silicone oil compared to salt solution: The absorption coefficient for sound in silicone oil according to Poujol and Massin [8] is 1 dB/mm of silicone oil. Verbeek, Bayer and Thijssen [12] found it to be 1.1 dB/mm. We found it to be 1 dB/mm of silicone oil with the foccused 10 MHz transducer. The sclera echo was diminished for 30 dB.

3. Higher reflection coefficient of silicone – water: the reflection coefficient of the surface of the silicone bubble in the vitreous cavity is 10 times higher compared to the boundary line of retina to vitreous. The surface of the silicone bubble represents the highest echo. In Kretz A-scan the peak is widened to 1.5 μsec, the form is symmetric, without steps. Its reflectivity is about that of sclera in normal eyes.

4. Small sectors in display. Because of the plan surface and the focussing of the oil bubble the displayed sector of the eye is smaller than normal. More single adjustments are necessary in which the phenomenons appear often in chronologic order. Water-bath coupling was not successful in these examinations.

5. Examination in cases of silicone bubbles smaller than vitreous cavity: Our employed silicone oil is lighter than physiologic salt solution and rises leaving sometimes a small unfilled compartiment at the bottom of the vitreous cavity. To avoid a diagonally striking at the end of the bubble and dispersion of ultrasonic energy, the patient should bend over so that the silicone bubble is in direct contact with the retina.

6. Cases of amotio retinae with direct contact and preretinal silicone oil: the peak in Kretz A-scan is widened to 2.5 μsec or more at tissue sensitivity and asymmetric with steps, several adjustments are necessary to evaluate the extent of the retinal detachment. Vector B-scan in Tri-Scan shows a higher reflecting membrane which is widened comparing with isolated bubble surface.

7. Amotio retinae with pre- and subretinal silicone oil: In Kretz A-scan the peak is widened to 2.5 μsec or more with a double peak sometimes showing a positive kinetic phenomenon and the end of the subretinal silicone bubble.

8. Asymmetric position of the silicone bubble to the vertical meridian: Here an amotio retinae has to be excluded. Lateral inclination of the patient's head may help bringing the silicone bubble closer to the retina and provide further information on the retinal detachment, quite similar to the bending over of the patient.

9. Vitreous strands and retinal folds: In Kretz A-scan the peak is widened to

2.5 μsec at its basis. Several adjustments are necessary.

10. Diagnosis of the posterior pole: Placing the transducer near the ora serrata causes a sound wave to strike the silicone bubble diagonally at the macula, leading to flattening of the silicone peaks. Directing the sound wave axially increases the diffusion and absorption by the lens.

References

1. Cibis PA, Becker B, Okun E, Caneary S. 1962. The use of liquid silicone in retinal detachment surgery. Arch Ophthal (Chicago) 68: 590–599.
2. Clemens S, Kroll P. 1984. Echographische Befunde nach intravitrealer Silikoninstillation. Klin Mbl Augenheilk 185: 17–21.
3. Coleman DJ, Lizzi FL, Jack RL. 1977. Ultrasonography of the Eye and Orbit. Lea, Febiger, Philadelphia.
4. Gonvers. 1983. Personal communication. Vitrectomy Simposium. Vail/Colorado, March.
5. Haigis W, Buschmann W. 1980. Die Bedeutung von Testreflektoren zur schnellen klinischen Überprüfung von Geräten für die ophthalmologische Ultraschalldiagnostik. In: Biomed Technik, Bd 25, Ergänzungsband, p. 53. Schiele, Schön, Berlin.
6. Leaver PK, Grey RHB, Garrer A. 1979. Silicone injection in the treatment of massive retinal retraction. II. Note: Complications in 93 eyes. Br J Ophthal 63: 361–367.
7. Ossoinig KC. 1979. Standardized Echography: Basic Principles, Clinical Applications and Results. In: Ophthalmic Ultrasonography: Comparative Techniques. R.L. Dallow (ed.). Internat Ophthal Clin 19: 4.
8. Poujol J, Massin M. 1979. L'examen échographique des yeux opérés de décollement de rétine avec injection de silicone. In: Diagnostika Ultrasonica in Ophthalmologia. H. Gernet (ed.). Remy, Münster.
9. Reibaldi A, di Pilato M, Tritto MM. 1983. Ultrasonographic Pattern of the eyeball operated on for Retinal Detachment. In: Ophthalmic Ultrasonography. J.S. Hillman, M.M. Le May (eds.). Dr W Junk Publishers, The Hague/Boston/Lancaster.
10. Scott JD. 1975. The treatment of massive vitreous retraction by the separation of preretinal membranes using liquid silicone. Mod Probl Ophthal 19: 285.
11. Till P. 1976. Solid tissue model for the standardisation of the echo-ophthalmograph 7200 MA (Kretz-Technik). Doc ophthal 41.
12. Verbeek AM, Bayer AL, Thijssen JM. 1981. Echographic diagnosis after intraocular silicone oil injection. In: Docum Ophthal Proc Series Vol 29. Thijssen JM, Verbeek AM (eds.). Junk, The Hague.
13. Watzke RC. 1967. Silicone Retinopiesis for Retinal Detachment. A Longterm Clinical Evaluation. Arch Ophthal (Chicago) 77: 185.
14. Zivojnović R, Mertens RE, Baarsma GS. 1981. Das flüssige Silikon in der Amotiochirurgie. Klin Mbl Augenheilk 179: 17.
15. Zivojnović R, Mertens DAE, Peperkamp E. 1982. Das flüssige Silikon in der Amotiochirurgie (II). Bericht über 280 Fälle – weitere Entwicklung der Technik. Klin Mbl Augenheilk 181: 444.

An experimental study of the ultrasonic characteristics of intravitreally injected sodium hyaluronate

H. HAYASHI, Y. TAKAO, K. OSHIMA and S. KYONO
Fukuoka, Japan

Introduction

Sodium hyaluronate is a substance of very high viscosity and is considered to be almost non-stimulating and non-toxic to living tissues (Balazs and Sweeny, 1966). On the basis of these characteristics, the substance has been injected into the anterior chamber and the vitreous cavity in order to preserve intraocular space during intraocular surgery. In cases of keratoplasty (Miller and Stegman, 1981), intraocular lens implantation (Miller and Stegman, 1980), and surgery for glaucoma (Pape and Balazs, 1980), favourable results of the use of sodium hyaluronate have been reported.

In retinal detachment and vitreous surgery, on the other hand, the injection of sodium hyaluronate into the vitreous cavity may induce such complications as transient vitreous opacification. No definite evaluation of the substance has thus been obtained yet (Pruett, Schepens and Swann, 1979; Stenkuls et al., 1981).

When vitreous or intraocular tamponade is undertaken in patients with severe vitreoretinal disease, opacification of the media may occur soon after surgery, necessitating postoperative intraocular examination by ultrasonography (Hayashi, Oshima and Takao, 1983). The presence of substances like gas or silicon oil in the vitreous cavity, whose ultrasonic characteristics differ from that of living tissues, frequently causes severe distortion of the ultrasonogram, interfering with its reading. Therefore, substances used for intraocular tamponade, in particular silicon oil, have been studied in terms of their ultrasonic characteristics and their influence on the ultrasonogram (Verbeek et al., 1981). However, no reports exist to date on sodium hyaluronate.

In this study, the ultrasonic characteristics of sodium hyaluronate and the ultrasonograms obtained when this substance was injected into the vitreous cavity of rabbits were examined prior to the clinical application of sodium hyaluronate into the vitreous cavity.

K.C. Ossoinig (editor), Ophthalmic Echography, ISBN 978-94-010-7988-4

Experimental methods

Materials and equipment

For the experiment, a 1% intraocular injection solution of Sodium hyaluronate (Pharmacia AB) as supplied by the Green Cross Corporation was used. The sound velocity in 1% sodium hyaluronate was determined using the axial length measurement unit of the Ophthalmoscan-Model 200 made by Sonometrics Inc. with a 10-MHz probe (Coleman et al., 1969). A ZK 2560 instrument made by General Corp. (Tane et al., 1983) was used for other parts of the experiments. A- and B-mode images were displayed using 10-MHz and 7.5-MHz probes at sensitivities of −6 dB and −12 dB, respectively.

Measurement of the sound velocity in 1% sodium hyaluronate

The ultrasonic probes were connected to a vertical micromanipulator according to the method described by Thijssen et al. (1981). The tips of the probes were immersed in 1% sodium hyaluronate in a glass vial. The probes were aligned so that the bottom of the container was reached by a perpendicular sound beam; they were moved in 0.5 mm steps over a range of 10 mm from the bottom to measure the echo return time of the sound waves from the bottom of the vial at each point. The distances between the glass bottom and the probes, and the echo return times were plotted to calculate the sound velocity. These experiments were undertaken at 35° C.

Internal echoes from 1% sodium hyaluronate

Degassed pure water was gently poured into the glass vial containing 1% sodium hyaluronate according to the superposition method. The 10-MHz probe was saturated in the mixture and echoes were observed. The pure water was then removed and allowed to remain at 4° C overnight or was subjected to vacuum degassing, after which echoes were observed. Furthermore, 1% sodium hyaluronate was taken into a syringe and was observed in the same vial. After being allowed to stand, the echoes were observed. Finally, 1% sodium hyaluronate and pure water were placed in separate vials, and silicon oil was added to each of them by superposition for observation.

Observation of ultrasonograms from rabbit eyes given intravitreal injections of 1% sodium hyaluronate

According to the previously mentioned method (Hayashi and Oshima, 1980), 1% sodium hyaluronate was injected into the vitreous cavities of 10 mature

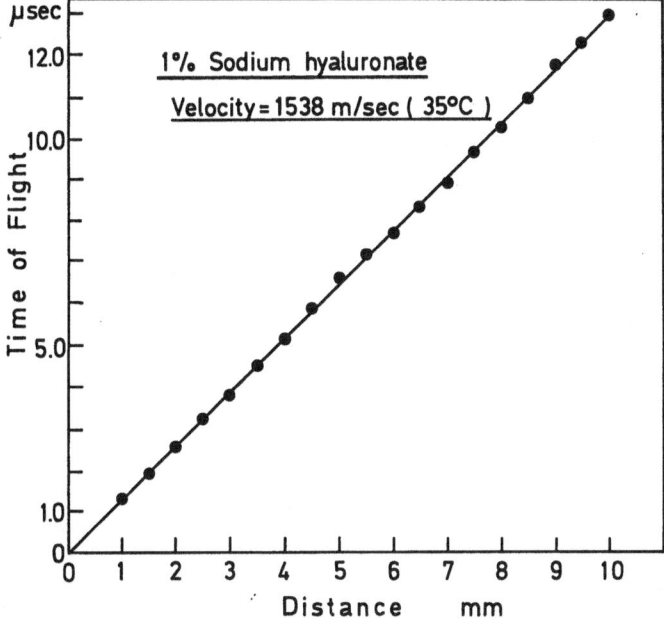

Fig. 1. Sound velocity curve in 1% sodium hyaluronate. Longitudinal axis: Time of flight. Horizontal axis: Distance between the probe and the reflection source.

rabbits. Ultrasonic A- and B-mode images were observed and photographed just before, and immediately after, injection. On the first day, and 1, 2, 3, and 4 weeks following the injections, changes were evaluated. The untreated fellow eyes as well as rabbit eyes that underwent plain vitrectomy were used as controls and were examined in the same fashion.

Results

Sound velocity in 1% sodium hyaluronate

The sound velocity in 1% sodium hyaluronate was calculated as 1538 m/sec at 35°C (Fig. 1). The sound velocity in water, determined under the same conditions, was 1539 m/sec.

Internal echoes in 1% sodium hyaluronate

Many air bubbles were observed macroscopically in 1% sodium hyaluronate immediately after it was placed into the glass vial. At this point in time, the

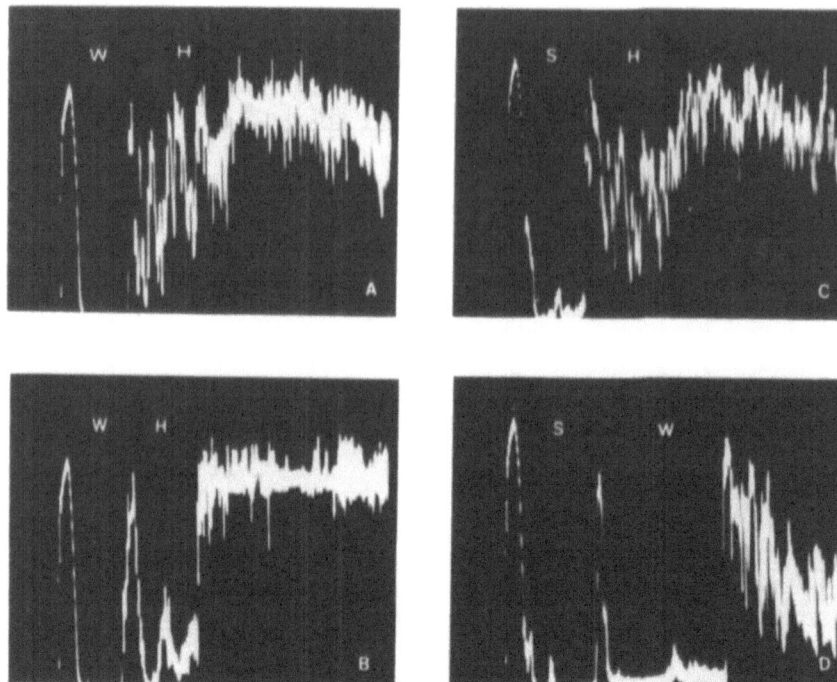

Fig. 2. Internal echoes (10 MHz probe) in 1% sodium hyaluronate in glass vials. A: pure water (W) immediately after injection of 1% sodium hyaluronate and 1% sodium hyaluronate (H). B: 1% sodium hyaluronate after standing overnight (H) and pure water (W). C: silicon oil (S) and 1% sodium hyaluronate (H). D: silicon oil (S) and pure water (W).

A-mode image revealed echoes of various intensities from the 1% sodium hyaluronate (Fig. 2). When the 1% sodium hyaluronate was allowed to remain undisturbed at 4° C overnight, or was subjected to vacuum degassing, the air bubbles disappeared macroscopically and, at the same time, the echo intensity in the A-mode display decreased (Fig. 3). When the 1% sodium hyaluronate was placed back into the glass vial using an injection syringe, air bubbles re-appeared and numerous echoes similar to those observed at the beginning were seen in the A-mode display. After leaving the container undisturbed overnight another time, the air bubbles disappeared and the echo intensities decreased again. The residual echoes persisted, however, even after the overnight rest period or following a vacuum degassing. Although no echoes (but a ringing artifact) appeared in the pure water superpositioned with silicon oil, many echoes were observed in 1% sodium hyaluronate under the same conditions (Fig. 2).

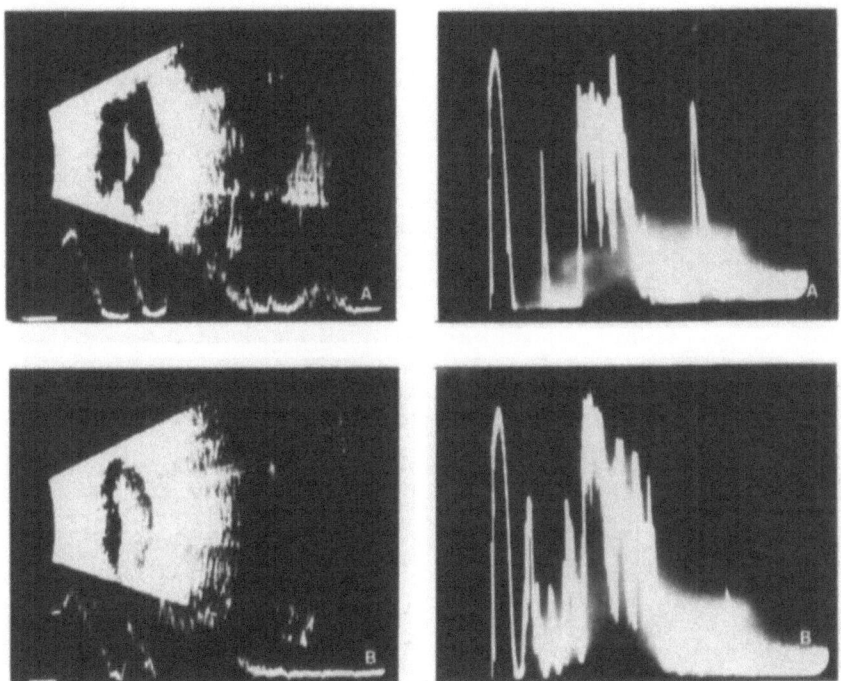

Fig. 3. Echograms of rabbit eyes before and after intravitreous injection of 1% sodium hyaluronate after vitrectomy. A: before injection. B: after injection.

Echograms of rabbit eyes with intravitreous injection of 1% sodium hyaluronate

Air bubbles were observed ophthalmoscopically in the vitreous cavity of the rabbit eyesimmediately after the injection of 1% sodium hyaluronate, and numerous scattered echoes appeared in the vitreous cavity in the ultrasonic A- and B-mode displays although none of them were observed prior to the injections (Fig. 3). However, there were no differences in the axial length or the curve of the retrobulbar wall in the ultrasonograms obtained before and after the injections. There were no echographic changes noted such as a weakening or a disappearance of the retrobulbar echoes as they are observed following the injection of silicon oil and gas. When plain vitrectomy alone was performed, no scattered echoes were noted like those observed in the eyes with an injection of 1% sodium hyaluronate (Fig. 4). These scattered echoes disappeared 1 to 2 weeks after the injections; simultaneously, the air bubbles in the vitreous cavity also disappeared (Fig. 5).

270

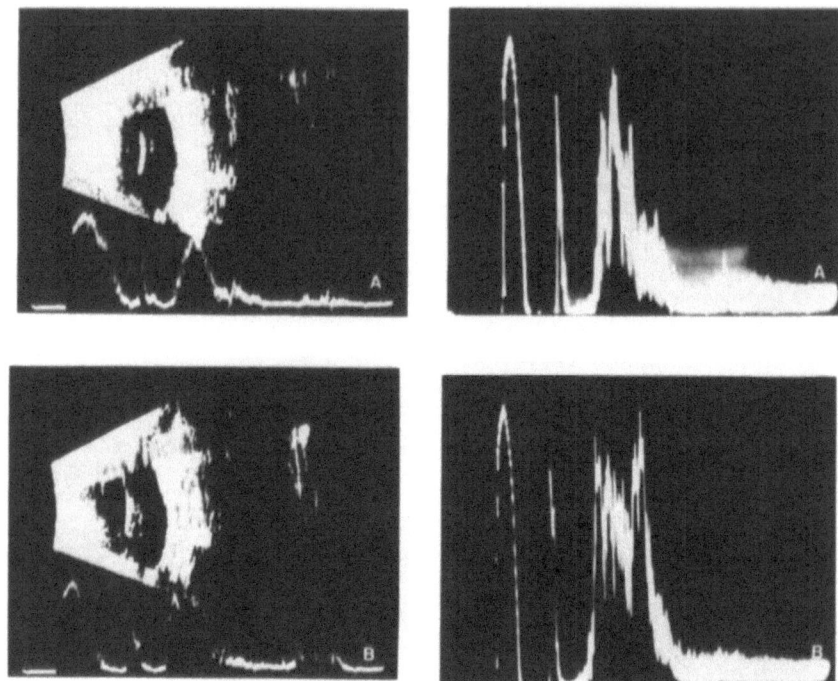

Fig. 4. Echograms of rabbit eyes after vitrectomy. A: before surgery. B: after surgery.

Discussion

The sound velocity of 1538 m/sec (35° C) in 1% sodium hyaluronate as determined in this study did not differ significantly from the sound velocity of 1539 m/sec (35°) in water determined by the same method. Both velocities are almost identical to the sound speed of 1532 m/sec (37° C) as known for the vitreous body (Jansson & Cock – 1962). For this reason, there is practically no change in intraocular sound velocity when the vitreous is replaced by 1% sodium hyaluronate. Unlike the injection of silicon oil which has the very slow sound velocity of 982 m/sec, the axial eye length in the echogram does not appear increased and the retrobulbar wall does not become flat, when 1% sodium hyaluronate is injected (Fig. 6). In fact, the morphological appearance of eyeballs in the echograms from rabbit eyes which had been injected with 1% sodium hyaluronate following vitrectomy did not differ from that before injection and was almost the same as that after replacement of the vitreous body with physiological saline solution following plain vitrectomy.

Numerous scattered echoes appearing in the vitreous cavity immediately after injections, were a definite change in the ultrasonograms induced by the

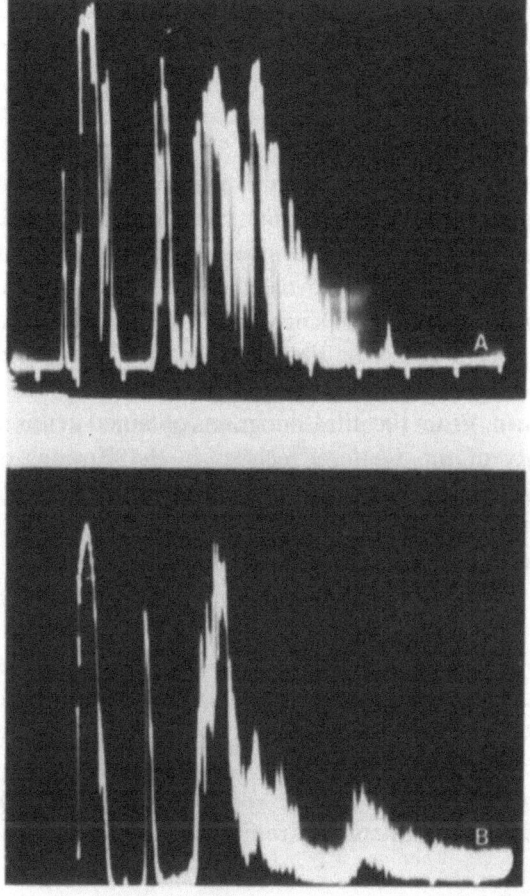

Fig. 5. Changes in A-mode echograms of rabbit eyes after intravitreous injection of 1% sodium hyaluronate. A: immediately after injection. B: one week after injection.

injection of 1% sodium hyaluronate. Although similar echoes are observed in the echograms before the injection of 1% sodium hyaluronate, they are considered to be scattered echoes due to air bubbles, because they are induced by the injection itself and they disappear like the air bubbles in 1% sodium hyaluronate after standing for some time or after vacuum degassing. Also, the air bubbles were ophthalmoscopically confirmed after intravitreal injection.

Scattered echoes are also observed to occur in water (in vitro). However, the echoes do not appear in ultrasonograms even if the vitreous is replaced. Therefore, the echoes appearing in the vitreous cavity seem to be specific to sodium hyaluronate. They should reflect the uptake of a large number of air bubbles in sodium hyaluronate because of its very high viscosity.

The present experiment did not explain the reason for the remaining echoes after degassing where air bubbles in sodium hyaluronate disappeared. It is believed that the gaseous components in 1% sodium hyaluronate cannot be removed completely even by vacuum degassing (personal communication from Pharmacia Laboratory, 1983). Therefore it is possible that invisibly small air bubbles remain.

The attenuation coefficient in sodium hyaluronate has not been defined in this series since the air bubbles in sodium hyaluronate change the density and distribution in each experiment. However, the ultrasonograms from eyes with intravitreal sodium hyaluronate revealed no attenuation of posterior pole and retrobulbar signals as seen with silicon oil. The sound attenuation in sodium hyaluronate is considered to be similar to that of water or vitreous.

The process of absorption of sodium hyaluronate from the vitreous cavity remains unknown. From the ultrasonograms obtained in this study, it appears that the density of the scattered echoes in the vitreous cavity decreases markedly, indicating a decrease in concentration. Further studies should be done in the future.

From the results of this study, the following knowledge may be deducted for the reading of ultrasonograms from eyes after intravitreal injection of sodium hyaluronate:

1. 1% sodium hyaluronate in the vitreous cavity does not influence the ultra-sonographic axial length measurement or the globe contour appearance.
2. Scattered echoes appearing after injection are very possibly due to sodium hyaluronate itself.
3. The membranous echoes in the vitreous cavity after injection suggest vitreous membrane or detached retina, as in usual findings.

Summary

We studied the ultrasonic characteristics of sodium hyaluronate and its influence on ultrasonograms when used for intravitreal injection. The sound velocity in 1% sodium hyaluronate for ophthalmic use was 1538 m/sec at 35° C (similar to the sound velocity in water and vitreous). Numerous scattered echoes appeared in the sodium hyaluronate after syringe injection into a container. The echoes disappeared after vacuum treatment or when leaving the container undisturbed overnight, leading to the assumption that the echoes were produced by air bubbles.

Intravitreal injection of sodium hyaluronate after vitrectomy in the rabbit eye had no effect on axial length or globe contour ultrasonically. Scattered echoes were observed in the vitreous cavity after injection which disappeared one to two weeks later.

References

Balazs EA, Sweeney DB. 1966. Replacement of the vitreous body of monkeys with reconstituted vitreous and hyaluronic acid. Streiff (ed.), Modern Problems in Ophthalmology, Surgery of Retinal Vascular disease and Prophyractic treatment of Retinal Detachment. Amersfoort, 1963, 230–232, Karger, Basel.

Colman DJ, Konig WF, Katz LA. 1969. A hand-operated ultrasound scan system for ophthalmic evaluation. Am J Ophthalmol 68: 258–265.

Hayashi H, Oshima K, Oshio Y, Nakamura M. 1982. Continuous in vivo measurement of intravitreous carbon dioxide tension and pH in normal rabbit eye and in the eye of rabbit and human during vitrectomy. Acta Soc Ophthalmol Jpn 86: 1184–1190.

Hayashi H, Oshima K, Takao Y. 1983. Use of ultrasonography in the management of eyes following vitrectomy. Jpn J of Clin Ophthalmol 37: 631–637.

Jansson F, Cock E. 1962. Determination of the velocity of ultrasound in the human lens and vitreous. Acta Ophthalmol 40: 420–425.

Miller D, Stegman R. 1980. Use of Na-hyaluronate in anterior segment eye surgery. Am Intra-Ocular Implant Soc J 6: 13–15.

Miller D, Stegman R. 1981. Use of Na-hyaluronate in corneal transplantation. J of Ocular Ther and Surg 1: 28–35.

Pape LG, Balazs EA. 1980. The use of sodium hyaluronate (HEALON) in human anterior segment surgery. Ophthalmol 87: 669–675.

Pruett RC, Schepens CL, Swann DA. 1979. Hyaluronic acid vitreous substitute. A six-year clinical evaluation. Arch Ophthalmol 97: 2325–2330.

Stenkula S, Ivert L. 1981. The use of sodium-hyaluronate (HEALON) in the treatment of retinal detachment. Ophthalmic Surgery 12: 435–437.

Tane M, Horikosi J, Shimizu Y. 1983. The studies on the ultrasonic diagnosis in ophthalmology (Report 16) The development and the clinical application of the home produced ophthalmic High-speed mechanical scanning ultrasonic diagnostic equipment. Acta Soc Ophthalmol Jpn 87: 79–84.

Verbeek AM, Bayer AL, Thijssen JM. 1981. Echographic diagnosis after silicon oil injection. In Docum Ophthal Proc Series ed. by Thijssen JM, Verbeek AM, Vol 29: 59–66, Dr W Junk Publishers, The Hague.

Detached retina versus dense fibrovascular membrane. Standardized A-scan and B-scan criteria

K.C. OSSOINIG, G. ISLAS, G.E. TAMAYO and C. TAMBURRELLI*
Iowa City, USA

Introduction

Simple rhegmatogenous retinal detachments and simple fibrovascular strands or membranes can be differentiated from each other with either B-scan or Standardized A-scan to a high degree of accuracy. However, in most complicated cases, particularly in ocular trauma and in diabetic retinopathy, a number of Standardized A-scan and B-scan criteria must be combined to arrive at a safe diagnosis [1]. Some of the more important as well as some of the lesser known echographic criteria will be explained and discussed in this report.

B-scan criteria

The topography and shape of membranous signals in B-scan echograms have been stressed as important differential criteria in most publications dealing with this subject. It should be noted here that the B-scan finding of a funnel-shaped membrane inserting into the disk is frequently, but by no means always, indicative of total retinal detachment. Quantitative A-scan echography [2] is definitely needed to make the diagnosis of a total retinal detachment a safe one. Quantitation includes the funnel-shaped membrane as well as the prescleral layer in these cases. The strongest and most reliable B-scan evidence of retinal detachment is produced by certain characteristic shapes of signals such as a triangular appearance, a tent-like elevation (Fig. 3), and a cyst formation.

*From the Echographic Service in the Department of Ophthalmology, University of Iowa Hospitals and Clinics. This research was supported in part by an unrestricted grant from Research to Prevent Blindness.
Offprint requests to Karl C. Ossoinig, M.D., C.S. O'Brien Library, Department of Ophthalmology, University of Iowa Hospitals, Iowa City, Iowa 52242, U.S.A.

K.C. Ossoinig (editor), Ophthalmic Echography, ISBN 978-94-010-7988-4

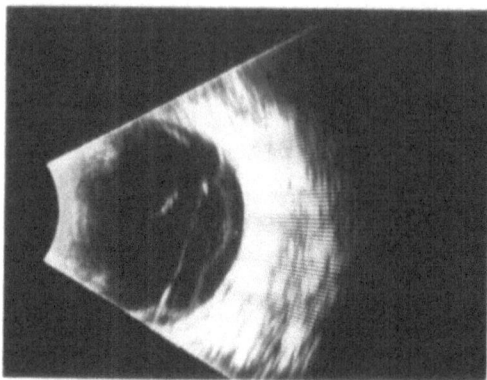

Fig. 1. B-scan echogram from eye with tractional retinal detachment displaying typical hammock shape.

Another lesser known, but very helpful, B-scan finding in non-total retinal detachments is the continuity of the detached surface line with the fundus signal where the retina is clearly on (Figs. 2 and 3). In order to enhance and safeguard this criterion, the echographer must make the effort to center the transition area between the detached and attached surfaces in the B-scan echogram. Only then the echographic resolution is sufficient to clearly show the continuity of the surfaces, and only then artifacts are prevented from interfering with this important echographic sign.

A frequent, though less reliable, B-scan sign of detached retina is the presence of 'macro-folds' as illustrated in Figs. 4, 5, and 8. Such folds, combined with a stiffness of the structure as indicated by the total absence of

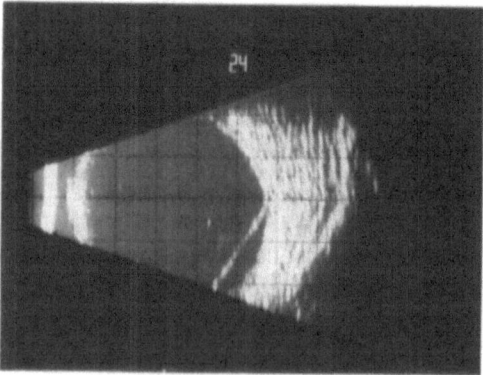

Fig. 2. B-scan echogram from eye with partial retinal detachment. Note the continuity of the detached retinal signal with the attached retinal line. System sensitivity was decreased and the transition area between the detached and attached portions of the retina were centered in the echogram for optimal resolution and clear indication of this differential criterion.

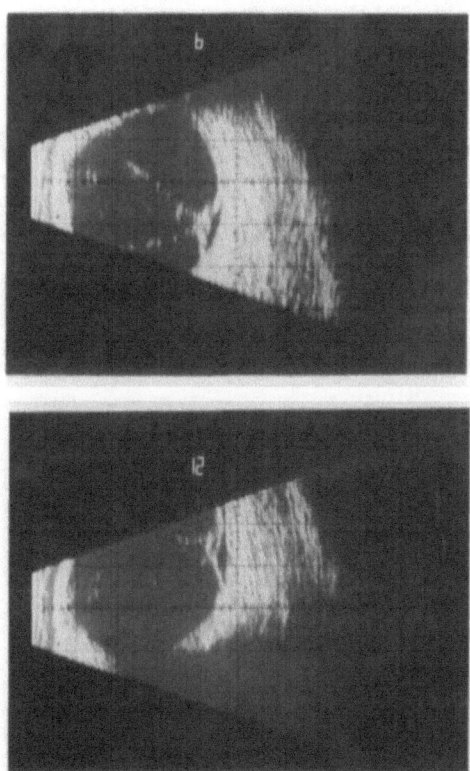

Fig. 3. B-scans from eye with tractional retinal detachment (tent-like elevation of retina). The transition zones between detached and attached portions of the retina on either side of the detachment were centered in the echogram in order to utilize this continuity criterion for the differential diagnosis (in addition to the typical shape). Note that the system sensitivity was adjusted differently in each situation to optimize resolution.

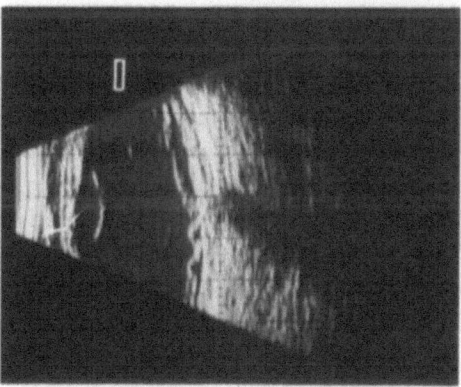

Fig. 4. B-scan from eye with shallow retinal detachment. Note the large (and stiff, as evidenced during kinetic echography) folds of the detached retina (PVR).

278

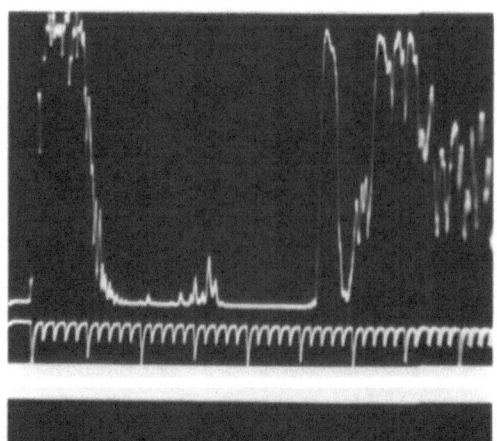

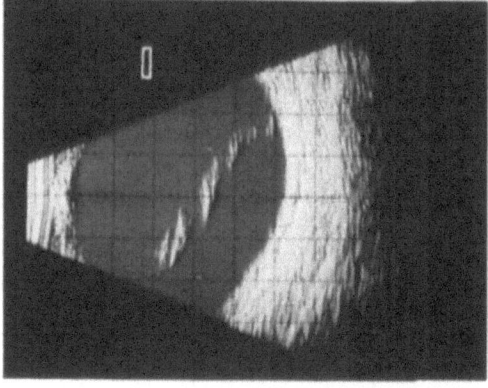

Fig. 5. A-scan and B-scan from eye with retinal detachment. The A-scan spike from the detached retina is high and overloaded. Its left ascending limb typically rises in a sharp and steep fashion with only very few long-stretched high-frequency nodules throughout its course. The B-scan displays typical macro-folds of the detached surface.

aftermovement in kinetic B-scan echography [3] and the absence of horizontal aftermovement in kinetic A-scan echography, indicate proliferative vitreo-retinopathy (PVR). If the retinal surface continues to be very smooth despite these proliferative changes, the B-scan line appears interrupted (Figs. 5, 8). While macro-folds often indicate a detached folded retina, they also may occasionally occur in posterior vitreous detachment (Fig. 6). In this case, the posterior vitreous surface is folded, whereas the underlying detached retina produces rather straight echo lines (folds appear much less obvious in this retinal signal than in the posterior vitreous membrane line).

A-scan criteria

The safest and most reliable echographic criterion is the specifically high

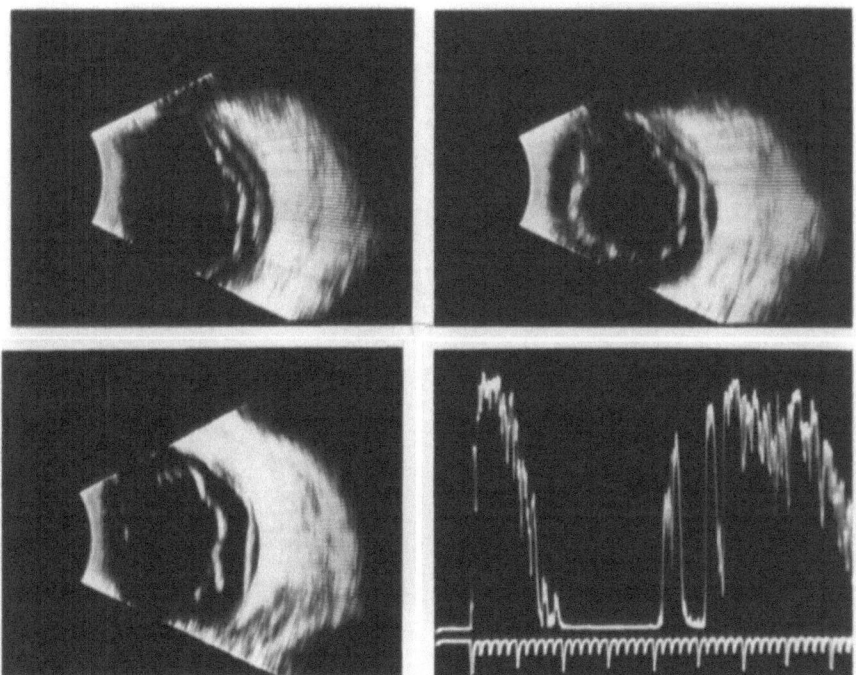

Fig. 6. B-scans and A-scan from eye with funnel-shaped posterior vitreous detachment and dense posterior vitreous membrane as well as localized retinal detachment. Note that in this case it is the posterior vitreous membrane that displays macro-folds rather than the detached retina which, for the most part, appears fairly stretched. Also note the difference in the ascending limbs of the maximal spikes from the vitreous membrane (interrupted by peaks) and the retina (sharply rising without any interruption and with few, hardly visible, long-stretched high-frequency nodules) in the much more diagnostic A-scan in this case.

reflectivity of a detached retina as compared to even the densest fibrovascular membranes [2]. When comparing the maximal signal from a detached surface with that from the inner scleral surface of the same eye, the difference in decibels (delta db) indicates whether the detached surface surely is the retina (delta db is equal to, or smaller than, 15), is most likely not the retina, at least not a viable retina (delta db>20), or whether this quantitative measurement alone is insufficient to differentiate between the two conditions (delta db between 16 and 19).

When performing this quantitative echography, one should keep several rules in mind:

Only the strongest maximal signals from the detached surface and from the sclera are to be used. The measurement requires Standardized A-scan (Kretz 7200 MA, Ophthascan S, or Sonokretz units). The measurement is initiated by screening the detached surface at Tissue Sensitivity and searching for a par-

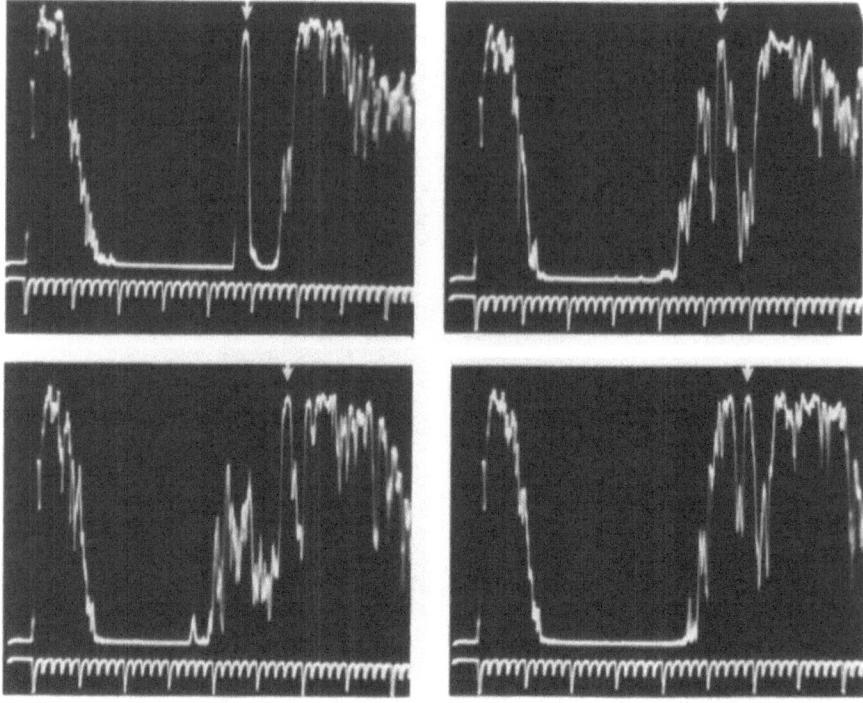

Fig. 7. A-scans from eye with dense vitreous membranes and extensive tractional retinal detachment. Note how sharply the left limbs of the high, overloaded retinal spikes (arrows) rise and how few long-stretched high-frequency oscillations are contained wihin these limbs. By contrast, even the maximized spike of the fibrovascular membrane overlying the retin rises only slowly with many interruptions by peaks (right bottom echogram).

ticularly strong, overloaded signal from this surface. Then system sensitivity is decreased while the probe and sound beam are slightly angled and minimally shifted in order to produce a maximal signal of the height indicated by the measuring line. Maximal signals (ideally perpendicular sound-beam exposures of rather even portions of the surface which is centered in the beam) are recognized not only from their height, but also from their sharp rise – a sharply rising left ascending limb of the spike either devoid of, or containing only a minimal number of, thinned high-frequency nodules along that limb. The strongest maximal signal from the inner scleral surface is usually obtained from the inferior meridians and a fairly anterior periphery of the globe. A maximal scleral signal at medium spike height is usually solitary. The signals from the prescleral layer, the outer scleral surface and the orbit (except for bony signals) are then below threshold. When quantitating a surface near the ora serrata in a phakic eye, the critical value is 18 rather than 15 decibels due to sound attenuation of part of the oncoming beam by the lens. In eyes with

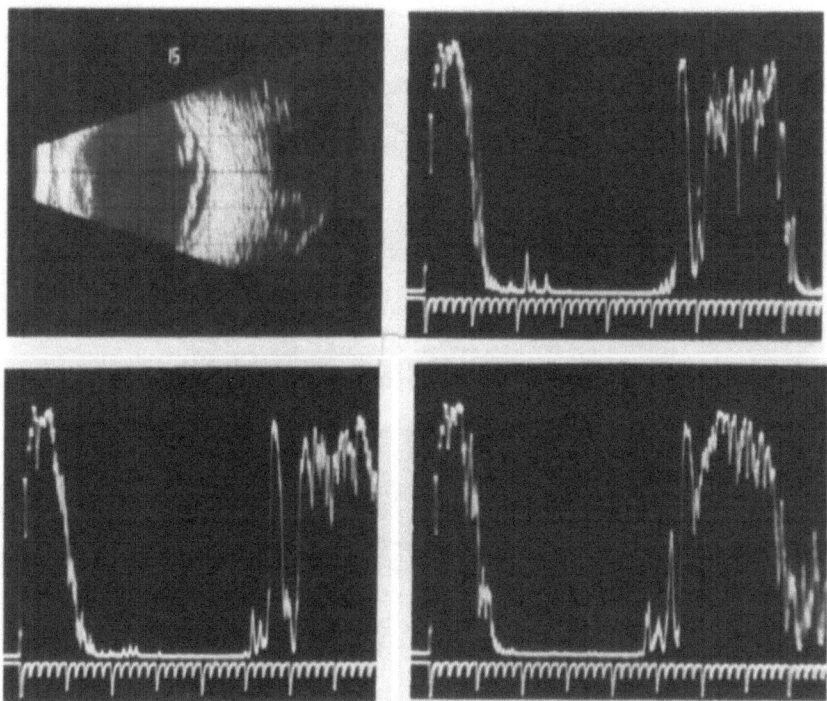

Fig. 8. B-scan and A-scans from eye with extensive tractional retinal detachment. Despite the (typical) macrofolds evidenced in the B-scan, the maximized (very high and overloaded) retinal spikes display the specific sharp rise of their left limbs with few thinned (long-stretched) high-frequency nodules. Because of rather oblique sound-beam incidence at the pigment epithelium behind the detached retina (tractional detachments usually are not parallel to the fundus), the narrow subretinal space seems to contain reflective sources (artifact).

severe hypotony (smaller size, shrunken sclera), in perforated globes, in microphthalmic eyes and also in the eyes of newborns or very young infants, the sclera cannot be used for such quantitation. In such cases, a normal fellow eye or the lowest decibel reading from a sclera known for the instrument and probe utilized in such quantitation, may be applied for the calculation of delta db values.

The same quantitative procedures are also applied to determine the delta db between the strongest maximal signal from the inner scleral surface and the maximal signals obtained from the prescleral layer surface. This is the surface of the pigment epithelium behind a detached retina (delta db equals 14 or more), or the inner retinal surface if the retina is attached and the detached surface belongs to a fibrovascular membrane (delta db equals 12 or less in this case). Again, there is a borderline range (delta db of 13) that does not allow differentiation between the two conditions on the basis of such measurement.

282

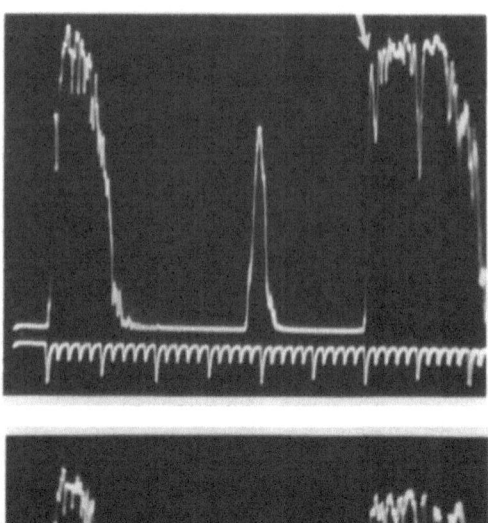

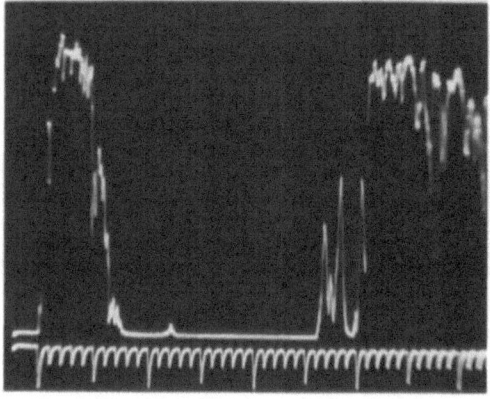

Fig. 9. A-scans from eye with total, funnel-shaped retinal detachment (top) and from eye with funnel-shaped, dense fibrovascular membrane (bottom). Both echograms were obtained from the most anterior fundus (ora serrata, top echogram; vitreous base, bottom echogram). The retinal spike (arrow) rises sharply and highly near the ora (may be low and multi-peaked and thus non-characteristic posteriorly where the retina is folded in a narrow funnel). The vitreous membrane becomes fluffy and produces several low spikes (bottom echogram) near the vitreous base, while it is much denser (producing high spikes) posteriorly. The membrane spike 'falls apart' when the beam shifts anteriorly, whereas the retina spike 'builds up' as the beam approaches the ora serrata.

Finally, the maximal echoes from the detached surface and the prescleral layer are compared to each other. If the detached surface is as reflective as, or more reflective than, the surface of the prescleral layer, a detached retina is indicated.

While the results of this quantitative echography provide the single most reliable and most accurate echographic criterion for the differentiation between a detached retina and a dense fibrovascular membrane in approximately two-thirds of all cases, the measurements are either borderline (and thus not that useful), or quantitative echography is not applicable, in another one-third of the cases. Such quantitative echography may be unnecessary in a number of cases when other more easily and quickly obtained A-scan and B-scan criteria enable the echographer to safely diagnose or rule out retinal detachment. Also, quantitative echography requires a meticulous approach and is a time-consuming effort. But in about one third of all cases, quantitative A-scan ecography remains the key to a reliable and safe differential diagnosis between retinal detachments and dense fibrovascular membranes.

Although it has thus far been insufficiently stressed in the literature, the easiest as well as very accurate Standardized A-scan criterion for determining a detached retina versus a dense fibrovascular membrane is the appearance of the left ascending limb of the maximized spike from a detached surface when evaluated at Tissue Sensitivity. Detached retinas produce sharply rising ascending limbs of their 100% high maximal spikes, which contain only minimal numbers of, thin and long-stretched high-frequency nodules (Fig. 5–9). In contrast, even the strongest signals received from dense fibrovascular membranes rise much more slowly containing several high-frequency nodules and often peaks which interrupt their left ascending limbs (Figs. 6 and 7). This particular criterion is always used by us first (in an initial screening of the posterior segment of an eye with opaque media) as a prompt and easy indicator of whether retinal detachment is present or not.

Another important, and often very helpful, A-scan criterion is the appearance of the maximal surface spike near the periphery of the fundus. If a detached surface extends toward the far periphery (toward the ora serrata or the vitreous base), the sound beam is shifted along this surface toward the periphery in an attempt to display the maximal height of the surface signal. Retinal detachment is indicated if, during the shift, the surface spike begins to rise steeply and high as it approaches the fundus signals (Fig. 9, top echogram). A membrane is indicated if, during this procedure, the surface signal falls apart and splits into several lower spikes (the membrane becomes fluffy as it inserts into the wide vitreous base; see bottom echogram in Fig. 9), or if the surface signal disappears before fusing with the fundus spikes (the membrane fades out).

Conclusion

With Standardized Echography, retinal detachment can be safely diagnosed and differentiated from dense fibrovascular membranes. Several A-scan and B-scan criteria must be combined in order to arrive at a reliable and accurate diagnosis. These important criteria, as discussed in this paper and as indicative of retinal detachment, are: a sharp rise of a 100% high maximal surface spike with only a few high-frequency nodules appearing along its left ascending limb; formation of such a spike when the sound beam is shifted toward the ora serrata; specifically high reflectivity of the surface; typical shape of the surface; continuity of the detached surface with the fundus plane; and macrofolds. None of these criteria are necessarily specific and always present. However, a majority of these criteria usually apply; these enable the echographer to make a safe and accurate diagnosis.

References

1. Ossoinig KC. 1985. Standardized Ophthalmic Echography of the Eye, Orbit and Periorbital Region. A comprehensive Slide Set (774 Slides) and Study Guide, third ed., p. 44, Goodfellow Co., Iowa City.
2. Ossoinig KC. 1974. Quantitative Echography – The Basis of Tissue Differentiation. J Clin Ultrasound 2 (1): 33.
3. Ossoinig KC. 1979. Standardized Echography. Basic principles, clinical applications, and results. Int Ophthalmol Clin 19 (4): 127.

Intraocular cysticercosis: migratory

M. FISHMAN, B. KERMAN and S. FOXMAN
Los Angeles, USA

Introduction

Cysticercosis has been recognized as a lesion occurring in childhood that is often difficult to distinguish from retinoblastoma both clinically and ultra-sonographically. Also known as the 'bladderworm', cysticercosis cellulosae has a predilection for the central nervous system and eyes. It induces no inflammatory reaction when alive.

History

On April 25, 1984 a 33 year old hispanic male presented with marked intraocular inflammation, a retinal detachment and presumed intraocular cysticercosis.

The ultrasound on that date showed a structure compatible with cysticercosis in the superotemporal quadrant. The pattern consisted of a retinal detachment, sub-retinal cyst formation and a very high-reflective echo source contained within the lesion that showed moderate mobility, consistent with the scolex or head of the parasite (Figs. 1 and 2).

Ultrasound examination was repeated on May 16, 1984. The cystic structure was acoustically hollow indicating that the presumed scolex had disappeared, leaving the residual cystic lesion (Figs. 3 and 4).

Trans-scleral removal of the cyst was performed on May 16, 1984. The cyst was identified and removed with the help of a cryo-probe. By observation the cyst appeared clear and fluid filled. However, during the surgical procedure the cyst ruptured and the contents were lost.

K.C. Ossoinig (editor), Ophthalmic Echography, ISBN 978-94-010-7988-4

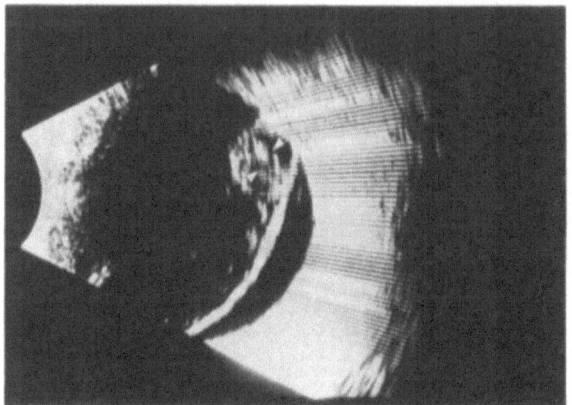

Fig. 1.

Discussion

According to various sources the cystic structure and scolex of cysticercosis can be easily identified ultrasonographically. We were able to document a clinically suspected cysticercosis echographically. Less than one month later we were able to document a major change in the ultrasonographic appearance of the sub-retinal cyst. This finding is consistent with either reabsorption or migration of the parasite.

Conclusion

In patients presenting with intraocular cystic lesions, with or without retinal detachment, the examiner must consider the possibility of intraocular cysticercosis, even if no scolex is seen.

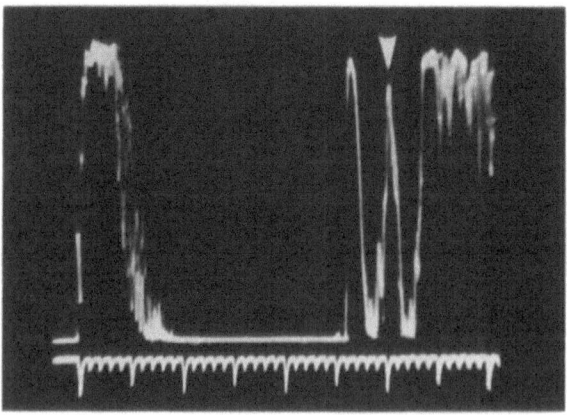

Fig. 2.

287

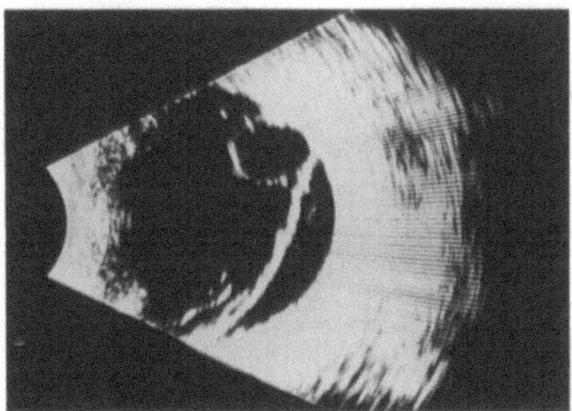

Fig. 3.

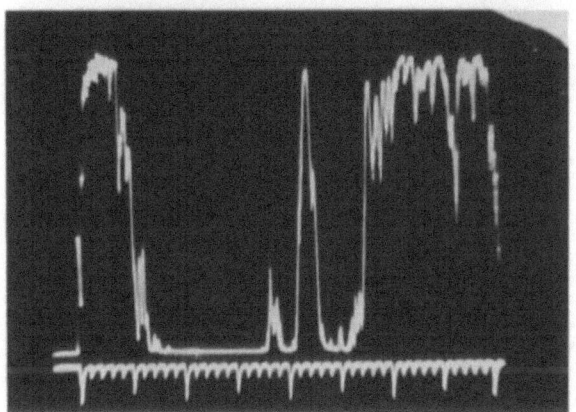

Fig. 4.

References

Hogan MJ, Zimmerman LE. 1962. Ophthalmic Pathology: An atlas and textbook. New York WB Saunders.

Moragrega E. 1983. Ultrasonic diagnosis of intraocular cysticercosis. Proceedings of the 9th Siduo Congress. Hillman JS & Le May MM (eds). The Hague: Junk.

Reese AB. 1976. Tumors of the Eye. Hagerstown Harper and Row.

Shammas HJ. 1984. Atlas of Ophthalmic Ultrasonography and Biometry. St. Louis CV Mosby.

Yanoff M, Fine B. 1975. Ocular Pathology. A Textbook and Atlas. Hagerstown Harper & Row.

Detection of macular disease in patients with opaque media

A.M. VERBEEK
Nijmegen, The Netherlands

Summary

Macular lesions with elevations or depressions to the surrounding tissue of 0.5 to 1.5 mm are detectable in patients with opaque media with accurate B-mode scanning. Often a combination of the patient's history, the clinical possibilities and the echographic findings can result in a probable diagnosis.

Introduction

According to the experience of several authors (Ossoinig 1972, Ossoinig et al. 1975, Coleman et al. 1977, Oksala 1977, Till and Hauff 1981, Dorn 1983) the lesions of the ocular fundus must be elevated at least 0.75 mm to be detectable and must be of more than 1.5 mm thickness to be differentiated by echography. Sometimes we can still diagnose a less prominent lesion because of the specific acoustic characteristics like e.g. the very high reflectivity of an optic nerve druse or of a choroidal osteoma. But in most cases the reflectivity of the pathologic tissue differs not so much from the surrounding tissue.

Materials and methods

Most of the lesions we studied – with exception of senile macular degenerations and tumours – had elevations or depressions to the directly surrounding tissue of 0.5 to 1.5 mm. Because the lesions are mostly of a small extension, they are very difficult to detect with the A-mode equipment. Topographic echography by using B-mode equipment (we used the Bronson-Turner contact B-scan) is the best way of examination while using the optic nerve as a landmark. During the scanning procedure we must give the patient a fixation point temporal to the examined eye to bypass the lens to avoid the lens artifact.

K.C. Ossoinig (editor), Ophthalmic Echography, ISBN 978-94-010-7988-4

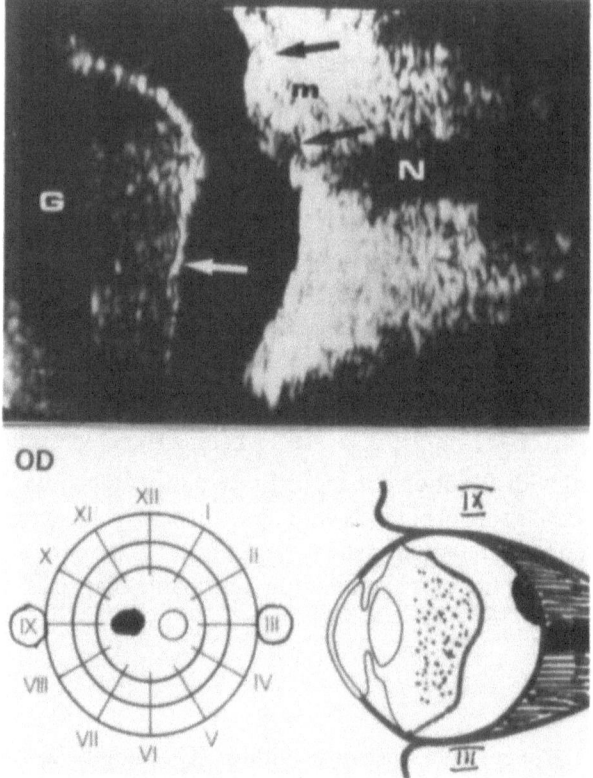

Fig. 1. B-mode echogram of a patient with S.M.D. (M: black arrows) with posterior vitreous detachment (white arrow) and disperse vitreous opacities (G). N = optic nerve.

Different sensitivity settings must be employed during the examination. If the macula area shows an abnormal aspect in B-mode topographic echography three possibilities can be distinguished: the macula area is smoothly elevated, shows an irregular surface or is depressed. An elevated macula area can be seen e.g. in edema, cystic lesions, degenerations, active chorioretinitis or tumours. An irregular surface of the macula area can be seen e.g. in macular pucker or choroidal rupture. A depressed macula area can exist e.g. in case of atrophic macular scar after a toxoplasmosis chorioretinitis.

Results

In 8 patients out of 45 with a sudden and dense vitreous hemorrhage of unknown etiology the probable diagnosis of fresh senile hemorrhagic macular degeneration was made and confirmed (Fig. 1). We found like Tani et al.

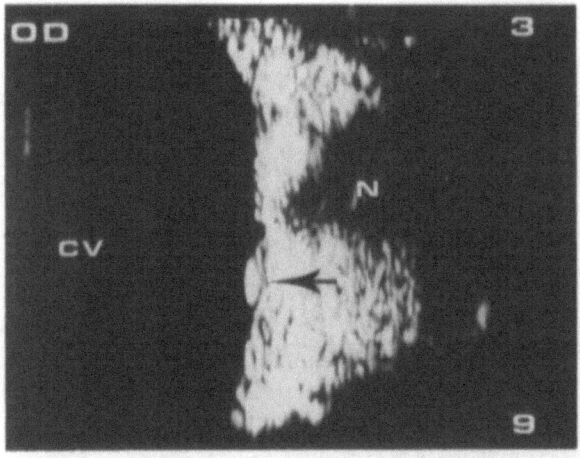

Fig. 2. B-mode echogram of a patient with cystoid macular edema (black arrow) in the meridian 3–9 o'clock. CV = vitreous cavity, N = optic nerve.

(1980) and Shields et al. (1976) a broad based elevated macula area with the elevation variable from 2.0 to 6.0 mm. So in these patients also the A-mode equipment was used. The internal reflectivity varied from low to medium while a choroidal excavation and signs of 'vascularity' were absent. In 4 patients a thick mobile posterior vitreous detachment was visible in 2 patients with a connection to the lesion. Growth during follow-up was never detected; regression could sometimes be seen during the following months. All fellow-eyes showed some degree of macular degeneration. In 12 patients with anterior segment opacities a smoothly elevated (0.5–1.0 mm) macula area was found suggestive, together with the patients history, for edema (Fig. 2) and they were all confirmed. In 2 patients the diagnosis of central serous retinopathy or serous detachment of the retinal pigment epithelium was suggested (Fig. 3) because the lesion was more prominent (1.5 mm). In 3 patients with opaque media after globe contusion the existence of a choroidal rupture was suggested based on the irregular aspect of the macula area and they were confirmed. In 4 patients the existence of a macular pucker was suggested based at the B-mode pictures seen at the lower sensitivity levels (Fig. 4). They suggest a pre-macular quite high reflective structure. In 2 patients with anterior segment opacities and an old history of toxoplasmosis chorioretinitis a depressed macula area especially at the low sensitivity settings was seen (Fig. 5) suggestive for an atrophic scar in the macula area.

292

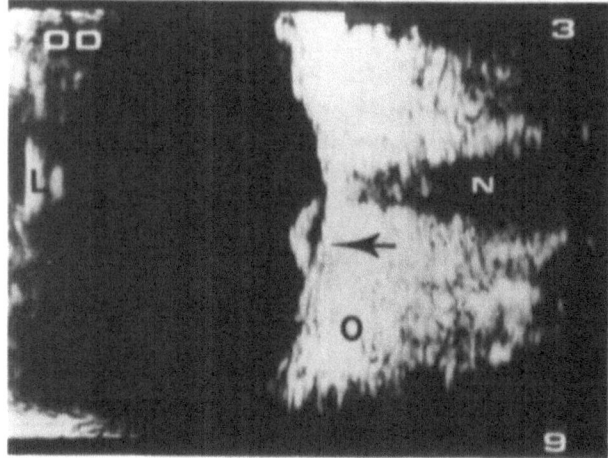

Fig. 3. B-mode echogram of a patient with a serous detachment of the R.P.E. (black arrow) L = lens, O = orbital fat, N = optic nerve.

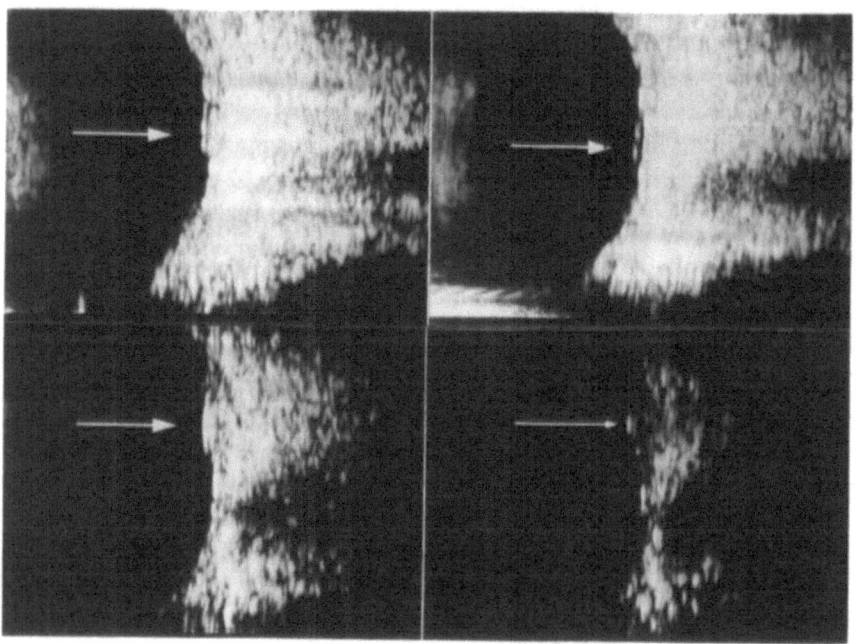

Fig. 4. B-mode echogram of a patient with macular pucker (white arrow). Sensitivity setting top right, top left: 90 dB, bottom left: 80 dB, bottom right: 70 dB.

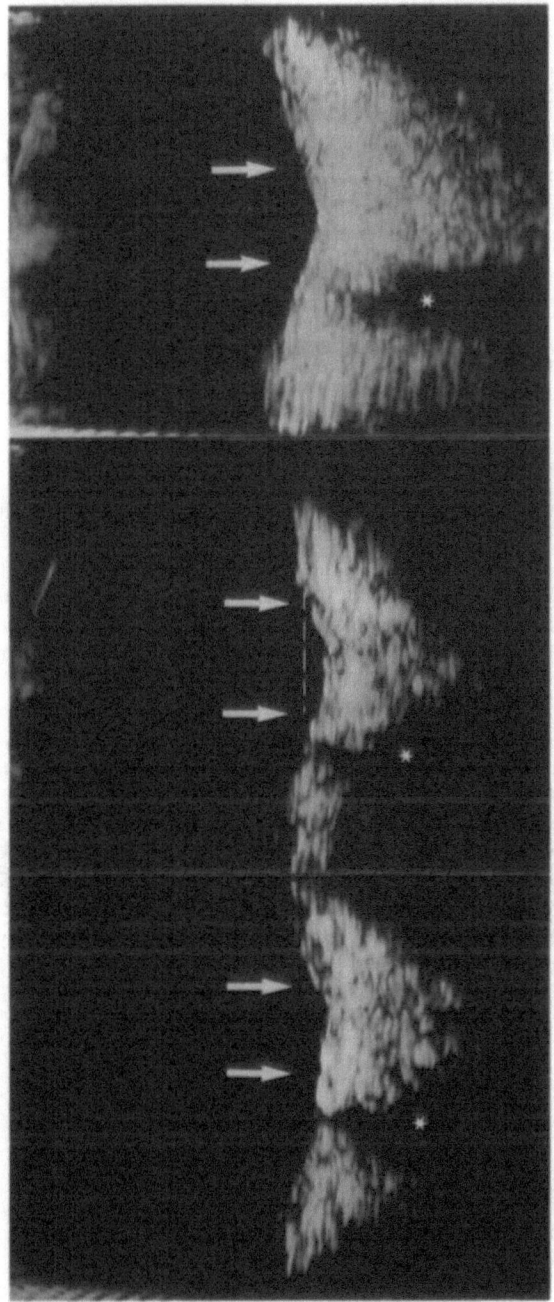

Fig. 5. B-mode echogram of a patient with an atrophic macular scar after toxoplasmosis chorioretinitis (white arrows) at different sensitivity settings.

Discussion

We are *not* suggesting that an accurate prospective diagnosis of macular lesions less prominent than 1.5 mm can be made with B-mode echography. What we have tried to show is that:
- with a good scanner.
- accurate scanning of the macula area.
- combining the history of the patient with the B-mode findings and some phantasy more often.
- a probable diagnosis can be made.

At least it can warn us in not promising the patient too much.

References

Coleman DJ, Lizzi F, Jack RL. 1977. Ultrasonography of the Eye and Orbit. Philadelphia, Lea and Febiger.

Dorn V. 1983. Experimental Imitations of the Less Prominent Lesions of the Fundus and their Echographic Analysis. In: Docum Ophthal Proc Series, Vol. 38 (Hillman JS, Le May MM, eds.) The Hague, Junk, p. 63–68.

Oksala A. 1977. Ultrasonic Findings in the Vitreous Space in Patients with Detachment of the Retina. Albrecht v. Graefes Arch klin exp Ophthalmol 202: 197.

Ossoinig KC. 1972. Clinical Echo-ophthalmography. In: Current Concepts in Ophthalmology III, (Blodi FC, ed.), St. Louis, Mosby, p. 101.

Ossoinig KC, Bigar R, Kaefring SL. 1975. Malignant Melanoma of the Choroid and Ciliary Body. Bibl Ophthal 83: 141.

Shields JA, McDonald PR, Leonard BC. 1976. Ultrasonography and [32]Ptest in Diagnosis of Malignant Melanomas in Eyes with Hazy Media. Tr Am Ophth Soc Vol LXXIV. p. 262–281.

Tani PM, Buettner H, Robertson DM. 1980. Massive Vitreous Hemorrhage and Senile Choroidal Degeneration. In: Am J Ophthalmol 90: p. 525–533.

Till P, Hauff W. 1981. Differential Diagnostic Results of Clinical Echography in Intraocular Tumours. In: Docum Ophthal Proc Series, Vol. 29 (Thijssen JM, Verbeek AM, eds.) The Hague, Junk, p. 91.

Ultrasonographic characteristics of Eales' disease

H. HAYASHI, Y. KITAGAWA, Y. TAKAO and K. OSHIMA
Fukuoka, Japan

Introduction

Most of the clinical studies of Eales' disease have been aimed at the changes of the retinal vasculature [1–4]. However, up until now little has been known about the gross structural changes of the vitreous and retina at the terminal stage of the disease, because of the obscuring properties of non-absorbing vitreous hemorrhage. Evaluation of the vitreo-retinal condition is necessary for planning the surgical treatment of the cases. In the present report we will describe the ultrasonographic characteristics of Eales' disease.

Subjects and methods

Diagnostic criteria

In eyes with clear media, the diagnosis of Eales' disease is based upon the presence of peripheral retinal vascular obstruction detected by ophthalmoscopy and IlsDlt fluorescein angiography. However, ophthalmoscopic examination was impossible in our cases due to vitreous hemorrhage before surgery.

Therefore, the cases in our study were selected according to the following criteria:
1) The cases with a history of recurrent vitreous hemorrhage.
2) Obliteration of the peripheral retinal vessel was found in healthy fellow eyes, in diseased eyes at the period with relatively clear vitreous during the course, and in the eyes during or after the vitrectomy.
3) Absence of systemic disease causing vessel obliteration and vitreous hemorrhage, e.g., diabetes, hypertension, sarcoidosis.

K.C. Ossoinig (editor), Ophthalmic Echography, ISBN 978-94-010-7988-4

Subjects

From May 1980 to November 1983, 18 eyes of 14 patients with long-standing vitreous hemorrhage were diagnosed in our department as Eales' disease according to the aforementioned criteria. The cases included 10 males ranging in age from 29 to 72 years (average 41.5 years).

Equipment and method

Combined A- and B-mode equipment of Ocuscan 410 (Sonometrix Systems, Inc.) and Ultrascan II (Xenotech, Inc.) was used for ultrasonic examination. As previously reported, the examination was performed with the contact method, and also the immersion method in several cases.

Ultrasonographic findings were confirmed by careful observation during the surgery. The results were compared with the ultrasonic findings of the cases with retinal vein occlusion and diabetic retinopathy.

Results

Table 1 presents the prevalence of the abnormalities diagnosed by ultrasonography in our series.

Hemorrhage in the vitreous cavity. Hemorrhage within the vitreous cavity could be detected in 17 of 18 eyes of the subject cases (94.4%). In 14 of the 17 eyes (77.8%), the hemorrhage was observed in the formed vitreous as scattered, point-like echoes (Fig. 1). The density of the intravitreous hemorrhage varied in each case. Hemorrhage behind the detached vitreous was seen in the remaining 3 eyes (16.6%).

Posterior vitreous detachment. Detachment of the formed vitreous was detected in fifteen (83.3%) of the 18 eyes. In one (6.7%) of the 15 eyes, the

Table 1. Prevalence of ultrasonic abnormalities on cases of Eales' disease.

	Retinal vein occlusion	Diabetic retinopathy	Eales' disease
none	4/25 (16.0%)	0/38 (0%)	1/15 (6.7%)
extensive	0/25 (0%)	20/38 (52.6%)	1/15 (6.7%)
posterior	21/25 (84.0%)	14/38 (36.8%)	7/15 (46.7%)
peripheral	0/25 (0%)	0/38 (0%)	3/15 (20.0%)
multiple	0/25 (0%)	4/38 (10.5%)	3/15 (20.0%)

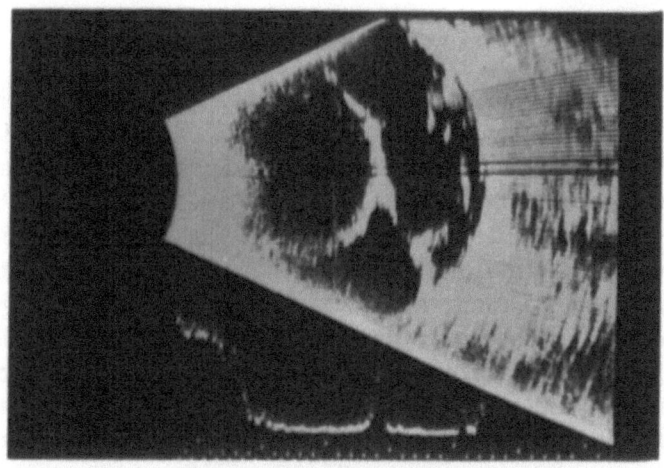

Fig. 1. Multiple, longitudinal vitreous adhesion associated with traction retinal detachment (Bridge & Girder).

posterior vitreous face was completely detached from the posterior ocular wall and formed a mobile membrane in the mid-vitreous cavity. In the other 14 eyes (93.3%), the detached posterior vitreous adhered to the ocular wall in various locations and to various extents, and formed a cone-shaped structure in the vitreous cavity. The mobility of the posterior vitreous varied from rigid to mobile in the cases examined. Adhesion was extensive in one (7.4%) of the 14 eyes and localized in 10 eyes (71.4%) (Fig. 2, 3). In the remaining 3 eyes (21.4%), adhesions were multiple, and arranged longitudinally from the peripheral to the posterior (Fig. 4), (Fig. 1). In the eyes with a single adhesion, the location of the adhesion was at the periphery in 3 eyes (21.4%), and at the posterior in 7 eyes (50%).

Retinal detachment. Retinal detachment was detected in 9 (50%) of the 18 eyes. An extensive detachment covering the posterior half of the ocular wall was seen in one eye (11.1%). In 8 eyes (88.9%), the detachment was localized in various positions on the posterior ocular wall. The retinal detachment was always associated with incomplete posterior vitreous detachment. On dynamic testing, the movement of the detached retina was either restricted or absent. The detachment was frequently tent-shaped and not convex. In addition to the findings above, the relationship between the detachment and vitreoretinal adhesion was found to be tractional in nature.

Discussion

The vitreous configuration in Eales' disease was markedly different from those in retinal vein occlusion and diabetic retinopathy (Table 2). In our series of 38 eyes with diabetic vitreous hemorrhage, detached posterior vitreous adhered extensively to the posterior retina in 63.2% of the cases, while one (6.7%) case of Eales' disease showed extensive adhesions. The vitreous pathology in Eales' disease also differed from the findings in 25 eyes of vitreous hemorrhage due to retinal vein occlusion where multiple peripheral adhesions were not found and where the incidence of complete posterior vitreous detachment was significantly high. A different pathology in the retinal vessels among the various diseases should contribute to the difference in the vitreous. Progressive occlusion of the peripheral vessel in Eales' disease should cause localized vitreous adhesions at the peripheral retina in contrast to the adhesion at the posterior retina in retinal vein occlusion in which the retinal vein occludes at the posterior pole, and to extensive vitreous adhesions in diabetes which induces concurrent extensive changes in the vessel.

The most important finding in Eales' disease was considered to be the multiple, longitudinal configurations of vitreous adhesion. In 3 eyes with multiple adhesions, longitudinal traction retinal detachment was associated along the adhesions as a 'bridge-girder' or 'monorail' (Fig. 1). During vitrectomy of these cases, a rigid retinal fold was observed extending from the

Table 2. Prevalence of vitreous abnormality detected by ultrasound in cases of retinal vein occlusion, diabetic retinopathy or Eales' disease.

Vitreous hemorrhage	Intravitreal	14/18 (77.8%)
	Sub-vitreal	3/18 (16.6%)
	Not detected	1/18 (5.6%)
Vitreous detachment	Detected	15/18 (83.3%)
	Not detected	3/15 (16.7%)
	Complete detachment	1/15 (6.7%)
	Incomplete detachment	14/15 (93.3%)
	Extensive adhesion	1/14 (7.4%)
	Posterior adhesion	7/14 (50.0%)
	Peripheral adhesion	3/14 (21.4%)
	Multiple adhesions	3/14 (21.4%)
Retinal detachment	Detected	9/18 (50.0%)
	Not detected	9/18 (50.0%)
	Extensive	1/9 (11.1%)
	Localised	8/9 (88.9%)

periphery toward the posterior pole. A schematic drawing of the eyes is presented in Figure 5. This phenomenon is probably due to progressive occlusion along one of the vessels and particularly to Eales' disease. Special attention must be given to the 'bridge-girder' shape since the retinal fold is difficult to flatten without using unusual techniques in vitrectomy, including intentional retinotomy.

References

1. Eales H. 1882. Primary retinal hemorrhage in young men. Ophthalmol Rev 1: 41–46.
2. Renie WA, Murphy RP et al. 1983. The evaluation of patients with Eales' disease. RETINA 3: 243–248.
3. Wadsworth OF (Summary by Jackson E). 1967. Recurrent retinal hemorrhage followed by the development of blood vessels in the vitreous. Ophthalmol Rev 6: 222–233.
4. Spitznas M, Meyer-Schwickerath G, Stephen B. 1975. The clinical picture of Eales' disease. Albrecht Von Graefes Arch Klin exp Ophthalmol 194: 73–85.

Ophthalmic ultrasound with a real-time small parts scanner

A.L. MABERLEY
Vancouver, Canada

Ophthalmic B-Scan echography was introduced and pioneered by G. Baum and I. Greenwood [1, 2] in the late 1950's and early 1960's. Coleman [3], Purnell [4] and others advanced the use and application of immersion B-Scan echography during the 1960's. Bronson [5] introduced the use of contact B-Scan ultrasonography and this has been followed by other contact B-Scan units during the 1970's. The commercially available units at least in North America include the Ocuscan 400 (Sonometrics), Ultrascan 2 (Cooper) and the Renaissance (Storz). All of these later units have utilized the B-Scan display and included the simultaneous or alternate use of A-Scan echography.

Since March of 1983 at the University of British Columbia we have used a Real Time Small Parts Unit for ocular and orbital evaluation. Initially, this was used as a stop gap measure when several of our other units wee not available. It is now however our preferred method for B-Scan echography.

This system was primarily designed as a peripheral vascular unit and is manufactured by Diasonics (DS-10) from Milpitas, California (Fig. 1). With little or no adjustment this unit can readily be used on the globe and the orbit. It provides simultaneous imaging and Doppler spectral analysis. The probes are either 7.5 or 10.0 MHz (Fig. 2), and the probe itself consists of a soft conforming membrane which acts much like a portable contact immersion system. Other features consist of a 26 bit microcomputer, a digital scan converter and an image memory $512 \times 512 \times 16$ bits. In addition, there is overlying and graphics memory.

The imaging system consists of a sector size of 28 degrees with approximately 2.5 cc width at skin surface. The frame rate at 20 frame 20 frames per second (FPS) in imaging only and 4 frames per second in Doppler mode. The overall system sensitivity is approximately 106 decibels.

The axial resolution with the 7.5 MHz transducer is .4 mm and with the 10 MHz transducer is .3 mm. The latter resolution with the 7.5 MHz transducer is .8 mm and with a 10 MHz units .6 mm. The penetration depth with 7.5 MHz transducer is 7.5 cc and with the 10 MHz transducer it is 3.8 cc.

K.C. Ossoinig (editor), Ophthalmic Echography, ISBN 978-94-010-7988-4

302

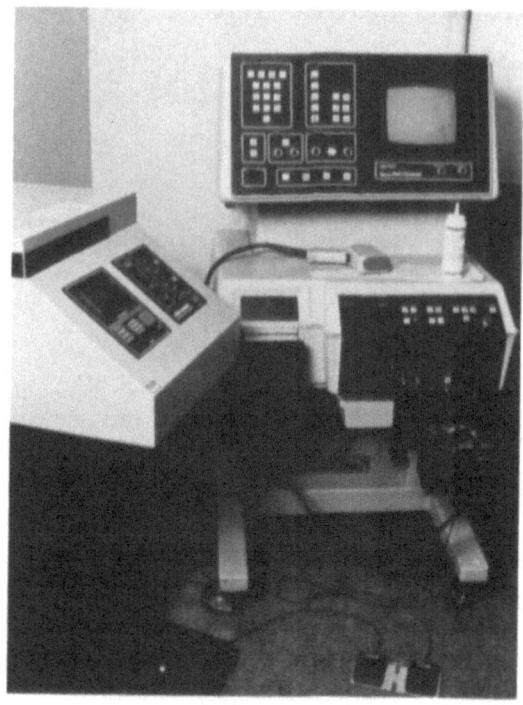

Fig. 1. Diasonics unit (DS-10) with screen, keyboard, multiformat processer, Polaroid camera and probe.

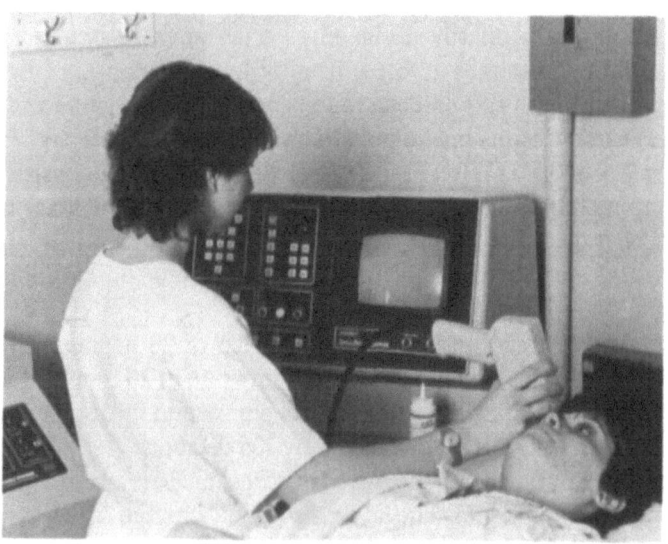

Fig. 2. Diasonics probe.

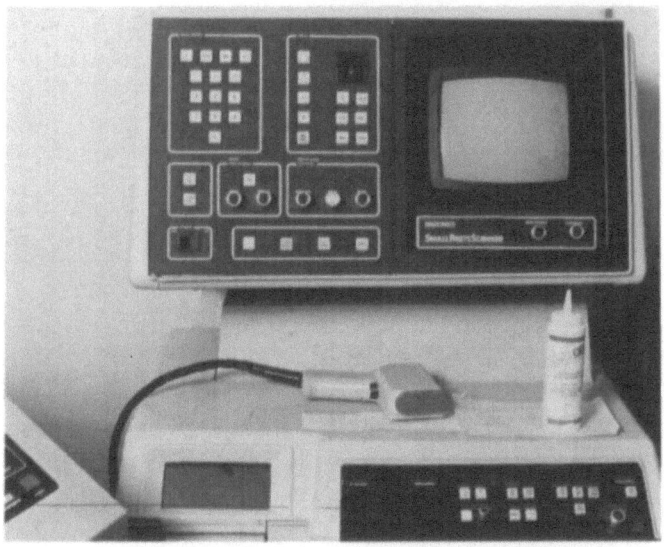

Fig. 3. Diasonics unit-close up of probe, screen and keyboard.

The image display has 64 shades of gray. There are five user selectable preprocessing curves and there is also post processing of the image gray scale. The 10 cm and 6 cm fields of view provide two times zoom magnification. There is freeze frame image storage and five different display modes.

a) The display modes consist of: Imaging only, imaging with Doppler beam cursor, a mixed mode display, a multigated spectrum and analyzer display #1 and a multigated spectrum analyzer display #2. The image only display is all that is required for ophthalmic work.

b) The on-screen display of the system parameters consists of (Fig. 3).

1. Pobe selection.
2. Field of view and magnification.
3. Transmitted power.
4. Compression curve selected.
5. Scan orientation either horizontal, oblique or vertical.
6. Depth gain control (DGC) settings.

Other features which we have found very useful on measuring approximate axial lengths or size of mass lesions consists of an electronic caliper for point to point distances, circumference area and area ratio measurement. There is in addition simultaneous polaroid photography, multi-formate and video systems available.

Up until November 1984 we had used this on a total of 1147 cases. These consisted of 987 ocular cases and 160 orbital cases (Figs. 4, 5, 6 and 7).

We have found it to be of excellent value when assessing complex vitreo-

304

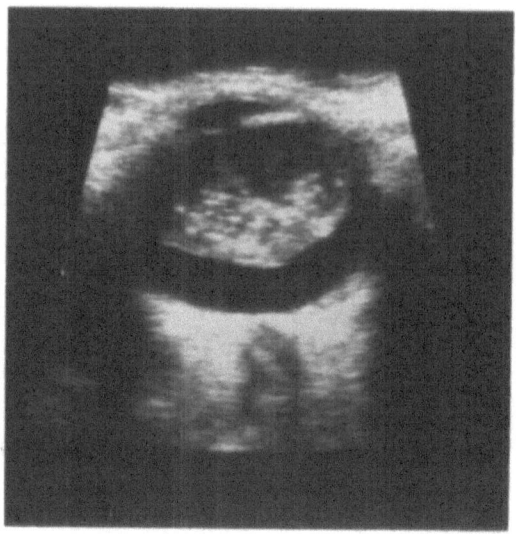

Fig. 4. Aphakic eye with diffuse vitreous hemorrhage and asteroid hyalosis.

retinal cases and in cases with severe trauma. It is also our preferred method to examining for intraocular mass lesions.

It very clearly delineates orbital mass lesions.

By virtue of the size of the transducer some lesions involving the floor and the roof of the orbit are somewhat difficult to evaluate. In addition it does have limitations when scanning for minimal enlargement of rectus muscles. A new

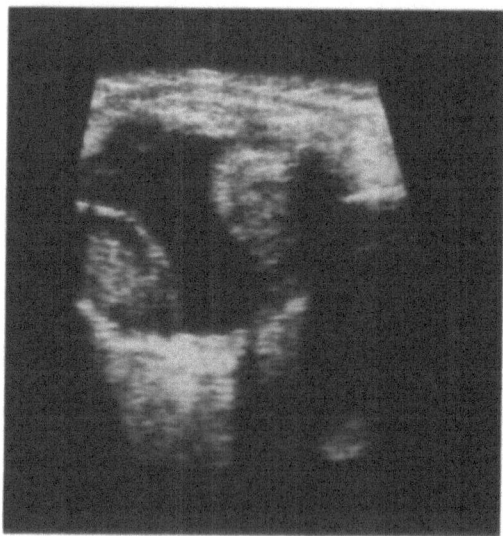

Fig. 5. Eye with large choroidal detachment – serous and hemorrhagic.

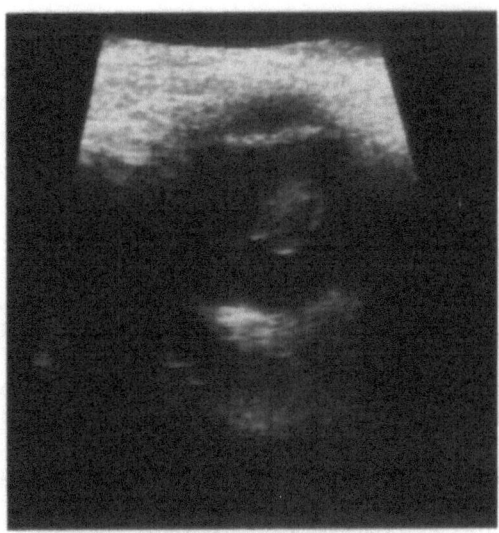

Fig. 6. Eye with dislocated cataractous lens.

smaller transducer is now available with this unit and this has certainly increased its overall versatility.

The major disadvantage of such a unit is its cost – double that of conventional ophthalmic units. If used in association with a large general ultrasound department this becomes less of a problem.

In summary, of the cases that we have evaluated this unit is certainly

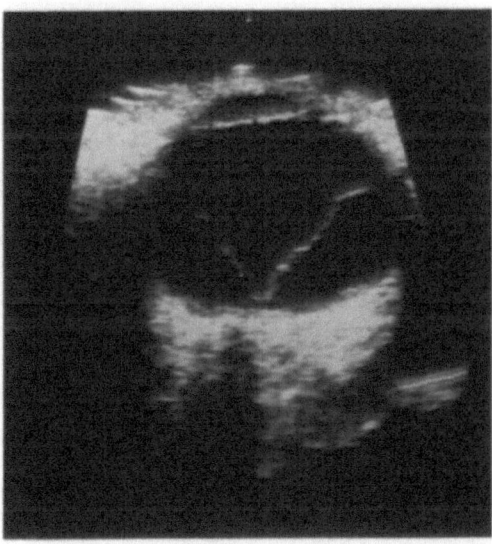

Fig. 7. Aphakic eye with vitreous hemorrhage and total retinal detachment.

superior to the other commercially available ophthalmic B-Scan units. It is hoped that with improved imaging systems and with more accurate tissue differentiation i.e. shades of gray, more units of this nature which are primarily ophthalmic in orientation will become available in future years.

References

1. Baum G, Greenwood I. 1958. The application of ultrasound locating techniques to ophthalmology: theoretic considerations and acoustic properties of ocular media. Part I Reflective Properties American Journal of Ophthalmology: 46 (Part II): 319–329.
2. Baum G, Greenwood I. 1958. The application of ultrasonic locating techniques to ophthalmology Part II Ultrasonic slit lamp in ultrasonic visualization of soft tissues. Arch Ophthalmology 60: 263–79.
3. Coleman DJ. 1973. Reliability of ocular tumour diagnosis with ultrasound Trans Am Acad Ophthal and Otolaryngol 77: OP 677–OP 686.
4. Purnell EW. 1966. Ultrasound in ophthalmological diagnosis. Grossman CC et al. eds. Diagnostic Ultrasound: proceedings of 1st International Conference of University of Pittsburgh 1965 New York Plenum Press, 95–110.
5. Bronson NR, Turner FT. 1973. A simple B-Scan ultrasound scope. Arch Ophthal 90: 237–.

Tissue characterization by computerized ultrasonic spectral analysis. Ocular tissues

S. TANE, J. KOHNO, A. KOMATSU, J. SUZUKI and J. HORIKOSHI
Kawasaki, Japan

Summary

Mathematical evaluation techniques to determine the calibrated power spectrum of reflected ultrasonic echoes from tissues involved by various ocular diseases can be used with a clinical computer system to objectively classify retinal detachment and vitreous hemorrhagic membrane. Tissue tructures can be acoustically stained in B-mode images to define the specific anatomic and structural properties that provide the acoustic differentiation. These data are obtained under in vivo conditions, and allow a noninvasive differentiation of intraocular membranes in a way not previously possible, aiding in the definitive diagnosis of intraocular diseases as well as in the planning and monitoring of treatment.

Although A-scan and B-scan imagings of ocular diseases are clinically important for differential diagnosis, much useful diagnostic information is not yet available through these procedures. However, wave spectral analysis by computer can gather much of the missing information, thereby providing material effective for diagnosis. Figure 1 shows a diagram of the experimental conditions.

In this study, we conducted spectral wave analysis of ultrasonic information from the eye by using a computeried wave form analyzer and attempted to make a differential diagnosis by wave form analysis, which is regarded as acoustic staining in the living body. B-mode images of ocular diseases were first obtained by a 10-MHz probe using the immersion method, and an A-mode beam was applied to the portion showing the most marked lesion. The radio-frequency signal of this portion was captured by oscilloscope and was then submitted to wave spectral analysis with a DATA 6000-Universal wave form analyzer.

According to the results of basic experiments in rabbit eyes, analysis of the reflected spectral echo-wave range of experimental retinal detachment re-

K.C. Ossoinig (editor), Ophthalmic Echography, ISBN 978-94-010-7988-4

308

(Block diagram of the data acquisition system)

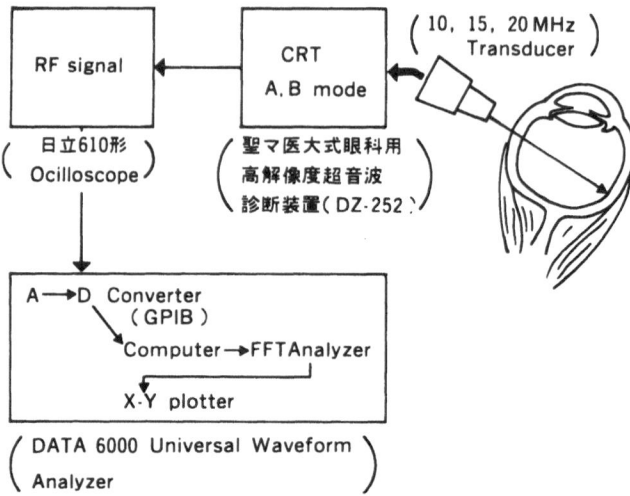

Fig. 1. Block diagram of the data acquisition system.

vealed a convex pattern with the maximum point of reflected spectral waves at 10 MHz, the same frequency as that of the transducer used. There was also a weak spectral echo-wave reflex between 10 and 50 MHz (Fig. 2).

Figure 3 shows the results of reflected spectral echo-wave analysis of rabbit eyes with experimental vitreous hemorrhage and experimental uveitis. The vitreous hemorrhage case on the left shows the maximum peak at about 10 MHz and a general, slightly flat pattern between 10 and 50 MHz. The uveitis case on the right shows marked peaks at about 10, 25 and 50 MHz in the whole

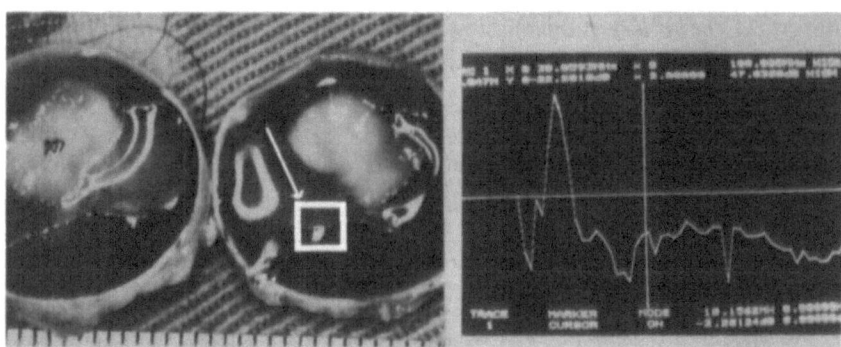

Fig. 2. The spectral analysis of RF signal of the A-scan ultrasonogram of a retinal detachment in rabbit eye. The contrasting overlay (BOX) outlines the area that can be digitized and displayed for computer analysis.

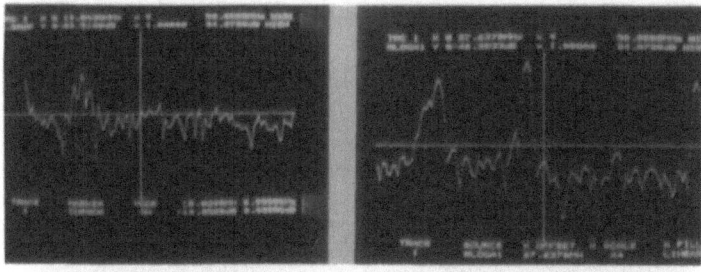

Fig. 3. The spectral analysis of the A-scan ultrasonograms of the experimental vitreous hemor-rhage (left) and vitreous opque due to experimental uveitis (right) in rabbit eyes.

range of reflected spectral echo-waves, which is due to the presence of multiple vitreous membrane formation inside the vitreous body (Fig. 3).

Next we examined human eyes with various ocular diseases. We examined 22 eyes with retinal detachment, 34 with vitreous hemorrhage and 16 with other ocular diseases, totaling 72 eyes.

As in the analysis using animal eyes, an analysis of human retinal detach-ment shows a convex pattern with the maximum point at around 10 MHz (the frequency of the transducer used), and a slightly flat pattern at the other frequencies (Fig. 4). Similar to previous cases, the maximum point of reflected waves was obtained at around 10 MHz, and a gradually increasing pattern was seen in the spectral range higher than 10 MHz.

Eyes with vitreous hemorrhage were examined as controls. There were no

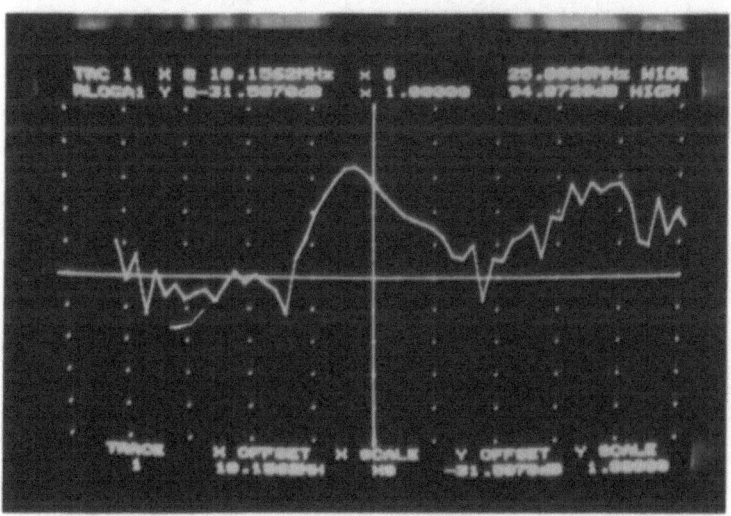

Fig. 4. The spectral analysis of the A-scan ultrasonogram of a case of retinal detachment.

310

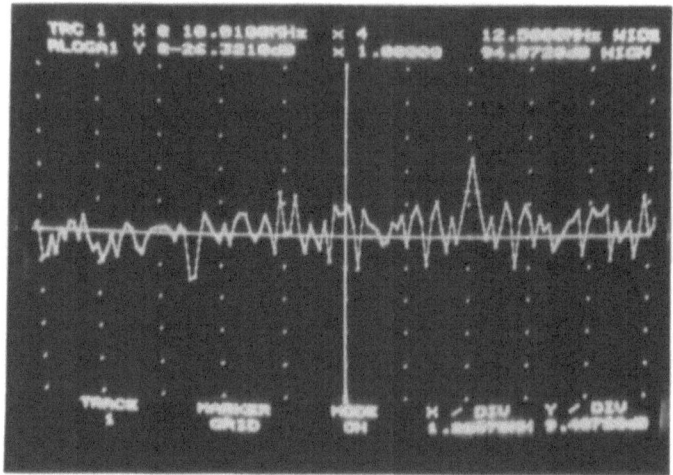

Fig. 5. The spectral analysis of the A-scan ultrasonogram of a case of fresh massive vitreous hemorrhage.

marked variations in the intensity of reflected spectral echo waves throughout the entire range. Thus, the pattern shown is flat (Fig. 5).

Next, a case of massive preretinal proliferation sowing vitreous hemorrhage accompanied by funnel-shaped proliferations of the vitreous membrane was examined. Large spectral waves representing diffuse reflection are seen throughout the entire range of reflected spectral echo waves (Fig. 6). Spectral analysis of a case of retinoblastoma showed a strong reflex at around 10 MHz.

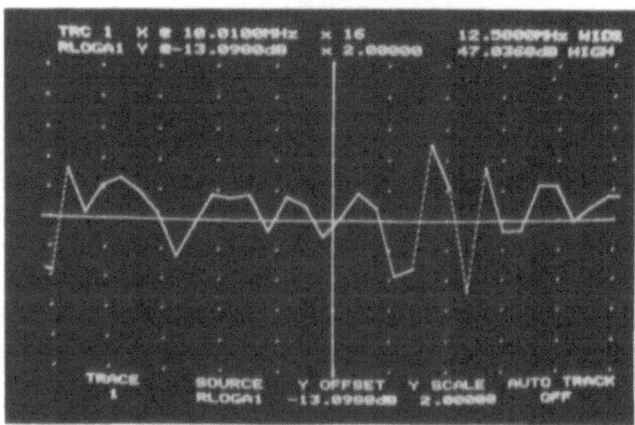

Fig. 6. The spectral analysis of A-scan ultrasonogram of a case of massivevitreous hemorrhage accompanied by funnel-shaped proliferation of the vitreous membrane.

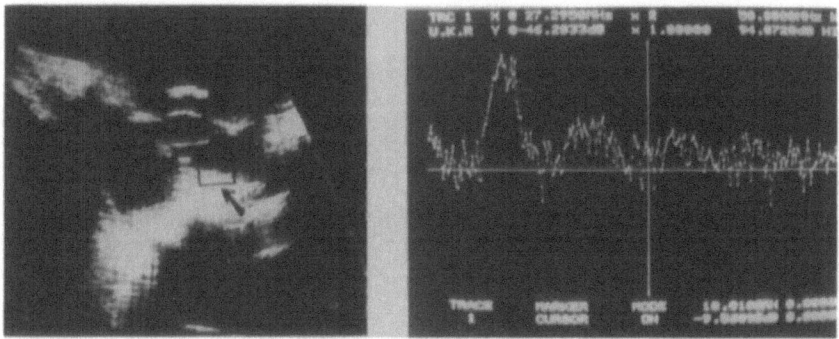

Fig. 7. The spectral analysis of the A-scan ultrasonogram of a case of retinoblastoma.

A somewhat strong but flat pattern, similar to that in other cases, was obtained at the other frequencies (Fig. 7).

In cases of retinal detachment, echo-wave reflex is strongly oriented to one direction because the surface of the detached retina is smooth, and therefore echo waves around the frequency used in the wave spectral analysis are particularly enhanced, producing a convex pattern. In contrast, cases of fresh hemorrhage show a flat pattern of reflected spectral waves, probably because uniform absorption attenuation or fine diffuse reflection of echoes in all direction occurs. Cases showing vitreous membrane formation show large wave patterns of reflected spectral waves. This is presumably because surface irregularities cause an almost diffuse reflection of echoes.

Conclusion

Spectral analysis of wave forms of A-scan radio-frequency signals by a computerized wave form analyzer has provided simpler differential diagnosis of tissues in living human eyes. Thus, this method, in addition to A-scan and B-scan, has enabled us to conduct analytic diagnosis of ocular diseases more readily than before.

Ultrasonographic evaluation of hemorrhagic choroidal detachments

L.A. BERLIN and Z.N. ZAKOV
Cleveland, USA

Introduction

The rare choroidal hemorrhage resulting in expulsion of the ocular contents during surgery is justifiably dreaded due to the devastating consequences for the patient. These cases understandably have drawn a lot of attention in the literature (Jaffe, 1976). A closely related, but less widely discussed entity is the choroidal hemorrhage that is controlled by the surgeon to avert expulsion of the ocular contents or one that occurs within hours to two weeks after surgery (Yanoff and Fine, 1982; Samuels, 1931). The increased frequency of referral of these cases of surgically related choroidal hemorrhages to our ultrasound laboratory led us to study the characteristics that describe the entity and to identify factors that may be predictive of visual outcome for these patients.

Patients and methods

A retrospective study was performed on all patients presenting to the ultrasound laboratory of the Department of Ophthalmology, Cleveland Clinic Foundation between June 1980 and June 1984, with subchoroidal hemorrhages. These hemorrhages had occurred either intra- or post-operatively. Patients with actual expulsive hemorrhages, clear choroidal effusions and spontaneous or traumatic choroidal hemorrhages were excluded. Remaining was a series of ten consecutive patients for whom adequate follow-up could be obtained.

The patient population included a five-year-old and then ranged between 49 and 85 years of age with a median of 72. There were six females and four males. Seven right eyes and three left eyes were involved. Predisposing factors for expulsive hemorrhages suggested by the literature were evaluated. All patients had at least one systemic disease in addition to an eye problem, as would be expected in an older population. Seven had cardiovascular disease, three had diabetes, two had lung disease and one had kidney stones. The child had otitis media and was febrile at the time of presentation with choroidal hemorrhage. Three had undergone previous surgery in the affected eye, two had glaucoma, and one had senile choroidal macular degeneration.

The types of surgery with which the choroidal hemorrhages were associated included one trabeculectomy, one retinal detachment repair, one medial rectus recession (the child), one IOL replacement operation, and six cataract extractions (two intracapsular cataract extractions, three aborted IOL insertions, and one successful IOL insertion). Seven cases were done under local anesthesia and three under general. Six of the patients suffered vitreous loss.

The subchoroidal hemorrhages were noted during surgery in six of the cases and within one to six days after surgery in the other four cases, although the exact time of onset of the latter hemorrhages could not be ascertained. The patients were referred for ultrasonography from one day to six weeks after surgery for a variety of reasons including differentiation of a pigmented choroidal tumor in two cases and opacification of the media or limited view of the fundus in the others.

All patients were examined by combined A- and B-mode ultrasonography with the Sonometrics Ophthalmoscan Model 200. Immersion technique was used in order to evaluate the anterior segment of the eye. Certain aspects of anatomy were assessed on all patients: the presence and extent of choroidal detachment, the clarity of the suprachoroidal space, the presence and extent of retinal detachment, the presence and density of vitreous opacities and any other abnormalities.

Results

Ultrasonographic findings in the ten cases included six vitreous hemorrhages, eight retinal detachments, and ten choroidal detachments ranging in elevation from eight to 20 mm. Two cases exhibited 'kissing choroidals' (Fig. 1). The acoustic characteristics of these entities are well known and so will not be discussed here (Coleman – 1974). In these cases where the hemorrhage stops short of being expulsive, the normal ocular architecture remains identifiable. Diagnostic difficulties, however, were encountered when on B-mode, the shape of the bullae of the choroidal detachments simulated malignant melanoma (Fig. 2). The A-mode pattern varied considerably across all the cases, most probably related to the varying densities of the blood clots as they formed and were resorbed. Six cases had more than one scan to document chronologic changes in position of detachment and density of hemorrhage.

Follow-up for these patients ranged from three to 36 months with a mean of 12 months. The shorter time periods were in patients who developed phthisis

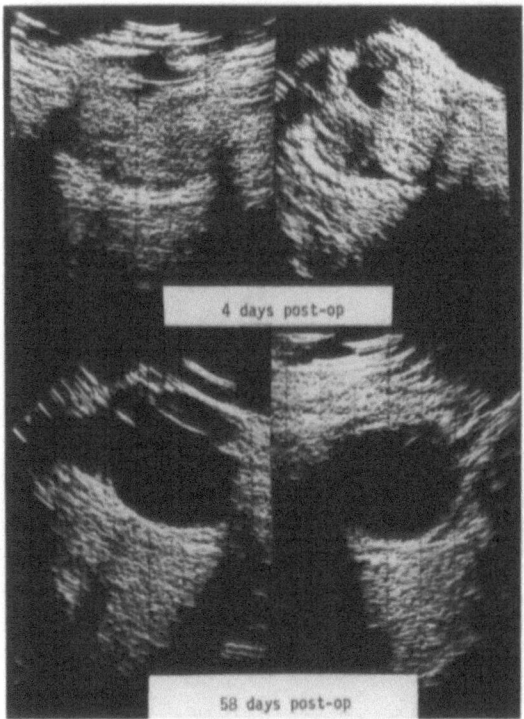

Fig. 1. (Top left) B-scans four days after trabeculectomy show a shallow anterior chamber and a totally detached choroid in the 'kissing choroidal' pattern with a dense subchoroidal hemorrhage. (Top right) At the inferior limbus with the eye gazing nasally, the vitreous appears clear. (Bottom) Fifty eight days after surgery only a residual choroidal thickening remained in the temporal periphery. The vision was 20/80.

bulbi. Treatment for all ten cases was solely medical to control inflammation and intraocular pressure; no surgical drainage of the subchoroidal space was performed.

The final visual acuities ranged from 20/40 to no light perception (NLP). We grouped them according to useful vision (three cases with 20/40 to 20/80 vision), ambulatory vision (two cases with 20/200 and 20/400 vision), and poor vision (five cases with count fingers at five feet to NLP vision).

Correlations were sought between the various predisposing factors as summarized by Jaffe, and the ultrasonographic findings in order to identify factors predictive of final visual acuity. No consistent relationship could be seen between size or extent of the choroidal hemorrhage (Fig. 1), density of the subchoroidal hemorrhage, presence or extent of retinal detachment, age or sex of the patient, eye involved, type of surgery, type of anesthetic, presence of systemic disease, time of occurrence of the hemorrhage whether during or

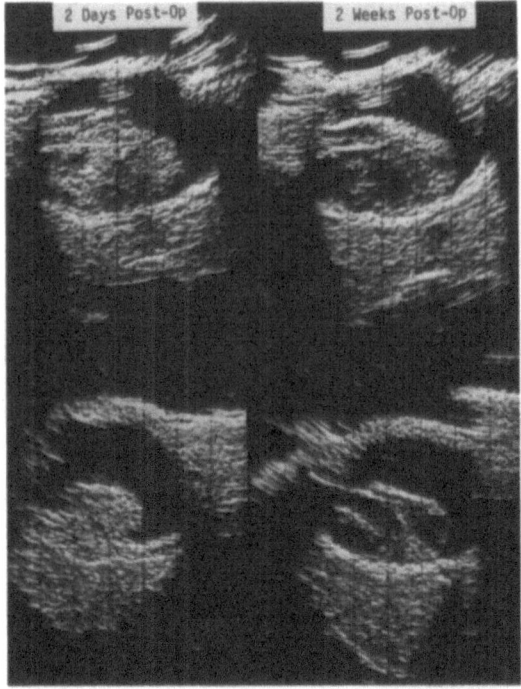

Fig. 2. (Top left) Two days after an IOL replacement procedure a large choroidal mass was seen in the temporal hemisphere. (Bottom left) Inferiorly, the mass assumed the typical mushroom shape of a malignant melanoma. (Top right) Two weeks later the subchoroidal hemorrhage was resorbing, appearing less echogenic. (Bottom right) The mushroom shape can now be seen to be the result of overlapping bullae of the choroidal detachment. The final vision, after the hemorrhage resorbed, was ambulatory at 20/400.

after surgery, and incidence of previous surgery on the eye. The subchoroidal hemorrhages that cleared did so within six to ten weeks, but the length of time did not correlate with visual acuity.

The presence of vitreous hemorrhage was the only factor that demonstrated a relationship to final visual acuity. All of the patients with poor visual acuity had experienced moderate to dense vitreous hemorrhages. One of the cases with ambulatory vision had experienced a light density vitreous hemorrhage. All of the patients with useful vision and the second patient with ambulatory vision experienced no clinically or ultrasonographically detectable vitreous hemorrhage.

Discussion

The entity of surgically related hemorrhagic choroidal detachment is serious

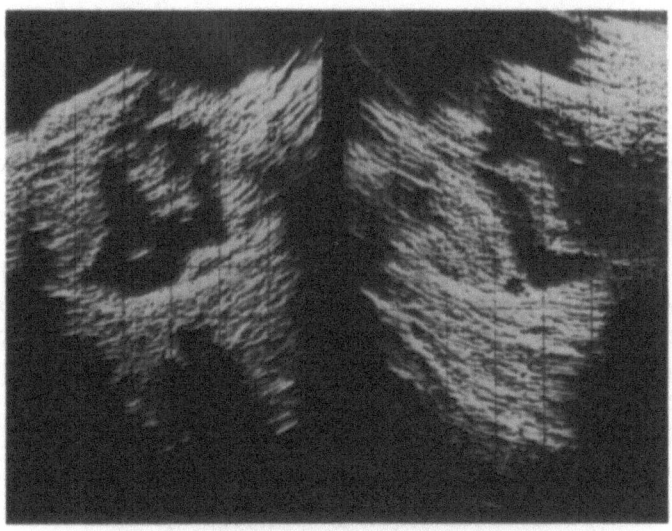

Fig. 3. (Left) Vitreous loss and a vitreous hemorrhage were seen clinically when this patient bucked under general anesthesia during a cataract extraction. B-scan of the eye gazing nasally shows a dense subchoroidal hemorrhage, vitreous hemorrhage and a retinal detachment nasal to the disk. (Right) The eye gazing temporally. This eye went to phthisis.

but not always devastating to the eye. In this series, half of the patients achieved ambulatory to useful vision with no surgical treatment, exceeding our initial expectation based on the uniformly bad prognosis for eyes that suffer expulsive hemorrhages. We, therefore, retrospectively reviewed our series to ascertain what factors, if any, were related to the cases with good visual results. The characteristics and distribution of our patient population and the predisposing factors in our series closely matched those described by other investigators (Jaffe, 1974 and Manschot, 1955). No strong correlations or trends were noted between the proposed predisposing factors or the characteristics of the patient population and visual outcome.

The only factor consistently indicative of poor visual outcome was vitreous hemorrhage. When vitreous hemorrhage was observed clinically and/or ultrasonographically, the final visual acuity ranged between 20/200 and NLP (Fig. 3). We can only speculate as to the role of vitreous hemorrhage in these particular cases with the deleterious effects. Since it is well known that even massive chronic hemorrhage from retinal sources such as diabetes may produce no apparent long term complications, we can postulate that additional factors must have been present in these cases. Migration of retinal pigment epithelial cells or ciliary body epithelial cells through retinal or ciliary body breaks may lead to secondary proliferation and organization along the path of the breakthrough bleeding. These proliferative and organizational processes may contribute to the poor visual and anatomic results.

None of the cases in this small series received surgical treatment, such as drainage of the subchoroidal hemorrhage or vitrectomy for the vitreous opacities. Since the prognosis for the eyes with both vitreous hemorrhage and subchoroidal hemorrhage was so uniformly poor, we would recommend considering surgical intervention in the future. Those cases of subchoroidal hemorrhage without vitreous hemorrhage seemed to fare better, and a more conservative medical course may be entertained.

Acknowledgement

We thank the ophthalmologists who referred these most difficult patient problems and kindly provided follow-up information.

References

Coleman DJ, Lizzi FL, Jack RL. 1974. Ultrasonography of the Eye and Orbit. Lea and Febiger, Philadelphia, pp. 242–245.

Jaffe NS. 1976. Cataract Surgery and its Complications. C.V. Mosby Co., St. Louis, pp. 326–340.

Manschot WA. 1955. The pathology of expulsive hemorrhage. Am J Ophthalmol 40: 15–24.

Samuels B. 1931. Postoperative nonexpulsive subchoroidal hemorrhage. Arch Ophthalmol 6: 840–851.

Yanoff M, Fine BS. 1982. Ocular Pathology. Harper & Row, Hagerstown, pp. 144–150.

Retinal and choroidal blood flow measurement in monkeys using implantable ultrasonic Doppler flow probes

R.H. KARDON, T.A. WEINGEIST and J. CUTCOMB
Iowa City, USA

Abstract

Retinal and choroidal blood flow were recorded simultaneously with an ultrasonic pulsed Doppler flow meter system. Miniature Doppler flow probes were surgically placed around the central retinal artery and lateral posterior ciliary artery. The probes emit a pulsatile 20 MHz signal and receive reflected sound waves from passing blood cells in the interval between ultrasonic pulses. The frequency shift of the reflected sound is proportional to the velocity of blood. Intraocular pressure, blood pressure, and KHz shift from the choroidal and retinal vascular beds were all continuously recorded. Choroidal and retinal vascular resistances were determined by dividing the perfusion pressure by the relative blood flow.

Introduction

This investigation was undertaken to develop the methodology for measuring blood flow simultaneously in both the choroidal and retinal microvascular beds in the monkey. In addition, uninterrupted continuous measurements were made in order to better understand the temporal aspects of blood flow in these two ocular microcirculatory beds.

The method employed consisted of pulsed Doppler ultrasonic velocimetry (Hartley and Cole, 1984). In this method, small piezoelectric crystals fashioned into probes are surgically implanted around the artery supplying a microvascular bed of interest. Because the sound waves are emitted at a fixed angle to the velocity of the blood stream, blood velocity can be quantitated and continuously recorded through the application of the Doppler principle. Such measurements have been shown to correlate well with volumetric blood flow (Haywood et al., 1981; Marcus et al., 1981). When blood pressure is also recorded, relative changes in vascular resistance can be calculated.

K.C. Ossoinig (editor), Ophthalmic Echography, ISBN 978-94-010-7988-4

Through the use of pulsed Doppler velocimetry applied to the ocular circulation it was hoped that differences between the behavior of the choroidal and retinal microcirculation under different conditions could be better understood.

Methods

Vascular probes for implantation were made from 1 mm diameter 20 MHz piezoelectric crystals (Valpey-Fisher, Hopkinton, Massachusetts) with two lead wires, each soldered onto opposing faces of the crystal. A vascular cuff containing the crystal was made by first positioning the crystal at a 45° angle to a segment of silastic tubing stretched to an outer diameter of approximately 300 microns. An epoxy resin (Hysol Hardener, H-W 796; the Dexter Corporation, Olean, New York) was then applied to the junction between the crystal and tubing to form a lens, following its polymerization. A silicon polymer (Medical Grade Silastic Elastomer 382; Dow Corning, Midland, MI.) was then used to surround the crystal, lens, and silastic tubing. Following polymerization of the silicon, a groove was cut through the silicon down to the silastic tubing which was then removed. This left a silicon vascular cuff containing the crystal positioned at a 45° angle to a 300 micron lumen within the cuff. The epoxy lens separated the crystal from the lumen.

The two channel directional pulsed Doppler velocimeter unit was constructed at the University of Iowa Bioengineering Resource Facility. A Beckman dynograph was used to make continuous recordings of the KHz shift, arterial blood pressure, and intraocular pressure.

Cynomolgus monkeys, 5 to 7 kilograms in weight were preanesthetized with 50 mg of ketamine IM and 0.2 mg of atropine IM and an intravenous line was established. After intubation, Halothane and nitrous oxide were used to maintain anesthesia with an inhalation system coupled to a Harvard mechanical ventilator pump and humidifier. A catheter was placed in the femoral artery for continuous monitoring of blood pressure. A lateral orbitotomy was then performed and a 3 mm length of the central retinal artery was dissected free from the optic nerve. One of the vascular cuff probes was then placed around this segment of the artery and secured in position using 7–0 silk sutures after an adequate audible and visible tracing of the Doppler signal had been obtained. The second probe was placed around the lateral posterior ciliary artery and secured in place in a similar manner.

For intraocular pressure measurements, two cannulas were placed through the limbus into the anterior chamber. One cannula was connected to a Statham pressure transducer and the other was connected to a reservoir of normal saline which was used to change intraocular pressure by varying its height.

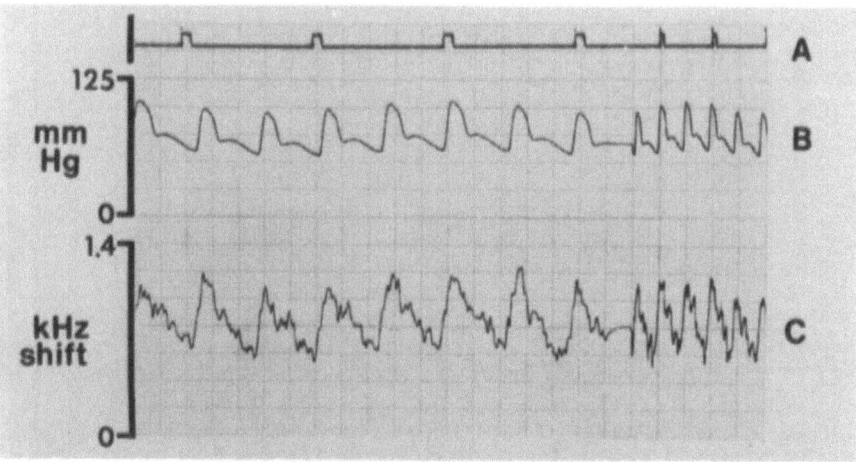

Fig. 1. Time course in seconds (A, top) of pulsatile arterial blood pressure (B, middle) compared to choroidal blood velocity (C, bottom) recorded simultaneously.

Reactive hyperemia of the retinal microcirculation was studied by mechanically occluding the central retinal artery with a vascular clamp for specific time periods.

Results and discussion

Doppler signals recorded in KHz shift from the choroidal and retinal circulations produced pulsatile velocity profiles which correlated well with simultaneous recordings of systolic and diastolic blood pressure (Fig. 1). Consistently, the velocity measured in KHz shift was much lower for the retinal vasculature compared to the choroidal circulation. The choroidal velocity was approximately 20 times higher in magnitude agreeing with previous measurements made by the radioactively labeled microsphere method (Alm et al. 1973).

The relative vascular resistance of the choroidal and retinal vascular beds at any specific time was obtained by dividing the perfusion pressure (mean arterial blood pressure – intraocular pressure) by the KHz shift. KHz shift is proportional to the velocity of flow according to the Doppler principle. In addition, the velocity of flow measured can be assumed to be proportional to volume flow providing the radius of the vessel at the segment being interrogated by the sound waves is constant. This is most likely the case considering that the tight vascular cuff containing the piezoelectric crystal restricts the diameter of the artery. Using a similar system, the KHz shift has been shown to be proportional to volume blood flow in the renal vascular bed of the rat (Haywood et al., 1981).

322

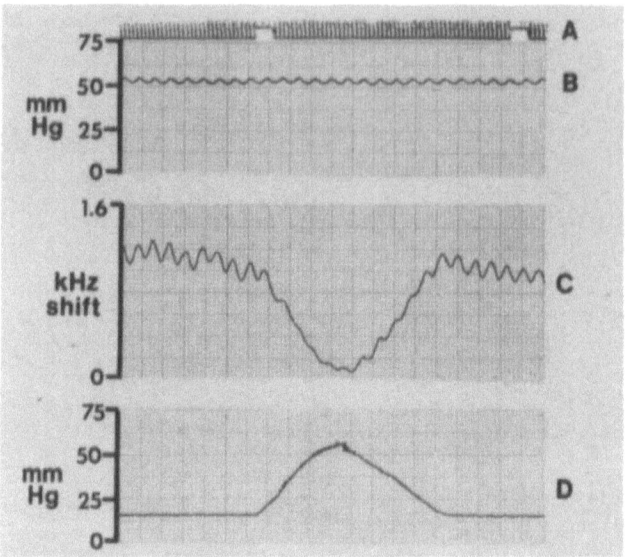

Fig. 2. Time course in seconds (A) of mean arterial blood pressure (B) and mean choroidal blood velocity (C) during changes in intraocular pressure (D).

The effect of changes of intraocular pressure on the mean KHz shift in the retinal and choroidal microcirculation is shown in Figs. 2 and 3. Choroidal blood velocity responded rapidly and inversely to even the smallest changes in intraocular pressure. The retinal blood velocity, however, showed much less change compared to the choroidal blood velocity in proportion to the same degree of change in intraocular pressure, while mean arterial blood pressure was constant. For example, in Fig. 3, when the intraocular pressure was abruptly raised to a higher level, the mean choroidal velocity also abruptly decreased and remained at the decreased level until the intraocular pressure was lowered to its baseline level. At this time the choroidal blood velocity immediately returned to its baseline level. The response of the mean retinal blood velocity was quite different during the same interval of change in intraocular pressure. Initially, when the intraocular pressure was abruptly increased, the mean retinal blood velocity decreased but within seconds began to increase back towards its baseline level in spite of the higher intraocular pressure. This indicated a decrease in vascular resistance. When the intraocular pressure was abruptly returned to its baseline level, the mean retinal blood velocity abruptly increased above its baseline level, due to the decreased vascular resistance which had resulted from the previously elevated intraocular pressure. The mean retinal blood velocity then responded by returning toward its baseline level within seconds. This indicated an increase in vascular resistance toward the original baseline resistance. Such changes in vascular

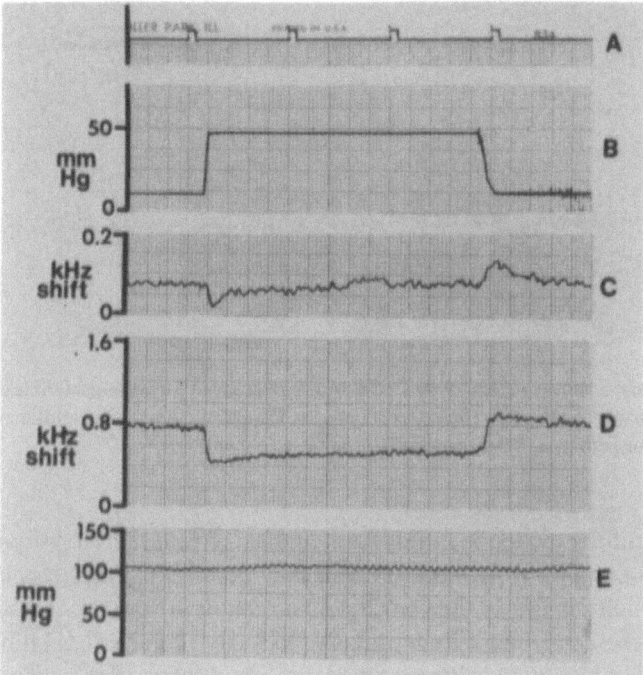

Fig. 3. Relationship of mean retinal blood velocity (C) and mean choroidal blood velocity (D) during a stepwise increase and decrease of intraocular pressure (B). Mean arterial blood pressure (E) is relatively constant. Time course (A) is recorded in minutes during this simultaneously recorded segment.

resistance with changing intraocular pressure indicated the existence of auto-regulation within the retinal vascular bed compared to relatively little auto-regulation of the choroidal vasculature. Furthermore, the autoregulatory response occurred within seconds.

Changes in vascular resistance of the retinal vascular bed were also brought about by occluding the central retinal artery for short periods of time. Figure 4 shows a tracing of mean retinal blood velocity and response to mechanical occlusion times of 40, 15 and 17 seconds. The low frequency pulsatile change in the mean retinal velocity corresponded to the similar changes in the mean arterial blood pressure caused by mechanical ventilation. When the ventilation was momentarily stopped this component of the tracing was eliminated. During central retinal artery occlusion the retinal blood velocity dropped to zero. Following release of the vascular clamp, the velocity initially increased to a higher level then returned to baseline velocity with time. Repeated occlusions of differing times seemed to indicate that with increasing time of vascular occlusion the magnitude and duration of the hyperemic response increased. The shortest occlusion time which produced a response was 4 seconds.

324

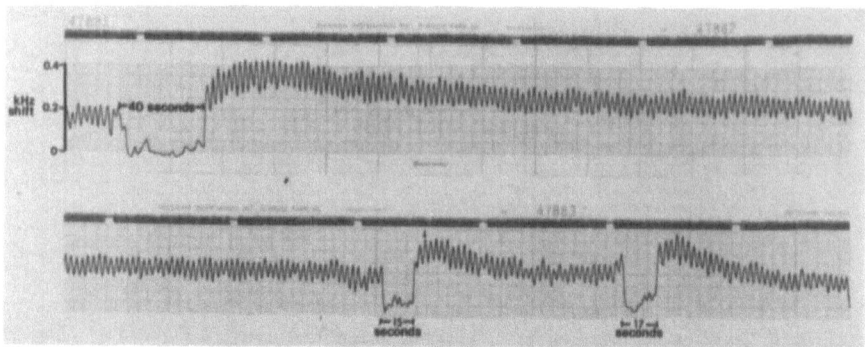

Fig. 4. Hyperemic response of the mean retinal blood velocity after mechanical occlusion of the central retinal artery. Divisions in time (seconds) are shown at the top of this continuous tracing consisting of three different occlusion times.

The preliminary evidence in this study indicated that the directional ultrasonic pulsed Doppler flow meter system may be a very sensitive method of measuring small changes in the velocity of blood flow in both the choroidal and retinal microvascular beds. Recordings of velocity of each circulation made simultaneously will allow differences in the physiology of the two vascular beds as well as their interaction to be studied in the future. In addition, since continuous recordings are possible, the temporal behavior of any vascular changes will be amenable to study. Through simultaneous measurement of the intraocular pressure and mean arterial blood pressure, relative changes in vascular resistance can be quantitated. Further characterization and testing of this methodology is needed, but the application of the technique to the understanding of the physiology of the ocular circulation appears to be promising.

References

1. Alm A, Bill A, Young FA. 1973. The effects of pilocarpine and neostigmine on the blood flow through the anterior uvea in monkeys. A study with radioactively labelled microspheres. Exp Eye Research 15: 31–36.
2. Hartley CJ, Cole JS. 1974. An ultrasound pulsed Doppler system for measuring blood flow in small vessels. J Appl Physiology 37: 626–629.
3. Haywood JR, Shaffer RA, Fastenow C, Fink GD, Brody MJ. 1981. Regional blood flow measurement in the conscious rat with pulsed Doppler flowmeter. Am J Physiol 241: H273–H278.
4. Marcus M, Wright C, Doty D, Eastman C, Laughlin D, Krumm P, Fastenow C, Brody M. 1981. Measurements of coronary velocity and reactive hyperemia in the coronary circulation of humans. Circ Res 49: 877–891.

The ultrasonographic evaluation of severely traumatized eyes

G.K. STERNS
Rochester, New York, USA

The complementary use of ultrasonography and computerized tomography has enabled the ophthalmologist to more accurately assess the extent of damage caused by ocular trauma. Ocular trauma includes concussion and contusion injuries, penetrating wounds, foreign body injuries and orbital and periorbital fractures. These injuries often cause cloudy or opaque media, making adequate ophthalmoscopic evaluation of the eye impossible. A series of 25 patients who sustained severe trauma were reviewed. Twenty of these patients had ultrasonographic evaluation, ten had computerized tomographic evaluation and five had both ultrasound and CT scanning performed. Thirteen patients had perforated globes, six had intraocular foreign bodies and four had severe periorbital trauma, resulting in visual disturbances.

Results

Ocular injury

The ultrasonographic examinations were accurate in 18 of the 20 patients scanned. This 90% accuracy rate is compatible with the results of previously reported series [2, 5, 8]. The ultrasound was accurate in evaluating extensive retinal and vitreous damage, as well as posterior perforations. Two cases are presented to illustrate the difficulties sometimes encountered in the use of ultrasound in this setting.

Case 1. A 34-year-old man, hit in the eye with an ashtray, sustained a corneal scleral laceration. The eye was repaired within the first 24 hours. An ultrasound performed 48 hours postoperatively demonstrated vitreous hemorrhage and a dense high amplitude echo posteriorly and inferiorly (Fig. 1). This finding was thought to be compatible with either a localized retinal detachment or a dense preretinal membrane. The patient underwent surgery and was

K.C. Ossoinig (editor), Ophthalmic Echography, ISBN 978-94-010-7988-4

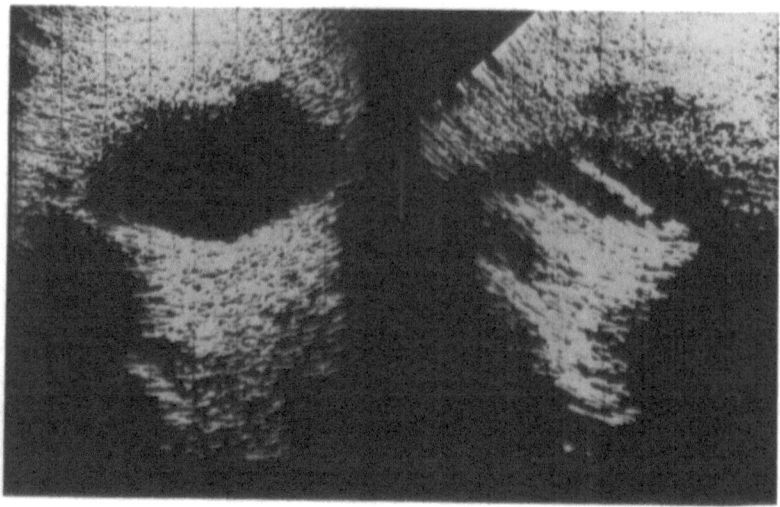

Fig. 1. Dense preretinal membrane showed high reflectivity on A-scan and resembled a traction retinal detachment.

found to have a dense preretinal membrane.

Case. 2. A 33-year-old man sustained a small self-healing perforation. Two days later he developed a severe endophthalmitis precluding ophthalmoscopic examination of the posterior pole. An ultrasonogram demonstrated a very high amplitude echo posteriorly compatible with either a small focal detachment or a dense preretinal membrane (Fig. 2). The patient underwent surgery for the endophthalmitis. A dense inflammatory membrane requiring surgical excision was found.

Foreign bodies

Six patients had intraocular or intraorbital foreign bodies following penetrating and perforating injuries. In all cases the foreign body was successfully located by CT scan. In two patients, repair and vitreous surgery to remove intraocular foreign bodies were performed within 12 hours of the injury, after CT scan and without ultrasound examination. The remaining four patients underwent primary repair of the penetrating wound and were subsequently examined with both CT and ultrasound. The intraocular damage was accurately assessed by ultrasound in all cases, and in one instance (case 3), the location of the foreign body was more precisely localized by ultrasound than by CT scan. Two cases are presented to illustrate the combined use of ultrasound and CT in this setting.

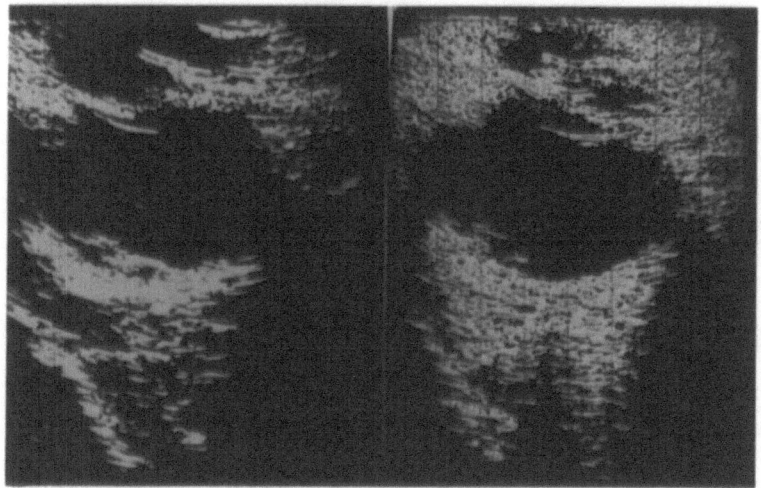

Fig. 2. Inflammatory membrane requiring surgical excision.

Case 3. A 30-year-old man was struck in the eye by a bullet fragment. A metallic foreign body was located by CT scan and was thought to be embedded in the sclera. On ultrasound exam, however, the correct location of the foreign body was identified, 1.5 mm within the globe surrounded by a vitreous hemorrhage. Magnification of the foreign body by CT scan explained its erroneous localization (Figs. 3 and 4).

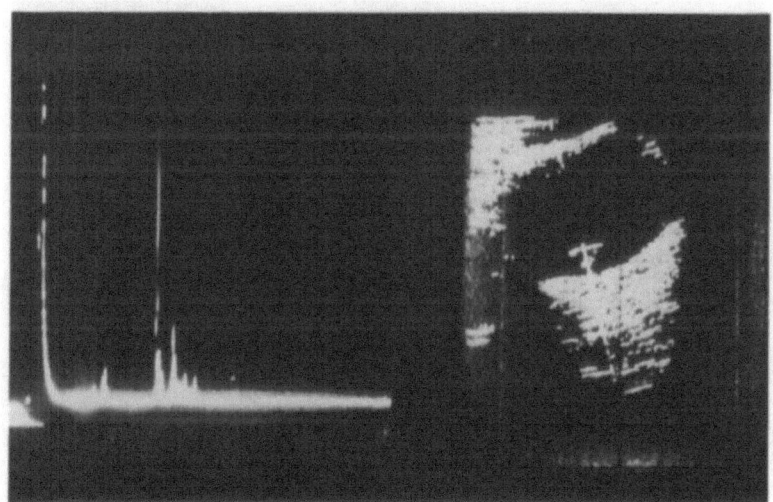

Fig. 3. The ultrasound places the foreign body within the eye anterior to the retina by approximately $1^{1}/_{2}$ mm.

328

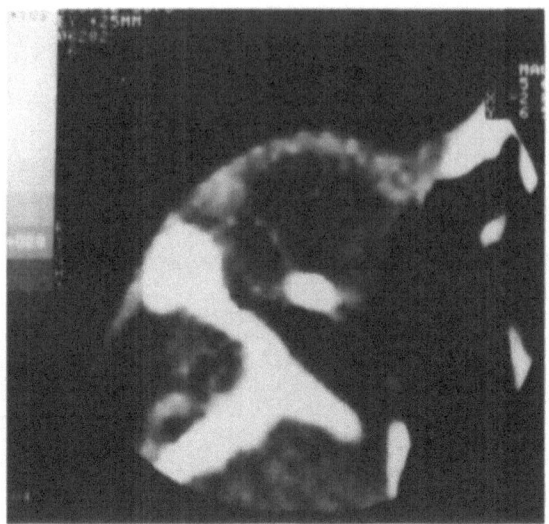

Fig. 4. The foreign body on CT scan appears adjacent to the sclera.

Case 4. A 40-year-old man was shot in the eye in a hunting accident. The ultrasound demonstrated a perforated globe, retinal detachment and vitreous hemorrhage (Fig. 5). The CT scan showed air in the eye and orbit and a foreign body in the orbital apex (Fig. 6).

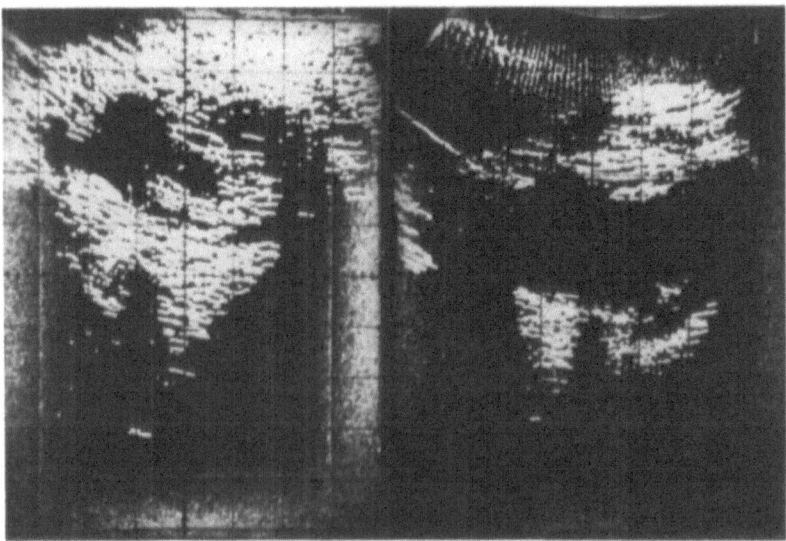

Fig. 5. Total retinal detachment and vitreous hemorrhage. The discontinuity of the posterior scleral wall suggests a posterior perforation.

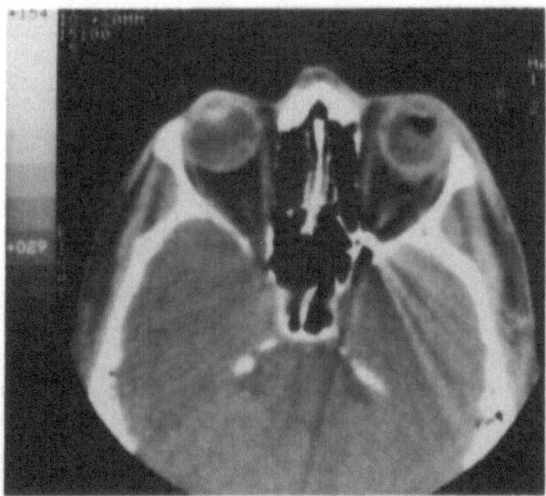

Fig. 6. The CT scan shows air within the eye and orbit suggesting perforation. A foreign body is lodged in the orbit.

Orbital and periorbital contusion injuries

Four patients sustained severe orbital and periorbital trauma. Two of these patients had sudden loss of vision. CT scanning in all of these patients yielded an accurate assessment of the orbital and periorbital injury. Two cases are presented to illustrate the use of the CT scan in this setting.

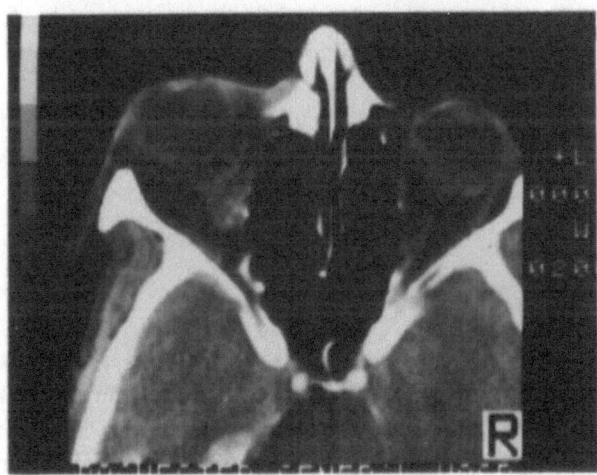

Fig. 7. CT scan demonstrates large retrobulbar hemorrhage compressing the optic nerve causing a central retinal artery occlusion.

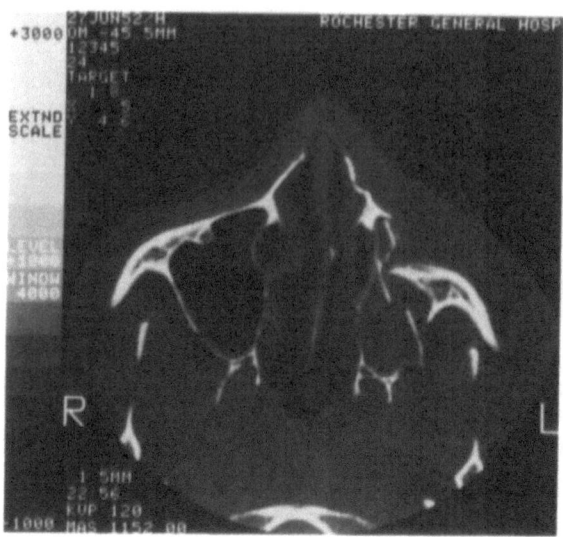

Fig. 8. CT scan demonstrating multiple fractures.

Case 5. A 35-year-old man fell on a screwdriver, penetrating his periorbital area just posterior to the globe. He presented to the Emergency Room with no light perception and a fixed dilated pupil in the affected eye. The lids were tense, the ocular motility was markedly limited and the globe was proptotic. A CT scan of the orbit (Fig. 7) clearly showed a large retrobulbar hemorrhage. The hemorrhage increased the intraocular pressure causing a central retinal artery occlusion and consequent loss of vision. Because of the delay between injury and treatment, vision could not be restored.

Case 6. A 35-year-old man lost consciousness after a severe beating. He had marked orbital and periorbital soft tissue damage. The CT scan demonstrated multiple fractures (Fig. 8).

Discussion

As has been previously reported [2, 5, 8], in our series, the ultrasonic examination could not always distinguish between dense preretinal membrane or organized hemorrhage and localized retinal detachment. Particularly in younger patients, a dense hemorrhage behind a formed vitreous can also mimic localized retinal detachment. In the two cases which gave us trouble (cases 1 and 2), dense preretinal hemorrhage and fibroplastic membrane formed by an ongoing endophthalmitis gave an ultrasonic appearance compatible with localized detachment. In both cases, the operating surgeon felt that the surgery was indicated and that the membrane had to be surgically excised. High amplitude echoes which mimic retina tend to be produced by highly organized membranes which require surgical removal. Thus, although the differential between these entities is difficult, both are indications for surgery. Several studies have assessed the importance of early vitreous surgery following trauma [1, 3, 5]. Each study has shown a better outcome with early intervention (although the benefit has not reached statistical significance in all cases). There have been no studies showing early surgery to be detrimental. Hence, no harm will be done if patients thought to have a localized detachment by ultrasound prove to have dense membranes at surgery.

We have used a combined approach using both CT scan and ultrasound in managing ocular and orbital foreign bodies and in assessing orbital trauma. A CT scan is indicated when a foreign body is suspected, in cases of suspected orbital and periorbital fractures and when unexplained loss of vision accompanies severe soft tissue injury [4, 7]. The CT scan allows accurate localization of a foreign body without manipulation of the globe and can detect occult posterior ruptures that are sometimes missed by ultrasound. The CT scan also provides a rapid and accurate assessment of the bony injuries caused by orbital trauma. Ultrasound may assist in localizing foreign bodies and provides the best means to accurately assess the topographic damage to the eye. It aids in planning appropriate surgery. When used together in select cases, the ultrasound and CT scan are mutually beneficial, providing the examiner with important information necessary in the management of these patients (Table 1).

Table 1.

	USG	CT
Ocular injury	++++	+
Orbital soft tissue injury	++	++++
Foreign bodies		
Ocular	+++	+++
Orbital	++	+++
Fractures		
Orbital and periorbital	0	++++

References

1. Brinton GS, Aaberg TM, Reeser FH, Topping TM, Abrams GW. 1982. Surgical results in ocular trauma involving the posterior segment. Am J Ophthalmol 93: 271–278.
2. Blumenkranz MS, Byrne SS. 1982. Standardized echography (ultrasonography) for the detection and characterization of retinal detachment. Ophthalmol 89: 821–831.
3. Coleman DJ. 1982. Early vitrectomy in the management of the severely traumatized eye. Am J Ophthalmol 93: 543–551.
4. Guyon, et al. 1984. CT demonstration of optic canal fractures. Am J Roentgenol 143: 1031–1034.
5. Hutton WL, Fuller DG. 1984. Factors influencing final visual results in severely injured eyes. Am J Ophthalmol 97: 715–722.
6. Jack RL, Hutton WL, Machemer R. 1974. Ultrasonography and vitrectomy. Am J Ophthalmol 78: 265–274.
7. Manfredi SJ, Raji M, Sprinkle PM, Weinstein GW, Minardi L, Swanson TJ. 1981. Computerized tomographic scan findings in facial fractures associated with blindness. Plastic Reconstructive Surg 68: 479–490.
8. Zakov ZN, Berlin LA, Gutman SA. 1983. Ultrasonographic mapping of vitreal retinal abnormalities. Am J Ophthalmol 96: 622–631.

Detection of posterior ruptures in opaque media*

J.R. HUGHES and S.F. BYRNE
Miami, USA

Abstract

The purpose of this paper is to highlight the echographic criteria for detecting and differentiating posterior ruptures in opaque media, many of which have been previously described [2, 3]. A retrospective study was performed in patients with a history of trauma by reviewing their medical records and echography findings. Only those patients with a posterior rupture confirmed at surgery, or later by histopathology or ophthalmoscopic follow-up were included in the study. The following echographic criteria were present in each case: (1) history of trauma, (2) vitreous pathology with vitreoretinal adhesion, and (3) thickening or detachment of the retino-choroid layer. In some instances, there were other useful signs: (1) scleral defect, (2) retrobulbar foreign body, (3) epi-bulbar hemorrhage and (4) hemorrhagic track through the orbital fat.

Materials and methods

The records of 115 trauma patients with opaque media and echography examination were reviewed. Twenty-five of these 115 patients were found to have scleral ruptures at the time of surgery or later by either histopathologic or ophthalmoscopic follow up. The patients had sustained various forms of blunt, penetrating or perforating trauma.

All patients were examined with standardized echography[5] (i.e. Kretz-technik 7200 MA and a contact, real-time B-scan instrument). The special techniques (e.g. topographic, quantitative and kinetic echography [1, 5] were performed during the dynamic examination. Photographic and written docu-

* This work has been supported in part by the Florida Lions Eye Bank

334

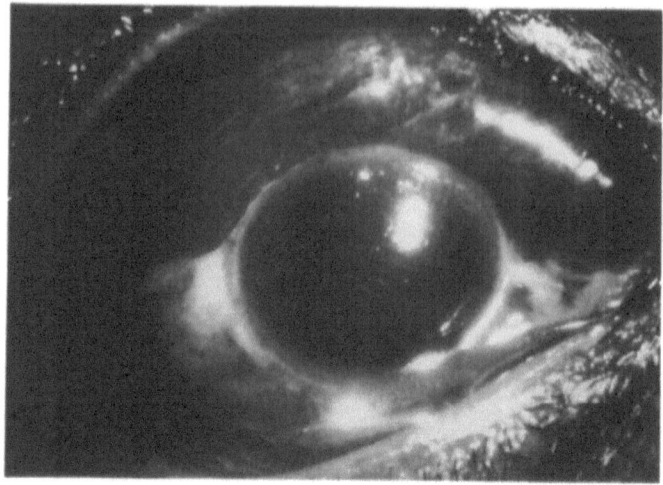

Fig. 1. This patient presented with a painful eye following being 'struck by a stick' three days before. There was marked ecchymosis superiorly and a total hyphema prevented fundus visualization. Visual acuity was light perception and the intraocular pressure was 16. A large posterior rupture was detected echographically (shown in Fig. 5).

mentation of the findings was made at the time of the examination; this data was compiled and analyzed at the onset of this study.

Clinical findings

Patients with posterior ruptures frequently present with a corneoscleral laceration, hyperemia and ecchymosis as well as opaque media and low intraocular pressure. All of these findings suggest the possibility of a posterior rupture clinically but require echography to confirm or exclude posterior rupture. In many instances, however, there is reasonable uncertainty as to whether or not a posterior rupture is present and the importance of echography is greatly enhanced (Fig. 1).

The significance of detecting a posterior rupture is in aiding the clinical management of these patients through indicating or obviating surgical intervention. The physician is also alerted to the possibility of endophthalmitis and/ or sympathetic ophthalmia.

Echographic findings

All 25 patients had opaque media, thus preventing ophthalmoscopic examination. Echography was employed to detect and localize vitreous hemorrhage,

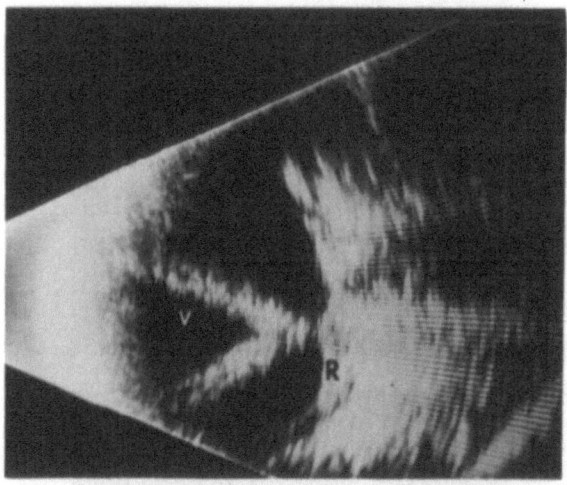

Fig. 2. This patient sustained a perforating injury from a gunshot wound through the cornea. Horizontal B-scan section at medium high sensitivity setting shows a posterior vitreous detachment (V) inserting into the macular region where the foreign body exited the globe. Note thickening of retino-choroid layer (R) in this region.

retinal or choroidal detachment, intraocular foreign body and scleral rupture.

Vitreous hemorrhage was present in all 25 cases and there was invariably some degree of vitreous organization and vitreoretinal adhesion (Fig. 2). Vitreous bands or membranes could often be traced from the region of injury anteriorly to insertion at the posterior rupture site.

Thickening or detachment of the retina and/or choroid was invariably seen in the area immediately surrounding the vitreoretinal adhesion and rupture (Figs. 2 and 3).

While vitreoretinal adhesions suggest a posterior rupture, the best indicator is demonstration of a scleral defect. The incarceration of viteous and retina into the wound is further evidence of rupture (Fig. 4). While high resolution contact, real-time B-scan may demonstrate large ruptures, topography may be confusing in the traumatized eye and standardized A-scan may help substantiate the presence of a rupture by demonstrating an irregular scleral spike during dynamic scanning of the suspicious region (Fig. 5).

Orbital foreign bodies occurring as a result of a perforating injury* may provide another clue to the presence of a posterior rupture. Retrobulbar foreign bodies are frequently associated with orbital hemorrhage (Fig. 6). On some occasions, the foreign body may travel through both the posterior eye wall and the orbital soft tissues leaving a hemorrhagic track through the orbital echogram (Fig. 7).

* *A perforating injury of the globe requires an entry and exit wound. Therefore, a projectile that enters the cornea and exits posteriorly into the orbital tissue causes a perforating injury [4, 6].*

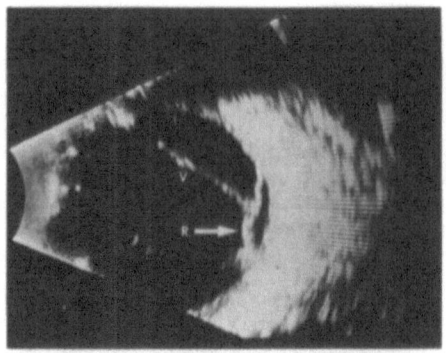

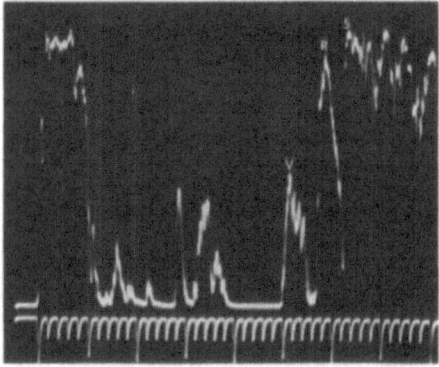

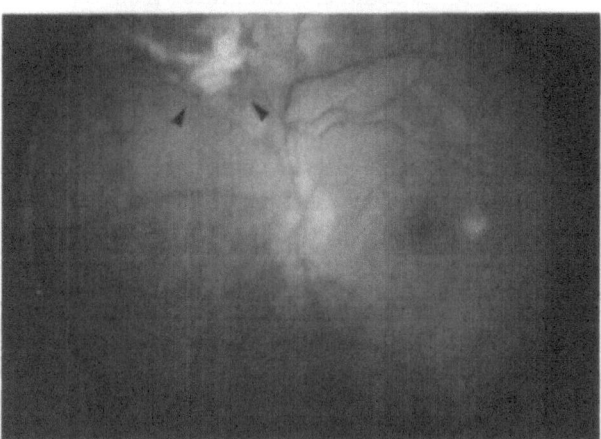

Fig. 3A. B- and A-scans show a dense vitreous band (V) inserting into a focal superonasal retinal detachment (R), S = sclera. The chain of spikes on the left of the A-scan are from vitreous hemorrhage.

Fig. 3B. Fundus examination several weeks after vitrectomy and scleral buckling procedure shows a posterior impact or exit site superonasal to the optic disc (arrows).

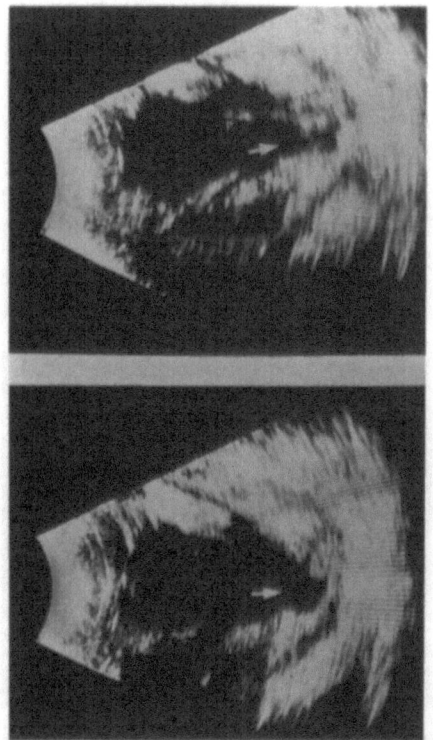

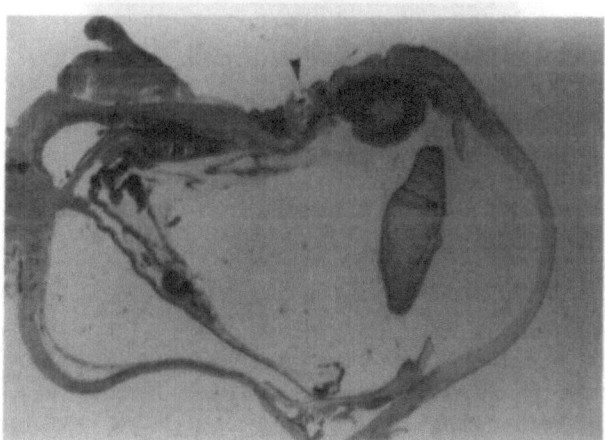

Fig. 4. This patient sustained blunt trauma by an air hose.

Fig. 4A. Vertical B-scans at high sensitivity setting (Top) and medium sensitivity setting (Bottom) through the temporal equatorial region. Extensive posterior vitreous detachment (P) and hemorrhagic retinal detachment (R) are incarcerated into large scleral rupture (arrow).

Fig. 4B. The globe was enucleated due to the grave prognosis. Macroscopic path specimen shows a full thickness scleral defect (arrow).

338

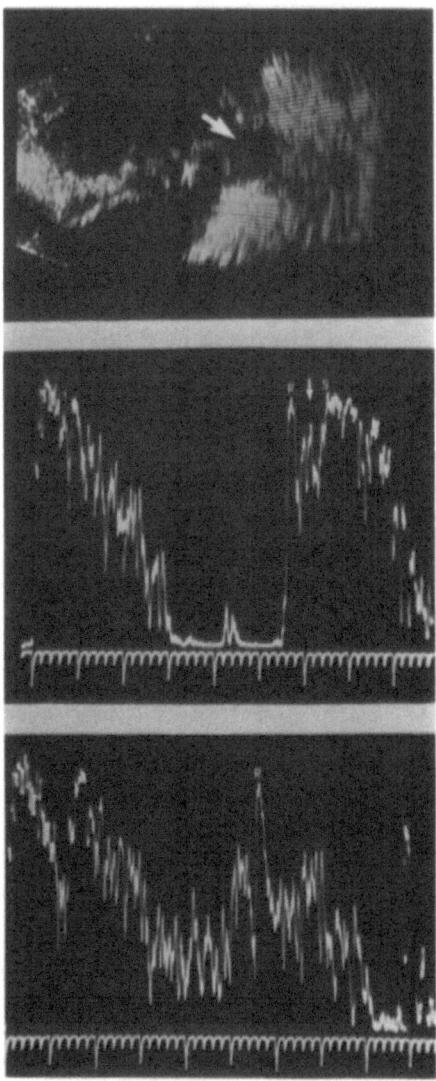

Fig. 5. Echograms of patient shown in Fig. 1. B-scan shows vitreous hemorrhage incarcerated into apparent scleral rupture (arrow). Center, A-scan shows subretinal hemorrhage (arrow) in area adjacent to scleral defect shown on B-scan. R = retina, S = slera. Bottom, A-scan taken with sound beam aimed partially into rupture area shows chain of spikes replacing vitreous baseline from dense vitreous hemorrhage, retina (R) and no distinct scleral signal.

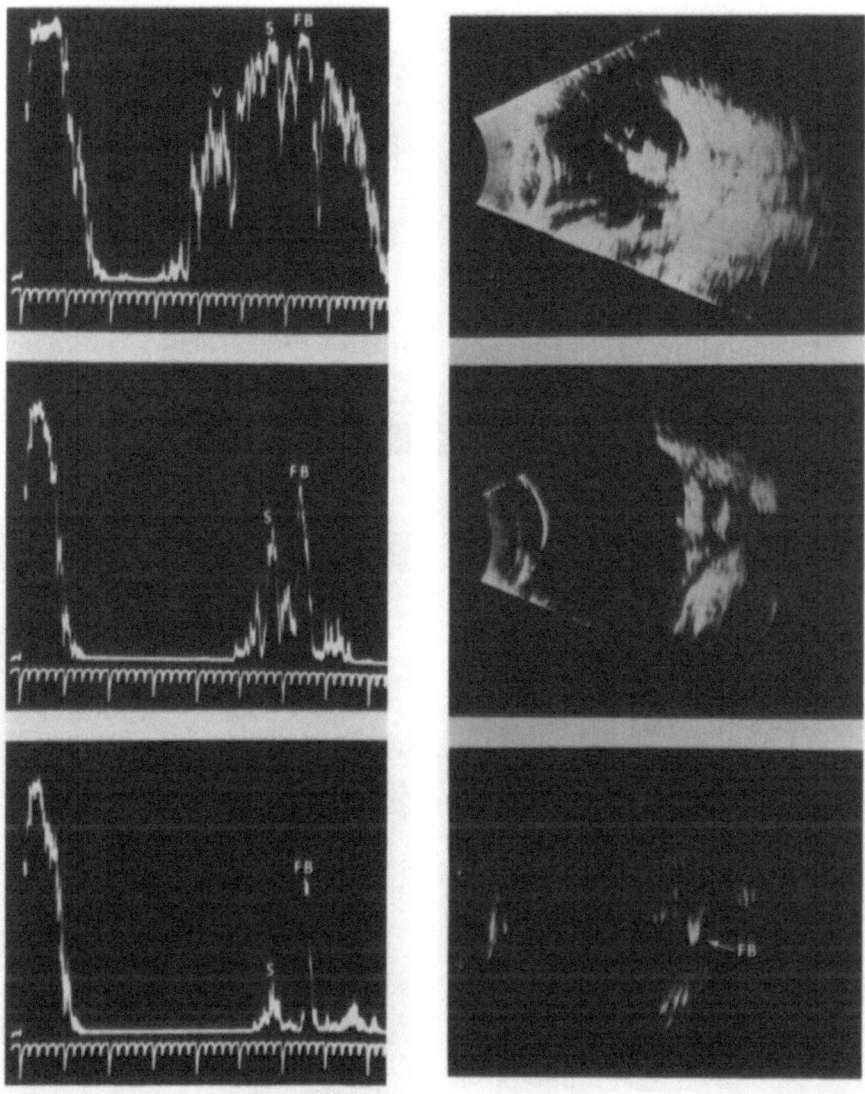

Fig. 6. This patient was pounding metal on metal and sustained a limbal scleral laceration with dense preretinal hemorrhage at the temporal posterior pole and an intraocular foreign body was suspected. Plane x-rays had diagnosed an intraocular foreign body. B- and A-scans at various sensitivity settings show dense vitreous hemorrhage inserting into the temporal fundus as well as retro-ocular foreign body and hemorrhage. Top, B-scan at high sensitivity and A-scan at the high tissue sensitivity setting show vitreous hemorrhage (V) inserting into the posterior fundus. A-scan also shows foreign body (FB) behind sclera (S). Center and bottom echograms at lower sensitivity settings show large epibulbar foreign body surrounded by hemorrhage. The highly reflective foreign body is most apparent in the bottom echograms which are at very low sensitivity settings.

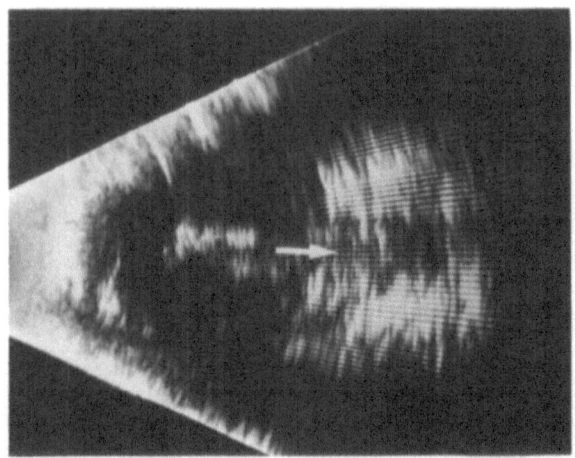

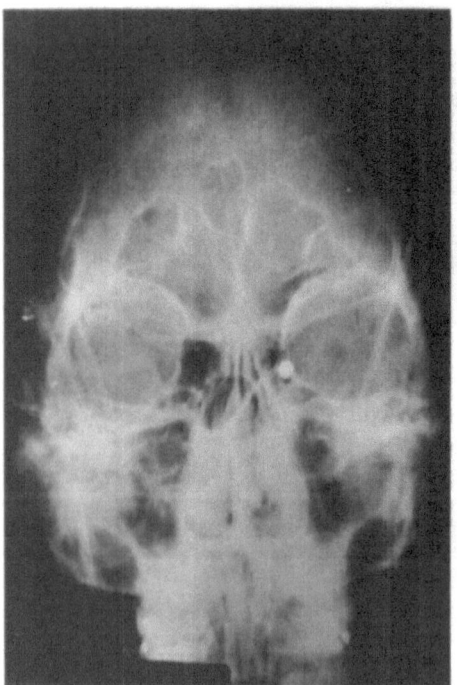
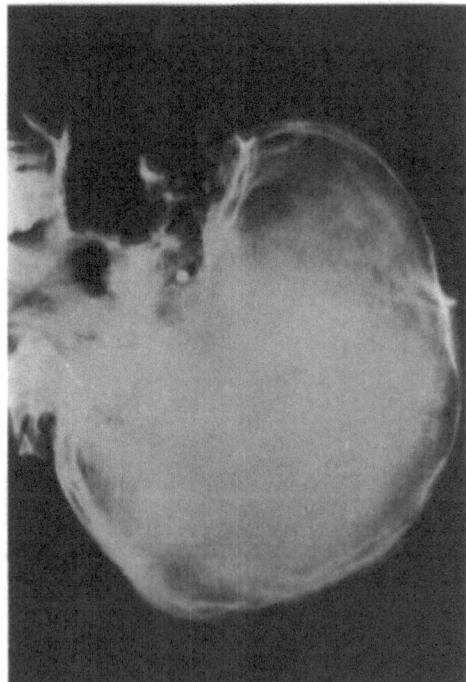

Fig. 7. This patient sustained a gunshot wound with large corneal laceration and perforating injury. 7A, B-scan shows dense vitreous hemorrhage streaming through vitreous cavity and incarcerated into posterior scleral rupture (arrow). Homogeneous track through orbital tissues behind scleral rupture is due to hemorrhage track as the foreign body passed through the orbit. Plane x-rays in frontal (7B) and lateral 7C views show pellet in sphenoid sinus.

Conclusion

Standardized echography should play an important role in the detection of a posterior rupture in patients with opaque media secondary to trauma. The identification of a posterior rupture may significantly influence management of the patient's injury.

The detection of vitreous hemorrhage, a vitreoretinal adhesion and thickening or detachment of the retino-choroid layer are clues as to the possibility of a posterior rupture. Additional findings of a scleral defect, retrobulbar foreign body and hemorrhage make the likelihood of posterior rupture even greater (Table 1).

Acknowledgement

The authors are grateful to Michele L. Fagin for typing this manuscript and for editorial assistance. Additional thanks are extended to the other Echography personnel: Eileen K. Novinski and Maria L. Rivera.

Table 1. Criteria necessary for diagnosing posterior ruptures with standardized echography.

Primary Criteria

History of trauma
Organized vitreous hemorrhage
Vitreoretinal adhesion
Thickening or Detachment of retina and/or choroid

Secondary Criteria

Scleral defect
Retrobular foreign body
Epibulbar hemorrhage
Hemorrhagic track through orbital soft tissues

342

References

1. Byrne SF. 1979. Standardized echography. Par 1: A-scan examination procedures. Int Ophthalmol Clin 19 (4): 267–81.
2. Coleman DJ, Lizzi FL, Jack RL. 1977. Ultrasonography of the Eye and Orbit. Philadelphia: Lea & Febiger, pp. 253–255.
3. Fuller DG, Hutton WL. 1982. Presurgical evaluation of eyes with opaque media. New York, Grune & Stratton, Inc: 168–72.
4. Fuller DG, Hutton WL. 1982. Presurgical evaluation of eyes with opaque media. New York, Grune & Stratton, Inc: 168–9.
5. Ossoinig KC. 1979. Standardized echography: basic principles, clinical applications, and results. Int Ophthalmol Clin 19 (4): 127–210.
6. Yanoff M, Fine BS. 1982. Ocular Pathology – A Text and Atlas (2nd edition). Philadelphia, Harper & Row: 185.

How to differentiate intraocular air bubbles from intraocular foreign bodies using standardized echography

K.C. OSSOINIG and K. CODY
Iowa City, USA

Abstract

Intraocular foreign bodies can be detected reliably and localized precisely with standardized A-scan. This method can be applied intraoperatively under sterile conditions and can be utilized to perform a non-invasive magnet test and to evaluate the vitreous, retina, choroid and sclera in the injured eye. Since such A-scan evaluation is non-traumatic and usually requires only a few minutes, it has proven very useful in the management of foreign body injuries of the eye.

In rare instances small air bubbles are introduced into the posterior segment by the intruding foreign body. Air is a perfect reflector and thus produces very strong echoes resembling those from foreign bodies. In order to retain the echographic reliability and accuracy, one must, therefore, be prepared to identify such air bubbles quickly and differentiate them from 'true' foreign bodies.

Intraocular air bubbles produce single-peaked, slim, sharply rising, 100% high spikes at Tissue Sensitivity. These spikes appear identical, or at least very similar, in all sound-beam directions as long as the air bubble is centered in the beam. By contrast, common foreign bodies (metallic splinters) produce clearly different, sometimes double-peaked signals in different sound-beam directions. Spherical foreign bodies (e.g., BB's), on the other hand, produce chains of multiple signals which are very different from both air bubbles and common foreign bodies. In addition to this initial acoustic difference, the signals from air bubbles weaken quickly and vanish within days as the air is being absorbed, whereas true foreign body signals persist.

K.C. Ossoinig (editor), Ophthalmic Echography, ISBN 978-94-010-7988-4

344

References

1. Ossoinig KC. 1979. Standardized echography: basic principles, clinical applications and results. In: Ophthalmic Ultrasonography: Comparative Techniques (Dallow, R.L. ed.) Int Ophthal Clin, 19/4: 127–210. Little, Brown & Co., Boston, 1979.
2. Ossoinig KC. 1982. Advances in diagnostic ultrasound. ACTA: XXIV International Congress of Ophthalmology (San Francisco), Paul Henkind, ed. Philadelphia: J.B. Lippincott Co., Vol. 1, pp. 89–114.
3. Ossoinig KC. 1985. Standardized ophthalmic echography of the eye, orbit and periorbital region. A comprehensive Slide Set (774 slides) and Study Guide, Third Edition. Iowa City, Iowa: Goodfellow Company, Inc., pp. 45–51.

The importance of Standardized Echography in the assessment of post-surgical choroidal detachments

A. NASR, K.C. OSSOINIG and T.A. WEINGEIST
Iowa City, USA

Abstract

Choroidal detachments following intra-ocular surgery in specific vitreo-retinal conditions occur in 15–20% of the cases. The management of these eyes depends on the accurate diagnosis and exact determination of the type, the extent, and the nature of the detachment. Standardized Echography is a non-invasive and specific modality in assessing and following these conditions.

Twenty-four eyes with post-surgical choroidal detachments were analyzed and divided ultrasonographically into three groups: serous, hemorrhagic-fluid, and hemorrhagic-coagulated.

Quantitative A-scan echography helps to differentiate these three types of choroidal detachments: at Tissue Sensitivity, the subchoroidal space produces no or hardly any (extremely weak) echoes in serous detachments; the hemorrhage spikes are low and equally distributed throughout the subchoroidal space in hemorrhagic detachments when the blood is fluid; and the blood spikes are high and often irregularly distributed when the subchoroidal blood is coagulated.

The following ultrasonographic equipment was used in this analysis: Standardized A-scan (Kretz 7200 MA) and contact real-time B-scan (Ocuscan 400 and/or Ultrascan II AB 404). Standardized Echography directs the surgeon to the site of best surgical approach for drainage and provides accurate follow-up assessments.

K.C. Ossoinig (editor), Ophthalmic Echography, ISBN 978-94-010-7988-4
© 1987, Martinus Nijhoff/Dr W. Junk Publishers, Dordrecht.

346

References

1. Hawkins WR, Schepens CL. 1966. Choroidal detachment and retinal surgery. American Journal of Ophthalmology. #5, Vol. 62, Nov., pp. 813–819.
2. Bellows RA, Chylack LT, Hutchinson BT. 1981. Choroidal detachment: clinical manifestation on therapy and mechanism. Ophthalmology, Vol. 88, #11, Nov., pp. 1107–1115.
3. Ossoinig KC. 1979. Standardized echography: basic principles, clinical applications and results from 'Ophthalmic Ultrasonography Comparative Techniques'. (Dallow RL, ed.) Int Ophth Clin, 19/4, 127–210. Little Brown and Co., Boston.

Acoustic analysis of the cytologic structure of malignant melanomas with standardized echography*

P.A. DIXON, G.W. ABRAMS and J.G. CAYA
Milwaukee, USA

Abstract

Twenty-seven consecutive choroidal malignant melanomas were prospectively classified by echographic criteria as predominantly spindle cell or predominantly epithelioid cell tumors. Histopathology of the enucleated eyes confirmed a correct echographic diagnosis in 15 eyes with predominantly spindle cell tumors which had a homogeneous to slightly heterogeneous internal structure, low to medium reflectivity, usually large angle kappas, and intense, diffuse spontaneous vascular activity in different sound beam directions. Three tumors echographically called predominantly spindle cell had no predominance of one cell type over the other. We correctly identified 5 predominantly epithelioid cell melanomas which displayed a markedly heterogeneous internal structure in 4 of 5, medium to medium-high reflectivity, little to no sound attenuation, and intense but less diffuse spontaneous vascular activity. Four other epithelioid cell tumors with echographic characteristics similar to the predominantly spindle cell tumors were misidentified. These tumors had only slightly heterogeneous structure on low power histopathologic examination in contrast to the more marked histopathologic heterogeneity of the correctly identified epithelioid cell lesions. This technique is valuable in identifying a certain group of highly malignant melanomas.

Differentiation of ocular tumors with echography is a common and reliable technique [1, 2]. Previous reports have described the principles of tissue characterization [1, 3, 4–11] and efforts have been made to differentiate the cell types of malignant melanomas with ophthalmic ultrasound [16]. Previous studies have demonstrated that the histologic classification of malignant melanomas is of prognostic significance: the more anaplastic the cell type, the more malignant the neoplasm [15, 17, 18]. The ability to differentiate the various

* This work is partially supported by an unrestricted grant from Research to Prevent Blindness, Inc.

K.C. Ossoinig (editor), Ophthalmic Echography, ISBN 978-94-010-7988-4

melanoma cell types with echography would allow the ophthalmologist to better predict the clinical course and decide the method of treatment.

We have noticed variations in the acoustic patterns of tumors diagnosed echographically as malignant melanomas, and these echographic variations correlate with variations in the histologic structure of ocular melanomas. We have undertaken a prospective study to classify melanomas echographically as either predominantly spindle or predominantly epithelioid cell prior to their enucleation. Pathologic correlations were obtained following removal of the affected eyes. We were able to accurately identify a specific group of epithelioid melanomas with our technique.

Materials and method

Twenty-eight consecutive eyes were enucleated which contained tumors diagnosed echographically as primary choroidal melanomas. Ciliary body and iris lesions were excluded to eliminate additional variables. All of the lesions were evaluated by one examiner (P.A.D.) with the Kretztechnik 7200 MA Standardized A-scan and the Ocuscan 400 Contact B-scan (Sonometrics Systems, Inc., New York, New York). Tissue sensitivity was established for the Standardized A-scan prior to the onset of the study with a silicone and glass bead tissue model developed by Till and Ossoinig [11, 12]. Tissue sensitivity was checked periodically throughout the study and noted to remain stable and consistent.

Lesions were evaluated according to topographic, quantitative, and kinetic echographic characteristics [5, 13]. Photographic documentation was obtained and all findings were recorded during the course of the examination.

Topographic information (i.e. shape, location and extension) was obtained primarily with the Contact B-scan. We elicited the shape of the tumor by scanning across the lesion from different sound beam directions. Location was noted by establishing the relationship of the lesion to normal intraocular structures. Special sections were obtained demonstrating the proximity of the tumor to the optic disc. The lateral dimensions were recorded with perpendicular B-scan sections through the middle of the tumor. The maximal elevation of these lesions was obtained with the Standardized A-scan at reduced sensitivity by measuring from the peak of the tumor surface signal to the inner scleral surface.

We obtained quantitative information with the Kretztechnik 7200 MA Standardized A-scan. We evaluated the internal structure of the lesion by directing the sound beam through the tumor in different sound beam directions. We took special care to aim the sound beam perpendicular to the surface of the tumor in each direction so that displayed echoes emanated from within the center of the mass and false readings from echoes striking the edges of the tumor were avoided. We graded the structure of the lesion as follows: homogeneous (consistent patterns in different sound beam directions with echoes basically of the same amplitude), slightly heterogeneous (slight variations noted in the multiple patterns), and heterogeneous (great variations noted in spike amplitude and pattern appearance in different sound beam directions).

We quantitated the internal reflectivity in homogeneous and slightly heterogeneous lesions [5, 13]. In those lesions which displayed a heterogeneous internal structure, the average or predominant reflectivity was recorded utilizing different sound beam directions.

We assessed the angle kappa (degree of sound attenuation) within the lesion by estimating the angle formed by an imaginary line at the top of the display and the slope of the internal lesion echoes [14]. In tumors which displayed extremely low internal reflectivity, we increased instrument gain to better quantitate the angle of sound attenuation.

We evaluated kinetic criteria with the Standardized A-scan. Solid consistency of the tumor was established if no aftermovement of the lesion's surface signal could be detected at reduced sensitivity. In those lesions with overlying retinal detachment, we placed emphasis on identifying both the echo emanating from the retinal surface and from the tumor surface. We graded spontaneous vascular activity, noting intensity (rate and amplitude of spontaneous vascular activity), and distribution (distribution throughout the mass in an anterior/posterior direction in different sound beam directions). We graded each criteria on a scale from one to three. Intensity graded 1 + was subtle, while intensity graded 3 + was quite marked. Distribution graded 1 + was localized, while grade 3 + was diffuse. Grade 2 + in both categories was intermediate between grades 1 + and 3 +. We obtained all kinetic criteria utilizing information from multiple sound beam directions.

We grouped homogeneous, low to medium reflective, highly vascularized tumors as predominantly spindle cell lesions and heterogeneous, medium to medium-high reflective lesions which displayed less vascularity (or irregularly distributed vascularity) as predominantly epithelioid cell tumors.

Following the enucleation of these eyes, the tumors were evaluated by an ocular pathologist (J.G.C.), masked to the echographic findings, and each tumor was graded as predominantly spindle or predominantly epithelioid cell type. Predominance of a cell type was called when a particular cell type exceeded 66%. Also noted was the caliber, number and distribution of vascular structures, variation in cellular arrangement, and variations within the tumor's structure such as necrosis and fibrous septa.

The tissue sections of each enucleated tumor were evaluated by another masked investigator (G.W.A.), blind of the echographic and histopathologic findings, who graded the homogeneity of the internal structure histologically

TECHNIQUE ACCURACY

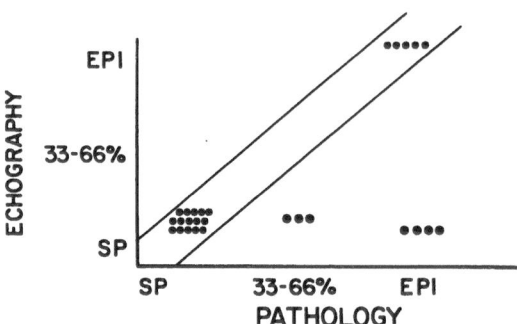

Table 1. Technique Accuracy: echographic Diagnosis vs. Histopathological Diagnosis of 27 melanomas. SP = Predominantly spindle cell, 33–66% = Intermediate cell group, Epi = Predominantly epithelioid cell.

at low power through the microscope. Those lesions which displayed a monotonous cellular appearance, void of fibrous septa and arrangement variability, were called homogeneous. Lesions with some fibrous septa or large vascular structures but otherwise with a monotonous cellular growth pattern were determined borderline heterogeneous. In cases where great variability or bizarre cellular patterns were noted, the structure was graded heterogeneous.

Results

Of the twenty-eight enucleated eyes suspected of harboring primary choroidal melanomas, twenty-seven of the lesions were melanomas and comprise the data of this study. The false positive lesion was an inflammatory granuloma in a blind painful eye in a patient later found to have Wegener's granulomatosis.

Of the twenty-seven enucleated tumors correctly diagnosed echographically as malignant melanomas, eighteen were in right eyes and nine in left. The patient age range was twenty-three to eighty-four years with a mean age of 63.4 years. Thirteen patients were male and fourteen female. Twenty-six patients were caucasian and one was black.

We called twenty-two melanomas predominantly spindle cell and five predominantly epithelioid cell echographically. On pathological evaluation, fifteen of the melanomas diagnosed with Standardized Echography as primarily spindle cell were predominantly spindle cell. All five diagnosed echographically as epithelioid cell tumors were composed predominantly of epithelioid cells. Of seven further tumors diagnosed as spindle cell melanomas by our echographic criteria, three fit into an intermediate zone (33–66% cellular mix)

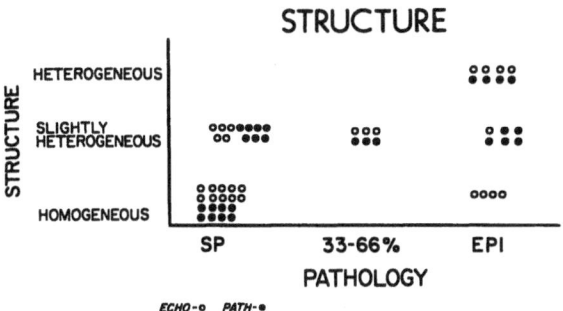

Table 2. Heterogeneity of structure determined by echography and low power microscopy vs. histopathological diagnosis.

and four were predominantly epithelioid (Table 1). The following results of the acoustic analyses of these tumors will indicate why our method worked in some instances but failed in others.

The tumors in our series had an average elevation of 10.86 mm ranging from 3.8 mm to 17.3 mm. Eighteen of the lesions were mushroom-shaped, seven were dome-shaped and two irregularly elevated. The tumors were scattered throughout the fundus with a predilection for the temporal fundus with fifteen occurring temporally, five nasally, four superiorly and three inferiorly.

Echographically, the internal structure was homogeneous in fourteen eyes, borderline heterogeneous in nine eyes and heterogeneous in four eyes. On pathological evaluation, internal structure was homogeneous in eight eyes, borderline heterogeneous in fifteen eyes and heterogeneous in four eyes (Table 2). All of the spindle cell tumors fell into the homogeneous or slightly heterogeneous groups both echographically and pathologically. The intermediate cell group were slightly heterogeneous on both pathologic and echographic evaluation. Those determined markedly heterogeneous echographically were noted to be heterogeneous pathologically. All four of these lesions were correctly diagnosed echographically as predominantly epithelioid cell tumors. One predominantly epithelioid tumor correctly diagnosed echographically had borderline heterogeneous structure by both echographic and pathologic examination. Four epithelioid melanomas misdiagnosed echographically as spindle cell tumors had homogeneous patterns ultrasonically. These tumors were noted to be slightly heterogeneous pathologically. The slight heterogeneity noted histologically within these four predominantly epithelioid lesions was secondary to scattered fibrous septa and/or large vascular channels. These pathologic interfaces did not appear to affect the homogeneity of the echographic patterns.

Nine of the tumors had low reflectivity, thirteen had low to medium reflectivity, and five had medium to medium-high reflectivity. All of the predomi-

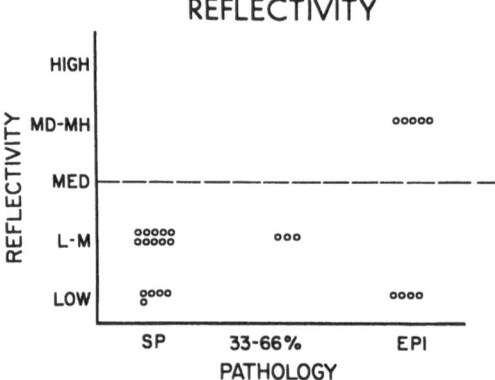

Table 3. Echographic tumor internal reflectivity vs. histopathological diagnosis. L–M = low to medium reflectivity, MD–MH = medium to medium high reflectivity.

nantly spindle cell tumors were of low to low-medium reflectivity (Table 3). The three intermediate lesions had low to medium reflectivity and four of the predominantly epithelioid tumors had low reflectivity. These last four tumors were the misdiagnosed tumors echographically and were also the same lesions which displayed a homogeneous internal structure. The five medium to medium-high reflective tumors were diagnosed echographically as predominantly epithelioid cell melanomas. This echographic prediction was shown to be correct pathologically.

Ten of the fifteen predominantly spindle cell tumors demonstrated significant signal attenuation (large angle kappa) (Table 4). Three predominantly spindle cell tumors had a small angle kappa, with two demonstrating no sound attenuation throughout the masses. The three tumors which fell into the

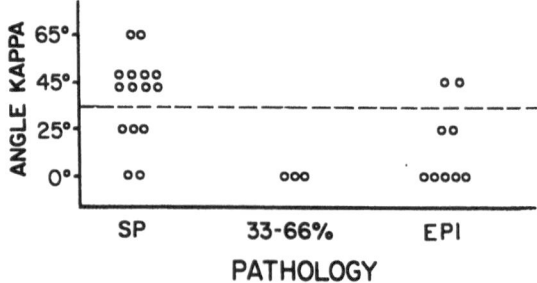

Table 4. Echographic tumor angle kappa vs. histopathological tumor diagnosis.

VASCULARITY

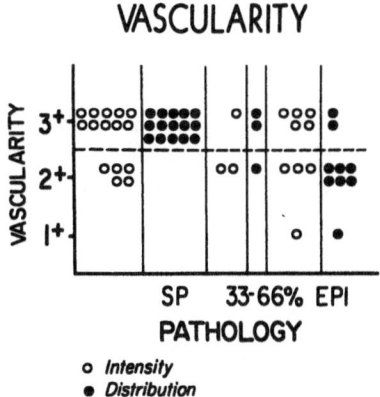

Table 5. Echographic tumor spontaneous vascular activity vs. histopathologic diagnosis.

classification of intermediate cell type showed no angle of attenuation. The five predominantly epithelioid tumors which displayed no angle kappa were the lesions diagnosed correctly echographically as predominantly epithelioid. The predominantly epithelioid masses which displayed a small angle kappa along with the two which demonstrated a large degree of sound attenuation were the tumors misdiagnosed echographically.

All twenty-seven of the lesions displayed acoustic characteristics of a solid consistency. Ten of the fifteen predominantly spindle cell tumors had spontaneous vascular activity of 3+ intensity with the remaining five of 2+ intensity. All fifteen of the predominantly spindle cell lesions were graded as 3+ on distribution (Table 5). The intermediate cell group was split between 2+ and 3+ on intensity and distribution. Five of the predominantly epithelioid masses were noted to demonstrate 3+ intensity of the spontaneous vascular activity, with three displaying 2+ and one 1+. Two demonstrated 3+ distribution, six showed 2+, and only one had 1+.

Discussion

All of the spindle cell tumors in our series had a homogeneous or slightly heterogeneous internal structure. They displayed low to low medium internal reflectivity, usually large angle kappas and intense, diffuse spontaneous vascular activity in different sound beam directions (Fig. 1). Our intermediate group of lesions were slightly heterogeneous, had low to medium reflectivity and displayed no angle of sound attenuation. Typically these lesions also demonstrated high degrees of diffuse spontaneous vascular activity. We detected two distinct groups of epithelioid lesions. The group that was correctly diagnosed

354

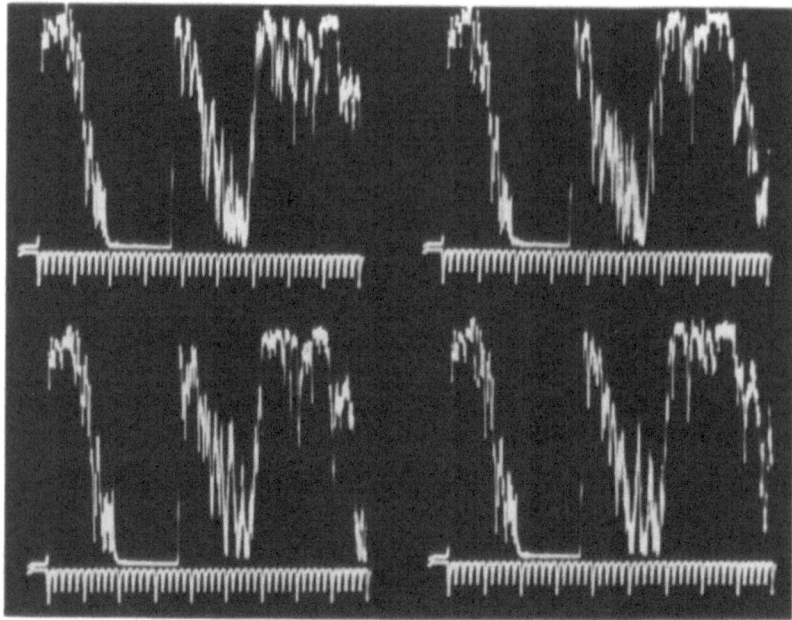

Fig. 1. Predominantly spindle cell tumor. Echograms in multiple sound beam directions. Note low to medium reflectivity, homogeneous internal structure, large angle kappa, and diffuse spontaneous vascular activity (blurred internal echoes).

echographically in each instance displayed a marked heterogeneous internal structure in four of five eyes, had medium to medium-high internal reflectivity, little to no sound attenuation and intense but less diffuse spontaneous vascular activity (Fig. 2). The group which we failed to identify correctly mimicked the acoustic characteristics of predominantly spindle cell tumors. This group displayed a homogeneous internal structure, low internal reflectivity, large angle kappa, and diffuse, intense spontaneous vascular activity in different sound beam directions.

We identified a specific group of predominantly epithelioid cell lesions which can be diagnosed accurately with Standardized A-scan. This group is characterized pathologically by great variation in cellular pattern. We believe that it is the interfaces created by these varying cellular patterns that yield the more irregular and highly reflective echographic patterns. Pathologically, these bizarre cellular patterns are indicative of a more highly malignant entity [15].

Noteworthy was the discovery of a group of predominantly epithelioid cell tumors which displayed a regular internal structure. Histologically the cellular patterns showed little variation, giving a monotonous appearance overall. We were unable to differentiate this group of epithelioid cell lesions from spindle

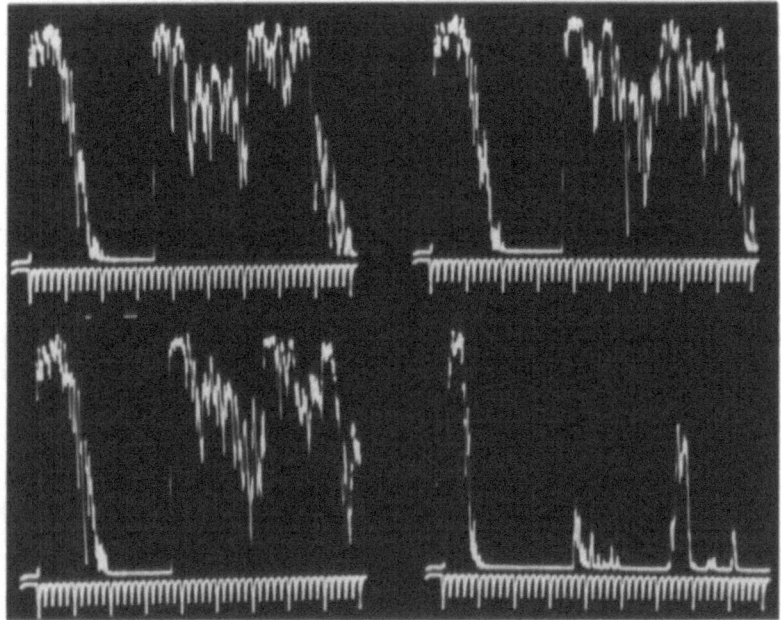

Fig. 2. Predominantly epithelioid cell tumor. Echograms in multiple sound beam directions. Note heterogeneous internal structure and medium to medium high reflectivity. Echogram in lower right corner at reduced sensitivity to demonstrate actual lesion elevation.

cell tumors with our current technique. Our series of tumors was too small and our patient follow-up insufficient to determine if there is a difference in the morbidity between these two groups of predominantly epithelioid cell tumors. The echographic differences between these two groups of predominantly epithelioid lesions was not due to the percentage of epithelioid cells.

No correlation could be drawn between our findings of intensity and distribution of the spontaneous vascular activity phenomenon noted with the Standardized A-scan and the caliber, number and location of the vascular structures which was described on pathologic evaluation.

This prospective study is significant in that we have shown that a specific group of predominantly epithelioid cell tumors can be identified utilizing our technique with the Standardized A-scan. This finding should be of value to the ophthalmologist in planning management of these more malignant tumors.

References

1. Ossoinig KC, Bigar F and Kaefring SL. 1975. Malignant Melanoma of the Choroid and Ciliary Body: A differential Diagnosis in Clinical Echography. In Ultrasonography in Ophthalmology. Bibl. Ophthalmol. 83: 141–154, Karger, Basel.

356

2. Ossoinig KD. 1983. Advances in Diagnostic Ultrasound. In ACTA: XXIV International Congress of Ophthalmology. Paul Henkind (Ed.) American Academy of Ophthalmology, JB Lippincott Co., Philadelphia.
3. Baum G. The Ultrasonic Characteristics of Malignant Melanoma. In Ultrasonics in Ophthalmology, Oksala and Gernet (Eds.), Karger, Basel, 1967a. pp 22–26.
4. Baum G. 1967. Ultrasonographic Characteristics of Malignant Melanoma. Arch. Ophthalmol. 78: 12–15.
5. Ossoinig KC. 1979. Standardized Echography: Basic Principles, Clinical Applications, and Results. Int. Ophthalmol. Clin. 19: 127–210.
6. Ossoinig KC. 1974. Quantitative Echography. The Basis of Tissue Differentiation. J. Clin. Ultrasound. 2: 33–46.
7. Ossoinig KC. 1974. Preoperative Differential Diagnosis of Tumors with Echography, Part I. Physical Principles and Morphologic Background and Tissue Echograms. Current Concepts in Ophthalmol, Vol. 4: Chapter 17, pp 264–280. CV Mosby Co., St. Louis.
8. Ossoinig KC. 1974. Preoperative Differential Diagnosis of Tumors with Echography, Part II. Instrumentation and Examination Techniques. Current Concepts in Ophthalmol., Vol. 4: Chapter 17, pp 280–296, CV Mosby Co., St. Louis.
9. Ossoinig KC, Blodi FC. 1974. Preoperative Differential Diagnosis of Tumors with Echography, Part III. Diagnosis of Intraocular Tumors. Current Concepts in Ophthalmol., Vol. 4: Chapter 17, pp 296–313, CV Mosby Co., St. Louis.
10. Ossoinig KC. 1974. Quantitative Echography. The Basis of Tissue Differentiation. J. Clin. Ultrasound. 2: 33–46.
11. Ossoinig KC, Patel JH. 1977. A-scan Instrumentation for Acoustic Tissue Differentiation, III. Testing and Calibration of the 7200 MA Unit of Kretztechnik. Ultrasound in Medicine, Vol. 3B: White D and Brown RE (Eds.) Plenum Publishing Corp., New York, pp 1955–1964.
12. Till P, Ossoinig KC. 1977. First Experiences with a Solid Tissue Model for the Standardization of A and B-scan Instruments in Tissue Diagnosis. In Ultrasound in Medicine, Vol. 3B: White D and Brown RE (Eds.) Plenum Publishing Corp., New York, pp 2167–2174.
13. Byrne SF. 1979. Standardized Echography Part I: A-scan Examination Procedures. Int. Ophthalmol. Clin., 19: 267–281.
14. Minning CA Jr., Davidorf FH. 1982. Ossoinig's Angle of Ultrasonic Absorption and its Role in the Diagnosis of Malignant Melanoma. Ann. Ophthalmol. 14: 564–568.
15. Callender GR. 1931. Malignant Melanotic Tumors of the Eye: A Study of Histologic Types in 111 Cases. Trans. Am. Acad. Ophthalmol. Otolarnygol. 36: 131–142.
16. Coleman DJ, Lizzi FL. 1983. Computerized Ultrasonic Tissue Characterization of Ocular Tumors. Am. J. Ophthalmol. 96: 165–175.
17. Paul EV, Parnell L, Fraker M. 1962. Prognosis of Malignant Melanomas of the Choroid and Ciliary Body Int. Ophthalmol. Cl. 2: 387–402.
18. Reese AB. 1976. Tumors of the Eye (Third Edition) Harper and Row, Hagerstown, New York, San Francisco, London, p. 196.

Is it possible to differentiate histological types of choroidal malignant melanoma with Kretztechnik 7200 MA A-scans?

V. MAZZEO, L. RAVALLI, M. SPETTOLI and A. ROSSI
Ferrara, Italy

Introduction

Two years ago Ossoinig and Till (1982) suggested the possibility of differentiating between the histological types of choroidal malignant melanoma. They
based their evaluation on A-scans obtained using the Kretztechnik machine.
However, their results were not published extensively and, if we remember
correctly, they chose internal tumor reflectivity and angle K as parameters. In
order to confirm their hypothesis, we have reviewed the A-scans obtained wih
Kretztechnik 7200 MA of choroidal malignant melanomas seen over the past
10 years. All of these tumors had been histologically evaluated by the same
pathologist in order to ensure a uniform answer.

Material and methods

We evaluated 33 eyes: 25 spindle and 8 epithelioid cell tumors. Mixed cell
tumors were not considered since their lack of homogeneity could create
difficulties in echographic classification. The parameters we chose for evaluation are summarized in Table 1. Reflectivity was choses because it is the main
parameter for differentiating pathologic tissues, although Noble, Findl et al.
(1984) found that this parameter alone is not sufficient to differentiate histological types of malignant melanoma. Angle K (Ossoinig, K.C., 1982) represents a clinical approximation of attenuation. The latter includes absorption,
reflection and diffusion. When frequency is constant, it is entirely dependent
on tissue characteristics and thickness. We considered angle K as positive, zero
and negative. We judged an echo trace as regular on the basis of height and
spatial distribution of the spikes. The latter seems to represent the spatial
distribution of the different tissue components (scattering areas vs. reflecting
areas). In order to choose the best traces in each patient's series, two physicians were employed to go through the traces. One was an expert with long

K.C. Ossoinig (editor), Ophthalmic Echography, ISBN 978-94-010-7988-4
© 1987, Martinus Nijhoff/Dr W. Junk Publishers, Dordrecht.

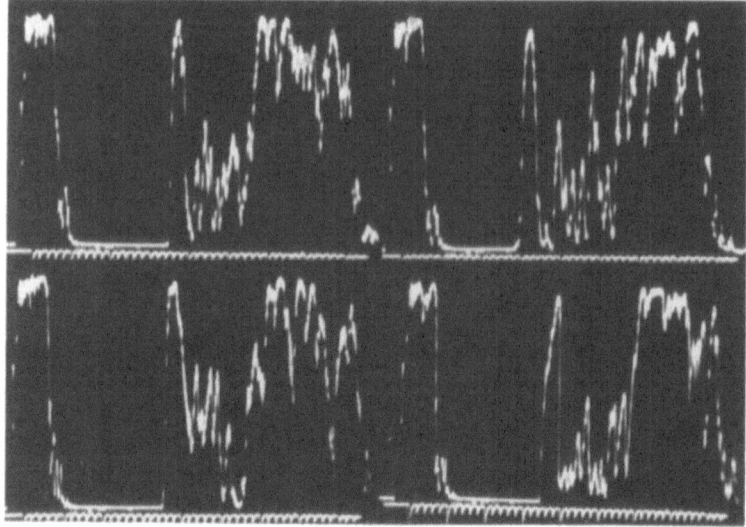

Fig. 1. A-scans of the same spindle cell malignant melanoma. The echo traces show different combination of relectivity, regularity and angle K.

experience in the field, and the other one was fairly new to this work. The A-scans belonging to the same histological type were evaluated on the basis of the above-mentioned parameters with a view to revealing common patterns. The second stage was performed by two different physicians (same criteria as physicians in stage 1) who, in a double-blind test, had to divide all the echo traces in the two histological classes on the basis of their previous colleagues' findings.

Results

Our results were entirely unsatisfactory. The choice of the most representative echogram in one patient's series was very difficult, the same case being regular

Table 1.

Reflectivity (average internal)	5–20%
	20–40%
	40–60%
Attenuation (angle K)	positive (+)
	absent (0)
	negative (−)
Regularity	homogeneous
	unhomogeneous

and irregular at the same time, as well as showing different K angles (Fig. 1). Among the images of an individual case, we chose the one which gave rise to the fewest problems for interpretation. The characteristics of the 33 echograms which were chosen are summarized in Table 2. It was impossible to find a common characteristic in the echo patterns of the different histological types (Fig. 2).

Table 2. Tabular presentation of cases.

Patient	Thickness	Average internal reflectivity	Regularity	Angle K
Spindle cell malignant melanomas				
B.N.	6 μsec.	30%	homogeneous	+30°
M.G.	14 μsec.	60%	homogeneous	+5°
S.D.	6 μsec.	5%	homogeneous	+5°
C.M.	3 μsec.	50%	homogeneous	neg.
B.B.	8,5 μsec.	50%	unhomogeneous	+50°
F.G.	13 μsec.	15%	homogeneous	+30°
Z.E.	9 μsec.	30%	homogeneous	+60°
M.R.	12 μsec.	50%	homogeneous	+40°
F.L.	3 μsec.	10%	homogeneous	+45°
G.L.	7,5 μsec.	20%	homogeneous	+35°
P.G.	11 μsec.	50%	unhomogeneous	+50°
Q.L.	14 μsec.	60%	unhomogeneous	+50°
R.M.	16 μsec.	50%	unhomogeneous	+45°
S.L.	4,5 μsec.	55%	homogeneous	neg.
Z.A.	10 μsec.	35%	unhomoeneous	neg.
M.G.	9 μsec.	60%	unhomogeneous	+50°
B.P.	9 μsec.	20%	unhomogeneous	neg.
S.G.	3 μsec.	40%	homogeneous	0
D.S.	11 μsec.	45%	homogeneous	+45°
C.L.	12 μsec.	60%	unhomogeneous	0
F.G.	4 μsec.	55%	homogeneous	+60°
G.E.	5 μsec.	40%	unhomogeneous	+50°
B.P.	3,5 μsec.	40%	homogeneous	neg.
A.E.	9 μsec.	30%	homogeneous	+55°
B.B.	9 μsec.	30%	homogeneous	+55°
Epithelioid cell malignant melanomas				
M.L.	6 μsec.	20%	unhomogeneous	0
B.G.	9,5 μsec.	15%	homogeneous	neg.
B.A.	12 μsec.	50%	unhomogeneous	+55°
P.D.	17 μsec.	45%	homogeneous	+45°
C.L.	5 μsec.	45%	homogeneous	+50°
T.M.	15 μsec.	40%	unhomogeneous	+25°
T.G.	7,5 μsec.	55%	homogeneous	0
B.E.	14 μsec.	70%	unhomogeneous	+25°

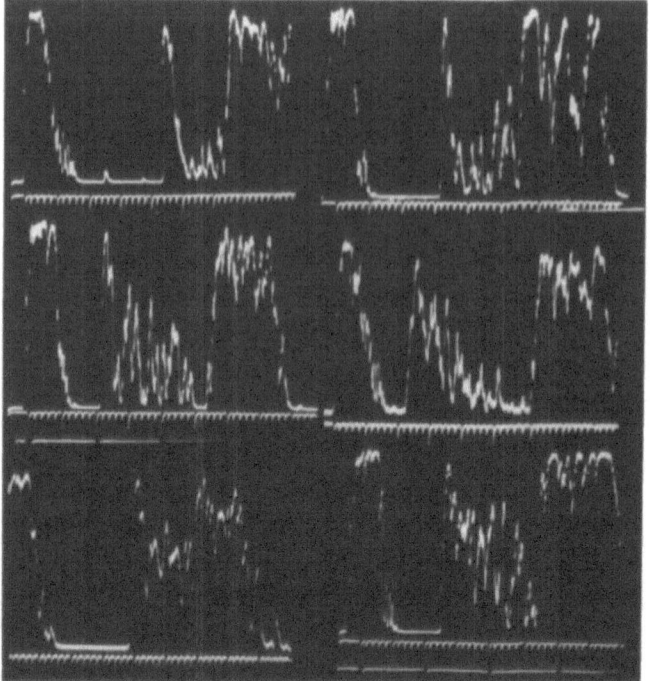

Fig. 2. A-scans belonging to 3 different spindle cell (left) and 3 different epithelioid cell (right) malignant melanoma. The traces are more similar in each row than in the two columns.

Conclusions

In the light of our study, it appears that average internal reflectivity, angle K and regularity have no significant correlation with histopathology. The cell type cannot, therefore, be differentiated by means of visual A-scan evaluation.

References

Ossoinig KC. 1982. Personal Communication. International School of Ultrasonology, Ettore Majorana Centre for Scientific Culture, Erice, Trapani, Italy 6–13 March.

Ossoinig KC, Till P. 1982. The echographic differential diagnosis of malignant melanoma of the uvea. SIDUO IX Abstract and program: 17.

Noble JL, Marsh IB. 1982. An analysis of 30 cases of proven malignant melanoma of the choroid; ultrasnographic and histological findings. Ophthalmic Ultrasonography. Proceedings of the 9th. SIDUO Congress, Leeds, 20–23 July: 29–36. Hilman & Le May (Eds.).

Acoustic tissue typing with computerized methods

D.J. COLEMAN, F.L. LIZZI, R.H. SILVERMAN, M. RONDEAU,
M.E. SMITH, J. TORPEY and P. GREENALL
New York, USA

Abstract

A retrospective review of 37 patients with histologically proven data indicates
a clear-cut differentiation of malignant melanoma into two separate entities
corresponding to the spindle B and the mixed-epithelioid staining model types
of the Calender classification. We have attempted to define the origin of tissue
differences by using an athymic nude mouse model which allows us to grow
tumors from human tissue cultures of the size and acoustic character that
simulate human intraocular tumors.

In a series of tumors including melanoma, metastatic carcinoma from lung,
breast and colon, the micro and macro architectural changes which relate to
spectral distinctions can be studied with light, electron, and acoustic microscopy. The effects of growth and treatment on the cell structure can thus be
monitored in a way not possible in human clinical studies. The clinical application of information from these studies can dictate pre-treatment differentiation and augment post-treatment evaluation of the effectiveness of treatment.

This work was supported by NIH Grants EY–01212 and EY–03183 and a
grant from The Dyson Foundation.

K.C. Ossoinig (editor), Ophthalmic Echography, ISBN 978-94-010-7988-4

Acoustic tissue differentiation with Standardized Echography in reference to melanomas and pseudomelanomas

K.C. OSSOINIG, D.S. RESHEF, R.P. HARRIE and G.C. HASENFRATZ
Iowa City, USA

Abstract

With Standardized A-scan, several acoustic properties of intraocular tumors can be determined and utilized for differentiation: the internal structure, as indicated by the lengths of the tumor spikes (regular and homogeneous, regular and heterogeneous, irregular); the reflectivity, as indicated by the height of the tumor spikes at 'Tissue Sensitivity' (extremely low, low, medium, high, and extremely high); the sound absorption as expressed by the angle kappa (no angle or minimal angle, medium angle, large angle); and the bloodflow within tumor vessels (intensity and distribution). These acoustic criteria are directly caused or influenced by the macroscopic and microscopic structures of the tumor tissues. Using certain combinations of those acoustic A-scan features – so-called tissue signatures – tissue diagnoses can be made from the Standardized A-scan echograms. So far, a reliable and accurate differentiation between melanomas and 'pseudomelanomas' (i.e., choroidal metastatic carcinomas, nevi, hemangiomas, disciform lesions, etc.) has been achieved. The detection of dense scleral infiltration and even of minute extraocular extension by melanomas has become routine. During the past few years, the differentiation of melanomas into various types was attempted on this basis. The correlation of these types with the histological cell types and the prognosis of patient survival is under investigation.

K.C. Ossoinig (editor), Ophthalmic Echography, ISBN 978-94-010-7988-4
© 1987, Martinus Nijhoff/Dr W. Junk Publishers, Dordrecht.

References

1. Ossoinig KC. 1979. Standardized echography: basic principles, clinical applications and results. In: Ophthalmic Ultrasonography: Comparative Techniques (Dallow RL, ed.) Int. Ophthal. Clin., 19/4 (1979): 127–210. Little, Brown & Co., Boston.
2. Ossoinig KC. 1982. Advances in diagnostic ultrasound. ACTA: XXIV International Congress of Ophthalmology, (San Francisco), Paul Henkind, ed. Philadelphia: JB Lippincott Co., Vol. 1: pp. 89–114.
3. Ossoinig KC. 1985. Standardized ophthalmic echography of the eye, orbit and periorbital region. A comprehensive Slide Set (774 slides) and Study Guide, Third Edition. Iowa City, Iowa: Goodfellow Company, Inc., pp. 29–36.

Use of pulsed Doppler ultrasonography to evaluate blood flow in intraocular melanomas

W.S. GRIZZARD, W.M. BLACKSHEAR, S.E. PAUTLER and S. LAMB
Tampa, USA

Abstract

Pulsed Doppler ultrasound was used to evaluate the eyes of 12 patients with ocular melanomas. Eight eyes were enucleated; one was lost to follow-up; three patients were treated with heavy ion radiation. In all patients flow could be detected using the pulsed Doppler technique. The location and character of the flow from within tumors was different than that detected in normal eyes.

Introduction

Ophthalmic ultrasound uses the reflective and absorptive properties of ultrasound in tissue but generally disregards the information available from the shift of ultrasound frequency caused by blood movement within the tissue scanned. Doppler ultrasound also uses a transducer composed of a piezoelectric crystal that emits a high frequency ultrasound wave. This wave is changed in frequency either above or below the base frequency as it is reflected from moving blood cells within arteries and veins. This signal is detected by a receiving crystal and is translated into an audible signal. The frequency shift is defined by the Doppler equation:

$$C\,F_D = 2VF_o\,\cos\theta.$$

C represents a constant related to the speed of sound in tissue, F_D is the frequency of the reflected Doppler signal, V represents the velocity of red blood cells, F_o is the frequency of the baseline Doppler signal, and theta is the Doppler angle between the axis of flow and the incident Doppler beam (Fig. 1).

A continuous wave Doppler uses two piezoelectric crystals within the scanning probe. One crystal acts as a sending crystal and the other crystal operates continuously as a receiver. The pulsed Doppler operates in a similar

K.C. Ossoinig (editor), Ophthalmic Echography, ISBN 978-94-010-7988-4

366

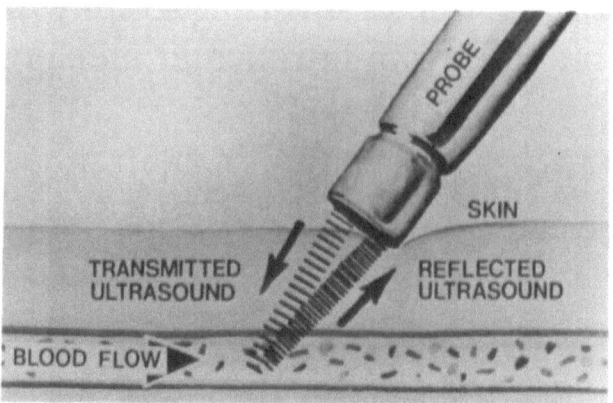

Fig. 1. Blood cells moving within arteries and veins cause frequency shift of ultrasound waves.

fashion but instead uses a single crystal which alternately sends and receives. By varying the time interval between transmission and reception of a pulse of ultrasound and by using a focused transducer, blood flow from within a small sample volume, a known distance from the transducer, can be evaluated (Fig. 2) (Grizzard et al., 1982).

The anatomy of the eye provides a uniquely informative setting for evaluation of abnormal masses with a pulsed Doppler probe. The eye generally has a fixed diameter with an avascular center. Blood flow within the vitreous is always abnormal and the direction of arterial flow within a tumor is always toward the apex from the base. The flow of blood in the choroid normally runs perpendicular to a probe scanning across the eye, which tends to minimize the signal received from normal flow.

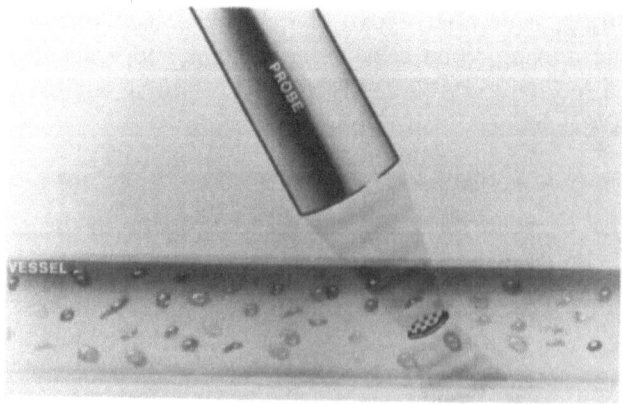

Fig. 2. Pulsed Doppler probe detects frequency shift from small coin shaped sample volume a known distance from the end of the probe.

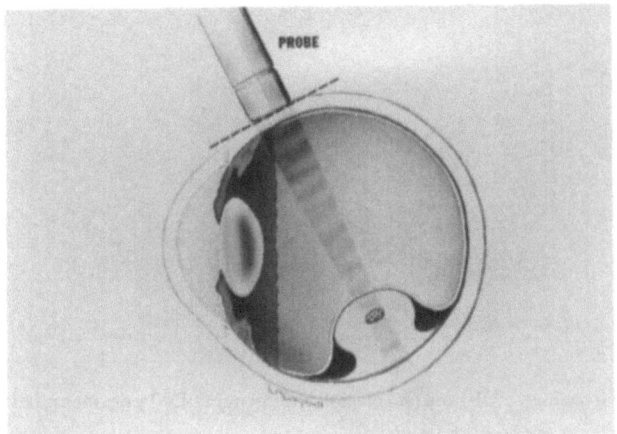

Fig. 3. Blood flow from ocular tumors is assessed by scanning across the eye.

Materials and methods

We used a pulsed Doppler probe with a base frequency of 5 megahertz focused 3 mm from the end of the probe.* The signal was processed in real time by fast Fourier transform spectrum analysis with a commercially available spectrum analyzer+ and spectral data was recorded on Polaroid film from an oscilloscope. The probe was used in a manner similar to that used in standardized echography by scanning from the limbus across the eye toward the tumor (Fig. 3). The probe position and location was determined by using a Kretz A-scan probe to locate the tumor and then positioning the Doppler probe in an identical manner.

Six normal eyes were scanned. Blood flow was detected from the optic nerve at 26 mm of depth. Choridal blood flow or ciliary artery blood flow was detected posteriorly at a depth of 22 to 24 mm. In the twelve patients with a tumor the depth of the scan was set at 22 mm and several additional depths were evaluated to locate the most intense signal.

All patients with a tumor greater than 4 mm in height were included in this study. The data from the twelve patients with a tumor were analyzed to see if peak systolic or peak diastolic frequency shift in ocular tumors were different from the blood flow detected from normal eyes. We also analyzed the frequency spectra to evaluate the flow in diastole as a function of systolic flow in a manner similar to that which Pourcelot described to measure the distal vascu-

* P–1 Ultrasonic arteriograph, D.E. Hokanson, Inc., Issiquah, Washington.
+ Angioscan, Union Industries, Inc., Mt. Vernon, New York.

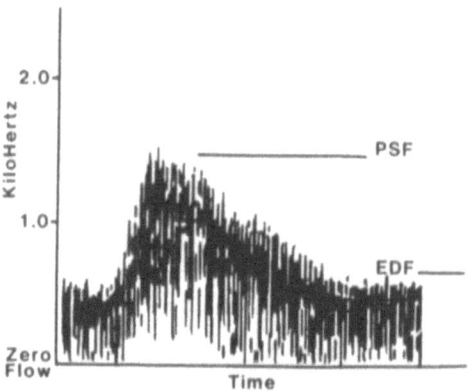

Fig. 4. Peak systolic frequency (PSF) and end diastolic frequency (EDF) were measured as shown.

lar resistance to flow in the common carotid artery (Planiol and Pourcelot, 1973). We measured the peak maximum systolic frequency (PSF) and the end maximum diastolic frequency (EDF) (Fig. 4) and constructed a frequency ratio:

$$FR = \frac{PSF - EDF}{PSF}.$$

We compared the ratio from our twelve patients with tumors with our normals. We also compared the four spindle cell tumors with the three mixed cell and one epithelioid tumor to see if the frequency shift data correlated with tissue type. All data was analyzed by the Student's T Test to evaluate statistical significance.

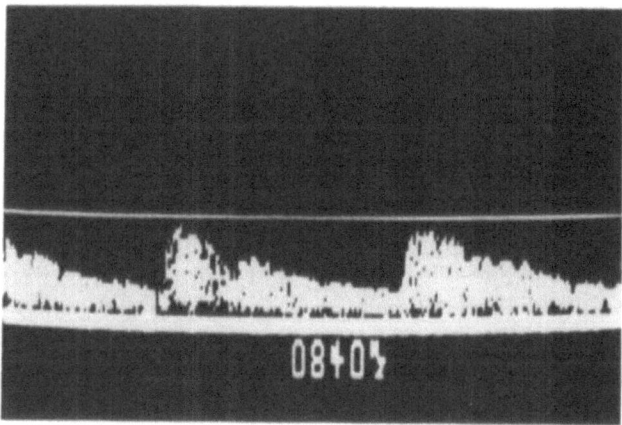

Fig. 5. Frequency shifts from 26 mm posterior to limbus scanning from the nasal limbus were presumed to be from central retinal artery within the optic nerve.

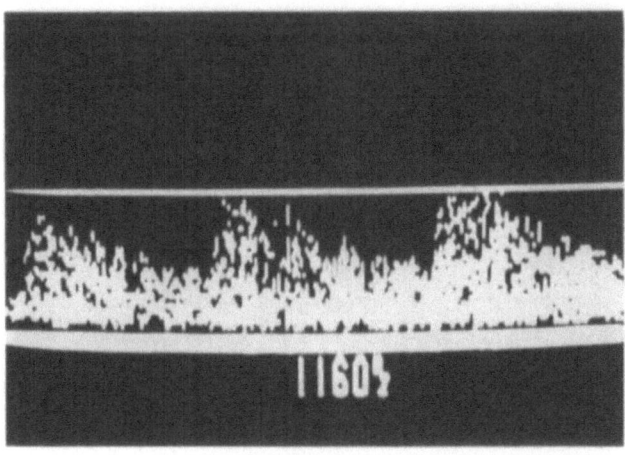

Fig. 6. Frequency shift from 22 mm posterior to limbus showed low FR which was thought to be caused by choroidal blood flow with low resistance.

Results

Normals demonstrated a characteristic pattern of optic nerve flow which showed a sawtooth pattern with diastolic flow approximately 25% of systolic (Fig. 5). This pattern is typical of a highly resistant vasculature and is caused, we think, by resistance within the retinal vascular system and the resistance to blood flow caused by intraocular pressure.

A normal choroidal blood flow could be found at 22 to 24 mm posteriorly, generally at 3 and 9 o'clock (Fig. 6). The characteristic flow pattern showed a diastolic flow usually about 50% of systolic. The frequency shift was minimal primarily because flow was perpendicular to the scanning beam. By angling the probe, the systolic and diastolic frequencies could be increased and readings could be obtained at less than 22 mm because the probe was no longer scanning across the diameter of the eye but across a shorter chord. False positive readings were thus possible when scanning technique was not meticulous.

In all patients with melanomas, flow was detected in the vitreous cavity where no flow was detected in normals (Fig. 7). Mean values for peak systolic fequency, end diastolic frequency, and frequency ratio are shown in Table 1. No significant difference was noted between normal patients and tumor patients with respect to PSF or EDF (P>0.2). FR was higher in the tumor patients suggesting an increased resistance to arterial flow than was present in the normal choroid. This difference was statistically significant (P<.05). The difference between mixed and epithelioid tumors (N = 4) and spindle B tumors (N = 4) was not significant for EDP, PSF, or FR.

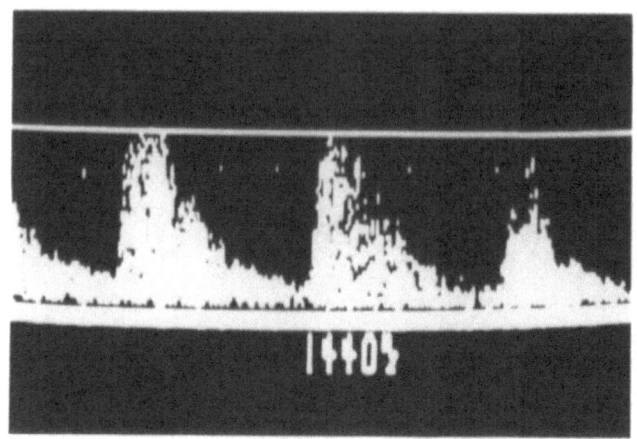

Fig. 7. Blood flow 21 mm posterior to limbus within mixed cell tumor shows marked increase in frequency ratio (FR).

The three patients who were treated have each behaved differently. One patient had flow which had been previously detected disappear nine months after treatment. Her eye subsequently developed rubeosis iridis and some diminution in tumor size. She is considered a therapeutic success. A second patient has shown increasing flow one year following treatment. His tumor has shown no change in size and still has subretinal fluid present. This tumor is still being followed but may represent a failure. The third patient has shown no response to treatment in ten months. Her tumor and Doppler findings have remained unchanged.

Discussion

Blood flow within eyes and ocular tumors can be detected using pulse Doppler ultrasound and offers yet another noninvasive confirmatory test in the evaluation of ocular masses. This may be helpful in evaluating ocular mass lesions, particularly in eyes with opaque media. Doppler flow spectra from within a

Table 1. Pulsed Doppler frequency data.

	PSF	EDF	FR
Normals (6)	880 ± 93	317 ± 55	0.645 ± 0.031
Tumors (12)	983 ± 105	250 ± 20	0.731 ± 0.021
$\pm$ SEM			

tumor gives information about blood flow over the entire cardiac cycle which is information not available by any other technique. This information may be helpful in the diagnosis of ocular tumors but may be of particular use in following patients who have been treated with radiation.

By combining a B-scan unit with a pulsed Doppler into what is called a duplex scanner, more precise localization of the sample volume can be obtained. The current technique used may allow blood flow from displaced retinal vessels over the tumor surface to contribute to the signal received. Such devices are now in use in noninvasive laboratories for carotid evaluation and we are in the preliminary stages of evaluating them for ophthalmic use.

The only similar work we are aware of is being done in England by Dr. Burns and coworkers (P.N.T. Burns et al, 1982). His group is using a duplex scanner with pulsed Doppler signal analysis in the evaluation of breast masses. He has noted abnormal flow characteristics in breast tumors. The use of pulsed Doppler flow has not, to our knowledge, been used to evaluate response to radiation therapy in cancerous tissue. This may prove to be a useful technique in the eye as well as in other parts of the body.

References

Burns PN, Virjee J, Halliwell M, Wells PNT, Webb AJ. 1982. On the Origin of Doppler Shift Signals from Malignant Breast Tumors. Third meeting of the World Federation for Ultrasound in Medicine and Biology. Brighton, England, 1982. Abstract in Volume 8: Supplement 1, Ultrasound in Medicine and Biology p27.

Grizzard WS, lackshear WM, Rush JA, Gordon SF. 1982. Noninvasive Carotid Evaluation Using Pulsed Doppler Imaging for Patients with Ophthalmic Disorders. Ophthalmology; 89: 1235–1240.

Planiol TH and Pourcelot L. 1973. Diagnostic des Thomboses et Stenoses Carotidenne: par esset Doppler. Second World Congress Ultrasonics in Medicine, Rotterdam.

Contact and immersion ultrasonography in the evaluation of topography of uveal melanomas

N. WEYER-HAAK, J.M. SEDDON, E. GRAGOUDAS and L. VERHEY
Boston, USA

Abstract

For the past 9 years, ophthalmologists from the Massachusetts Eye and Ear Infirmary in collaboration with the Department of Radiation Medicine at the Massachusetts General Hospital have been using proton beam irradiation at the Harvard University Cyclotron for the treatment of uveal melanomas. As part of their pretreatment evaluation, patients undergo ultrasound examinations. These examinations are of particular importance in the planning of the radiation treatments, specifically for defining the size and the three dimensional shape of the lesion and its relationship to the optic nerve, macula and anterior structures of the eye. To assist the ophthalmologists, radiation therapists and physicists in their planning efforts, immersion ultrasonography has been supplemented in recent months by the addition of a contact B scan. Advantages and disadvantages of the two techniques in regard to resolution, definition of tumor shape and direction into the vitreous and the ability to visualize the relationship of the optic nerve to the lesion will be discussed.

Introduction

From August 1975 to September 1984, a total of 520 patients with uveal melanoma have been treated with proton beam irradiation. High energy proton beams offer multiple advantages for the irradiation of selected tumors, particularly ocular tumors [3]. The advantages are based exclusively on the physical properties of the proton beam, namely minimal scatter, tissue sparing at the entry site, uniformly high dose throughout the tumor region, and a sharp fall-off of dose just beyond the tumor at the end of the beam [5]. All of these characteristics are ideal for highly localized dose distributions such as those necessary to irradiate uveal melanomas. Since a controlled tumoricidal dose can be delivered to the tumor, the surrounding ocular tissues can be spared from radiation.

K.C. Ossoinig (editor), Ophthalmic Echography, ISBN 978-94-010-7988-4

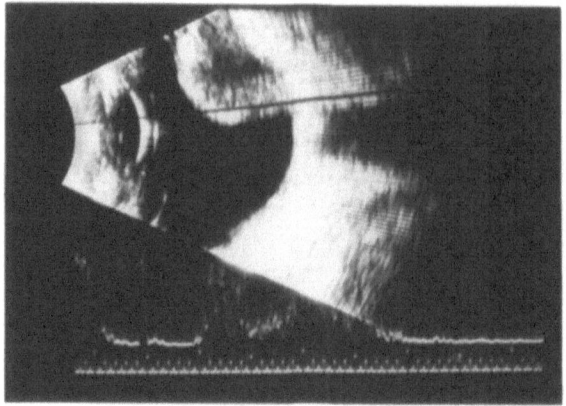

Fig. 1. Contact scan of uveal melanoma.

Patients with melanomas underwent pretreatment ultrasound examinations which included contact and immersion B scanning. The physicists depend on the ultrasound for the exact dimensions of the eye, the shape, location, and height of the tumor as well as the position of the optic nerve in different directions of gaze. The information obtained from the ultrasound together with the fundus photographs and the radiographically determined coordinates of four tantalum rings sutured to the sclera, which outline the edges of the tumor, is used in the treatment planning (Figs. 1 and 2).

Methods

Between June 1984 and September 1984, 50 patients with uveal melanomas were examined by contact and immersion B scan ultrasound. The instruments used were the Cooper Vision Ultrascan contact B scan and the Sonometrics Ophthalmoscan 200, an immersion system. Each examination was performed with a 10 MHz transducer. The examinations included axial length measurements, measurement of the height of the tumor, and scans taken through the optic nerve and lesion simultaneously.

The first portion of the examination was performed with the immersion system. The axial length was measured with the A scan biometry module of the Ophthalmoscan 200. Scans were taken in horizontal and vertical directions, displaying the optic nerve while attempting to simultaneously display the maximum height of the tumor. When this was not possible, scans were done to search for the maximum height of the tumor.

Contact B scan examination was performed following the immersion examination. Axial length measurements were obtained using the biometry module

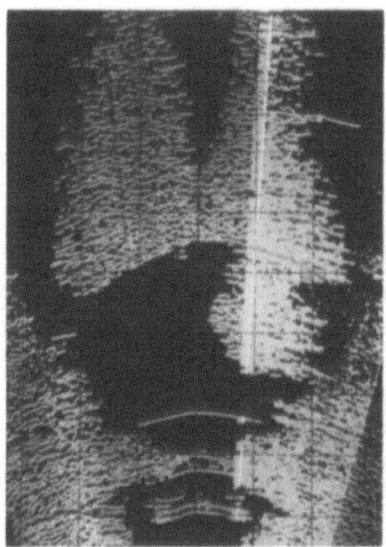

Fig. 2. Immersion scan of uveal melanoma.

and the immersion technique using a scleral shell. Again multiple scans were taken with the optic nerve and the lesion in the scan. Each scan was labeled as to the approximate orientation in the eye. Transverse scans were also taken displaying the maximal elevation of the tumor with the tumor centered in the photograph. The height of the tumor is obtained by measuring the greatest perpendicular distance between the surface of the retina and the base of the tumor. In contact scanning, the tumor height is measured by using the measuring scale provided on the A and B combined scan. In the future, the height of the tumors will be measured by the standardized A scan 7200 MA from Kretz.

Results

For the purposes of evaluation of the topography of uveal melanomas, we found contact B scanning to be superior to immersion scanning. The advantages of both techniques are listed in the table (Table 1).

The resolution of the contact scan was superior to that of the immersion scan and produced ultrasound photographs which provided more information to the physicists. Evaluation of the topography of lesions is the domain of B scanning. Through B scan evaluation, the shape, lateral extension and location of intraocular tumors can be determined [7]. The contact scan provided superior documentation of tumor extension into the vitreous, an important criteria in the treatment planning. During the examination sectional cuts were taken through the lesion maintaining the optic nerve in the scan. The patient maintained a straight gaze position during the procedure. Because the probe could be placed directly on the eye and controlled by the ultrasonographer, the orientation of the scan relative to the axes of the eye could be more precisely determined. Large melanomas often present with an irregular shape and the procedure of making serial cuts through the tumor was very helpful, thereby giving an accurate assessment of the tumor topography.

Since the height of the tumor is currently measured from B scan photographs, tumors that are located anteriorly are difficult to measure with immersion ultrasound. Because of the locaton of these tumors, the anterior retinal surface is not well defined. We believe that anterior tumors are inherently more difficult to differentiate from retina due to the tangential approach of the sound waves. We have found that the higher resolution of the contact unit and the absence of the lid speculum make the contact scan superior to the immersion scan in the evaluation of such lesions.

We found contact scanning to provide greater sensitivity. With contact scanning the subtle differences between interfaces was well appreciated. The ability to adjust the sensitivity buttons on the Cooper unit helped in the detection of more discrete pathology that was missed by the immersion examination. The sensitivity setting of the immersion scanner was kept at maximum for all examinations. Several patients have undergone evaluations where the vitreous appeared clear on immersion scanning and a vitreous hemorrhage was detected on contact scan evaluation. In patients who have developed cataracts or dense hemorrhage and no view of the fundus was possible, the greater sensitivity of the contact scan was a positive factor in the examination.

Contact B scan has the advantage of providing real time examinations. This is often helpful in cases of melanomas with associated vitreous hemorrhage where the aftermovement of the hemorrhage can be appreciated [1]. Reduplication artifacts and blurring of the signals received from the interior of the eye due to the irregularity of the surface of the eye are eliminated with

Table 1.

Contact	Immersion
1. Better resolution	1. Superior in anterior segment
2. Greater sensitivity	
3. Advantage of real time	
4. Elimination of artifacts	
5. More comfortable and easier for patients	

contact B scanning. Refraction and sometimes total reflection of the sound waves occurs at the surface of the eye causing significant blurring of the ultrasound image. The placement of the probe directly on the globe eliminates these artifacts [1, 6].

It has been our experience that patients are more comfortable with the contact examination than with the immersion examination. Due to this fact, we have found a greater level of cooperation from patients during these difficult ultrasonic examinations. In addition, the contact examination is shorter and easier for the patient to undergo.

The immersion scan does provide better resolution of the anterior segment and therefore is superior to the contact scan for the evaluation of iris melanomas. Due to the presence of a large electronic artifact, the first few millimeters adjacent to the transducer are obscured in contact scanning. In order to view the anerior segment, a water bath is used to provide the standoff.

Contact B scanning is now being used in the follow up ultrasounds of patients who have been treated with proton beam irradiation. For the reasons mentioned above we find that contact scanning provides the necessary information to evaluate tumor regression or growth.

References

1. Bronson NR. 1974. Contact B-Scan Ultrasonography. Am J Ophthalmol, February, 77/2: 181–191.
2. Kremkau F. 1980. Diagnostic Ultrasound, Physical Principles and Exercises. New York, Grune & Stratton, Inc., pp. 68–71.
3. Gragoudas ES, Goitein M, Verhey L, et al. 1982. Proton Beam Irradiation of Uveal Melanomas. Arch Ophthalmol, June, 100: 928–934.
4. Gragoudas ES, Goitein M, Koehler A, et al. 1977. Proton Irradiation of mall Choroidal Malignant Melanomas. Am J Ophthalmol, May, 83/5: 665–673.
5. Lou P and Gragoudas E. 1983. A- & B- Mode Ultrasound Biometry in the Proton Beam Irradiation f Uveal Melanomas. In Hillman JS, Lemay MM (eds): Ophthalmic Ultrasonography. The Hague/Boston/Lancaster, Dr. W. Junk Publishers, pp. 51–56.
6. Ossoinig KC. 1972. Clinical Echo-Ophthalmography. In Current Concepts in Ophthalmology. St. Louis, C.V. Mosby Co. Vol. III: pp. 101–130.
7. Ossoinig KC. 1979. Standardized Echography: Basic Principles, Clinical Applications, and Results. In Dallow RL (ed): In Ophthal Clin. Boston, Little Brown & Co., 19/4: pp. 127–285.
8. Seddon J, Gragoudas E, and Albert D. 1983. Ciliary Body and Choroidal Melanomas Treated by Proton Beam Irradiation: Histopathologic Study of Eyes. Arch Ophthalmol, September, 101: 1402–1408.
9. Verhey L and MunzenriderJE. 1982. Proton Beam Therapy. Ann Rev Biophys Bioeng, 11: 331–357.

Ultrasound characteristics of posterior uveal melanomas treated with cobalt plaque radiotherapy

H.J. SHAMMAS, D.S. BOYER and J.B. MILLER
Los Angeles, USA

Abstract

Five eyes harboring posterior uveal melanomas were examined before and one year after treatment with cobalt plaque radiotherapy. Post-operatively, B-scan ultrasonograms revealed a change in the tumor's size and shape, a decrease in the area of echolucency within the tumor and the formation of new areas of echolucency within the sclera and orbital tissues. Standardized A-scan echograms showed an irregular acoustic structure, a higher reflectivity and wide orbital echoes. The average decrease in height was 37%.

Introduction

Ultrasonography is a major diagnostic tool in presence of an intraocular tumor [1, 2]. A and B scan acoustic criteria are typical and allow a differentiation between posterior uveal melanomas and other choroidal tumors. These acoustic criteria change when the tumor is exposed to radiotherapy [1, 3]. We herein describe the ultrasound findings in five cases of posterior uveal melanomas treated with cobalt plaque radiotherapy.

Material and methods

We treated five eyes harboring uveal melanomas with cobalt plaque radiotherapy; each scleral cobalt-60 plaque delivered approximately 10,000 rads to the tumor's apex. One tumor (case 1) was located in the ciliary body and the other four tumors (cases 2-5) were choroidal. Each eye was evaluated with ultrasonography before and approximately one year after treatment; we used a contact B-scan unit and the Kretz 7200 MA standardized A-scan unit.

The tumor's thickness was measured before and one year after treatment; for this purpose, the system sensitivity of the Kretz unit was decreased by 20 decibels.

K.C. Ossoinig (editor), Ophthalmic Echography, ISBN 978-94-010-7988-4

380

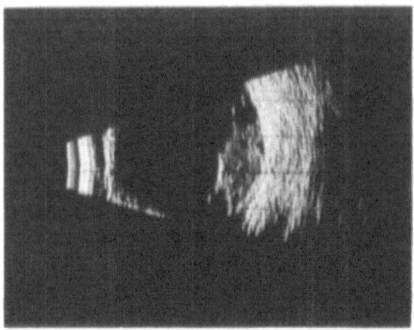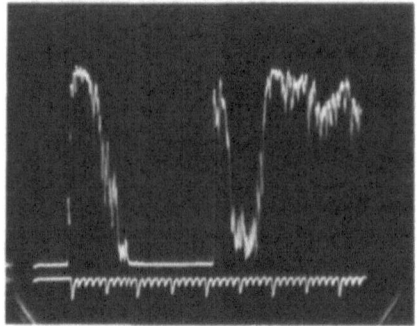

Fig. 1. Choroidal melanoma before treatment (case 5). *Left* (Fig. 1a) B-scan ultrasound. *Right* (Fig. 1b) A-scan ultrasound.

Results

Melanoma changes on B-scan ultrasonography

Treated melanomas (Figs. 2a and 4a) appeared as highly echogenic masses. Preoperative areas of echolucency within the tumors and areas of choroidal excavation (Figs. 1a and 3a) tended to disappear after treatment.

The tumors decreased in size with a change in shape. The regression pattern was regular in cases 2, 3, & 5 (Figs. 1a and 2a) and irregular in cases 1 and 4 (Figs. 3a and 4a). New areas of echolucency were noted within the sclera and orbit behind the tumor (Fig. 4a).

Table 1. Ultrasound changes of treated posterior uveal melanomas compared to the preoperative findings.

	Case 1	Case 2	Case 3	Case 4	Case 5
*B-scan changes**					
– variation in size and shape	++	++	++	++	++
– highly echogenic mass	+	–	++	+	+
– sclera echolucency	+	++	–	++	–
*A-scan changes**					
– Irregular acoustic structure	+	++	+	+	++
– high internal reflectivity	++	–	++	++	++
– widening of orbital echoes	+	++	++	++	–

* These changes were extreme (++), minimal (+) or absent (-).

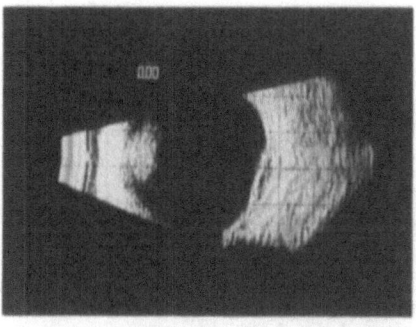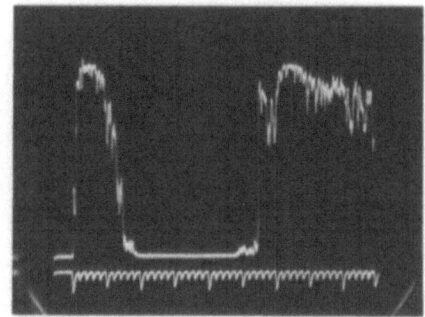

Fig. 2. Choroidal melanoma one year after treatment (case 5) showing a regular pattern of regression. *Left* (Fig. 2a) B-scan ultrasound. *Right* (Fig. 2b) A-scan ultrasound.

Melanoma changes on A-scan ultrasonography

The acoustic structure in treated choroidal melanomas became irregular and the internal reflectivity increased (Figs. 2b and 4b) compared to a regular structure and low internal reflectivity prior to treatment (Figs. 1b and 3b). Vascularity within the tumor remained present, however, the spontaneous movements of the lesion spikes were difficult to display. The orbital echoes became wider with a decrease in reflectivity. (Fig. 4b).

These B and A scan changes were variable. Their presence or absence in our five cases is noted in Table 1.

The tumor's height decreased in every case. The decrease varied from 14% to 60% during the follow-up period. The average decrease in height was 37%.

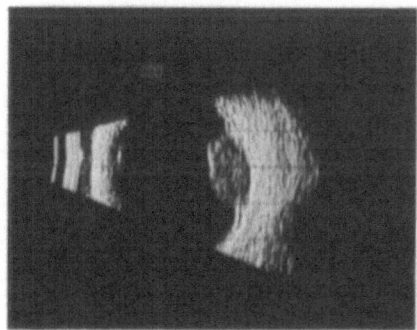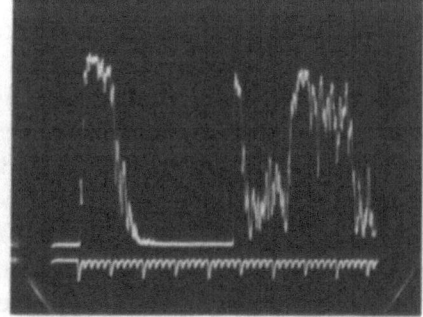

Fig. 3. Choroidal melanoma before treatment (case 4). *Left* (Fig. 3a) B-scan ultrasound. *Right* (Fig. 3b) A-scan ultrasound.

382

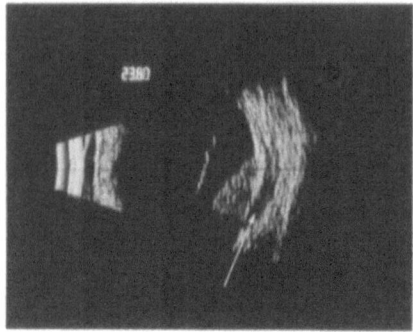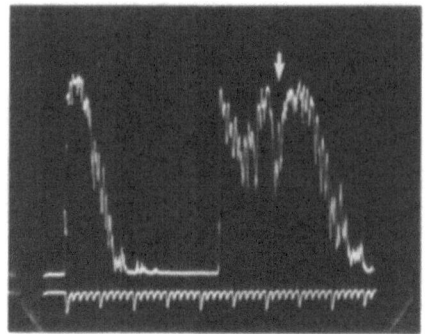

Fig. 4. Choroidal melanoma one year after treatment (case 4) showing an irregular pattern of regression. *Left* (Fig. 4a) B-scan ultrasound. *Right* (Fig. 4b) A-scan ultrasound.
Note the presence of an area of echolucency (arrow) with the scleral and orbital tissues on the B-scan and the widening of the orbital echoes (arrow) on the A-scan (arrow).

Vitreo-retinal changes

Vitreo-retinal changes were noted in three eyes. These included the clearing of a vitreous hemorrhage in case 1, a detached retinal in case 2, and vitreous opacities with a posterior vitreous detachment in case 4.

Discussion

For several years, enucleation was the treatment of choice of an eye harboring a posterior uveal melanoma. [4] In 1978, Zimmerman et al [5] questioned the value of enucleation leading to a more conservative approach in the management of posterior uveal melanomas; cobalt plaque radiotherapy is an alternative to enucleation. [3]

Ultrasonography is useful in making an accurate preoperative diagnosis. [1, 2] The major B-scan acoustic criteria include the presence of an echogenic subretinal mass and a moderate sound attenuation with areas of echolucency within the uveal mass. The major A-scan acoustic criteria include a regular acoustic structure and a low to medium internal reflectivity. Our article describes marked changes in these acoustic criteria following cobalt plaque radiotherapy. Variations in size and shape are noted in every case with either a regular (Figs. 1 and 2) or and irregular regression pattern (Figs. 3 and 4).

In most cases the uveal mass becomes highly echogenic on B-scan echography and displays a high internal reflectivity on A-scan echography. These ultrasound changes indicate the presence of multiple large interfaces; these interfaces separate fibrotic and necrotic areas within the uveal mass. Scleral and orbital changes are noted in four out of the five cases. Areas of echolu-cency are noted on B-scans and widening of the orbital echoes on A-scan; these changes are due to necrotic and inflammatory process within the sclera and adjacent orbital tissues, produced by the large dose of radiation. These scleral and orbital changes noted on ultrasonography should not be confused with an orbital extension of the tumor.

The tumor thickness decreased in every case; the decrease was minimal in cases 3 and 4 and substantial in cases 1 and 5. The average decrease in height was 37% after a one year follow-up. However these tumors can become active again. All treated eyes should be evaluated at regular intervals by indirect ophthalmoscopy and ultrasonography; an increase in tumor thickness and the formation of low reflective areas on A-scan echography are suspicious of tumor growth.

References

1. Shammas HJ. 1984. Atlas of ophthalmic ultrasonography and biometry. The C.V. Mosby Co., St. Louis. pp. 57–93.
2. Ossoinig KC. 1974. Preoperative differential diagnosis of tumors with echography, III: Diagnosis of intraocular tumors. In current concepts in ophthalmology, F.C. Blodi (ed), pp. 296–313, Vol. 4, St. Louis. The C.V. Mosby Co.
3. Shields JA. 1983 Diagnosis and management of intraocular tumors. The C.V. Mosby Co., St. Louis. pp. 224–238.
4. Shammas, HF and Blodi FC. 1977. Prognostic factors in chorial and ciliary body melanomas. Arch Ophthalmol. 95: 63–69.
5. Zimmerman LE, McLean IW and Foster WP. 1978. Does enucleation of an eye containing a malignant melanoma prevent or a accelerate the dissemination of tumor cells? Br. J. Ophthalmol. 62: 420–425.

Uveal melanomas before and after Ruthenium application therapy

A.M. VERBEEK
Nijmegen, The Netherlands

Summary

A- and B-mode echography play a major role in the planning and control of irradiation therapy in uveal melanomas by helping to make the accurate diagnosis, choosing the way of treatment (measurement of tumour size, ruling out of extraocular extension), controlling the applicator position and measuring the radiation effects.

Introduction

Concerning uveal melanomas before and after Ruthenium application therapy we can subdivide this subject into five heads:
– the accurate diagnosis
– measurement of the tumour size
– ruling out of extraocular extension
– checking of the applicator position
– evaluation of the irradiation effects
To start with the accurate diagnosis: in 1983 Ossoinig (Ossoinig, 1983) showed in a world wide study that with standardised investigation techniques and calibrated equipment a very high accuracy level in the echographic diagnosis of uveal melanomas is achieved. In the same year Coleman and Lizzi (1983) showed that with computerized tissue characterization a further differentiation in cell-type is even possible, so we will spend no more time to the diagnostic part.

Methods

Echography plays its second role in the choice of treatment. Because of the

K.C. Ossoinig (editor), Ophthalmic Echography, ISBN 978-94-010-7988-4
© 1987, Martinus Nijhoff/Dr W. Junk Publishers, Dordrecht.

386

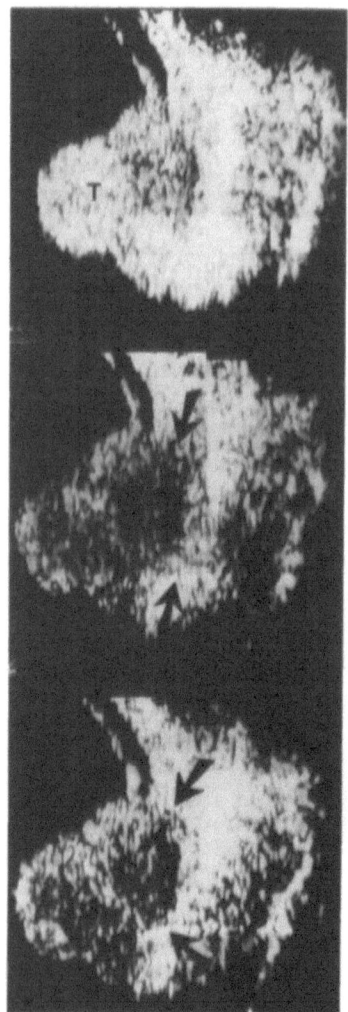

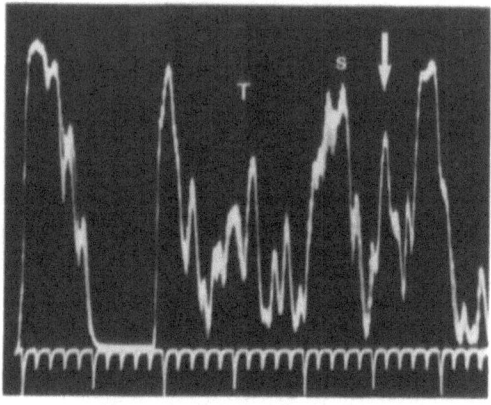

Fig. 1a. A-mode echogram of a 10.5 mm elevated choroidal melanoma (T) with extraocular outgrowth (white arrow) of 5 mm antero-posterior diameter.

Fig. 1b. B-mode echogram of the same melanoma. Black arrows indicate the extrascleral extension.

small penetration depth of Beta radiation into the tissue, only tumours with an elevation of 5 to 6 mm and a tumour base of 15 mm can be treated (Lommatzsch, 1983). So an exact measurement of the tumour size is needed and if treatment is possible echography will give the figures from which the application time can be calculated. This measurement is more accurate than when performed with the funduscope especially in case of a secondary retinal

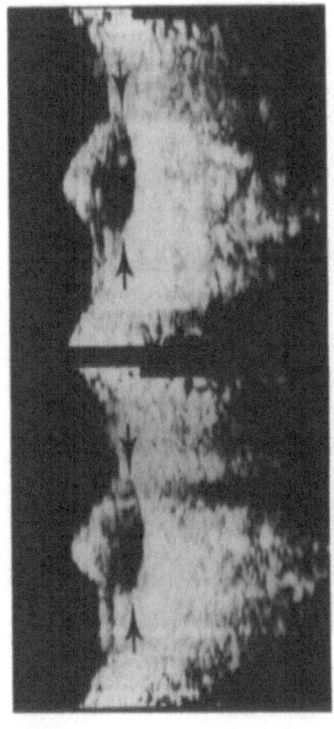

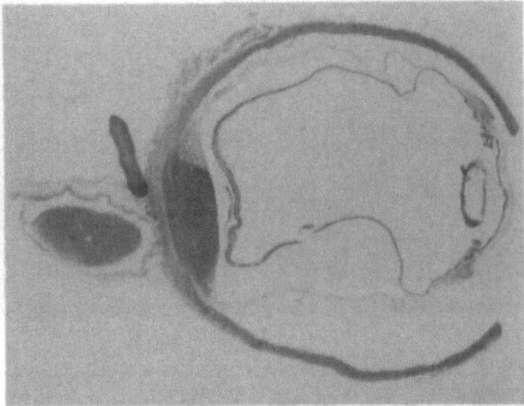

Fig. 2a. B-mode echogram of a choroidal melanoma with deep choroidal excavation (black arrows).

Fig. 2b. Histological section of this tumour shows a small extraocular extension.

detachment (Gutthof, 1980, Fried et al., 1982). With our equipment – the 7200 MA Kretztechnik A-scan, the Bronson-Turner and Triscan B-scanners – we think we are able to measure the tumour elevation with an accuracy of 0.3 mm and the tumour base with an accuracy of 2.0 mm. An even more important point in the planning of the treatment is to rule out an extraocular extension. In our experience, which is in accordance with the study of Noble and Marsh (1983), small extraocular outgrowth must be considered as a major problem of the pre-operative diagnosis. A real nodular extension with a minimum diameter of 2 mm can be detected (Martin et al., 1983) (Figs. 1 and b). Smaller extensions could not be detected as we experienced several times after histological examination (Figs. 2a and b). If radiotherapeutic treatment is decided on our next task is to control the right position of the applicator to the tumour base. Again, because of the small penetration depth of Beta radiation the application time depends much on a right apposition of the applicator. The last role for echography is the evaluation of the irradiation effect. In our

388

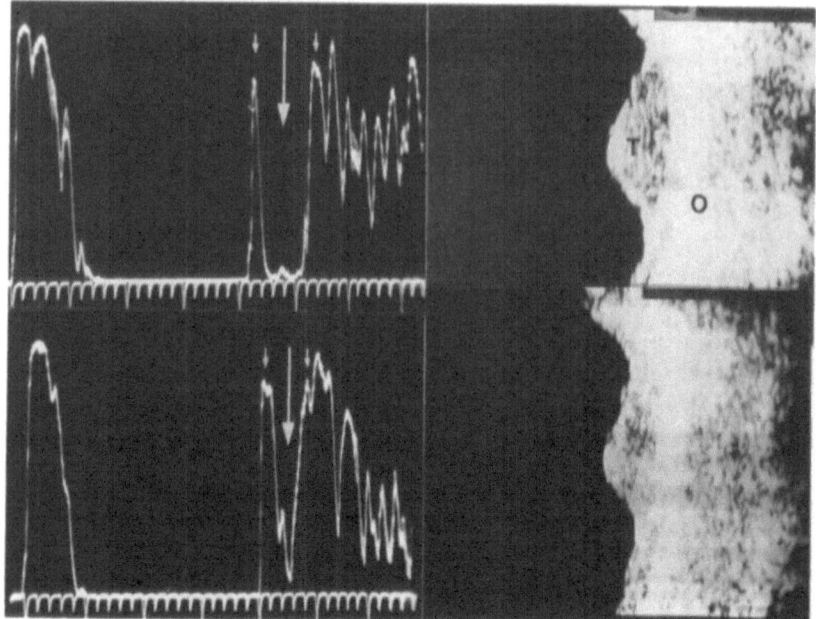

Fig. 3. Top: A- and B-mode echogram of a choroidal melanoma pre-radiation therapy. Bottom: The same process 9 months after Rutheniumapplication therapy. Note: the regression of the tumour elevation and the increase of internal reflectivity (white arrows).

relative small series we found like Shammas (1984) as signs of good effect:
– regression of the tumour size
– increase of the internal reflectivity
The increase of the internal reflectivity can be accompanied by the disappearance of the choroidal excavation and of the signs of vascularity (Figs. 3 and 4).

Results

Our patients were treated in the University Eye Clinics, Department of Ophthalmology Essen (Prof. dr. A. Wessing). We did the pre- and postoperative examinations. We are following 16 patients, 14 with a choroidal melanoma, 2 with a ciliary body melanoma. The follow-up time varies from 3 to 48 months. The media were clear in 13 patients of which 2 had a secondary retinal detachment. The media were opaque in 3 patients who came in after therapy. There was a mean tumour elevation of 4.25 mm (2.5–7.5 mm) and a mean tumour base of 8.4 mm (5.0–13.0 mm). We saw a reduction of the elevation in 5 patients from an average of 3.7 mm to undetectable in an average

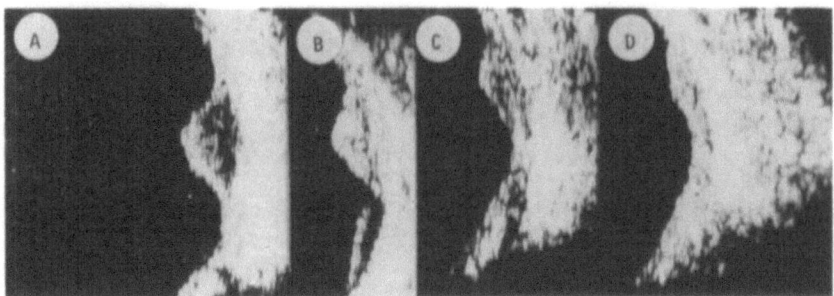

Fig. 4. B-mode sections of a choroidal melanoma pre- (A) and post (B, C, D) radiation therapy. The prominence of the tumour regresses, the internal reflectivity increases while a temporary exsudative retinal detachment existed (B).

period of 17.6 months (mean value: 0.2 mm elevation regression per month). In the 3 patients with opaque media no tumour residue could be detected. In the other 8 patients we found up till now a mean value of elevation regression of 0.1 mm per month. In 3 patients we saw after treatment an exsudative retinal detachment. We dit not find signs of regrowth or extraocular outgrowth in these patients. To summarize: we value echography as very positive in the planning and control of irradiation therapy in uveal melanomas. The measurements are sufficient accurate for the intended result. However, we have to realize that small extraocular extensions are not detectable.

References

Coleman JD, Lizzi FL. 1983. Computerized Ultrasonic Tissue Characterization of Ocular Tumours. Am. J. Ophthalmol. 96: p. 165–175.

Fried M, Foerster MH, Wessing A, Meyer-Schwickerath G. 1982. Echographische Größenbestimmung von Tumor und Lageüberprüfung des Applikators in der Ruthenium-Therapie beim Aderhautmelanom. Fortschr. Ophthalmol. 79: p. 193–198.

Guthoff R. 1980. Modellmessungen zur Volumenbestimmung des malignen Aderhautmelanoms. Albrecht von Graefes Arch. klin. Ophthalmol. 214: p. 139–146.

Lommatzsch PK. 1983. B-Irradiation of Choroidal Melanoma with $106_{Ru}/106_{Rh}$ Applicators. Arch. Ophthalmol. 101: p. 713–717.

Martin JA, Dennis F, Robertson M. 1983. Extrascleral Extension of Choroidal Melanoma diagnosed by Ultrasound. Ophthalmology. Vol. 90: p. 1554–1559.

Ossoinig KC. 1983. Advances in diagnostic Ultrasound. Acta: XXIV International Congress of Ophthalmology, American Academy of Ophthalmology (P. Henkind, ed.). J.B. Lippincott Company, Philadelphia.

Noble L, Marsh IB. 1984. An Analysis of 30 Cases of Proven Malignant Melanoma of the Choroid; Ultrasonographic and Histological Findings. In: Docum. Ophthalm. Proc. Series, Vol. 38 (J.S. Hillman and M.M. Le May, Eds.) The Hague, Junk: p. 29–36.

Shammas HJ. 1984. Atlas of Ophthalmic Ultrasonography and Biometry. C.V. Mosby Company St. Louis Toronto: p. 76–77.

Intraoperative use of ultrasound in the management of choroidal melanomas

C.J. PAVLIN, B. JAPP, D.G. PAYNE, A.M. DRYSDALE* and
B.L. GALLIE
Toronto, Canada

Introduction

We have used ultrasound intraoperatively as an adjunct in two types of therapy for choroidal melanoma. Ultrasound has been found useful as an aid in precisely positioning radioactive plaques in relation to the tumor base and confirming this relationship intra- and postoperatively. Ultrasound has also been used in cryo-enucleation to position the cryo-device and monitor the freezing process prior to enucleation.

Positioning radioactive plaques

Material and methods

A Cooper ultrascan (formerly Xenotec) combined A- and B-scan contact ultrasound unit is used. Preoperatively a radioactive plaque is constructed of concentric 192 iridium wire rings embedded in plastic and molded to the approximate curvature of the globe. Using a computer program, this plaque is individually designed to deliver an adequate radiation dose to the entire tumor [3]. Holes are made in the plaque edge for fixation to the sclera. At the same time a dummy plaque is constructed with the same dimensions and suture holes (Fig. 1).

The dummy plaque must provide good ultrasonic visibility for proper positioning. The ultrasonic characteristics found most useful for plaque visualization include the bright echoes from the surface of the plaque and the shadowing upon the orbital fat pattern secondary to reflection, scattering and absorption of sound by the plaque material. Several materials were tested in an

* Supported by A Gordon E. Richards Fellowship Grant from the Canadian Cancer Society, Ontario Division.

K.C. Ossoinig (editor), Ophthalmic Echography, ISBN 978-94-010-7988-4

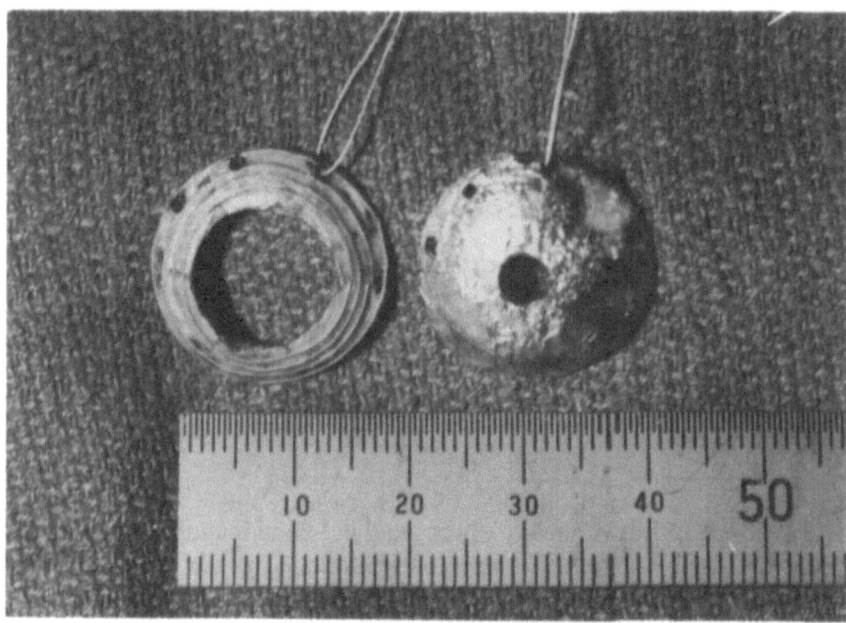

Fig. 1. Left: Radioactive plaque constructed of 192 iridium wires embedded in plastic. *Right:* Dummy plaque of identical dimensions constructed of aluminum foil embedded in plastic.

attempt to optimize these sonic characteristics (Figs. 2a, b and c). Most types of plastic, including hard acrylic, allow considerable passage of sound energy. Smooth metal produces confusing reverberation echoes behind it. Rough surfaced heavy duty aluminum foil was found to produce a bright echo from its surface and complete shadowing of structures behind it. The irregular surface scatters sound waves striking obliquely, improving visualization of the entire plaque at one time. The dummy plaque is, therefore, constructed of a sandwich of this material between two layers of plastic heat-molded to the approximate curve of the globe. A hole left in the centre of the dummy allows visualization of the orbital fat pattern at the centre of the plaque. This is an important aid in positioning the plaque below the centre of the tumor (Fig. 3).

Operative technique

The cord and most of the scanning head of the ultrasound unit is covered by a sterile sleeve (Fig. 4a). The transducer end is covered with a steridrape in which a sterile surgical lubricant (e.g. propylene glycol and hydroxy-ethyl cellulose gel) has been placed centrally (Fig. 4b). This produces good ultrasound transmission and prevents sticking of the drape to the membrane of the

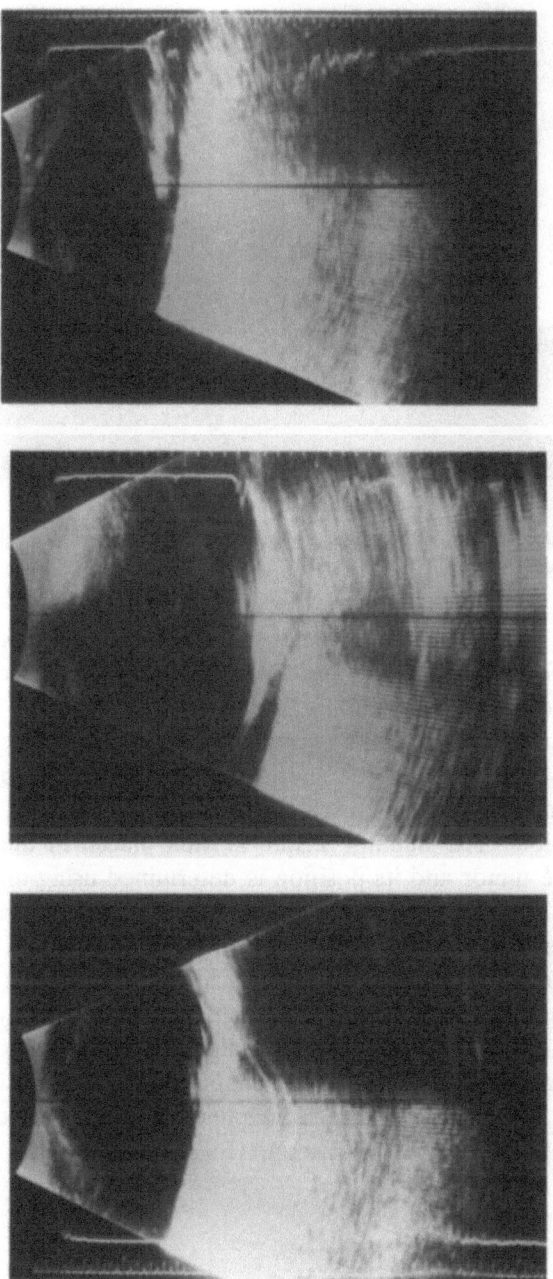

Fig. 2. Acoustic shadowing produced by various materials in a water bath, using a sponge to simulate the orbital fat pad. *Top:* Plastic produces poor shadowing. *Middle:* Metal produces reverberation echoes. *Bottom:* Aluminum foil produces almost complete shadowing.

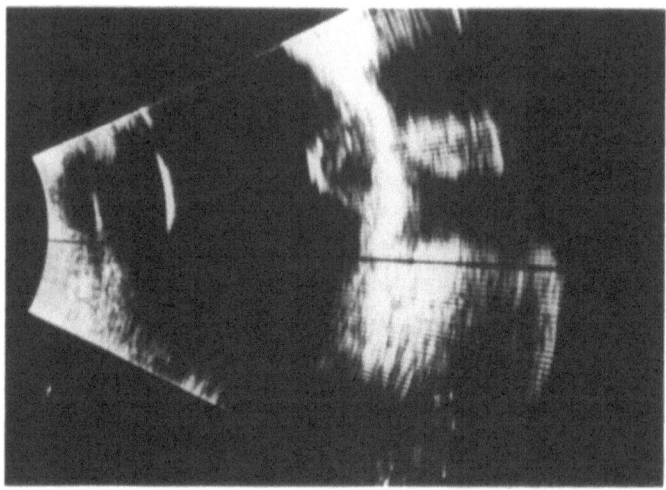

Fig. 3. A well centred dummy plaque. The orbital fat pattern visualized through the central hole aids in positioning.

scanning head. The same sterile, water soluble gel is used to provide contact with the eye. Scanning is done either through the lids or in direct contact with the eye depending on the location of the tumor (Fig. 4c).

The location of the tumor is known preoperatively from direct visualization and ultrasonic localization. Using a peritomy, the sclera in the tumor quadrant is bared. Transillumination is used to delineate the anterior aspect of the tumor if possible. The dummy plaque is then placed in the approximate position of the tumor and its position is determined using ultrasound. The plaque is then moved to the optimal position. During this process the plaque generally stays approximated to the globe by friction. When it is well placed two or three Dacron sutures are placed in sclera at the edge of the plaque and temporarily tied using a bow knot. The plaque position is then rechecked with ultrasound. The sutures are untied, the dummy plaque removed, and the radioactive plaque of identical size and shape is secured in position using the same sutures. The position of the radioactive plaque can be confirmed both intra- and postoperatively by ultrasound (Figs. 5a and b).

Results

This method has been used to position plaques in twelve patients with choroidal melanomas. Tumors ranged in height from 4.3 to 10.2 mm and in width from 9 to 18 mm.

For tumors close to the optic nerve the plaque was positioned eccentrically

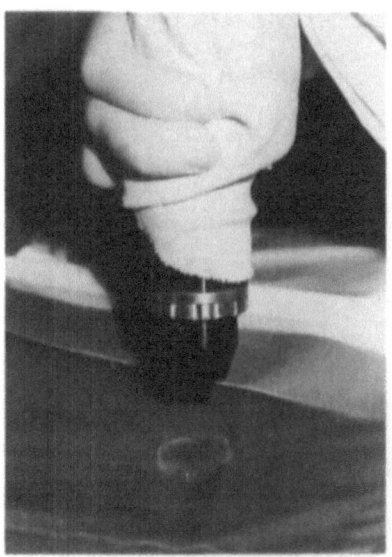

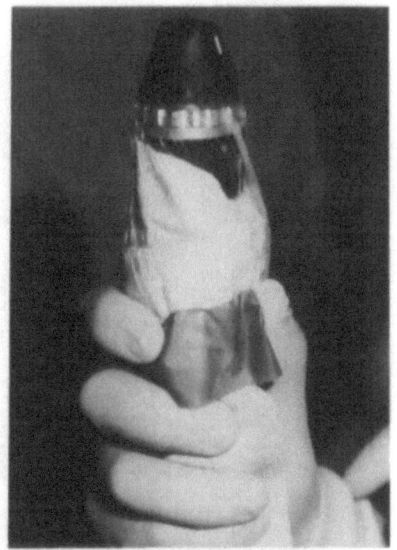

Fig. 4a. Sterile gel is placed on the steridrape and a sleeve placed on the transducer.

Fig. 4b. The drape covers that part of the transducer not covered by a sterile sleeve.

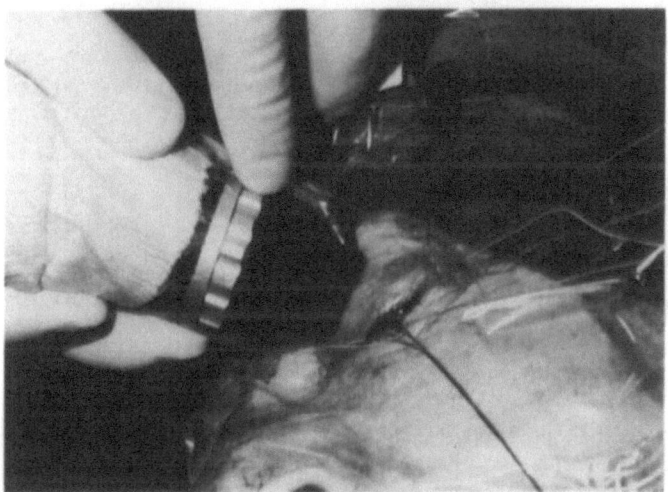

Fig. 4c. Scanning is usually done through the lids.

to allow maximal separation from the nerve while still placing the tumor within the optimal dose distribution.

All patients had postoperative ultrasound to confirm the position of the plaque. The iridium wires making up the plaque are quite well visualized ultrasonically. All plaques were found to be placed accurately in relationship to the tumor base.

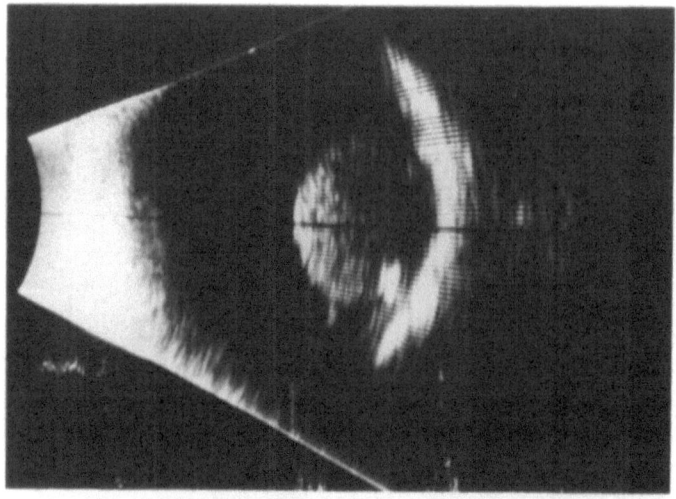

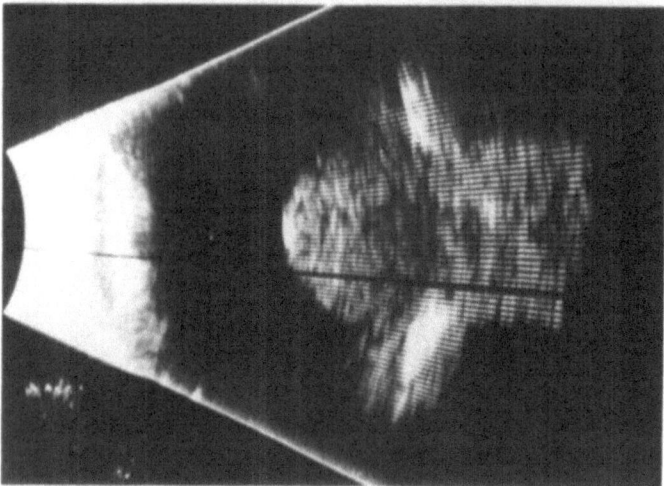

Fig. 5a. Intraoperative ultrasound shows a well positioned dummy plaque.

Fig. 5b. Postoperative ultrasound shows bright reflections from the iridium wires and confirms proper plaque positioning.

Cryo-enucleation

Cryo-enucleation had been recommended as a theoretical method of decreasing possibility of tumor spread during the process of enucleation by freezing the blood supply to the tumor base. In our institution we use a cryospoon designed by Dr. B. Gallie (Fig. 6). Ultrasound is used intraoperatively using similar techniques to those described for placing radioactive plaques. The

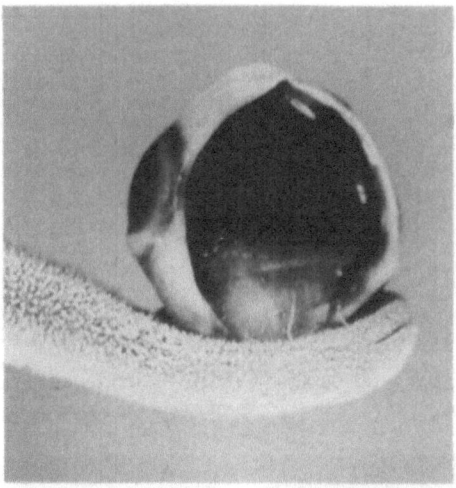

Fig. 6. The Gallie cryo-enucleator - formation of an iceball in an enucleated globe is illustrated.

position of the spoon behind the tumor can be well visualized. After proper positioning the cooling system is turned on. The formation of the iceball can then be monitored. When the iceball envelopes the tumor base, the enucleation process is completed. (Figs. 7a, b, c and d). This method has been used in 16 cases.

Discussion

The use of individually tailored plaques can theoretically produce an optimal radiation dose to the tumor, while minimizing the radiation dose to surrounding ocular structures. Some of this advantage is lost if the plaque is not accurately placed. Transillumination of the tumor base remains the main method of positioning radioactive plaques [4]. The anterior margin of the tumor can usually be located and the posterior margin assumed from pre-operative knowledge of tumor size. Occasionally however, transillumination can be difficult, especially with posteriorly located tumors, and tumors with excessive intraocular hemorrhage.

Ultrasound has been found to be a feasible method of radioactive plaque placement and an excellent method of confirming that the plaque was indeed placed correctly.

The relationship of the posterior margin of the plaque to the optic nerve can also be noted intraoperatively allowing one to place the plaque as far from the nerve as possible, while still maintaining the tumor in the proper isodose distribution.

398

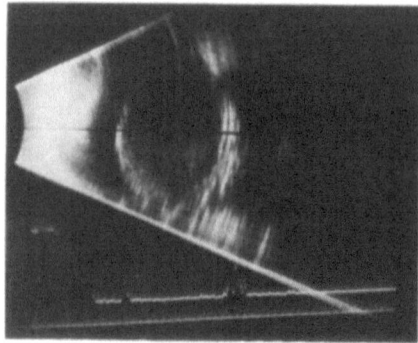

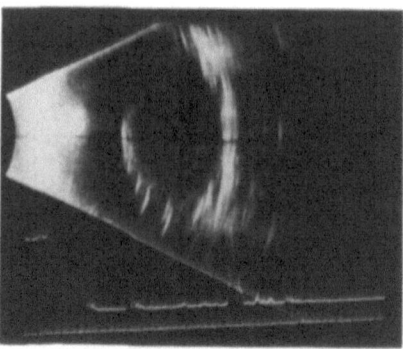

Fig. 7a. The shadowing of the cryospoon can be noted behind the tumor.

Fig. 7b. Shortly after turning on the liquid nitrogen the spoon profile flattens.

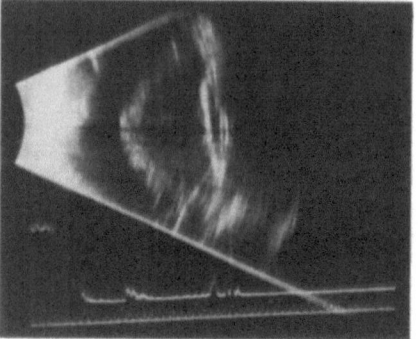

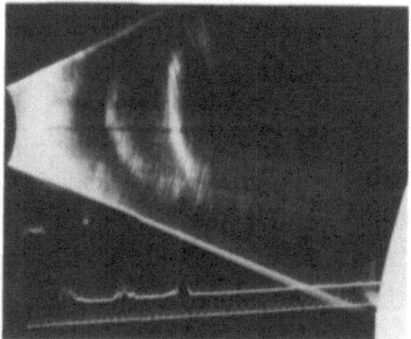

Fig. 7c. The beginning of an iceball in the tumor itself.

Fig. 7d. The iceball expands to envelope the tumor base.

Zimmerman et al. [6] noted that the incidence of metastatic disease rises sharply after enucleation. They hypothesized that dissemination of tumor cells into the systemic circulation at the time of surgery could account for this rise. To avoid this Fraunfelder and Wilson [1, 5] proposed a method of cryosurgical enucleation stressing gentle handling of the globe and freezing of the base of the tumor while the optic nerve is cut. This method has been modified in our institution by the use of a specially designed instrument, the 'Gallie cryo-enucleator' [2]. Intraoperative ultrasound assures accurate placement of the cryo-enucleator, and permits the depth of freeze to be monitored.

References

1. Fraunfelder FT, Boozman FW, Wilson RS, et al. 1977. No-touch technique for intraocular malignant melonomas. Arch Ophthalmol 95: 1616–1620.

2. Gallie BL, Drysdale AM, Pavlin CJ. A new instrument for cryo-enucleation, Ophthalmology, in press.
3. Japp B, Payne DG, Gallie BL. 1982. Individualized Ir–192 wire moulds for the treatment of large accessible malignant melanomas of the choroid. Proc of the 24th Annual ASTR, Abstracts. Int J Radiat Oncol Biol Phys Vol. 8 (Suppl.).
4. Shields JA. 1983. Diagnosis and management of intraocular tumors. St. Louis: CV Mosby Company p. 46.
5. Wilson RS, Fraunfelder FT. 1978. 'No-touch' cryosurgical enucleation: A minimal trauma technique for eyes harboring intraocular malignancy. Ophthalmol 85: 1170–11.
6. Zimmerman E, McLean IW, Foster WD. 1978. Does enucleation of the eye containing a malignant melanoma prevent or accelerate the dissemination of tumor cells? Br J Ophth 62: 420–425.

Regression patterns of choroidal malignant melanoma: standardized echography (A-mode) and immersion tomography (B-mode). (a comparative study)

R.D. STONE
San Francisco, USA

Introduction

Through cooperation with the Ocular Oncology Unit of the Department of Ophthalmology of the University of California, San Francisco, we have obtained long-term follow-up ultrasound data on the growth and regression of many intraocular tumors. We have followed, ultrasonically, many of these intraocular lesions prior to therapy and have observed their growth [2]. A most interesting subgroup of patients, however, is the group that has been treated through this institution using the external beam helium ion irradiation available at the Lawrence Radiation Laboratory, Berkeley. This is one of the treatment modalities that has, in recent years, been proposed as an alternative to enucleation for therapy of choroidal malignant melanomas [1]. This particular subgroup now numbers 181 patients irradiated using helium ion (U.C. Berkeley) as of the date of this communication. We would like to present the patterns of regression we have observed in this unique subgroup of treated malignant melanomas. We have undertaken this analysis of our data to answer the question: Is there a clinical ultrasound (or acoustic) feature of helium ion irradiated malignant melanomas that is characteristic for successful treatment?

Methods and materials

We researched the cross referenced files of the Ophthalmic Ultrasound Laboratory at the University of California, San Francisco, and noted those patients who were sent for our ultrasound evaluation of their eyes for the presence of an intraocular tumor. From a total of 3,556 patient records available in this Ultrasound Laboratory from March 14, 1977 to October 16, 1984, there have been 401 diagnoses of melanoma (of the ciliary body and choroid), 171 diagnoses of 'nevus versus melanoma' of the choroid who have been followed,

K.C. Ossoinig (editor), Ophthalmic Echography, ISBN 978-94-010-7988-4

subsequently, for evidence of growth, ultrasonically, and 21 diagnoses of nevus of the choroid who have also, for the most part, been followed here. The 181 patients who have been treated here using the helium ion irradiation modality have also been followed here, ultrasonographically, subsequent to their therapy. The ultrasonographic techniques consisted of serially scanned immersion tomography (B-mode) as described elsewhere [5] using the Sono-metrics Model 200 instrument and standardized echography (A-mode) utilizing techniques described elsewhere [6, 8] with the Kretz 7200 MA Echography instrument.

The data used in this communication were collected in a prospective manner. This means that an abstracting sheet was designed in 1976 for the purpose of computerized data analysis and this author abstracted each ultrasound examination on the day of examination and dictation of the ultrasound report from this laboratory. These computer data entry sheets were then stored for later analysis, and this presentation comprises a retrospective analysis of data which was accumulated in a prospective way. The abstracted information included the date of examination, the patient's name, the eye, and whether or not any of the following clinical ultrasound features were present or absent at the time of examination: choroidal excavation, collar button configuration, internal acoustic quiet zones, acoustic shadowing in the orbital fat echo pattern, retinal detachment extending away from the base of the mass, and internal spontaneous movement (vascular pulsation) of the A-scan echo spikes. This last item, internal spontaneous vascular pulsation, could only be evaluated by analyzing the echograms on the day of examination and abstracting the data prospectively. In addition, we measured the maximum height of the mass from the retinal surface echo spike (if the retina was attached) or from the tumor surface echo spike (retina detached) to the inner scleral echo spike. This is only possible with the Kretz 7200 MA Echography Unit in our opinion. This unit allows access to all lesions and the criteria for maximum spike height at maximum tumor thickness have been well established. This is the best estimation of maximum tumor thickness. In addition, we estimated the width of choroidal excavation from the Polaroid B-scan photographs utilizing calipers and millimeter measurements taken directly from the oscilloscope calibration marks which were already on the Poloroid photographs. All of this data collection took place in addition to and at the same time as the ultrasonograms were analyzed for their diagnostic information. The Sono-metrics 10 mega-Hertz B-scan transducer was utilized for all immersion tomography (B-mode) and the Kretz 8 mHz A-scan transducer was utilized for all standardized echograms (A-mode). This assisted in the diagnostic tissue pattern recognition which it is well known for. These data collection methods are summarized in Fig. 1. The B-scan measurement of the extent of choroidal excavation can only be used as a rough estimate of the maximum tumor

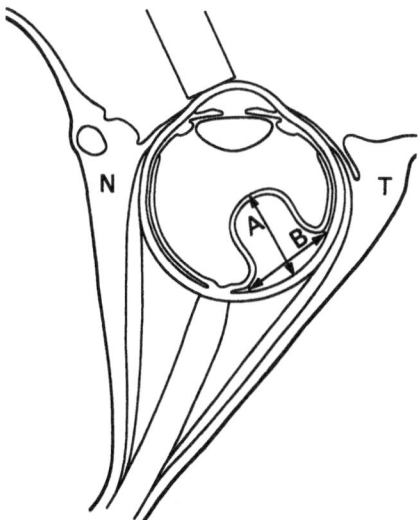

Fig. 1. A: Maximum thickness measurement is taken from the maximum echo spike distance from the retinal surface to the inner scleral surface obtained with the Kretz 7200 MA Echography instrument (8 mHz unfocused transducer). B: Maximum extent of choroidal excavation is esti-mated using calipers on the B-scan Polaroid photograph of the oscilloscope screen and the simultaneously photographed millimeter oscilloscope markings (10 mHz focused transducer). The method is discussed in the text.

diameter at its base since this technique suffers from certain sampling errors where large irregular tumors are involved [3] and certain acoustic errors in making measurements from B-scan photographs. Nevertheless we felt that the extent of choroidal excavation was the best estimate of the maximum width of a tumor at its base ultrasonographically.

Ultrasonography is only one of the diagnostic modalities available to the clinician in the evaluation of intraocular tumors. Therapeutic decisions were not based on the ultrasound findings alone. Therapeutic decisions were made in each individual case based on clinical, ultrasonographic, photographic, angiographic, and clinical laboratory information, as well as the other opin-ions of our Tumor Board members. Our experience with various diagnostic modalities in evaluation choroidal tumors has been communicated elsewhere [4, 7].

This retrospective analysis of data accumulated in a prospective way in-cludes those patients who have been irradiated using helium ion and who have been followed for a year or more. The mean length of follow-up is more than a year in this group of patients. In our verbal presentation at this meeting, we included in our statistical analysis the three patients who had been retreated for failure to initially respond to this therapy and three other patients who had been followed for 11 months but not exactly a full year. In this written

404

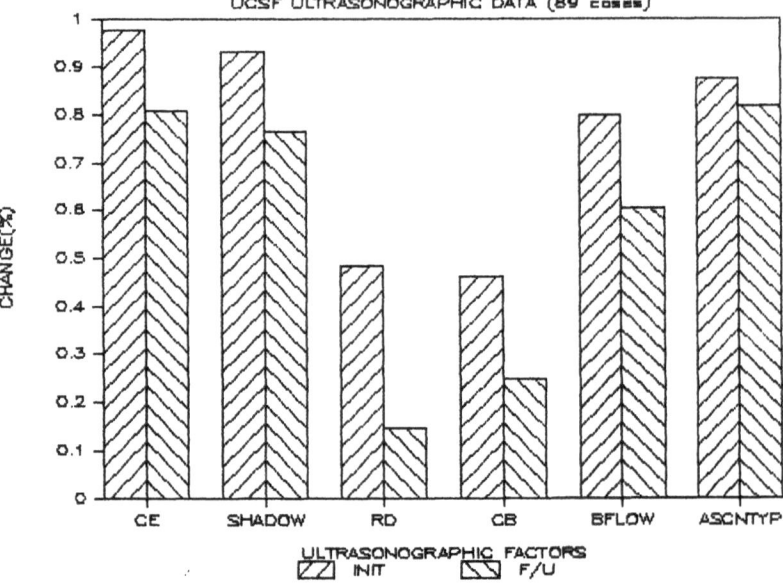

OPHTHALMIC MELANOMA
UCSF ULTRASONOGRAPHIC DATA (89 cases)

Fig. 2. Ultrasonographic factors present initially (INIT) and at the end of one year of follow-up (F/U) in 89 cases of malignant melanoma of the choroid and the ciliary body treated by helium ion irradiation. Vertical scae is in percent (present). Horizontal codes refer to: CE = choroidal excavation, SHADOW = acoustic shadow in the orbital fat echo pattern, RD = retinal detachment away from the base of the mass, CB = collar button configuration, BFLOW = spontaneous spike movement (blood flow, vascular pulsation), and ASCNTYP = A-scan typical form malignant melanoma tissue pattern (Kretz 7200 MA).

communication, however, we have excluded those six patients and re-calculated our data to include 89 cases that have been followed for a minimum of one year in our laboratory.

Results and discussion

Most of our findings are summarized in graphic form in Fig. 2 and Fig. 3. Figure 2 summarizes, for 89 patients followed for one year or more after therapy, the initial ultrasonographic factors present and accounted for at the time they were first examined in our laboratory and also demonstrates the summarized change for each factor at the end of one year of follow-up. This does not average all of the visits in between but only takes the initial examination and compares it to the examination at the end of one year. Choroidal excavation is a very sensitive initial diagnostic indicator in our hands, as is

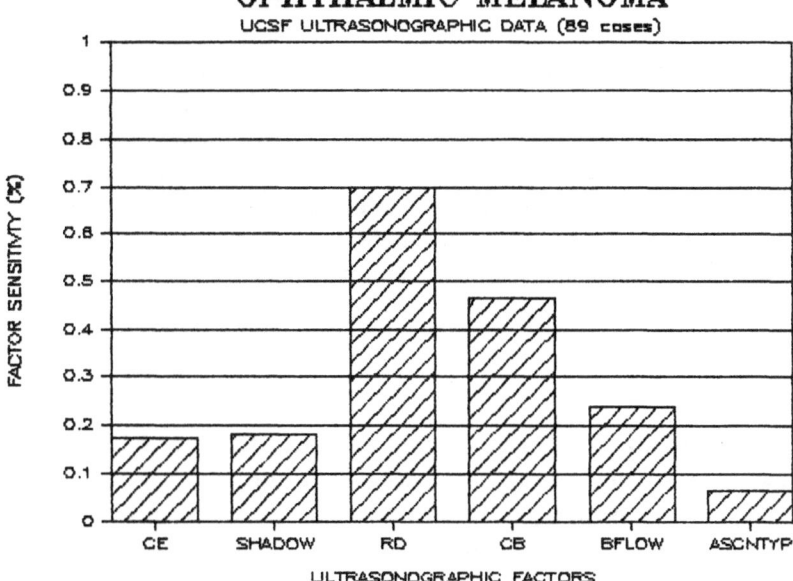

Fig. 3. Ultrasonographic factor sensitivity for response to helium ion irradiation therapy expressed for 89 cases of malignant melanoma of the choroid as percent change at the end of one year. Vertical scale in percent of cases changing at the end of one year. Methods of analysis are described in the text. Horizontal codes are explained in the legend of Fig. 2.

acoustic shadowing in the orbital fat echo pattern and the presence of spontaneous vascular pulsation (blood flow) and a typical A-scan tissue pattern as obtained with the Kretz 7200 MA instrument. Retinal detachments were not present in all tumors diagnosed as malignant melanomas. A collar button configuration was not an absolute criterion for this diagnosis either.

The sensitivity of each factor as an indicator of a satisfactory response to therapy was evaluated and is summarized in Fig. 3. It becomes readily apparent that the regression of a retinal detachment is the most sensitive indicator of satisfactory response to therapy at the end of one year in these cases. The next most sensitive factor indicating a response to therapy is the regression of the collar button configuration (to the point that it is indistinguishable to the ultrasonographer from a tumor which never exhibited a collar button configuration). The regression of spontaneous vascular pulsation to the point of being indetectable by the ultrasonographer was the next most sensitive factor. The most surprising finding was that the A-scan tissue pattern as determined by the Kretz 7200 MA in our hands, remained typical for the diagnosis of a malignant melanoma of the choroid for at least a year in a large number of patients and in our hands was the least sensitive clinical ultrasonographic predictor of a therapeutic response to this form of therapy.

406

It is, therefore, our recommendation that ultrasonographers having the opportunity to study a large number of patients undergoing this form of alternative therapy be particularly cautious in the future to determine accurately the presence or absence and extent of three major factors that we have shown as sensitive indicators of response to therapy, namely: retinal detachments, collar button configurations, and spontaneous movements (vascular pulsations or blood flow). The accurate initial assessment of patients undergoing these therapeutic modalities will benefit the ultrasonographer who is called upon to evaluate these patients after therapy.

Acknowledgements

Sharon Humphrey, R.D.M.S., Marvin Zielinski, C.O.T., Jane Rubatzky, B.S., and Larry Wong, were technicians in the Ultrasound Laboratory during this study. Nancy King typed the manuscript. The statistics were prepared utilizing an IBM PC XT computer and Lotus 123 and DBase III software programs.

References

1. Char DH, Castro JR, Quivey JM, et al. 1980. Helium Ion Charged Particle Therapy for Choroidal Melanoma. Ophthalmol. 87 (6): 565–570.
2. Char DH, Heilbron DC, Juster RP, Stone RD. 1981. Choroidal melanoma growth patterns. British J. Ophthal. 67 (9): 575–578.
3. Char DH, Stone RD, et al. 1980. Diffuse melanoma of the choroid. British J. Ophthal. 64 (3): 178–180.
4. Char DH, Stone RD, Irvine AR, et al. 1980. Diagnostic Modalities in Choroidal Melanoma. Am. J. Ophth. 89 (2): 223–230.
5. Coleman DJ, Lizzi FL, Jack RL. 1977. Ultrasonography of the eye and orbit. Lea & Febiger, Philadelphia, p. 353–357.
6. Dallow RL. 183. The eye. In Goldberg BB, Wells PNT (eds) Ultrasonics in clinical diagnosis. Churchill Livingstone, p. 167–179.
7. Irvine AR, Stone RD. 1979. Diagnostic tests and choroidal tumors. Trans. Pac. Coast Otoophth. Soc. 60: 121–124.
8. Ossoinig KC. 1979. Standardized echography: basic principles, clinical applications, and results. Ossoinig KC, course manual prepared for the American Academy of Ophthalmology; 127–210.

Echographic characteristics of a subpigment epithelial reticulum cell sarcoma*

B. BYRNE and W.A.J. VAN HEUVEN
San Antonio, USA

A characteristic funduscopic picture has been described [1] in cases of multifocal pigment epithelial detachments caused by reticulum cell sarcoma. The purpose of this report is to demonstrate the echographic characteristics of these bilateral, multiple, solid detachments of the pigment epithelium, which are typical of this disease. Of special interest is the spontaneous progression and regression of these lesions, which can be documented echographically and photographically.

Case report

On May 24, 1984, a 59-year-old white male came to our clinic complaining of slight bilateral blurring of vision with floaters of several weeks duration. In addition, the patient had pain in the left eye when reading. Past medical history was not significant. Past eye history was negative except for the need for reading glasses. The patient did not drink or smoke. There was no history of drug abuse. Family history indicated cataract in one grandmother and diabetes in the other grandmother. The eye exam showed a vision of 20/25 OD and 20/15 OS. Tensions were 15 mm Hg in both eyes. The anterior segments were normal with no cells or flare. Pupils were normally reactive with no afferent defect. The vitreous was slightly hazy in both eyes, with some vitreous cells peripherally. The fundus showed similar changes in the two eyes, consisting of multiple, mid-peripheral, subretinal lesions in all quadrants with various degrees of elevation, depigmentation and pigment clumping (Fig. 1). The pattern of pigmentation was a diffuse mottling and was not related to retinal vessels. The right eye was slightly more involved than the left. The macula was not involved by the lesions and blurring of vision was attributed to vitreous

* Supported in part by a Research Development grant from Research to Prevent Blindness, Inc., N.Y.

K.C. Ossoinig (editor), Ophthalmic Echography, ISBN 978-94-010-7988-4

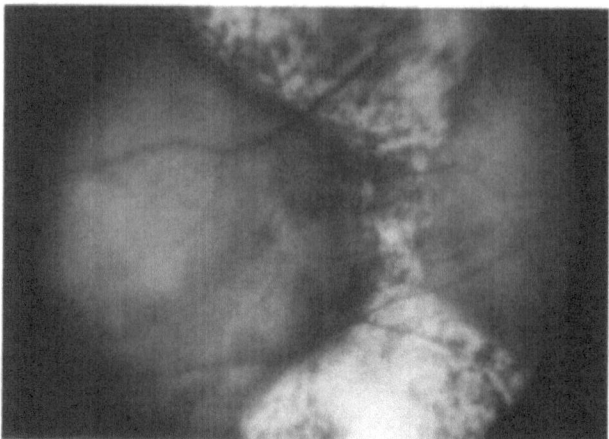

Fig. 1. Initial appearance of two of the multiple, midperipheral, elevated solid retinal detachments connected by a narrow isthmus of less elevation. These lesions have a yellow color with brown, mottled pigmentation. They fail to stain with fluorscein, suggesting that the subpigment epithelial material is cellular.

cells and flare. Diagnostic echography, using standardized A-scan (Kretz 7200 MA) and contact B-scan, was performed. B-scan demonstrated the topography of the multi-focal lesions with various amounts of elevation (Fig. 2). In the right eye, some of the more elevated lesions were connected to each other by a narrow isthmus of abnormality (Fig. 1). Vitreous opacities were seen in the posterior half of the vitreous and at times close to the surface of the lesions. Quantitative A-scan also demonstrated the vitreous opacities and indicated that the subretinal elevations were solid, with attached overlying

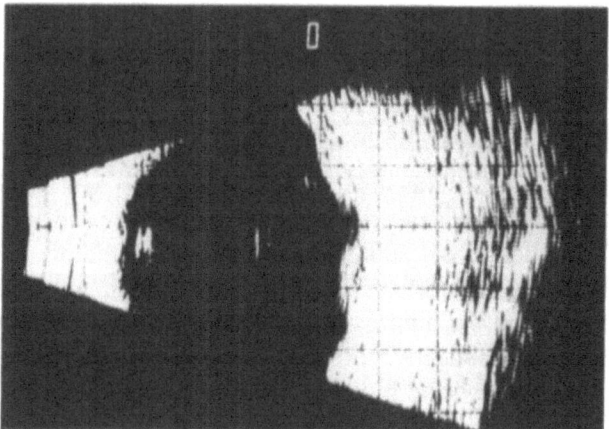

Fig. 2. B-scan echogram of the lesions in Figure 1 showing the vitreous opacities in front of the tumors.

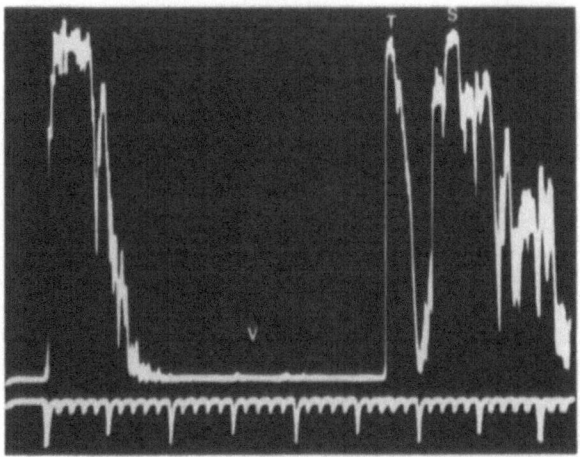

Fig. 3. Standardized A-scan echogram at tissue sensitivity showing mild vitreous opacities (V), tumor surface (T), and sclera (S). Note the very low internal reflectivity of the tumor.

retina (Fig. 3). The internal reflectivity of the elevated lesions was very low to low, i.e. less than 40%. The internal structure was regular, i.e. the spikes were of uniform length and height. No blood flow was detected within the lesions. The elevation from the retinal surface to the inner sclera of the most elevated lesion in the right eye was 3.8 mm.

The patient was presented at Grand Rounds where the diagnosis of reticulum cell sarcoma was discussed. Fundus photographs were also sent to J. Donald Gass, M.D., at the Bascom Palmer Eye Institute, who diagnosed reticulum cell sarcoma on the basis of the photographic appearance. On 7/9/84, the patient was admitted to the Audie Murphy V.A. Hospital for a vitreous biopsy. The specimen was studied by our eye pathologist, Marilyn Kincaid, M.D., and our cytologist, Ibrahim Ramzy, M.D., who agreed that the findings were typical of reticulum cell sarcoma [2] (Fig. 4). The patient was then transfered to the oncology service for further workup. A biopsy of a small subcutaneous abdominal mass showed lipoma. CT-scans of the head and orbit were normal. Lumbar puncture showed no malignant cells. Bone marrow aspiration and biopsy showed marrow with lymphocytic aggregates of small lymphocytes not representative of histiocytic lymphoma. The report stated that a small cell lymphoma could not be ruled out. CT-scan of the abdomen was normal except for a small heterogeneous area in the liver which could not be ruled out as metastatic carcinoma. An abdominal sonogram subsequently showed no discreet liver masses. During the following six weeks, repeat photographic and echographic examinations were done (Fig. 5). These showed no increase in elevation of the largest lesions but both an increase and a decrease in elevations of some of the smaller lesions. Finally, at the end of six

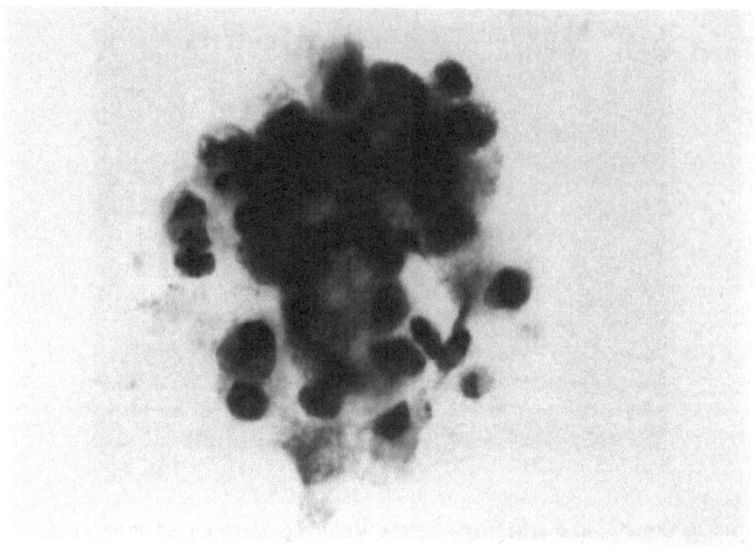

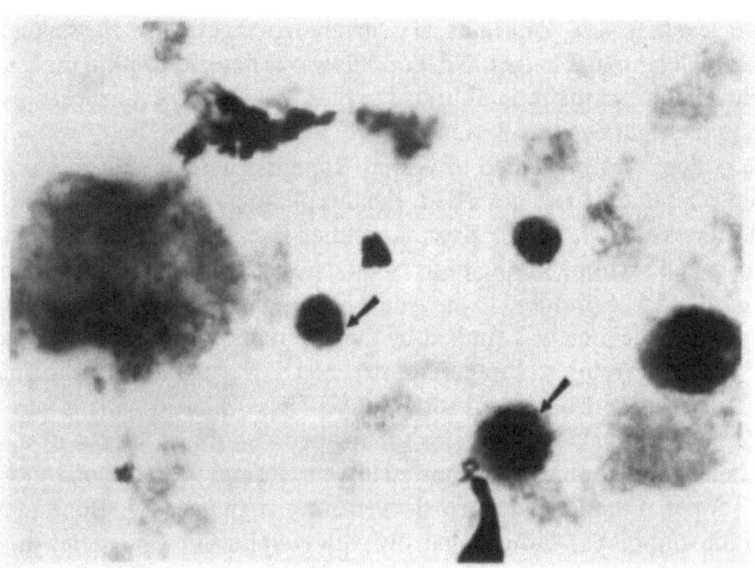

Fig. 4a. Vitreous biopsy specimen depicts cells of various sizes with irregular chromatin and nuclear molding, interpreted as typical for malignant cells.

Fig. 4b. The cells (arrows) show nuclear projections, typical of reticulum cell sarcoma.

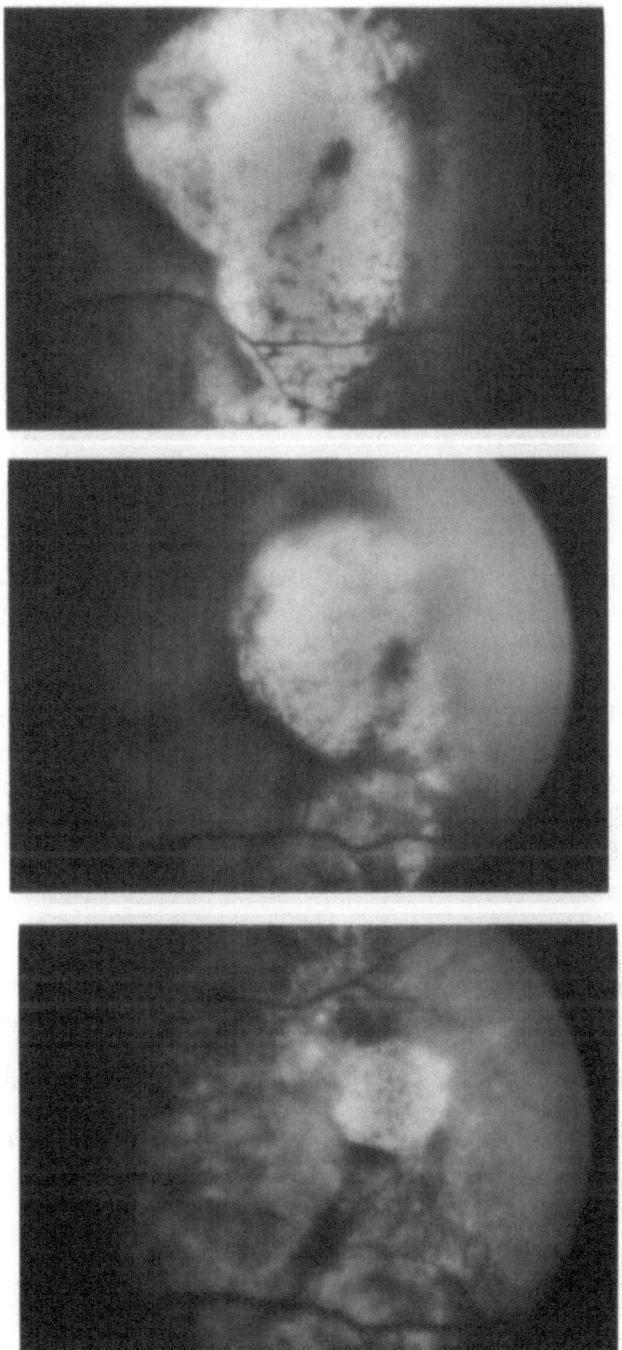

Fig. 5a, b and c. Demonstration of the spontaneous regresion of one of the lesions before any treatment was started.

412

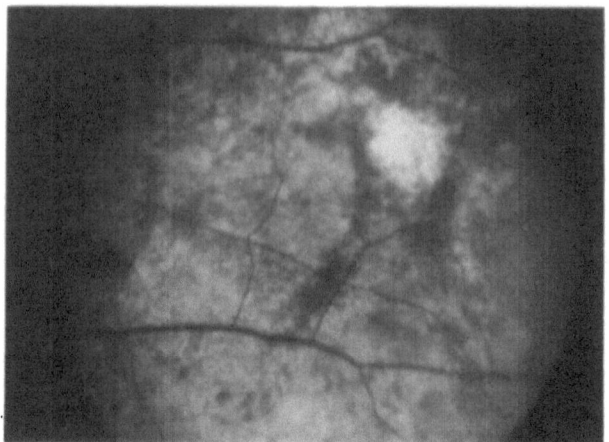

Fig. 5d. There is continued regression one month after irradiation treatment was begun.

weeks, the maximally elevated lesion also increased to 4.6 mm, while some other lesions almost entirely disappeared, leaving flat areas with mottled pigmentary changes.

At the suggestion of the oncology consultants, 'whole brain' irradiation, including orbits, was begun on 8/28/84. One month later CHOP chemotherapy was added and continued to date [3]. At last report in May, 1987, the patient's vision was 20/25 in both eyes. The vitritis had cleared, the tumors had decreased in size, and no systemic manifestations of reticulum cell sarcoma were as yet manifest.

References

1. Gass JD, Sever RJ, Grizzard WS, et al. 1984. Multifocal Pigment Epithelial Detachments By Reticulum Cell Sarcoma – A Characteristic Funduscopic Picture. Retina 4: 135–143.
2. Wagoner MD, Gonder JR, et al. 1980. Intraocular Reticulum Cell Sarcoma. Ophthalmol. 87: 724–727.
3. Char DH, Margolis LM, Newman AB. 1981. Ocular Reticulum Cell Sarcoma. Ophthalmol. 91: 480–483.

Non-melanomatous collar-button tumors

B.M. KERMAN and M.L. FISHMAN
Los Angeles, USA

Introduction

The ultrasonographic diagnostic criteria for malignant melanoma of the choroid include low internal reflectivity, strong sound attenuation, spontaneous internal spike motion indicative of vascularity, characteristic configuration, choroidal excavation and orbital shadowing (Coleman et al. 1974; Ossoinig, 1974; Fuller et al. 1979; Green, 1984). Of the B-scan criteria, the one thought to be most reliable for melanoma is the collar-button or mushroom-shaped configuration. This shape is not always present in melanomas, but when it is present, it is felt to be highly characteristic of melanoma. This paper will present three patients with collar-button shaped intraocular tumors which proved to be lesions other than malignant melanoma.

Case reports

Case 1. An 18 year old female presented in October, 1980 with headache and blurred vision in the left eye. Clinically, a nasal anterior choroidal mass was noted in the left eye. Ultrasonographic evaluation demonstrated a 12 mm elevation in the anteronasal choroid. The mass had a collar-button configuration on B-scan and showed high internal reflectivity without spontaneous spike motion on A-scan. Over the next 18 months, she developed an inferior retinal detachment and slight increase in the size of the lesion. The ultrasonographic characteristics of the tumor remained unchanged (Figs. 1 and 2). In June 1982, the left globe was enucleated. Histopathological examination of the tumor demonstrated a well-differentiated astrocytoma.

Case 2. In July, 1983, an 81 year old male underwent extracapsular cataract extraction. During the course of surgery, a dark bulge was evident in the superior ciliary body region, and vitreous presented in the wound. An anterior

K.C. Ossoinig (editor), Ophthalmic Echography, ISBN 978-94-010-7988-4
© 1987, Martinus Nijhoff/Dr W. Junk Publishers, Dordrecht.

414

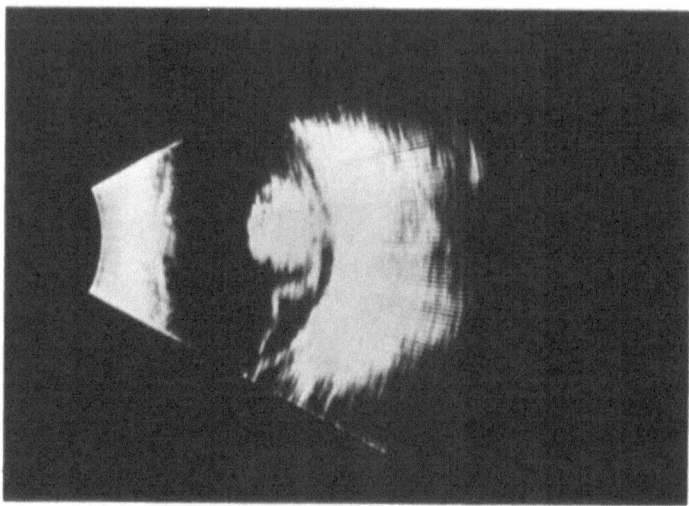

Fig. 1. Case 1: B-scan ultrasonogram showing mass lesion with collar-button configuration and inferior retinal detachment.

vitrectomy was performed, and the incision was closed. Ultrasound examination in September, 1983 showed an 11.6 mm elevation in the superonasal ciliary boy. The lesion had a mushroom-shaped configuration (Fig. 3). On A-scan evaluation the lesion showed high internal reflectivity without evidence of spontaneous spike motion (Fig. 4). In February, 1984, a right parotid mass was noted, and needle biopsy of the mass was read as showing a poorly

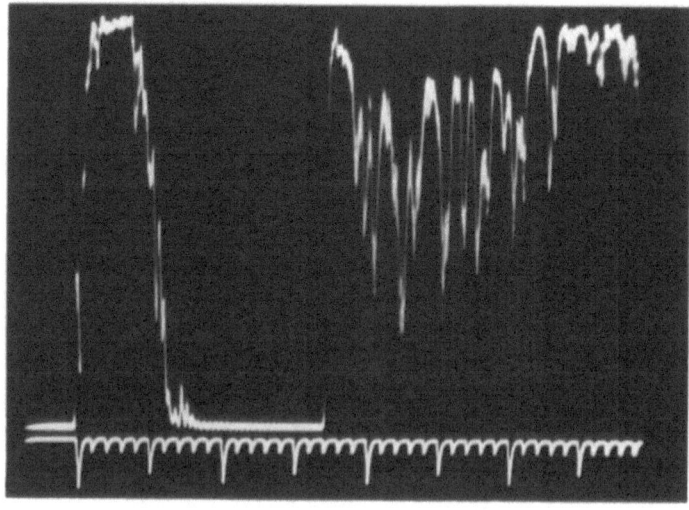

Fig. 2. Case 1: A-scan ultrasonogram showing high internal reflectivity within ocular mass without spontaneous spike motion.

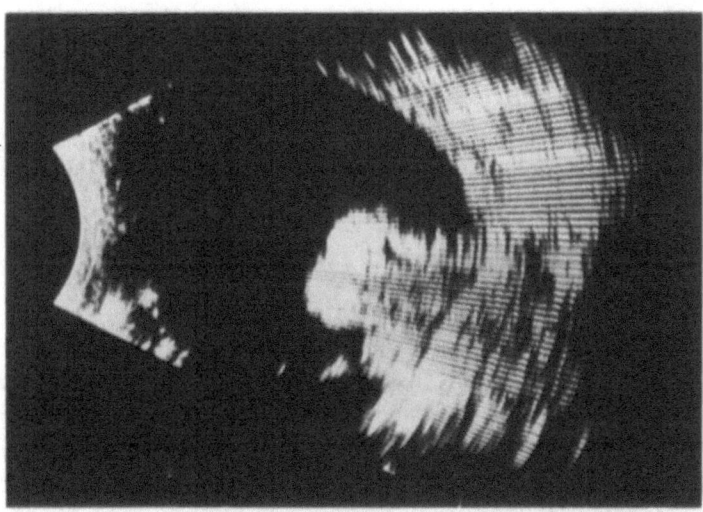

Fig. 3. Case 2: B-scan ultrasonogram showing mass lesion with collar-button configuration and associated orbital shadowing.

differentiated carcinoma of the parotid gland. Based on the A-scan appearance and the presence of a known malignancy, the ocular lesion was diagnosed as metastatic carcinoma.

Case 3. A 3 year old male was seen in November, 1983 because of bilateral leukocoria. Examination of the right eye showed a white superior tumor with

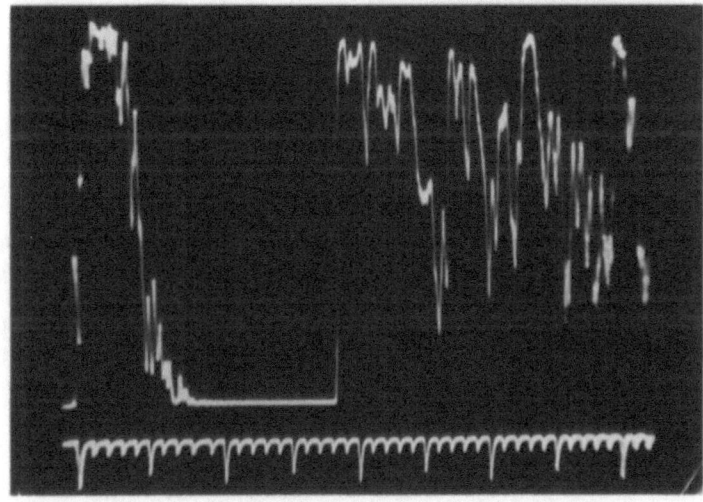

Fig. 4. Case 2: A-scan ultrasonogram showing ocular mass with high internal reflectivity without spontaneous spike motion.

vitreous seeding. Ultrasonographic evaluation demonstrated a superior mush-room-shaped mass consisting of high internal reflectivity. Dense central vitreous opacification was present, but no orbital shadowing could be demonstrated. The diagnosis of retinoblastoma was made and a course of 4500 rads to the right orbit was completed in January, 1984. Three months later, the tumor was noted to be clinically smaller.

Discussion

The collar-button or mushroom-shaped configuration of malignant melanoma of the choroid occurs when the tumor breaks through Bruch's membrane and, thus, assumes a bilobed configuration. This characteristic shape, when present, is thought to be highly useful in the differentiation of melanoma from simulating neoplasms. This paper has presented three cases of ocular neoplasms showing a collar-button configuration, none of which were malignant melanoma. One tumor was an astrocytoma of the ciliary body; the second was a presumed metastatic carcinoma; the third tumor proved to be a retinoblastoma. All lesions showed high internal reflectivity without spontaneous spike motion, features which would rule out the diagnosis of malignant melanoma. Therefore, even though the B-scan ultrasonographic configuration of these tumors was consistent with malignant melanoma, the A-scan features were not. When faced with an unknown ocular mass lesion, the examiner must utilize all diagnostic criteria in order to arrive at the correct diagnosis.

References

1. Coleman DJ, Abramson DH, Jack RL, Franzen LA. 1974. Ultrasonographic diagnosis of tumors of the choroid. Arch. Ophthalmol. 9:344.
2. Fuller DF, Snyder WB, Hutton WL, Vaiser A. 1979. Ultrasonographic diagnosis of choroidal malignant melanomas. Arch. Ophthalmol. 97: 465.
3. Green RL. 1984. Echographic diagnosis of large choroidal melanomas. Ophthalmic Ultra-sonography, Proceedings of the 9th SIDUO Congress. J.S. Hilman and M.M. LeMay (eds). The Hague: Junk: 15.
4. Ossoinig KC. 1974. Preoperative differential diagnosis of tumors with echography. III. Diagnosis of intraocular tumors. Current Concepts in Ophthalmology, Vol. 4. F.C. Blodi (ed). St. Louis: Mosby: 296.

Computerized ultrasonic analysis of uveal malignant melanomas and response to cobalt-60 plaque

M.E. SMITH, D.J. COLEMAN, F.L. LIZZI, R.H. SILVERMAN,
M. RONDEAU, R.M. ELLSWORTH and B.G. HAIK
New York, USA

Abstract

Radioactive cobalt-60 plaque has proved an effective means of treatment of malignant melanoma of the uvea. Intraocular tumors show a wide range of response to this treatment modality, ranging from complete regression to unabated growth. At present, tumor location relative to radio-sensitive intra-ocular structures and tumor size and growth are the leading indicators used to judge suitability of cobalt plaque therapy. Characterization of intraocular melanomas by computerized analysis of digitized ultrasound scan data, how-ever, provides a new set of parameters which we find related to tumor responsivity to treatment.

In a statistical analysis of tumor regression versus computer processing of digitized ultrasound scan data, Type B tumors (related to spindle cell mela-nomas) showed a significantly greater percentage decrease in anterior to posterior dimension than those tumors identified as Type E (related to mixed/epithelioid cell types). At both six and twelve months after treatment, Type B tumors demonstrated over twice the mean percentage decrease in height as Type E tumors.

In an overall evaluation relating pre-treatment tumor size, location and digital acoustic analysis with regression and complications, computer analysis of ultrasound scan data was found to be an important indicator of treatment outcome.

This work was supported by NIH Grants EY-01212 and EY-03183 and a grant from The Dyson Foundation.

K.C. Ossoinig (editor), Ophthalmic Echography, ISBN 978-94-010-7988-4

Retinoblastoma of the diffused type on the A- and B-scan

G. GALLI, P. PERRI and V. MAZZEO
Ferrara, Italy

The echographic term 'pathognomonic of retinoblastoma' has been widely described by Coleman et al. (1977) and Ossoinig et al. (1983).

Last year we examined a 6-year-old boy who clinically harbored a retinoblastoma, while the echographic examination with A- and B-scan absolutely showed no characteristic of retinoblastoma as described in the echographic literture.

Case report

The boy was sent to undergo an echographic examination in September 1983. He showed leucocoria in his left eye dating from about seven months. His family and personal history was negative. He was hospitalized in his city hospital for the first time in March 1983. At that time posterior uveitis was diagnosed. He was sent for therapy in a childrens department where he was treated with Azathioprine (Imuran) and corticosteroids for twenty days. The ocular situation got worse, so consultation with a uveitis expert was required. The diagnosis of retinoblastoma was made by the consulting ophthalmologist. When seen by us, his right eye was perfectly normal. Right eye visual acuity was 1.0, while his left eye had only light perception. Left eye intraocular pressure was 34 mm Hg (by applanation). A mild conjunctival injection was present. At the slit-lamp examination, the cornea was transparent and the anterior chamber had normal depth. White little masses were clearly visible in the anterior chamber angle and on the iris which was partly heterochromic because of rubeosis (Fig. 1).

A severe Tyndall phenomenon (+ + + +) was present. The pupil was slightly mydriatic but reacted to direct and indirect light reflex. The lens was transparent. The vitreous body appeared like a white brilliant thick liquid. A yellowish mass was seen on the nasal side. The fundus was not explorable.

Using a Kretztechnik 7200 MA (Zipf, Austria) and an Ophthalmoscan 200

420

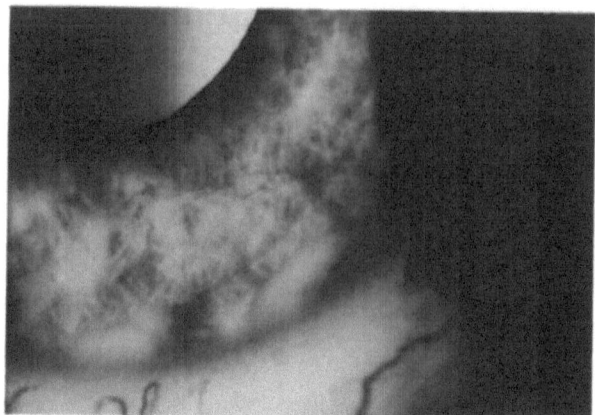

Fig. 1. Retinoblastoma. Anterior segment picture showing white nodules invading the iris and the anterior chamber.

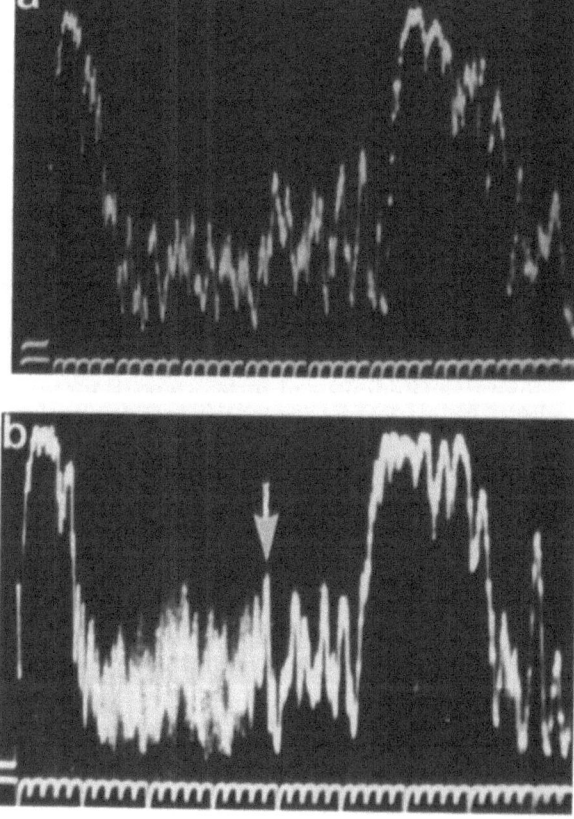

Fig. 2. A-scans of retinoblastoma. (a) The vitreous length is full of low- to medium-reflective echoes; (b) the anterior aspect of the echoes show clear after-movements.

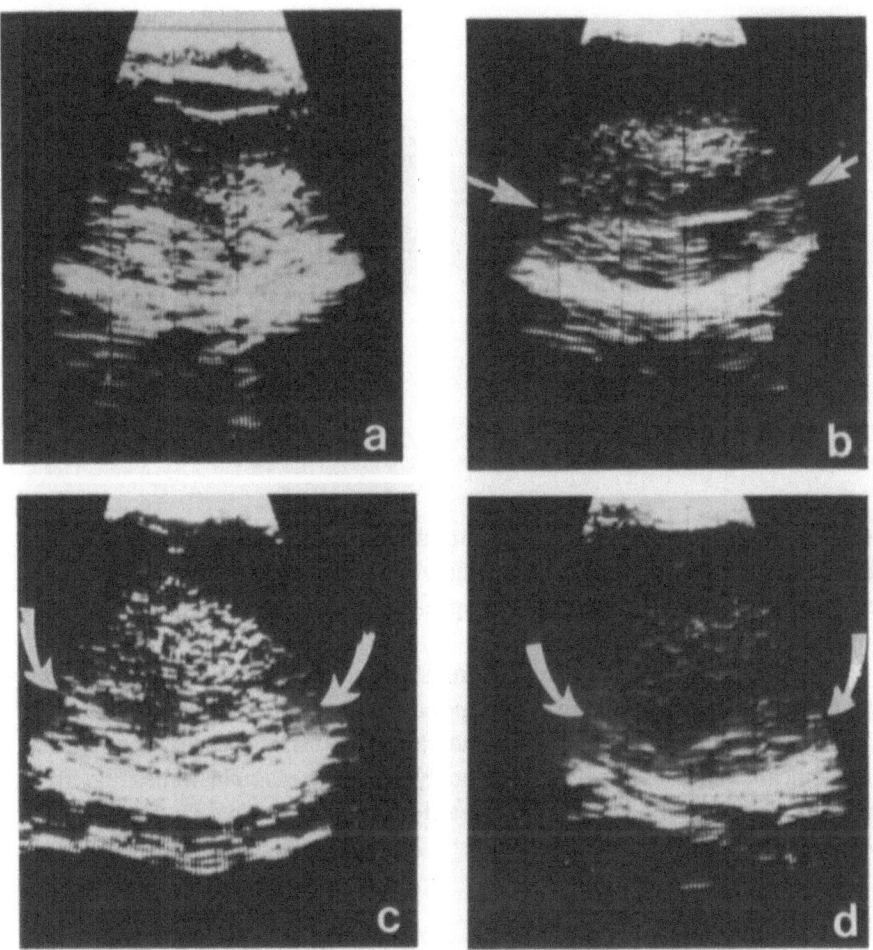

Fig. 3. Contact B-scans of retinoblastoma. The vitreous body is full of scattered echoes. A very thin membrane-like structure appeared in some sound-beam directions when the system sensitivity was reduced (b, c, d arrows).

S.S.I., NY., USA) an ultrasound examination was performed. On the A-scan, the whole vitreous length was full of low- to medium-reflective echoes (Fig. 2a). In some sound beam directions the anterior aspect of these echoes showed a clear motility only after many eye movements (Fig. 2b), while in other directions all the echoes were mobile.

Contact B-scan revealed a vitreous body full of scattered echoes. No solid or cystic mass was clearly visible. Only in the mid-periphery, a very thin and irregular membrane-like structure was evident when the sensitivity setting was lowered. It separated two zones with almost the same reflectivity (Fig. 3). An

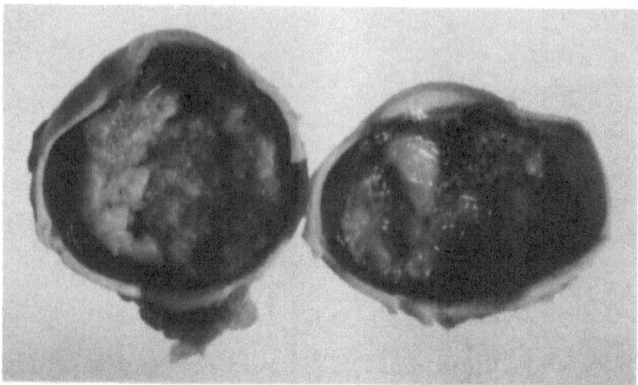

Fig. 4. Macroscopic picture of the eye.

anterior chamber tap was performed and neoplastic cells were found in the acqueous humor, so the eye was enucleated. The optic nerve was free of tumor cells. Intracranial and general tumor spread were excluded by CT and lumbar puncture.

At gross anatomy inspection, a creamish fluid and whitish seeds spread out when the globe was opened. The appearance of the retina was that of a whitish, folded mass that showed hemorrhages and friable areas (Fig. 4). The histological examination revealed a widely necrotic retinoblastoma (Fig. 5). It invaded the iris, the ciliary body, the anterior chamber angle, and the optic-nerve head.

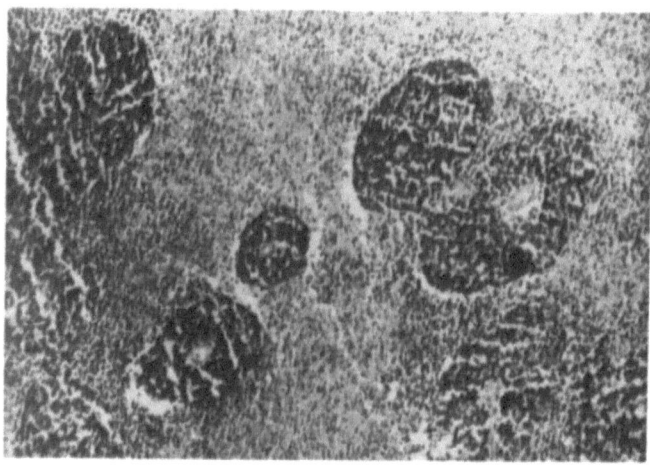

Fig. 5. Histologic section showing a widely necrotic retinoblastoma.

Comments

When the echographic examination was performed, we did not know that this kind of echographic behavior of retinoblastoma could exist. Fernandez-Vigo Lopez and Cueva Alvarez (1983) had described three cases of what they called 'diffused retinoblastoma', but we were unaware of their experience.

Another case of diffused retinoblastoma was found at the University Eye Clinic of Bari (Delle Noci, personal communication, 1984). It was even more puzzling because the clinical appearance was also that of a vitreous hemorrhage.

We do think that from now on this atypical echographic behavior of retinoblastoma should be considered as one of the possible echographic types of this tumor.

References

Coleman DJ, Lizzi FL, Jack RL. 1977. Ultrasonography in Ophthalmology, Lea & Febiger, Philadelphia.

Fernandez-Vigo, Lopez J, Cueva, Alvarez J. 1983. Formes echographiques typiques et atypiques des retinoblastomes. J Fr Ophthal 6/1: 43–49.

Ossoinig KC, Cennamo G, Green RL, Weyer NL. 1981. Echographic results in the diagnosis of retinoblastoma. Docum Ophthal Junk Proc Series, 29: 103–107.

Ultrasonography in the diagnosis of advanced Coats' disease

B.G. HAIK, M.E. SMITH, R.M. ELLSWORTH and D.J. COLEMAN
New York City, USA

Leukokoria, a white pupillary reflex, is an important clinical sign in ophthalmology since it is the most common presenting sign of retinoblastoma, a highly malignant pediatric intraocular tumor. Numerous simulating conditions need to be distinguished from retinoblastoma in order to insure prompt recognition and appropriate treatment of all conditions. The majority of cases can be diagnosed through careful clinical examination and correlation with pertinent historical data. Unfortunately, in approximately 20% of cases a secure diagnosis cannot be established through standard clinical techniques, and in these patients ancillary diagnostic testing is extremely valuable.

Coats' disease is a condition characterized by retinal telangiectases and secondary intraretinal and subretinal exudation, resulting in retinal detachment [1]. This condition is extremely difficult to differentiate from retinoblastoma on purely clinical appearance since both exophytic retinoblastoma and advanced Coats' disease can present with a total retinal detachment, superficial telangiectatic vessels and the appearance of a subretinal mass [2]. Since Coats' disease is a totally benign condition, and occasionally may be rectified by vitreo-retinal surgery, early diagnosis of this condition may result in successful retention of the eye with peripheral vision. Conversely, retinoblastoma in its advanced form is best treated by enucleation to ensure the least possibility of extraocular spread. If a retinoblastoma is misdiagnosed as Coats' disease and no therapy is indicated an undue delay in appropriate therapy can occur, therefore, risking increased mortality. If retinoblastoma is misdiagnosed as Coats' disease and surgical intervention is recommended, subretinal drainage can be performed in the course of retinal surgery and tumor seeding can occur, thus significantly increasing mortality. Lastly, in cases of Coats' disease misdiagnosed as retinoblastoma, and enucleated unneccessarily, the chance of preservation of the globe and potential peripheral vision is lost.

Ultrasonography appears to be a valuable adjunct in the diagnosis of Coats' disease and the differentiation of this entity from exophytic retinoblastoma

K.C. Ossoinig (editor), Ophthalmic Echography,

426

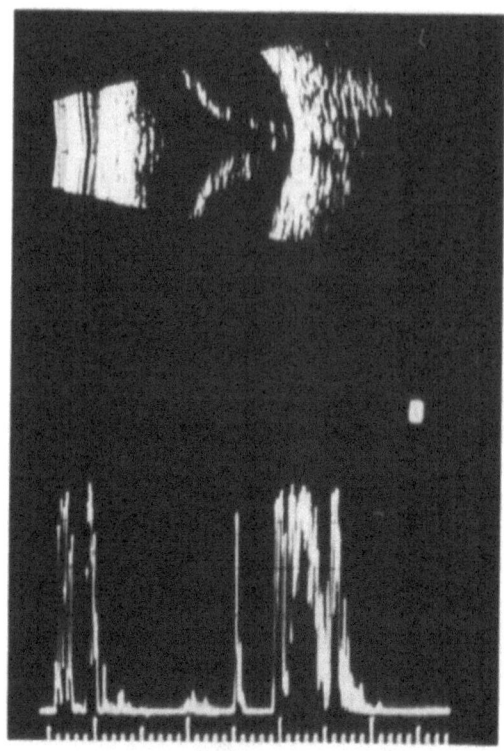

Fig. 1. Contact B- (top) and A-scan of a patient with advanced Coats' disease demonstrating a total retinal detachment and clear subretinal fluid.

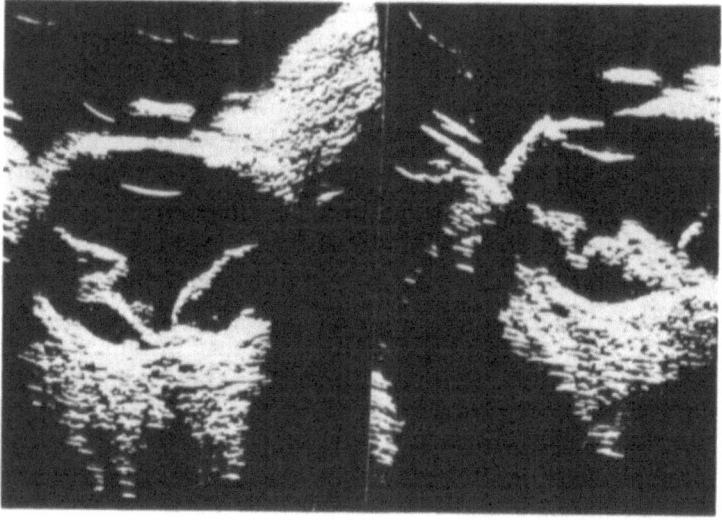

Fig. 2. Immersion B-scan demonstrating convoluted and thickened retinal detachment.

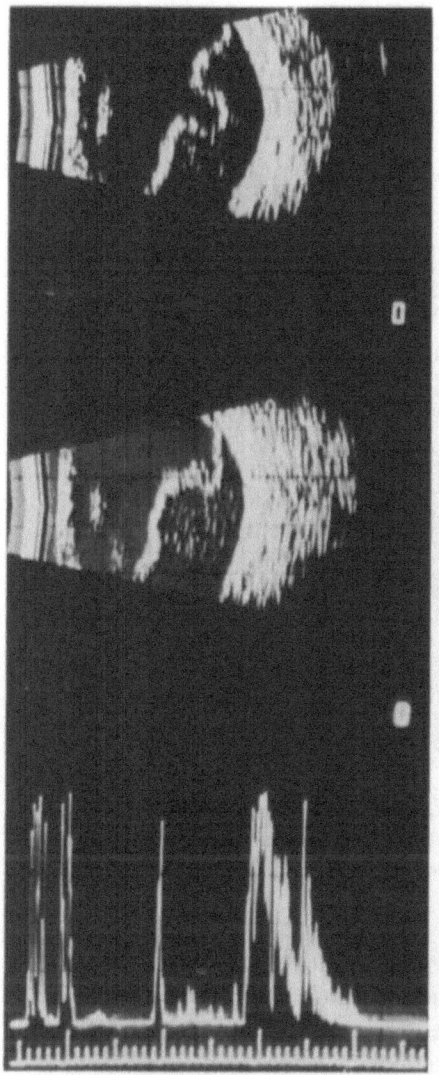

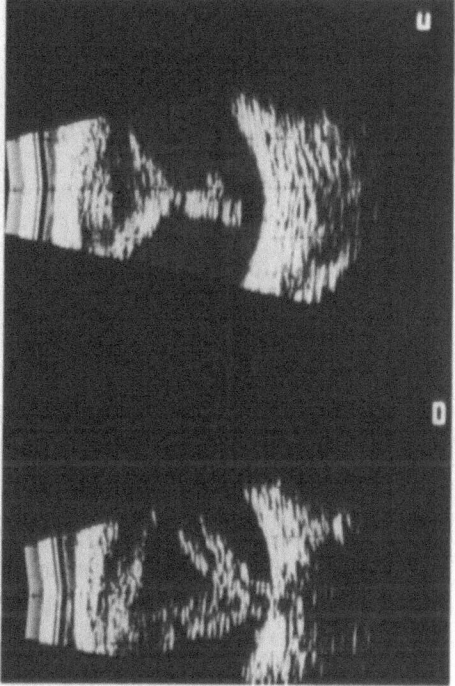

Fig. 3. Contact B- (top and middle) and A-(bottom) scan of the same patient in Fig. 1 demonstrating subretinal accumulations of cholesterol three months after presentation.

Fig. 4. Contact B-scan of patient with long standing advanced Coats' disease producing a contracted retinal detachment.

[3]. In the initial stages of advanced Coats' disease, a total retinal detachment is evident with retinal leaves extending from the optic nerve to the ora serrata (Fig. 1). The subretinal space is sonolucent on both B- and A-scan, and the retina is freely mobile without evidence of organization. In the intermediate stages of Coats' disease, the retina becomes more convoluted and thickened, with signs of focal organization (Fig. 2). The retina may undulate sluggishly on

428

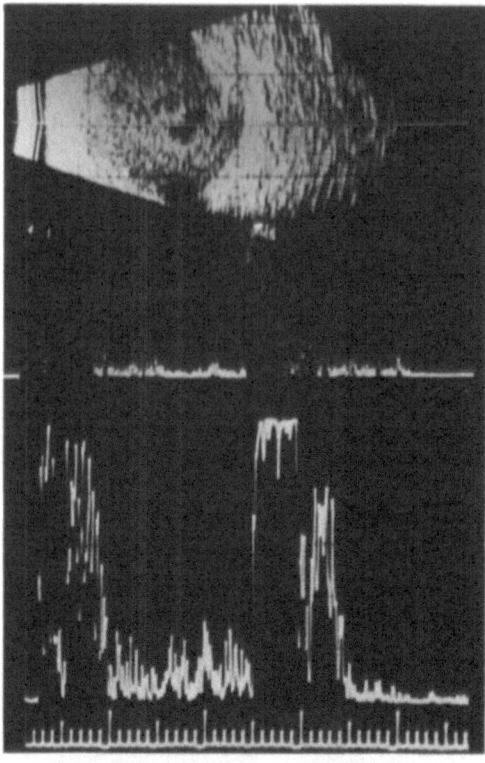

Fig. 5. Contact B- (top) and A- (bottom) scan of a patient in the late stage of advanced Coats'
disease. The retina is contracted and drawn anteriorly and only a small vitreous pocket remains.
Subretinal accumulations of cholosterol fill the globe.

eye movement. The subretinal space may present with low amplitude, diffuse
subretinal echoes, that arise from accumulation of subretinal cholesterol (Fig.
3). In contrast to retinoblastoma, isolated or multiple solid lesions are not
identified. Neither the retina nor the subretinal densities show persistence on
lower sensitivity settings or absorption defects in the posterior globe or retrobulbar fat, both acoustic findings strongly associated with retinoblastoma. In
the late stages of Coats' disease, the retina remains totally detached, with
rigidity of the retinal bullae, and contracture resulting from interretinal adhesions (Fig. 4). The subretinal space may show massive accumulations of
cholesterol and/or hemorrhage that are difficult to distinguish from poorly
calcified retinoblastoma (Fig. 5).

As in any other process where massive retinal detachment and disorganization occurs, the eye afflicted with Coats' disease may show changes associated
with phthisis, including a shortened axial length, a retrolenticular, or cyclitic
membrane, and scattered internal calcifications along the planes of normal

structures. At this stage, it may be more difficult to distinguish from phthisis of other etiologies including spontaneous regression of retinoblastoma.

In summary, ultrasonography is an extremely valuable imaging technique in the diagnosis of Coats' disease and its differentiation from other, potentially lethal causes of leukokoria. It is helpful in determining the stage of disease and in monitoring and documenting progression.

References

1. Coats G. 1912. Retinitis exudativa (retinitis haemorrhagica externa). Archives of Ophthalmol 81: 275–327.
2. Reese AB. 1976. Tumors of the Eye. Third Edition, New York: Harper & Row, 268–271.
3. Haik BG, Smith ME, Saint Louis L. 1983. Ancillary diagnostic testing in the differentiation of retinoblastoma and advanced Coats' disease. J of Ultrasound in Medicine, 2: 125.

B-scan in retinopathy of prematurity (ROP)

V. MAZZEO, L. RAVALLI, L. FALCO[1] and R. SCORRANO
Ferrara and Florence[1], Italy

Vitreo-retinal surgery has promoted new interest in the echographic examination of patients with retinopathy of prematurity (ROP). Until recently these eyes were only considered in the differential diagnosis of retinoblastoma. There are very few reports in the literature of such echographic imaging, particularly with reference to B-scan (Shammas, 1983).

The purpose of this report is to discuss the echographic B-scan images of ROP carried out over the past two years. Echographic patterns were reviewed and compared with clinical findings, then correlated on the basis of our knowledge. Some discussion will also be devoted to the comparison of the echographic findings with schemes published by several vitreo-retinal surgeons.

Materials and methods

Twelve children and two adolescents with cicatricial stage ROP were examined between January 1982 and July 1984 at the University Eye Clinic of Ferrara. All patients underwent contact B-scan examinations using an Ophthalmoscan 200 (S.S.I., N.Y., USA) equipped with a 10 MHz probe. Two of the oldest patients also underwent immersion B-scan examination. The 'mini-water-bath' technique was used when examining patients under general anesthesia (Coleman et al., 1979). No clear echographic patterns could be recorded in very uncooperative out-patients so, for this reason, these 'technically bad' images were excluded. The files and the phsysicians' recordings were reviewed to compare clinical pictures and echographic findings.

Results

The disease was clinically staged following Patz's classification. B-scan images

K.C. Ossoinig (editor), Ophthalmic Echography, ISBN 978-94-010-7988-4

Table 1. Echographic classification of ROP.

a	=	small mass of tissue in the periphery
b	=	more or less peripheric tractional detachment with complete or incomplete retrolental mass
c	=	complete retrolental mass without any apparent retinal detachment
d	=	complete retrolental mass with triangle-shaped or T-shaped retinal detachment
e	=	not interpretable echopattern

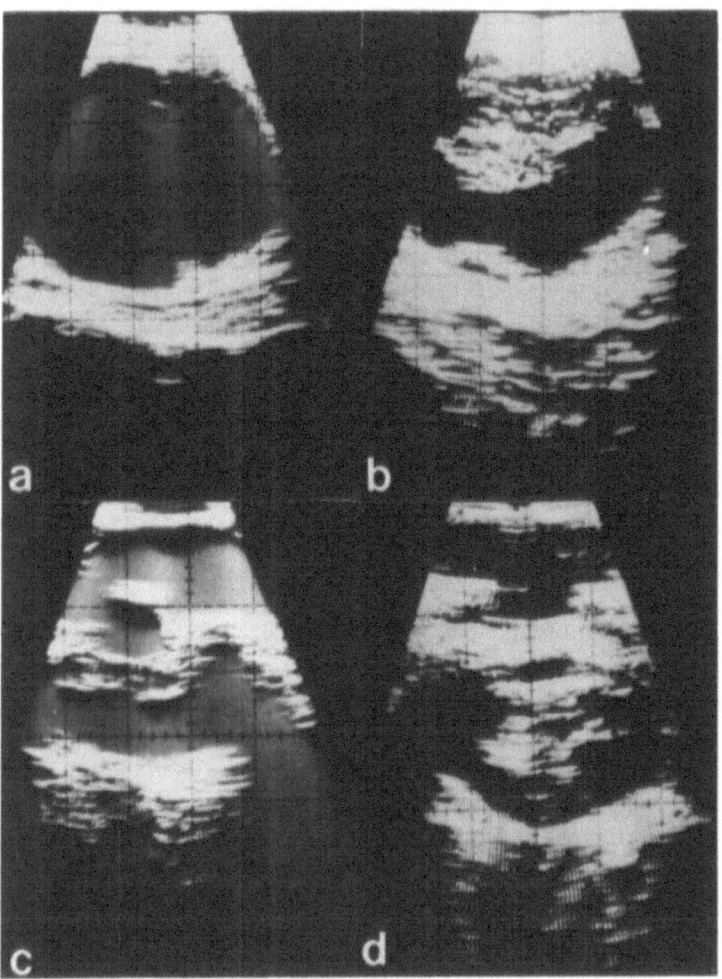

Fig. 1. For explanation, see Table 1.

were divided into 5 groups according to their appearance (Table 1, Fig. 1). Under item 'e' we put the echograms that could not be interpreted even when they were good technically. The clinical and echographic findings are summarized in Table 2.

Discussion

A few differences can be found in the clinical classification of ROP over the years (Reese et al., 1952; Patz, 1969; Tasman, 1983; Ausburger et al. 1983). Patz's classification best described our clinical cases. Our echographic classifications seem to adhere very well to the clinical staging. With the exception of case 5 where a very dense and white retrolental mass was present in the left eye, no clear retinal detachment was found at the echographic examination (Fig. 2). Our findings cannot be explained since it is well-known in pathology that cicatricial ROP is characterized by a partial or total retinal detachment. Technical errors may be excluded since the examination was repeated twice and also because partial or total retinal detachment, if present, was always clearly visible. Furthermore, Shammas (1983) described a case of ROP in which a retrolental mass was accompanied by a normal posterior pole. A few apparent discrepancies between clinical and echographic classifications were also present (Cases 1 and 7).

Table 2. Tabular presentation of patients.

Patient N°	Gestation Age (weeks)	Birth weight (grams)	Age at echo (months)	ROP grade RE	ROP grade LE	Echo classification RE	Echo classification LE	Axial length (μ sec) RE	Axial length (μ sec) LE
1	26	720	19	5	2	b	a	20	28
2	n.r.	900	24	5	5	d	d	20	22
3	26	1,040	8	5	5	d	b	20	19
4	27	1,100	3	5	2–3	d	a	20	21
5	30	1,490	6	1	5	a	c	17	11
			18	1	5			28	20
6	32	1,030	9	2	2	a	a	25	25
7	27	n.r.	72	5	5	b	d	21	21
8	28	1,500	180	5	5	d	d	–	–
9	29	n.r.	24	5	5	e	d	–	–
10	28	1,450	144	0	5	0	d	0	13
11	27	1,100	8	5	5	d	d	–	18

n.r. = not recorded; – = not measurable.

434

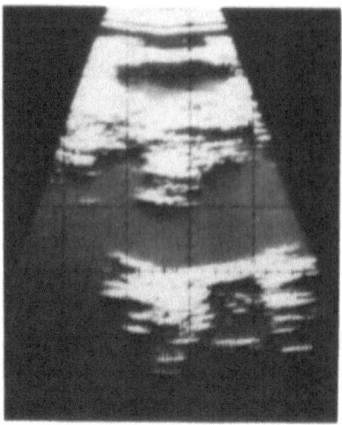

Fig. 2. Case 5. Contact B-scan. 'Mini water-bath' technique. A retrolental mass is clearly visible; the posterior pole appears normal.

Comments and conclusions

On comparison of our echographic images with drawings published by several vitreo-retinal surgeons, only partial agreement emerged. Trese (1984) stated that they were unable to predict by ultrasound which eyes had a partially closed retinal detachment and which had a totally closed retinal detachment. It is our opinion that these problems are due to the complexity of the anatomical condition of the vitreo-retina. Almost all standard echographic criteria used for diagnosing traction retinal detachment are of little use, particularly for the differentiation of membranes vs. retina. Most of these eyes are very small and their relationship with our contact B-scan probe dimensions does not lessen the difficulty of the examination.

References

Ausburger JJ, Goldberg RE, Margargal LE. 1983. Retinal and choroidal vascular abnormalities. In Pediatric Ophthalmology (R.D. Harley ed.), 627–740, W.B. Saunders Company, Philadelphia.

Coleman DJ, Dallow RL, Smith ME. 1979. A combined System of contact A-scan and B-scan. Int Ophthal Clinics 19/4: 211–224.

Lightfoot D, Irvine R. 1982. Vitrectomy in infants and children with retinal detachments caused by cicatricial retrolental fibroplasia. Am J Ophthal 94: 305–312.

Machemer R. 1983. Closed vitrectomy for Severe Retrolental Fibroplasia in the infant. Ophthalmology 90: 436–441.

Machemer R. 1984. Retrolental fibroplasia-pathogenesis of late stages. Basic and advanced vitreous surgery course. Abstract book. Rome, September 5–7.

Patz A. 1969. Retrolental fibroplasia. Surv Ophthal 14: 1–29.

Reese AB, Blodi FC, Locke JC. 1952. The pathology of early retrolental fibroplasia with an analysis of the histologic findings in the eyes of newborn and stillborn infants. Am J Ophthal 35: 1407–1426.

Shammas J. 1983. Atlas of Ophthalmic Ultrasonography and Biometry. The C.V. Mosby Co., St. Louis.

Tasman W. 1983. Disease of the retina and vitreous. In Pediatric Ophthalmology (R.D. Harley ed.) 599–625, W.B. Saunders Company, Philadelphia.

Trese MT. 1984. Surgical results of Stage V Retrolental Fibroplasia and timing of Surgical Repair. Ophthalmology 91: 461–466.

B-scan ultrasonographic findings in eyes with the rush-type of active retinopathy of prematurity (ROP)

Y. TAKAO, H. HAYASHI, K. OSHIMA and Y. KITAGAWA
Fukuoka, Japan

Introduction

Retinopathy of prematurity (ROP) is one of the leading causes of blindness in infants. Although low birth weight infant mortality is decreasing, this particular disease appears to be occurring more frequently [1].

The mechanism of retinal detachment in the cicatricial stage of ROP was considered to be a combination of a break in cicatricial retina and traction by proliferative changes in the vitreous [2–8]. These cases should be treated by vitreous surgery or routine retinal detachment surgery [9–11].

However, the mechanism of retinal detachment in the active stage of ROP is controversial. It has been thought to be due to exudation, traction, or a combination of both. Little is known about the advance of the rush-type or 'plus' type ROP in extremely low birth weight infants, since the ocular media become hazy in almost all cases and the disease process progresses rapidly. Presented in this report are the results of ultrasonographic examinations of rush-type ROP in its active stages. Also, the mechanism of retinal detachment and the value of ultrasonic examination in these cases are discussed.

Subjects and method

Twenty-two eyes in eleven cases of rush-type ROP were examined with ultrasonography during a recent five-year period. The cases included seven males and four females. Two cases underwent photocoagulation before examination. All examinations were done with contact real-time B-mode equipment, and no general anesthesia was employed during the examinations.

K.C. Ossoinig (editor), Ophthalmic Echography, ISBN 978-94-010-7988-4

438

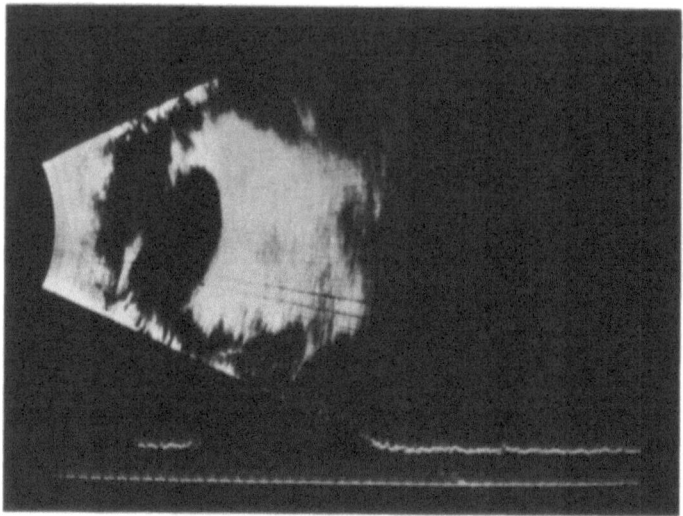

Fig. 1.

Results and discussion

In the early stage of rush-type ROP, a membranous structure in the vitreous cavity was frequently detected on B-scan ultrasonography prior to the appearance of retinal detachment. The membrane arose from the peripheral retina, and was perpendicular to the retinal plane. It appeared like a wedge whose base was attached to the retina and which sometimes bridged the vitreous cavity between opposite sides of the peripheral retina (Fig. 1). Although it seems most reasonable to conclude that this membrane-like structure represents an extraretinal fibrovascular proliferation growing from the ridge of the retina, ophthalmoscopic examination performed through an increased vitreous haze in these cases failed to reveal a definite fibrovascular proliferation. In contrast, the cases of non-rush-type ROP with apparent fibrovascular proliferation arising from the retinal ridge did not show the membranous structure during ultrasonic examination. Also, the membrane disappeared after adequate treatment with cryo- or photocoagulation. Therefore the membrane seen during ultrasonography should be conceived as an exudation into, or an infiltration of, vitreous rather than fibrovascular tissue per se.

In all cases, the detachment of the retina appeared first in the periphery. The retina detached steeply in the periphery and, from its highest elevation, sloped to the posterior. While the detachment might be localized early on, it expanded toward all quadrants later on. The retinal detachment may well be associated with the membrane which appeared to adhere to the retina at the retina's highest elevation. The B-scan picture resembles a shirt collar (Fig. 2).

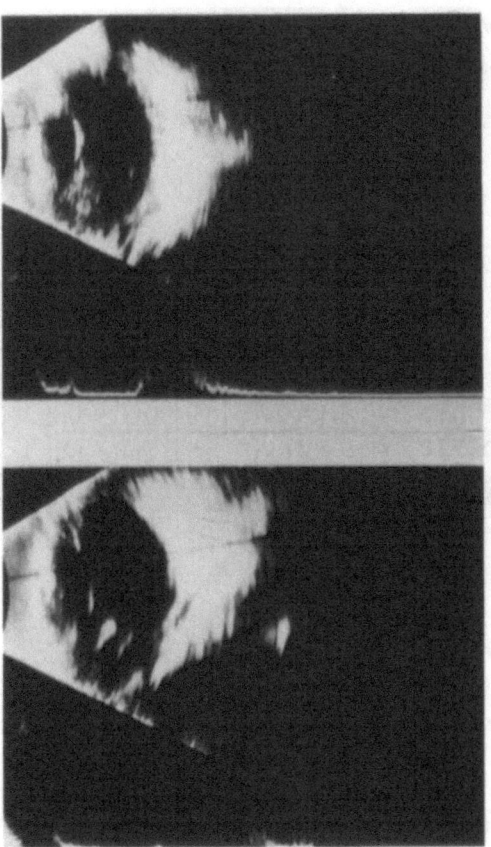

Fig. 2.

As a consequence of this traction, the retina is finally pulled along the posterior surface of the lens (Fig. 3). Occasionally the two retinal leaves from opposite fundus areas may be pulled toward each other and may thus unite behind the lens. As the height of the peripheral detachment increases, the posterior slope of the detachment reaches the posterior pole. In some cases, the detached posterior retina showed a 'table-top' configuration, so that the presence of tractional force on the posterior retina was considered. In two patients who underwent extensive photocoagulation, only the posterior retina detached (Fig. 3). This posterior retinal detachment also showed traction of the retina toward the optic disc with a 'table-top' configuration (Fig. 4). The Figure 5 presents schematic drawings of the ultrasonographic findings discussed above.

Finally several conclusions should be drawn from the ultrasonographic findings discussed:

1. The mechanism of retinal detachment in rush-type ROP is mainly tractional.

440

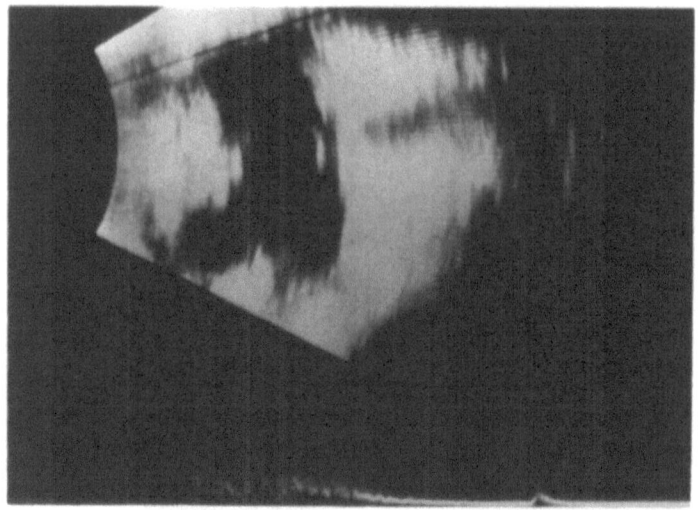

Fig. 3.

2. The presence of a wedge-shaped membrane in the eyes with hazy media suggests that ROP is rapidly progressing in these eyes.
3. The ultrasonographic findings are valuable in active stage ROP with extremely hazy media or with a miotic pupil, in determining if surgical intervention is indicated.
4. The state of the posterior retina, especially the macula, can be determined with ultrasonography even when highly elevated peripheral retina obscures the posterior view.

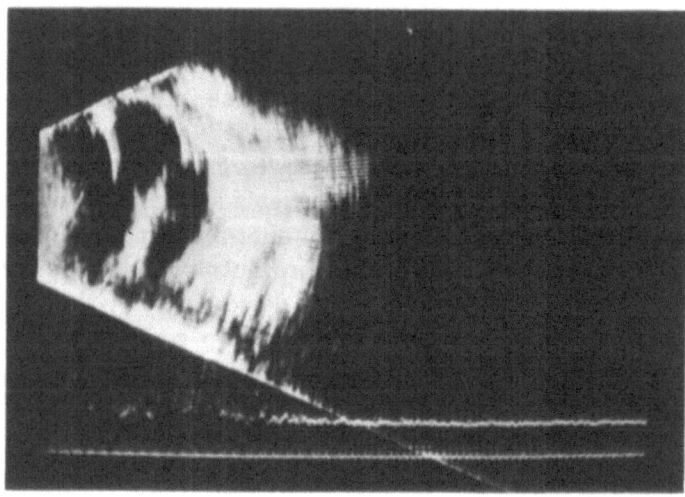

Fig. 4.

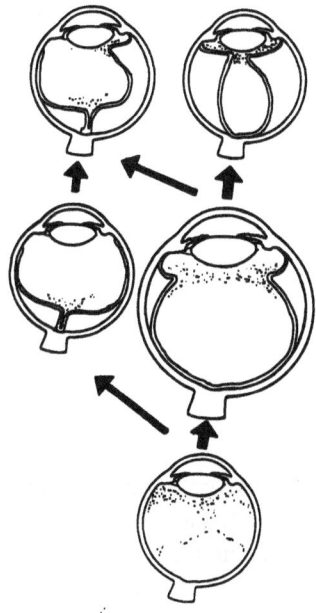

Fig. 5.

References

1. Pyne JW, Patz A. 1979. Current status of retrolental fibroplasia Ann Clin Res 11: 205–221.
2. Winslow RL, Tasman W. 1978. Juvenile Rhegmatogenous retinal detachment. Ophthalmology 85: 607–616.
3. Tasman W. 1979. Late complications of retrolental fibroplasia. Ophthalmology 86: 1724–1740.
4. Tasman W, Annesley W. 1966. Retinal detachment in the retinopathy of prematurity. Arch Ophthalmol 75: 608–614.
5. Tasman W. 1975. Retinal detachment in retrolental fibroplasia. Albert v. Graefes Arch Klin exp Ophthalmol: 129–139.
6. Faris B, Tolentino FI, Freeman HM, Brockhurst RJ, Schepens CL. 1971. Retrolental fibroplasia in the cicatricial stage. Fundus and vitreous findings. Arch Ophthalmol 85: 661–668.
7. Patz A, Payne JW. Retrolental fibroplasia. Clinical Ophthalmol: Vol. 3 Chap 20: 1–10.
8. Bertenyi A, Yebi M, Fodor M. 1980. A-mode ultrasonography and Oculometry in Retrolental fibroplasia. Ultrasound in Medicine & Biology 5: 19–24.
9. McPherson A, Hittner HM. 1979. Scleral buckling in 2¹/₂ to 11-month-old premature infants with retinal detachment associated with acute retrolental fibroplasia. Ophthalmol 86: 819–835.
10. Lightfoot D, Iruine AR. 1982. Vitrectomy in infants and children with retinal detachments caused by cicatricial retrolental fibroplasia. Am J Ophthalmol 94: 305–312.
11. Machemer R. 1983. Closed Vitrectomy for Severe Retrolental Fibroplasia in the Infant. Ophthalmol 90: 436–441.

The acoustic differentiation of retinoblastoma and various other causes of leukokoria

R.L. GREEN
Los Angeles, USA

Abstract

Standardized Echography has proven to be extremely useful in differentiatir retinoblastoma from other intraocular lesions. This paper reviews the echc graphic criteria used in establishing this diagnosis. The key echographic finc ings in retinoblastoma are produced by the calcium deposits within the tumo. The characteristic pattern of this calcification can clearly be distinguished fro calcification seen in other conditions, such as a phthisical globe. Studie presented will show that Standardized Echography has correctly diagnose calcification within retinoblastomas in 98% of those cases examined. In ac dition to retinoblastoma, Standardized Echography is extremely helpful ' differentiating other causes of leukokoria, such as RLF, PHPV, and Coat. disease.

References

1. Ossoinig KC. 1982. Advances in Diagnostic Ultrasound. ACTA: XXIV International Congre of Ophthalmology, (San Francisco), Paul Henkind, ed. Philadelphia: J.B. Lippincott Co., Vc 1, pp. 89–114.
2. Ossoinig KC. 1985. Standardized Ophthalmic Echography of the Eye, Orbit and Periorbit Region. A Comprehensive Slide Set (774 slides) and Study Guide, Third Edition. Iowa Cit Iowa: Goodfellow Company, Inc., pp. 37–38.

K.C. Ossoinig (editor), Ophthalmic Echography, ISBN 978-94-010-7988-4

Ancillary diagnostic testing in the differentiation of retinoblastoma and advanced Coats' disease

B.G. HAIK, R.M. ELLSWORTH, M.E. SMITH and L. SAINT LOUIS
New York, USA

Abstract

Leukocoria is an important clinical sign in ophthalmology characterized by a white pupillary reflex resulting from an intraocular mass or retrolental opacity. Although a number of developmental, inflammatory, neoplastic, and hemorrhagic conditions can result in this clinical sign, the most important condition in which it occurs is retinoblastoma. Retinoblastoma is a primary malignant retinal tumor that if left untreated will eventually lead to destruction of the globe followed by extraocular spread with resultant mortality. Its diagnosis and differentiation from other leukocoria conditions is important in order to permit appropriate specific therapy. Many clinical findings are helpful in delineating the cause of leukocoria and in differentiating retinoblastoma from simulating conditions. However, in other cases, diagnosis cannot be established on purely ophthalmoscopic grounds. Advanced Coats' disease is a condition characterized by congenital retinal telangiectasias with associated massive subretinal exudation and retinal detachment that can closely mimic the clinical appearance of retinoblastoma. We have found that certain ancillary diagnostic tests are helpful in establishing a secure diagnosis. The synergistic use of ultrasonography, computerized tomography and magnetic resonance imaging has aided in this important clinical distinction.

K.C. Ossoinig (editor), Ophthalmic Echography, ISBN 978-94-010-7988-4

The echographic diagnosis of non-calcified retinoblastoma

K.C. OSSOINIG and K.M. ITANI
Iowa City, USA

Abstract

Most retinoblastomas (94% among 49 consecutive cases seen in the Ey
Department at the University of Iowa) are calcified and can be reliably an
accurately diagnosed with Standardized Echography. Most of them produc
echographic patterns that are pathognomonic for retinoblastoma.

In only three of our cases the retinoblastomas lacked any calcification. Eve:
in these rare cases, echography at least suggests the presence of this tumor
The echographic findings in such non-calcified retinoblastomas include: tu
mefaction with irregular internal structure, medium reflectivity and typica
signs of vascularity, and retinal detachment with part of the retinal surfac
being destroyed.

References

1. Ossoinig KC. 1982. Advances in Diagnostic Ultrasound. ACTA: XXIV International Congres
of Ophthalmology, (San Francisco), Paul Henkind, ed. Philadelphia: J.B. Lippincott Co., Vc.
1, pp. 89–114.
2. Ossoinig KC. 1985. Standardized Ophthalmic Echography of the eye, Orbit and Periorbitz
Region. A comprehensive Slide Set (774 slides) and Study Guide, Third Edition. Iowa City
Iowa: Goodfellow Company, Inc., pp. 37, 38.

K.C. Ossoinig (editor), Ophthalmic Echography, ISBN 978-94-010-7988-4
© 1987, Martinus Nijhoff/Dr W. Junk Publishers, Dordrecht.

Standardized echography of the orbit (review)

R.P. HARRIE
Salt Lake City, USA

The orbit is a 28 cubic millimeter space that can harbor a tremendous amount of pathology. The list of disease processes is a very long one and is being added to constantly. The major categories of orbital disease include (Henderson, 1980):
– Congenital abnormalities
– Trauma
– Infections
– Inflammatory processes
   Grave's disease
   Tumors
      malignant and benign
      primary, secondary, and metastatic

The evaluation of the orbit includes a careful history and physical examination, radiographic imaging techniques, and echography. New modalities such as nuclear magnetic resonance are on the immediate horizon. The problem with all of these techniques except for echography is that they are relatively sensitive for something being abnormal in the orbit but are generally nonspecific as to the exact nature of the orbital pathology. The tremendous value of standardized echography of the orbit is its ability to noninvasively differentiate different disease entities. Whether the echographer is an ophthalmologist working in a general practice setting or an academician concerned with research of unusual problems, the technique is of immense value.

I will illustrate the value of standardized echography of the orbit by several case examples. Several of these are typical problems seen in a general ophthalmology office and others are more unusual referral cases. The first case is that of a 21-year-old woman who was 4 months pregnant when she noticed the sudden onset of a sharp pain in the area of her left eye after a sneezing episode. She complained of the pain to her obstetrician but he could find no obvious clinical signs except for some mild upper lid swelling. She was referred for

K.C. Ossoinig (editor), Ophthalmic Echography, ISBN 978-94-010-7988-4
© 1987, Martinus Nijhoff/Dr W. Junk Publishers, Dordrecht.

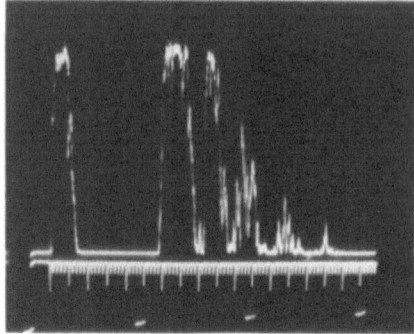

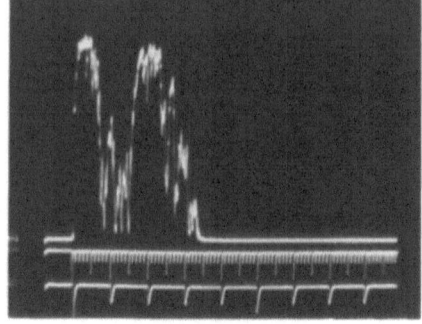

Fig. 1. Subperiosteal effusion.   *Fig. 2.* Lacrimal pseudotumor.

ophthalmological examination which only revealed a mild amount of left upper lid edema and some slight tenderness to palpation in the brow area. An ultrasound examination was performed of the periorbital area and a sharply defined very low reflective area was identified in the anterior nasal orbit. This was quite consistent with subperiosteal fluid and was felt to be an effusion, possibly forced into the subperiosteal area by the pressure of the patient sneezing. The echogram is illustrated in Fig. 1. The patient was treated with sinus decongestants but the pain and symptoms persisted so a subperiosteal exploration under local anesthetic was performed and a straw colored fluid was obtained. Postoperative ultrasound examination revealed only a slight residual swelling of the subperiosteal space.

Case 2 is that of a 70-year-old woman who complained of intermittent right eye pain for several weeks. She stated that at times the pain had become so bad that it had awakened her from sleep. She had also experienced a moderate amount of lid swelling and a mild conjunctival injection of the right eye. She was evaluated by an ophthalmologist and was felt to have a chronic blepharitis which was treated with a topical combination antibiotic and steroid ointment. Her symptoms persisted and, in fact, became somewhat worse. She was referred for echographic evaluation and was found to have a low medium reflective area in her right lacrimal gland. This finding was felt to be most consistent with a dense cellular infiltrate of the lacrimal gland and in light of her fairly recent onset of symptoms with signs of inflammation it was elected to treat her with high dose prednisone. This was done and her symptoms rapidly abated over several days. They then leveled off and she did have some moderate persistent tenderness and swelling in spite of continued steroids. At this time it was elected to perform an orbital biopsy and lacrimal gland tissue was obtained. The pathological diagnosis was that of lacrimal pseudotumor. The patient was continued on tapering doses of prenisone and her symptoms completely resolved after an additional two weeks. The A-scan is illustrated in Fig. 2.

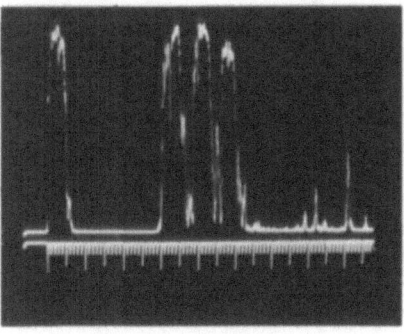 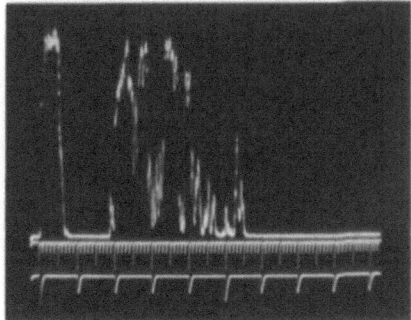

Fig. 3. Subperiosteal hemorrhage.   *Fig. 4.* Infantile hemangioma.

Case 3 is that of a 25-year-old medical student's wife who presented with 'a bloody left eye'. She experienced a marked amount of pain in conjunction with the vascular engorgement of her eye. Her ophthalmologist evaluated her and referred her for echographic evaluation. She was in a marked amount of discomfort at the time of the evaluation and was noted to have engorgement, especially of the nasal palpebral conjunctiva. A-scan revealed a sharply defined area in the anterior and mid nasal orbit. This area was so well delineated both anteriorly and posteriorly at its borders that it was felt to be in the subperiosteal space. A careful search was made to identify a source for this subperiosteal hemorrhage. No intraorbital mass lesion could be identified. The patient later underwent a CT scan and an angiogram both of which failed to reveal any arteriovenous malformation. On careful questioning the patient admitted to having a less severe but similar episode several years previously. Her symptoms abated over several days after treatment with cold compresses and analgesics. Her ultrasound is illustrated in Fig. 3.

Case 4 is that of a 3½-month-old infant in whom the parents noted rapidly increasing proptosis. This occurred in a period of less than one week and seemed to increase in size daily. A CT scan was performed by the ophthalmologist and showed an intraorbital mass lesion felt to be consistent with a rhabdomyosarcoma. Standardized echography of the orbit was performed and revealed a multireflective lesion. In one portion of the lesion the reflectivity was rather high and in another area several large cystic spaces were seen with rapid spontaneous pulsations consistent with arterial blood flow. The lesion was moderately soft to compression. The diagnosis of an infantile hemangioma was made and it was elected to treat the child with high dose steroids because of the marked lid swelling with the danger of occlusive amblyopia. The child responded rapidly to this regimen with marked decrease in swelling and clearing of the visual axis. The ultrasound is demonstrated in Fig. 4.

Case 5 is that of an eight-year-old child who was referred with rapidly

448

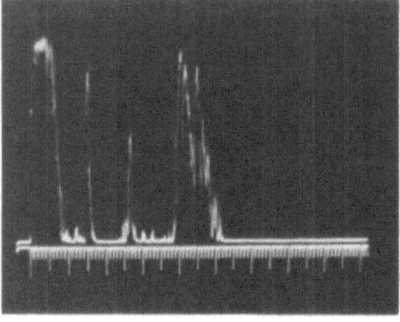 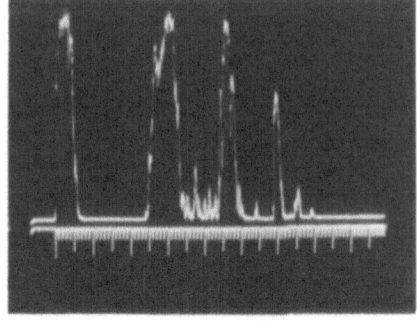

Fig. 5. Lymphangioma with hemorrhage into huge cyst.

Fig. 6. Orbital myositis of right lateral rectus.

increasing proptosis of his left eye over a period of several days. A CT scan had been performed and had been interpreted as an orbital mass lesion consistent with a rhabdomyosarcoma and this was the diagnosis of the referring ophthalmologist. Standardized echography was performed and revealed a multicystic lesion with very low internal reflectivity in the cystic spaces. One of them was quite large and filled at least one half of the orbit. The diagnosis of a lymphangioma that had spontaneously bled into itself was made and the child was observed over two weeks with marked resolution of his proptosis spontaneously. He has been seen on one occasion since that episode with a similar occurrence although of a less severe degree. The ultrasound is illustrated in Fig. 5.

Case 6 is that of a nine-year-old child who was left at a daycare center with a mildly swollen right eye. When his mother returned after work to pick him up she noticed a marked increase in swelling of the eye and the child complained of a moderate amount of pain. He was seen by an ophthalmologist who was very concerned about the diagnosis of a malignant process and obtained a CT scan. This showed a large orbital mass lesion. He scheduled surgery for that evening and was prepared to do a frozen section biopsy with the possibility of enucleation or orbital exenteration. Before he went to the hospital the child was examined by standardized echography and was seen to have a huge right lateral rectus muscle with low to medium internal reflectivity. The muscle was swollen all the way to its insertion on the globe. The diagnosis of an orbital myositis was made and the patient was placed on 100 mg. of prednisone that evening. The referring ophthalmologist was still prepared to perform surgery the following day but the child responded so dramatically to the prednisone that surgery was cancelled. Over a several day period the symptoms almost completely resolved. Follow-up ultrasound examination revealed marked decrease in swelling of the muscle. The ultrasound is illustrated in Fig. 6.

Case 7 is that of a 58-year-old woman who was seen by her internist with

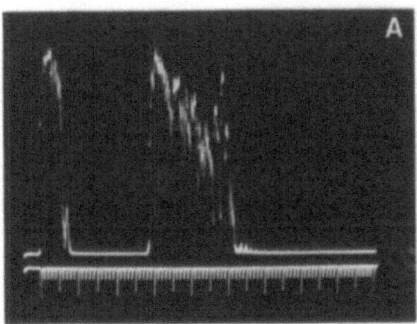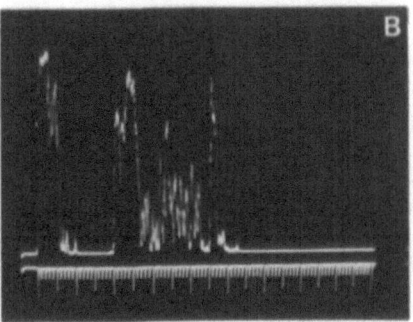

Fig. 7. Orbital apex syndrome. (A) normal left apex and (B) infiltrate in right apex.

symptoms of marked pain in the eye and with a mild amount of lid swelling. His initial diagnosis was that of acute closed angle glaucoma because of the severity of her pain. She was seen by her ophthalmologist who found normal intraocular pressure and an open angle. Her symptoms had increased some-what when he saw her and there was more lid swelling. There was a mild amount of pain on moving the eye. He requested an ear, nose, and throat consult and sinus x-rays were obtained which were read as normal. The patient was given analgesics and told to go home. Her symptoms became so much worse in the following few hours that she sought a second opinion. Her clinical symptoms had increased at that time with ptosis of the right lid and restriction of extraocular movement consistent with a third nerve palsy. There was also a mild amount of dilation of her right pupil. Standardized echography was available in the office and was performed prior to obtaining a neurosurgical consult with the thought that she was undergoing an expanding aneurysm intracranially. The ultrasound surprisingly showed a low reflective area in the orbital apex and some mild swelling of her right medial rectus muscle. There were also some weak signals obtained from the ethmoid sinus area. The diagnosis of an inflammatory orbital apex syndrome was made and the patient was hospitalized and placed on intravenous antibiotics. A CT scan was per-formed in the hospital and did not reveal any intracranial pathology. The patient's symptoms markedly improved over a several day course of antibio-tics. Interestingly, however, her right medial rectus muscle increased dramat-ically in size and gave the classic appearance of an orbital myositis. A moderate dose of prednisone was added to her regimen at this point and over several days her symptoms completely abated and she has been symptom free for two years. The ultrasound is illustrated in Fig. 7.

Case 8 is that of a very active 45-year-old businesswoman who had persistent symptoms of scratchiness, irritation and dryness, in both eyes but worse in her right eye. She had been seen by a number of ophthalmologists and presented in

450

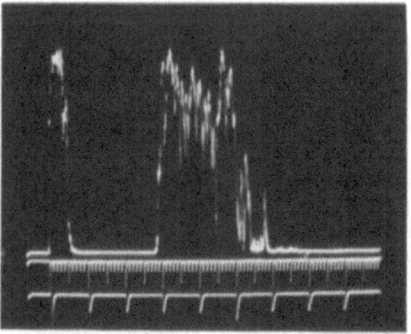

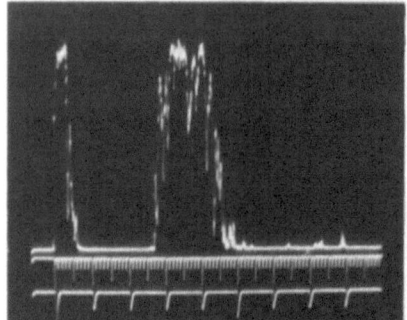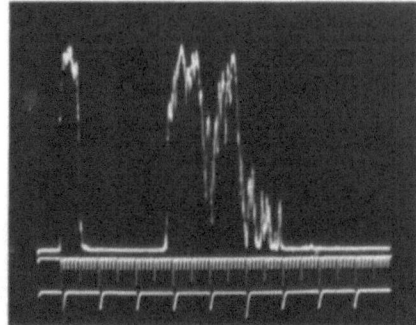

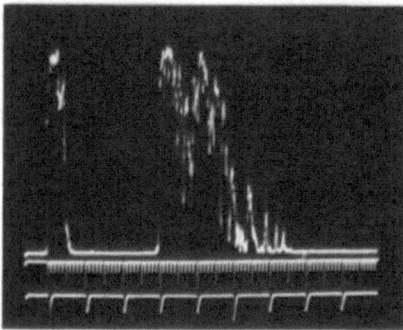

Fig. 8. Grave's disease (right superior, lateral, inferior, medial rectus muscles in clockwise direction).

the office with a large bag of ocular medicines of various types. She had been given the diagnoses of blepharitis, keratitis sicca, allergic conjunctivitis, and infectious conjunctivitis. Standardized echography was performed and revealed typical muscle swelling and irregular internal reflectivity consistent with Grave's disease. This disease was discussed at length with her and suggestions were given for symptomatic treatment which has helped her greatly. The ultrasound is illustrated in Fig. 8.

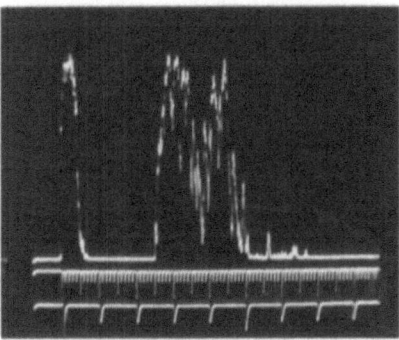
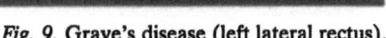
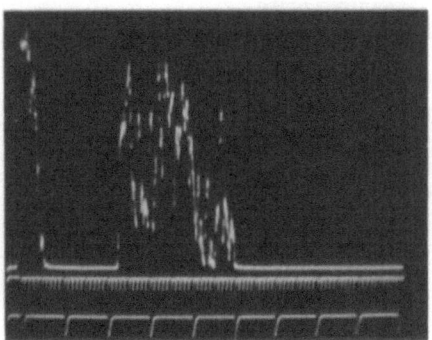

Fig. 9. Grave's disease (left lateral rectus).   *Fig. 10.* Optic nerve sheath meningioma.

Case 9 is that of a gentleman in his mid-60's who was noted to have incrasing proptosis over several months. He was evaluated by his ophthalmologist and a CT scan was performed which revealed a mass lesion of the orbit. He was referred for further consultation by a neuro-ophthalmologist. Standardized echography was performed and revealed no intraorbital mass lesion but did reveal diffuse muscle thickening, especially near the apex, consistent with Grave's disease and giving the false appearance of a mass lesion on CT scan. His medical course has been consistent with this diagnosis since that time. The ultrasound is illustrated in Fig. 9.

Case 10 is that of a 34-year-old patient who was 2-months pregnant and had noticed a sudden decrease of vision in her right eye. Her ophthalmologist had made the diagnosis of optic neuritis but had hesitated to put her on prednisone because of her pregnancy. Also, radiological studies had not been obtained for the same reason. Standardized echography was performed in the office and revealed typical nerve involvement of an meningioma of the optic nerve. She was referred to a neurosurgeon for follow-up care during her pregnancy. The ultrasound is illustrated in Fig. 10.

These cases represent only a small portion of the wide spectrum of orbital pathology that can be accurately diagnosed by standardized echography. (Ossoinig, 1979)

References

Henderson JW. 1980. Orbital Tumors, Brian C. Decker, a Divion of Thieme-Stratton, Inc., New York, pp. 68–70.

Ossoinig KC. Winter 1979. Standardized Echography; Basic Principles, Clininal Applications, and Results. Intl. Ophthalmol. Clin.; 19(4): 127–133.

The accuracy of ultrasonic and other methods in orbital diagnosis demonstrated on selected pathological cases

H.G. LÜNEBORG and H.G. TRIER
Bonn, FRG

In this presentation we will try to demonstrate the value of different diagnostic methods used in orbital diseases. The cases were selected from patients of the Bonn University Eye Clinic. The sonographic examinations were performed with Kretz 7200 MA A-scan, Cooper Vision Ultrascan 404 B-scan, and Delalande directional continuous-wave Doppler. Other methods included conventional X-rays, computerized tomography, and carotid angiography. The examination by A- and B-scan was performed first. The orbital diseases were divided into four groups:

1. tumors of the optic nerve;
2. mass lesions of the orbit, without tumors of the optic nerve and vascular anomalies;
3. vascular anomalies of the orbit;
4. extraocular muscle disease.

Due to the limited amount of time, only the first three groups will be discussed. Cases representative for each group will be demonstrated.

Group 1. The first case of this group was a 45-year-old male patient who presented with a loss of vision of the left eye over a period of 8 months. Other findings were: visual field loss with only a temporal field remaining, papilledema, and congestion of retinal veins.

The standard B-scan examination was supplemented by a special scanning plane to display the optic nerve (Fig. 1). We define this scanning plane as 'DOT', where D stands for diameter, O for oblique scanning plane, and T for temporal gaze. With a sector scanner of 45 to 60°, a simultaneous display of the optic nerve and extraocular muscles (M. superior rectus, superior oblique, and medial rectus) is achieved. The B-scan showed a widening of the optic sheath with no internal echoes (Fig. 2). Moving towards the centre of the nerve, a loud echo representing the border between the optic sheath and the actual nerve fibres could be recognized. Moving further towards the centre, there was an echo which probably came from the optic nerve vessels. The echofree

K.C. Ossoinig (editor), Ophthalmic Echography, ISBN 978-94-010-7988-4
© 1987, Martinus Nijhoff/Dr W. Junk Publishers, Dordrecht.

454

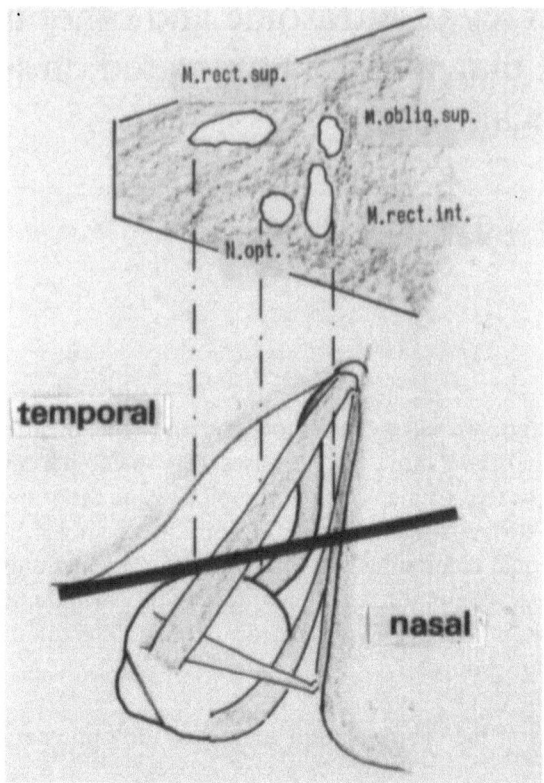

Fig. 1. Illustration of DOT sector scan plane for display of optic nerve and muscle cross-section.

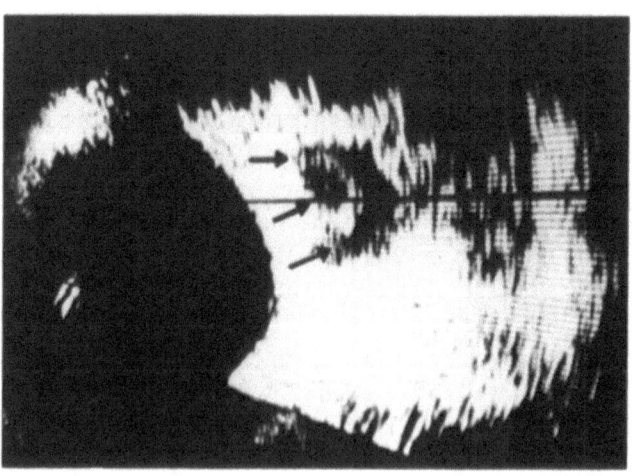

Fig. 2. B-mode echogram in DOT scan plane showing fluid distension of optic nerve sheaths and echo compatible with optic nerve central vessel (case 1).

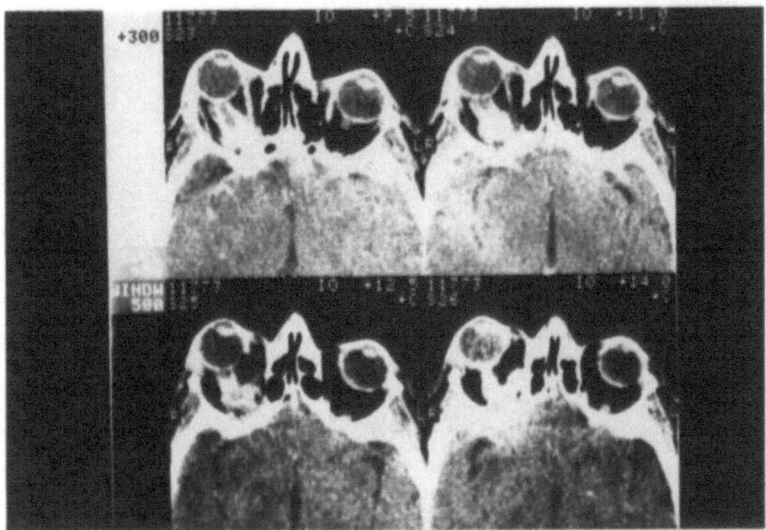

Fig. 3. X-ray computer tomography of case 1 showing on OD enlargement of optic nerve sheath (anterior part) and solid tumor of the optic nerve (posterior part) in a case of optic nerve sheath meningioma (Courtesy of Dr. Greeven, Elisabeth-Krankenhaus Neuwied).

zone was interpreted not as being the actual tumor, but as an increased amount of subarachnoid fluid caused by the tumor. The computerized tomography (CT) (Fig. 3) showed an enlargement of the optic sheath on its course through the orbit. Histopathology of the resected optic nerve tumor verified the diagnosis of an optic nerve sheath meningioma.

The second case was a 48-year-old female patient with proptosis of the right eye for three years, and a slight blurring of the optic disk margin (Fig. 4). As in

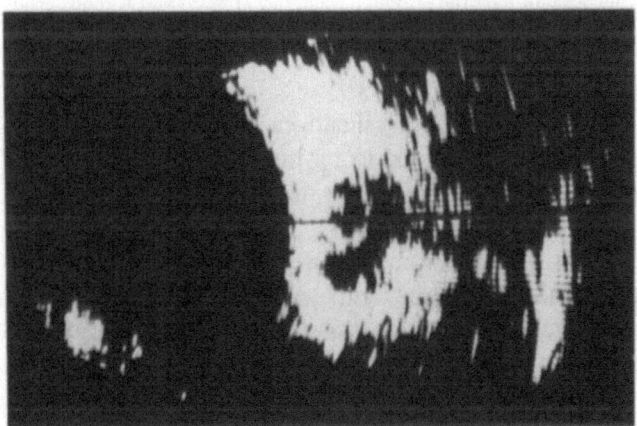

Fig. 4. B-mode echogram (case 2) in DOT scan plane showing the same findings as Fi. 2.

456

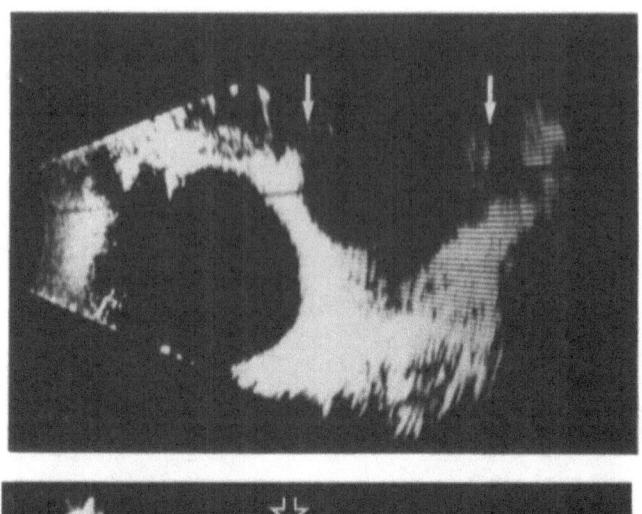

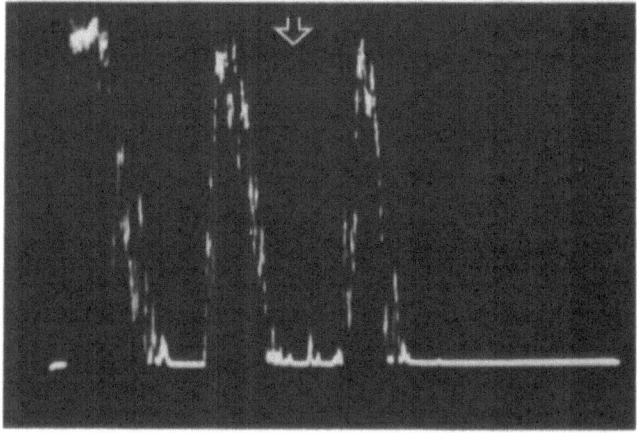

Figs. 5 and 6. Mucocele of the orbit, B-mode echogram (Fig. 5) and A-mode echogram (80 dB amplification) (Fig. 6).

the latter case, the congested optic sheath can be differentiated from the optic nerve fibres. What we presumed to be the optic nerve vessels can also be noted. CT revealed a large optic nerve tumor.

Group 2. A 45-year-old male patient presented with a downward displacement, proptosis, and ptosis of the right eye. At maximal sensitivity, the B-scan showed a round, well-defined mass lesion (Fig. 5). The superior rectus muscle was displaced downwards. Figure 6 gives the A-scan display of the lesion at 80 dB. Conventional X-rays showed a destruction of the superior-lateral orbital rim. CT revealed a mass lesion in the lateral orbit with destruction of the orbital roof. Histologically, this lesion proved to be a mucocele.

Table 1 (a and b) gives a survey of the patients of group 2, and the examinations performed, table 2 the combination of techniques and their value in detecting and characterizing a lesion. p is defined as the probability of correct diagnosis and is calculated by 1/n, wherein n is the number of equally probable diagnosis.

In all cases, the lesion was detected by A- and B-scan. Using ultrasonography only had a 37% probability, whereas combined ultrasonography and CT showed 100% probability.

Table 1a. Mass lesions of the orbit without optic tumors and vascular anomalies.

Pat.	Sex	Age	Symptoms	
B.K.	f	79	downward displacement, protrusion	OD
R.J.	m	75	swelling of parotid gland, protrusion	OD
K.K.	f	58	palpable tumor on lower nasal orbital rim, ptosis	OD
P.K.	f	56	upward displacement, protrusion	OS
T.A.	m	65	swelling of upper lid, ptosis	OD
P.O.	m	45	downward displacement, protrusion, ptosis	OD
P.P.	m	3	amaurosis	OD
			amaurosis	OS
S.D.	f	10	palpable tumor on nasal orbital rim	OS
K.L.	f	35	pain, protrusion, blurring of disk margin, retinal folds	OS

Table 1b. Clinical evaluation methods.

Pat.	Ultrasound (A+B)	CT	Con- vent. X-ray	Biopsy	Diagnosis (a: histolog., b: clinical)
B.K.	+	+	+	−	b sphenoid meningioma with penetration into the orbit
R.J.	+	+	+	+	a epipharynx carcinoma with penetration into the orbit
K.K.	+	−	+	+	a lymphoma
P.E.	+	+	−	+	a meningioma
T.A.	+	+	−	−	b lymphoma
P.O.	+	+	−	−	a mucocele
P.P.	+	+	−	−	a meningo-encephalocele
S.D.	+	−	+	−	b dermoid cyst or mucocele
K.L.	+	−	+	−	a granulomatous fibrinous inflammation
n =	9	6	5	3	

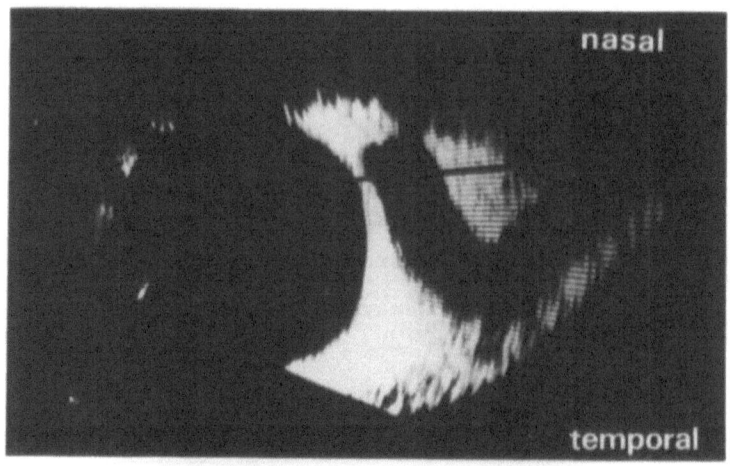

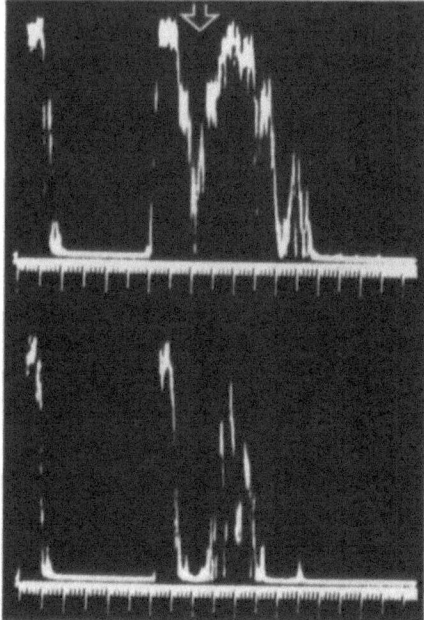

Figs. 7 and 8. Congestion of superior orbital vein. B-mode echogram (horizontal plane), A-mode echogram at different amplifications.

Table 2. Combination of examination techniques and their diagnostic value.

	n	Detection of lesion	Differentiation of lesion (p)
Ultrasound (A+B)	11	11	0.37
Ultrasound + orbit CT	6	6	1.0
Ultrasound + X-ray	3	3	0.37
Ultrasound + X-ray + orbit CT	2	2	1.0

Group 3. A 22-year-old male patient with previous brain trauma suffered of a VIth nerve palsy and proptosis (6 mm) of the right eye. Episcleral and retinal veins were congested. B-scan examination revealed a tube-shaped echofree space with a constant diameter of about 5 mm, which could hardly be compressed (Fig. 7). Enlarged ocular muscles, especially the superior rectus, can be seen. The tube-shaped echo courses from the superior anterior nasal part of the orbit towards temporal posterior. This course corresponds anatomically to the superior orbital vein.

Figure 8 demonstrates that the blurring of internal echo spikes can clearly be seen. During Doppler examination a 'machine murmur' was heard. CT of the orbit indicated an orbital fracture, CT of the brain proved normal. Seldinger's angiography showed carotid cavernosus fistula with congestion of the superior orbital vein.

Tables 3 (a and b) summarize the patients of group 3, and the examinations performed. Table 4 gives the techniques used in detecting and characterizing the vascular anomalies. The use of A- and B-scan only achieved a probability of 44%, whereas combined A-, B-, and Doppler sonography gave a 77% probability.

Table 3a. Vascular anomalies of the orbit.

Pat.	Sex	Age	Symptoms	
K.H.	f	80	protrusion, impaired motility of all muscles	OD
H.D.	m	1	swelling of the upper and lower lid, hypotropia	OS
K.D.	f	1	protrusion	OD
E.F.	m	25	protrusion, impaired motility of all muscles, hypotropia	OD
D.B.	f	37	pain on motility	OD
S.P.	m	22	protrusion, VI nerve palsy, veins congested	OD

Table 3b. Clinical evaluation methods.

Pat.	Ultrasound (A+B)	Doppler	CT	Angiography	Convent. X-ray	Diagnosis
K.H.	+	+	+	+	−	carotid cavernosus fistula
H.D.	+	+	−	−	+	hemangioma
K.D.	+	+	−	−	−	hemangioma
E.F.	+	+	+	+	+	dura angioma
D.B.	+	−	+	−	−	varicosis or venous anomalies
S.P.	+	+	+	+	−	carotid cavernosus fistula
n =	6	5	4	3	2	

Table 4. Combination of examination techniques and their diagnostic value.

	n	Detection of lesion	Differentiation of lesion (p)
Ultrasound (A+B)	6	6	0.44
Ultrasound (A+B) + Doppler	5	5	0.77
Ultrasound (A+B) + orbit CT	1	1	0.50
Ultrasound (A+B) + Doppler + angiography	3	3	1.0

In conclusion, we believe the method of choice in diagnosing orbital mass lesions to be a combination of A- and B-scan ultrasonography with CT. As found by BIGAR et al., sufficient diagnostic accuracy in the anterior third of the orbit is obtained by A- and B-scan only. In the middle third, ultrasound and CT are of equivalent accuracy. In the posterior third, CT gives the better results. NOVER et al. prefer CT to other methods, if diagnosing flat tumors.

CT offers the surgeon a better understanding of the exact anatomical relationships, as described by CHAR and NORMAN. We believe that a combination of ultrasound and CT is helpful in minimizing the number of biopsies, and that it enables the surgeon to perform these with greater precision. In AV-fistula angiography is indispensable for diagnosis and surgery.

According to BIGAR et al. cavernous hemangioma cannot be evaluated by means of angiography. Table 5 shows a proposal for non-invasive examination techniques in orbital disease, which developed from our studies and from

Table 5. Proposal for non-invasive diagnostic evaluation of the orbit.

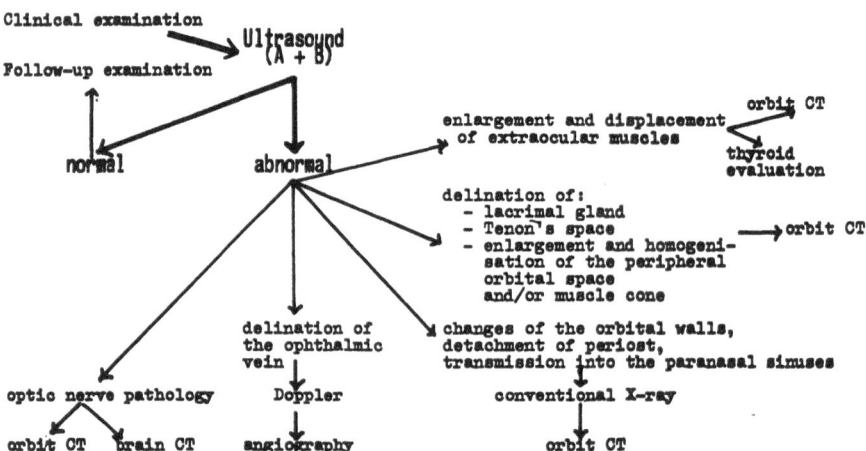

studies of other authors, especially GUTHOFF. Our clinical experience reveals that A-scan, B-scan, and Doppler ultrasonography play a central role in the diagnosis of orbital disease, which corresponds to the findings of other authors (OSSOINIG 1979).

References

Bigar F, Spiess H, Gruber HU 1979. Kombinierte Anwendung der Computer-Tomoraphie und Echographie in der Ophthalmologie. Klin. Mbl. Augenheilk. 174: 806–815.

Char DH and Norman D. 1982. The use of computed tomography and ultrasonography in the evaluation of orbital masses. Survey Ophthal. 27: 49–63.

Guthoff R. 1983.Der Beitrag der Kontakt-B-Bild-Echographie für die Differenzierung einer oritalen Raumforderung. Skriptum 7. Fortbildungskurs 'Ophthalmologische Ultraschalldiagnostik', Bonn, 3. 8.10.1983.

Nover A, Rochels R, Queckenstedt N und Wende S. 1982. Vergleich echographischer, computertomographischer und histologischer Befunde bei Orbitatumoren. Fortschr. Ophthalmol. 79: 22–24.

Ossoinig KC. 1979. Standardized echography: Basic principles, clinical applications, and results. In: Ophthalmic Ultrasonography. Comparative techniques. R.L. Dallow, ed., Intern. Ophthal. Clinics 19: 127–210.

Ultrasound diagnoses of orbital masses and intraocular tumors

HAROLD W. SKALKA

Birmingham, Al., USA

We have reviewed our recent experience with orbital mass lesions and intra-ocular tumors referred for ultrasound examination. All patients were evaluated by the same examiner, and many had more than one ultrasound examination – for example, serial measurements to evaluate tumor growth or response to therapy. Most examinations were performed utilizing Kretz-technik 7200 MA A-scan and Bronson-Turner B-scan units. Twenty-six ultrasound diagnoses are included in this compilation of 787 patients.

Excluded from this tabulation are orbital entities such as cellulitis, edema, hemorrhage, and orbital foreign bodies. Intraocular exclusions include foreign bodies, scleritis, hemorrhage, nevi, retinal cysts, choroidal osteoma, choroidal detachment, chorioretinal scars, fibrous vitreous lesions, Coats' disease, sub-retinal or choroidal hemorrhages, etc.

The vast majority of the ultrasound diagnoses were confirmed by histo-pathology or clinical course. In several cases, the initial ultrasound diagnosis was determined to be incorrect; and in these instances, the final diagnosis was used in the tabulation.

As may be seen in Table 1, orbital masses accounted for 77.6% of the cases studied, with ocular tumors representing less than a quarter of the total cases (Table 2).

Twenty-one orbital diagnoses are included in this tabulation, of which the most common by far is endocrine orbitopathy, accounting for 31.1% of the total cases, and 40.1% of the orbital cases. The other common orbital diagnosis was the pseudotumor/lymphoma/sarcoma group of orbital masses, representing 13.1% of all cases and 16.9% of orbital cases. All other orbital diagnoses were significantly less common.

Ocular malignant melanoma represented 15.4% of all cases, but 68.8% of the ocular tumors (Table 2).

Together, metastatic carcinomas of the orbit and eye accounted for 72 patients – 38 orbital and 34 intraocular; representing 9.1% of all referred cases. There were 23 periorbital malignancies invading the orbit, and therefore

K.C. Ossoinig (editor), Ophthalmic Echography, ISBN 978-94-010-7988-4

Table 1. Orbital masses.

Diagnosis	#	%
Endocrine orbitopathy	245	31.1
Pseudotumor/lymphoma/sarcoma	103	13.1
Carcinoma of orbit	38	4.8
Dermoid cyst	29	3.7
Cavernous hemangioma/lymphangioma	28	3.6
Abscess	25	3.2
Mucocoele	23	2.9
Periorbital malignancy	23	2.9
Serous cyst	19	2.4
Lacrimal gland tumor	14	1.8
Supraorbital meningioma	12	1.5
A-V fistula	10	1.3
Meningioma of optic nerve	9	1.1
Glioma of optic nerve	8	1.0
Neurofibroma	8	1.0
Varix	5	0.6
Encephalocoele	4	0.5
Neurilemmoma	4	0.5
Fibroma	2	0.3
Fibrous dysplasia	1	0.1
Amyloidosis	1	0.1

secondary orbital (or ocular) invasion by malignant disease accounted for 12.1% of the total series (95 cases).

The relative frequencies of the diagnoses encountered likely reflect some bias due to referral factors (we provide tertiary, as well as primary eye care and surgery), in addition to the personal interests of the examiner (e.g. endocrine orbitopathy). Nonetheless, they probably represent a fair reflection of true regional disease incidence; at least of those entities where physicians feel ultrasound evaluation to be helpful.

Table 2. Ocular tumors.

Diagnosis	#	%
Malignant melanoma	121	15.4
Metastatic carcinoma	34	4.3
Retinoblastoma	12	1.5
Choroidal hemangioma	8	1.0
Tumor of RPE	1	0.1

Orbital dermoid cysts

S.F. BYRNE and J.R. HUGHES
Miami, USA

Abstract

Because of their diverse contents, orbital dermoid cysts may produce vastly different echograms which may make differentiation from other orbital lesions challenging. [3, 4] This paper addresses six cases of orbital dermoid cyst where standardized echography [5] was performed preoperatively.

Echographic findings (photographic and written documentation) were retrospectively analyzed and compiled with emphasis on the special examination techniques developed by Ossoinig (e.g. quantitative, topographic and kinetic echography). [1, 2] Acoustic similarities and dissimilarities between the six lesions were stressed in an attempt to provide better detailed criteria for improved differentiation.

Introduction

Standardized echography was performed on six patients just prior to surgical removal of their dermoid cysts. The Kretztechnik 7200 MA, a contact real-time B-scan and a Doppler instrument were utilized.

The six patients had a fairly routine clinical course with a history of slowly progressive, painless proptosis with globe displacement but without visual disturbance or diplopia (Fig. 1). The duration of symptoms spanned six months to thirty years. Four were males and two were females, ranging from age eight to forty-two. In the eight year old, signs of symptoms of the lesion only emerged after trauma to the orbit six months previously.

This work has been supported in part by the Florida Lions Eye Bank.

K.C. Ossoinig (editor), Ophthalmic Echography, ISBN 0-89838-873-2.

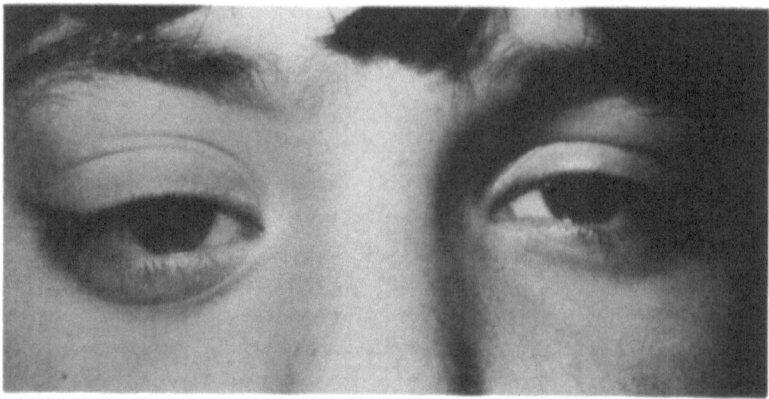

Fig. 1. Typical young patient with superotemporal orbital dermoid cyst where globe is proptosed and displaced inferiorly.

Echographic findings

Location

Five of the six lesions were located in the superotemporal quadrant of the orbit. The surrounding bony wall was found to be abnormal at surgery in all five of the superotemporal lesions. Three of these were primarily in the lacrimal gland region, whereas two were mainly retrobulbar.

One of the three lacrimal gland lesions caused marked reformation of the surrounding bony wall but there was no dehiscence (Fig. 2). In the other two lacrimal gland lesions, a small bony defect and slight extension into the fossa temporalis was discovered at surgery which had not been detected with either standardized echography or CT scan (Fig. 3).

Each of the two retrobulbar dermoids extruded into the fossa temporalis through a larger bony defect; this extension was detected preoperatively by both CT scan and echography (Fig. 4). The only case in which the adjacent bony wall was found to be normal at surgery was in the eight year old boy with the superonasal lesion.

Shape, borders, sound attenuation

All of the dermoids were oval shaped, measuring more in depth than in width. Three of the lesions were well outlined with a distinct, double-peaked posterior border spike ranging in height from 40% to 90% of display height.

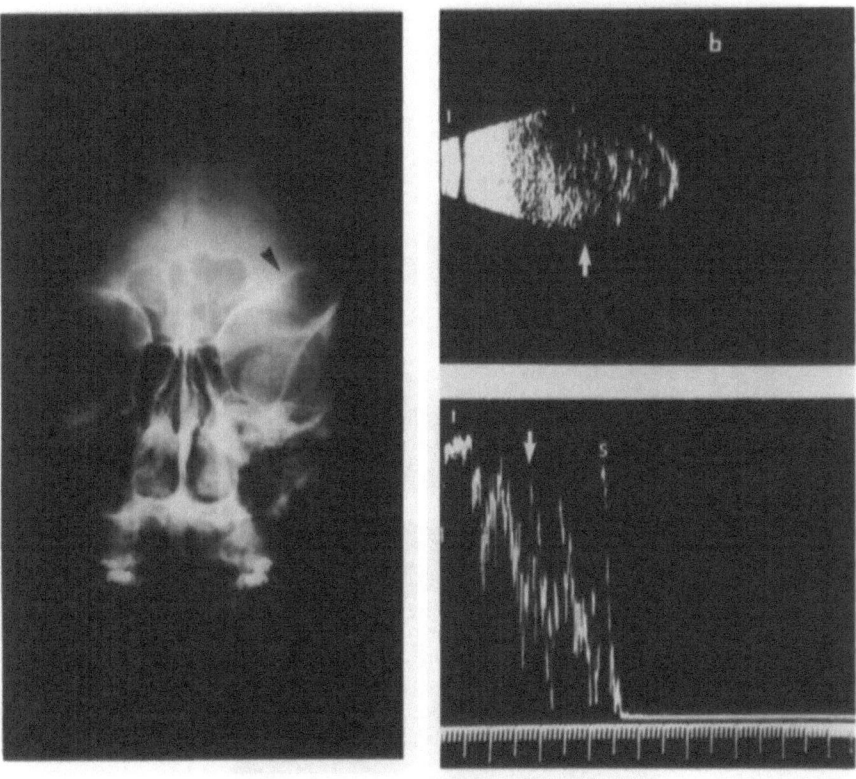

Fig. 2a. Plane x-ray shows marked reformation of bone surrounding lesion (arrows).

Fig. 2b. Paraocular B-scan (top) and A-scan (bottom). Bone reformation was suspected echographically since this extensive lesion was best displayed with the probes directed toward the adjacent bony roof rather than toward the orbital apex. I = initial probe signal, Arrows = lesion contents, S = posterior border spike.

A judgement of the degree of angle kappa* was made in each case, although this was more difficult in the irregularly structured lesions. It was interesting that the angle kappa was medium or high in the two lesions with posterior border spike height of 60% and 40% respectively (Fig. 5), whereas it was low to medium in the third lesion with a 90% high posterior border spike and low or variable in the other three lesions with a 100% tall, steeply rising, thick double-peaked posterior border spike (Fig. 6). These findings suggest a correlation between the degree of sound attenuation and height of the posterior

---

* Angle Kappa, produced by sound attenuation, is the angle formed by an imaginary line drawn through the peaks of the lesion spikes and the baseline.

468

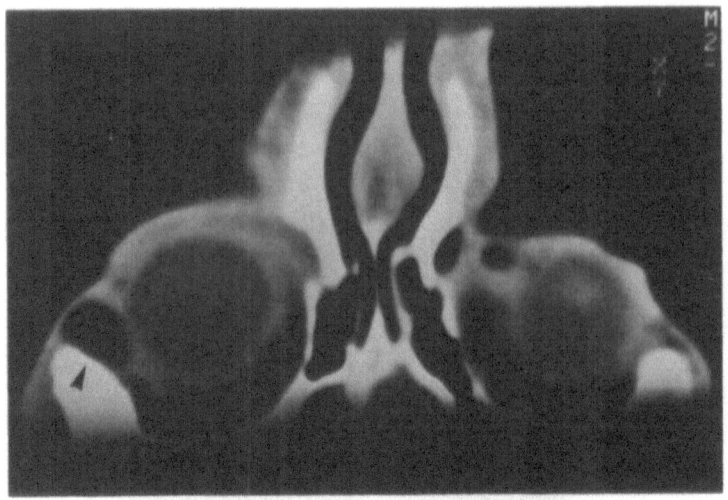

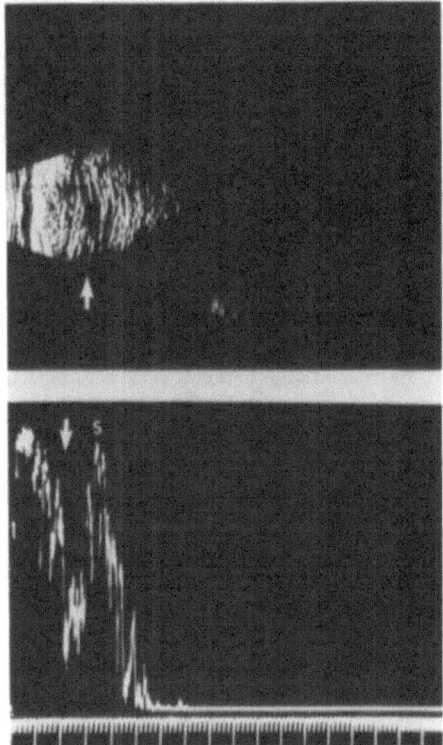

Fig. 3a. Coronal CT-scan shows small mass in lacrimal gland region (arrow).

Fig. 3b. Paraocular B- and A-scans of same anterior dermoid. Arrows = lesion contents, S = posterior border spike.

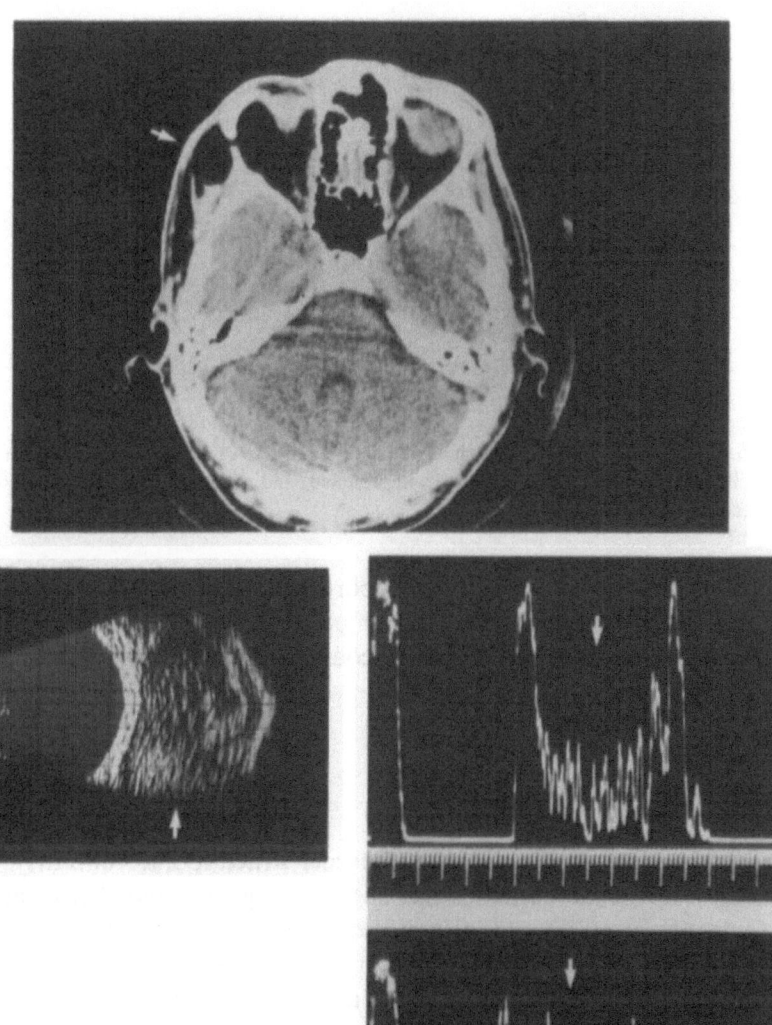

Fig. 4a. Axial CT-scan shows dumb-bell shaped dermoid in temporal orbit extending through bony defect into temporal fossa (arrow).

Fig. 4b. Transocular B- and A-scans of lesion (closed arrows). The A-scan echograms, taken in different sound beam directions, show irregular structure. Center, A-scan shows low reflectivity. Bottom, another sound beam direction shows variable reflectivity (open arrows).

470

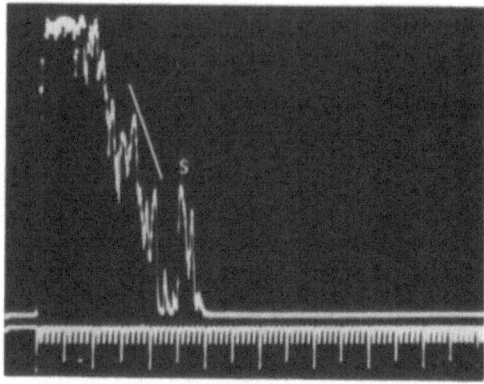

Fig. 5. Paraocular A-scan shows high angle kappa indicative of strong sound attenuation (indicated by oblique line and angle formed with baseline) and only 40% high, distinct of posterior border spike (S).

border spike (Table 1). While most reports in the literature have stated that a cystic mass invariably has a 100% high posterior border spike [6], this study shows that sound attenuation may account for lower height of the posterior border spike.

Internal structure and reflectivity

Careful analysis was made of the internal structure and reflectivty of the lesions. Two of the dermoids had slightly irregular internal structure (i.e. reflectivity was uniform in most directions but varied slightly in one or two areas). One of these two lesions was mainly high reflective and the other was mainly low reflective. Figure 7 shows a large retrobular dermoid cyst which was mainly high reflective with only one or two areas of low reflectivity. In

Table 1. Angle kappa and posterior border spike height*

Case	Angle kappa	Spike height of posterior border
1	Strong	40%
2	Medium	60%
3	Low-Medium	90%
4	Low/Variable	100%
5	Variable	100%
6	Variable	100%

* Determined with standardized A-scan instrumentation.

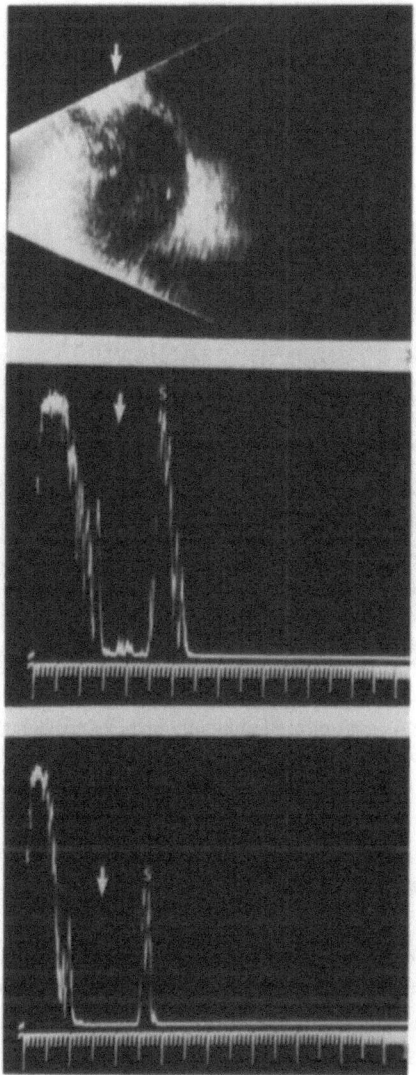

Fig. 6. Paraocular B- and A-scans of dermoid (arrows) with sharp outline. Posterior border spike (S) is steeply rising, 100% tall at tissue sensitivity (center) with thick double peak better shown at low sensitivity (bottom).

contrast, the superonasal lesion was predominantly low reflective but a few medium high internal spikes were found in one area (Fig. 8). Four of the lesions had irregular internal structure where reflectivity was too erratic to be classified as primarily high or low (Fig. 4b). Such irregularity was undoubtedly due to the lesion's variable contents as well as to the bony defects.

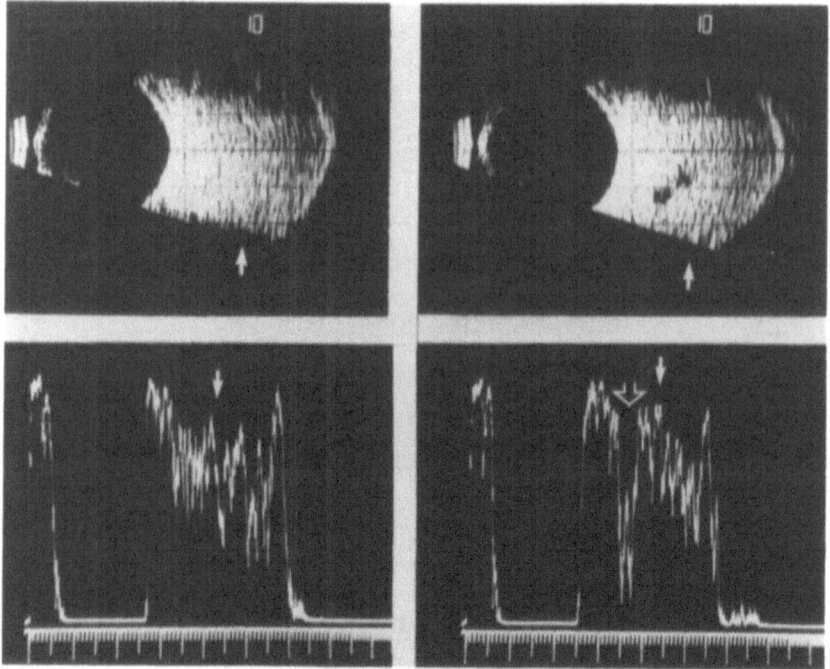

Fig. 7. Transocular B- and A-scans of predominantly high reflective dermoid (closed arrows). Montage on right shows low reflective area (open arrow).

Vascularity, compressibility, mobility

Kinetic echography indicated no vascularity with either A-scan or Doppler. On compression testing, three of the lesions were firm or slightly deformable, while three were hard with no deformability and none were soft. None of the lesions were significantly mobile.

Pathology

Histopathology of the six lesions indicated their cavities to be filled with various substances ranging from hair shafts, follicles, glands, inflammatory cells and red blood cells to fat, keratin and caseous material. No direct correlation between contents of the individual masses and their reflectivity could be made retrospectively. In all cases, the cyst wall was comprised of keratinized squamous epithelium (Fig. 9).

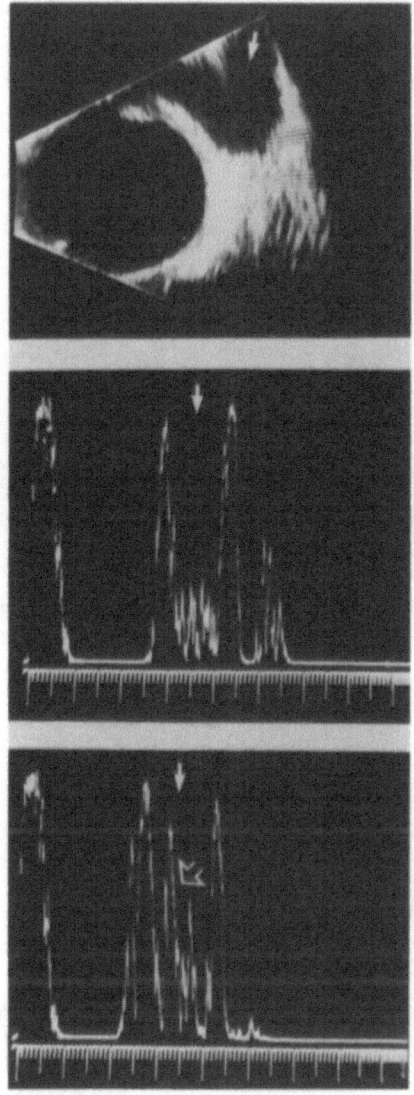

Fig. 8. Transocular B- and A-scans of superonasal dermoid (solid arrows) show predominantly low reflectivity (center) but one area with medium high spikes (open arrow) (bottom).

Conclusion

Table 2 itemizes the acoustic characteristics of dermoid cysts based on standardized echography of these six cases. Dermoid cysts are most frequently located in the superotemporal quadrant of the orbit and are oval shaped. The surrounding bony wall is abnormal, either by reformation or dehiscence (but

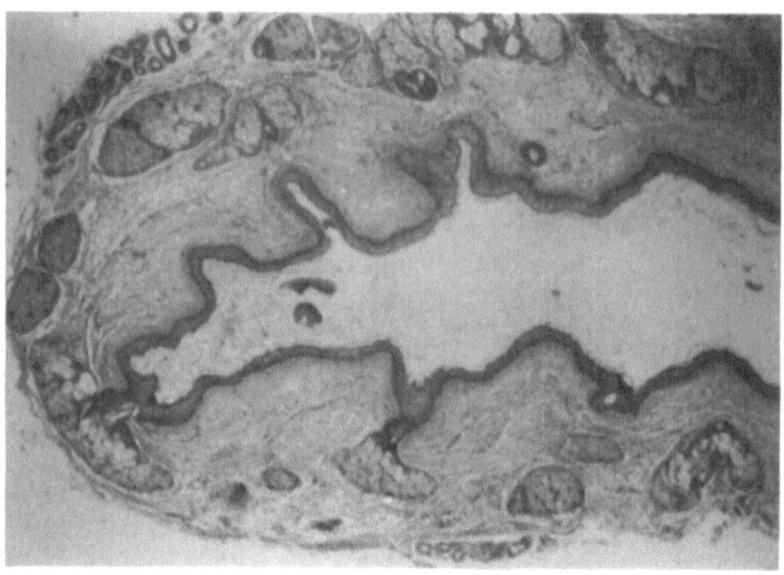

Fig. 9. Histopathology of wall of dermoid show keratinized, squamous epithelium. This was found in all six lesions.

Table 2. Acoustic criteria for dermoid cysts.*

Topographic

1. Location:	superotemporal orbit (B, A**)
2. Shape:	oval (B, A)
3. Borders:	well or sharply outlined (A)
4. Bone:	erosion (dehiscence or reformation) (A, B)

Quantitative

5. Structure:	variable (A, B)
6. Reflectivity:	variable (A)
7. Angle Kappa:	variable (A)

Kinetic

8. Vascularity:	none (A, D)
9. Compressibility:	firm to hard (A)
10. Mobility:	none (A)

---

* Based on instrumentation and techniques of standardized echography. Criteria based on six cases of orbital dermoid cyst.
** A: Standardized A-scan; B: Contact, Real-time B-scan; D: Doppler.

small bony erosion may be difficult to detect). When a bony defect is present, the lesion communicates with the fossa temporalis. These cystic lesions are well outlined with medium to strong angle kappa or are sharply outlined with low angle kappa. They have varying degrees of irregular internal structure but are predominantly high reflective. They are completely avascular as opposed to many solid, encapsulated tumors which contain some degree of vascularity. On compression testing the lesions are firm to hard in consistency.

Acknowledgement

The authors are grateful to Michele Comella for typing this manuscript and for editorial assistance. Additional thanks are extended to the other Echography personnel: Eileen K. Novinski and Maria L. Rivera.

References

1. Byrne SF. 1979. Standardized echography. Part I: A-scan examination procedures. Int Ophthalmol Clin; 19(4): 267–81.
2. Byrne SF, Glaser JS. 1983. Orbital tissue differentiation with standardized echography. Ophthalmology; 90(9): 1071–1090.
3. Ossoinig KC. 1973. A-scan echography and orbital disease. In: Proceedings of the 2nd International Symposium on Orbital Disorders, Amsterdam (Karger, Basel 1975): 224.
4. Ossoinig KC. 1978. The role of clinical echography in modern diagnosis of periorbital and orbital lesions. In: Proceedings of the 3rd International Symposium on Orbital Disorders, Amsterdam, September 5-6, 1977. The Hague: Junk: 517.
5. Ossoinig KC. 1979. Standardized echography: basic principles, clinical applications and results. Int. Ophthalmol Clin; 19(4): 127–210.
6. Ossoinig KC. 1978. The role of clinical echography in modern diagnosis of periorbital and orbital lesions. In: Proceedings of the 3rd International Symposium on Orbital Disorders, Amsterdam, September 5-7, 1977. The Hague: Junk: 510.

Orbital malignant melanoma with ipsilateral intraocular pathology

B.M. KERMAN and M.L. FISHMAN
Los Angeles, USA

Introduction

Involvement of the orbit with malignant melanoma can occur via direct extension of a malignant melanoma of the ipsilateral choroid or ciliary body or metastatic spread from a skin melanoma or contralateral uveal melanoma (Kerman et al. 1984).

In patients harboring known uveal malignant melanoma, the ophthalmic ultrasonographer is often asked to rule out orbital extension of the tumor. However, in patients with known or suspected orbital mass lesions, the sonographer rarely searches for coexisting intraocular pathology. This paper presents three patients demonstrating the combination of low-reflective orbital mass lesions and intraocular pathology in the ipsilateral globe. All cases proved to have malignant melanoma of the orbit.

Case reports

Case 1. A 57-year-old female with Nevus of Ota presented in December, 1977 with an elevated intraocular mass lesion temporal to the optic nerve of the right eye. Ultrasonographic evaluation demonstrated a 4.6 mm thick mass showing low internal reflectivity and no spontaneous spike motion (Fig. 1). There was no evidence for orbital pathology. Repeat evaluation in September, 1978 demonstrated a slight increase in the height of the lesion to 5.4 mm and evidence of infiltration of the orbital pattern adjacent to the optic nerve (Fig. 2). Enucleation was performed, and pathologically the eye showed an epithelioid cell malignant melanoma of the choroid with extraocular extension (Fig. 3).

Case 2. A 54-year-old male presented in February, 1984 with proptosis of the left eye. Two choroidal nevi were noted within the globe. Ultrasound evalua-

K.C. Ossoinig (editor), Ophthalmic Echography, ISBN 978-94-010-7988-4

478

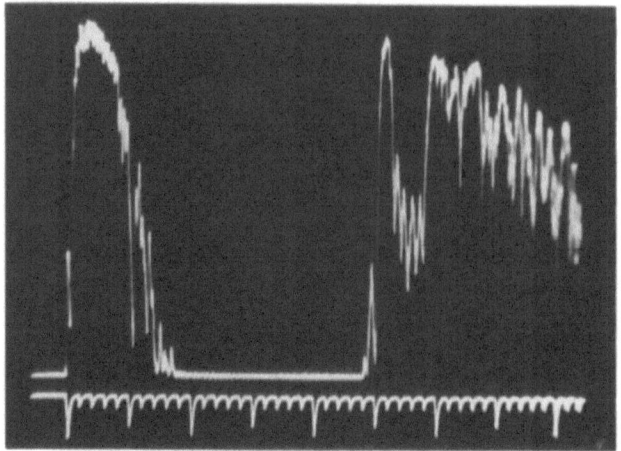

Fig. 1. Case 1: Ocular A-scan ultrasonogram showing mass lesion with low internal reflectivity.

tion showed a large low-reflective orbital mass posterior to the globe. No spontaneous spike motion was present (Fig. 4). Two minimally elevated intraocular lesions were seen, and the B-scan demonstrated communication through the sclera between the orbital tumor and the intraocular pathology (Fig. 5). Biopsy of the orbital mass showed epithelioid cell malignant melanoma. Orbital exenteration was performed and demonstrated flat epithelioid cell malignant melanoma of the choroid with extrascleral extension via the posterior ciliary vessels and nerves.

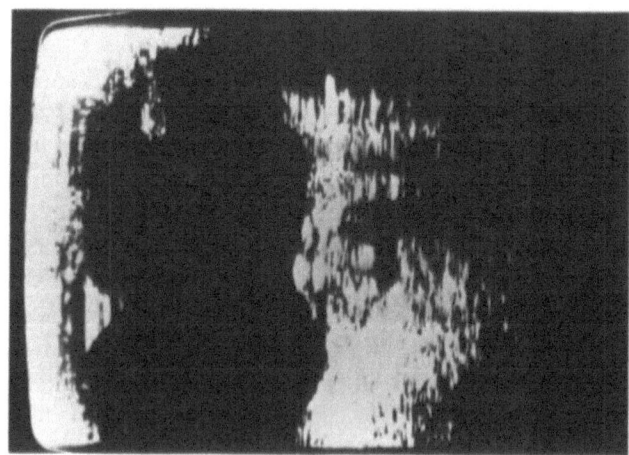

Fig. 2. Case 1: B-scan ultrasonogram showing intraocular mass lesion near optic nerve and orbital infiltration adjacent to optic nerve.

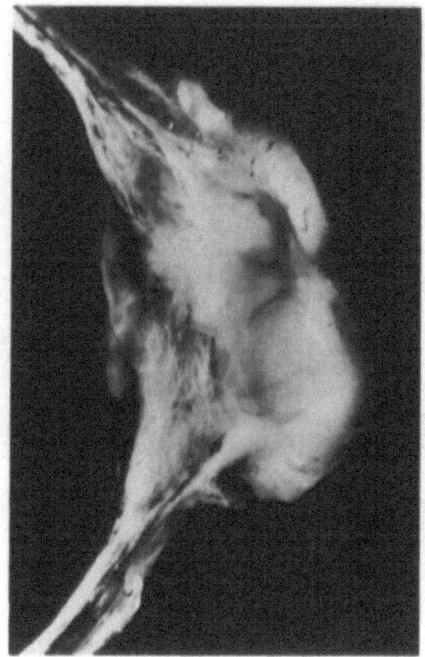

Fig. 3. Case 1: Gross pathological specimen showing intraocular and extraocular portions of tumor.

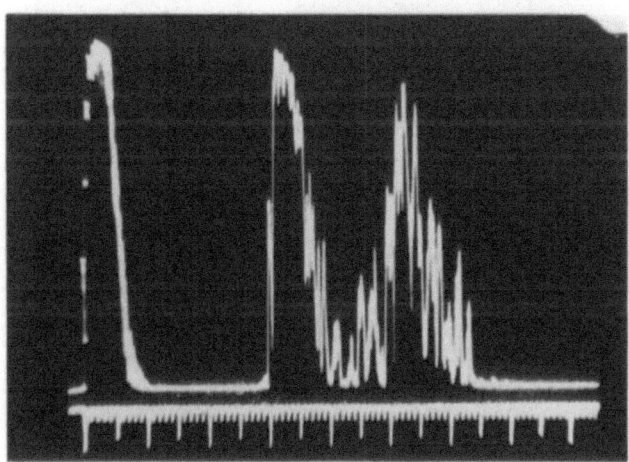

Fig. 4. Case 2: Orbital A-scan ultrasonogram showing large low-reflective orbital mass lesion.

480

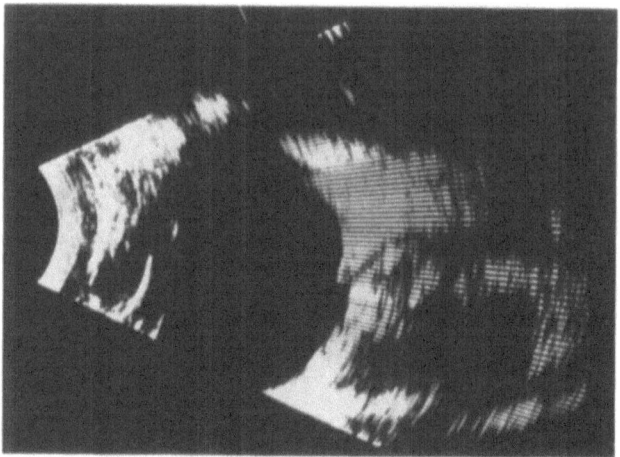

Fig. 5. Case 2: B-scan ultrasonogram showing communication of orbital mass lesion with interior of globe.

Case 3. A 69-year-old male presented in December, 1983 with proptosis of the left eye. Twelve years previously, this eye had sustained a branch retinal vein occlusion with subsequent blindness. Ultrasonographic evaluation demonstrated a low-reflective nasal orbital mass lesion without evidence of spontaneous spike motion (Fig. 6). The ipsilateral globe showed a dislocated lens and organized total retinal detachment (Fig. 7). No intraocular tumor was seen. Biopsy of the orbital mass showed mixed cell malignant melanoma. Aspiration of subretinal fluid demonstrated cells consistent with melanoma

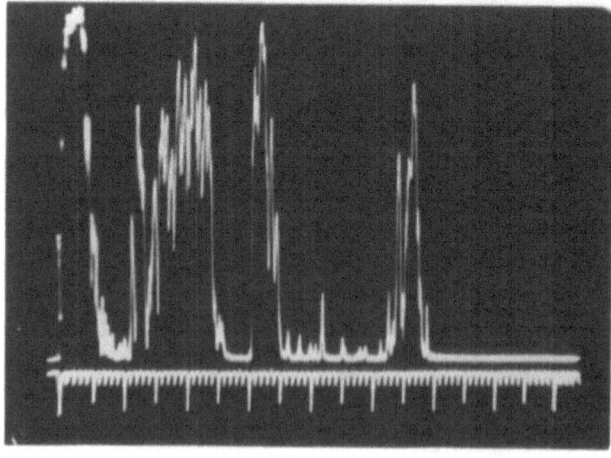

Fig. 6. Case 2: Orbital A-scan ultrasonogram showing high reflective echo source within the globe (retinal detachment) and large low-reflective orbital mass lesion.

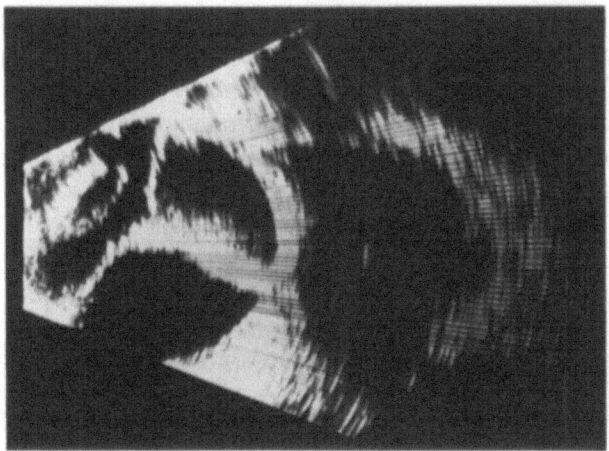

Fig. 7. Case 3: B-scan ultrasonogram showing dislocated lens, organized retinal detachment and large, low-reflective orbital mass.

cells. Orbital exenteration was performed, and the globe contained a flat, heavily pigmented choroidal malignant melanoma continuous with a large spindle cell orbital malignant melanoma.

Discussion

The criteria for differentiation of orbital mass lesions by ultrasound have been well described by previous authors (Coleman, 1972; Coleman et al. 1977; Ossoinig, 1974; Ossoinig, 1983). Many orbital lesions fall into the category of low reflective masses. These lesions include the lymphoma/sarcoma/pseudotumor group, orbital abscess, dermoid cyst, mucocele, arteriovenous fistula, hematoma, capillary hemangioma and malignant melanoma. Within this group of low-reflective lesions, other diagnostic criteria such as location, borders, compressibility and vascularity are helpful in tumor differentiation. In addition to the above features, which relate to the tumor itself, there may be associated pathological conditions which suggest a specific diagnosis. For example, associated orbital inflammatory signs are suggestive that the low reflective mass is an abscess, while the presence of an associated bone defect is highly characteristic of mucocele.

This paper has demonstrated three patients with low reflective orbital mass lesions who had associated intraocular pathology. In one case, the patient was suspected to have an intraocular malignant melanoma; in the second case choroidal nevi were clinically seen; in the third case no intraocular tumor was suspected, but the patient had a total organized retinal detachment and past history of retinal vascular occlusion. All patients proved to have intraocular malignant melanoma with direct transscleral connection to a large orbital melanoma. These findings suggest that the presence of associated intraocular pathology in patients with low-reflective orbital mass lesions be considered strong presumptive evidence that the orbital mass is a malignant melanoma arising from direct spread from an intraocular melanoma.

References

1. Coleman DJ. 1972. Reliability of ocular and orbital diagnosis with B-scan ultrasound: II. Orbital diagnosis. Am. J. Ophthalmol. 74: 704.
2. Coleman DJ, Lizzi FL and Jack RL. 1977. Ultrasonography of the Eye and Orbit. Philadelphia: Lea & Febiger.
3. Kerman BM, Findl ML. 1984. Spectrum of manifestations of metastatic malignant melanoma. Ophthalmic Ultrasonography, Proceedings of the 9th SIDUO Congress. J.S. Hillman and M.H. LeMay (eds). The Hague: Junk: 21.
4. Ossoinig KC. 1974. Preoperative differential diagnosis of tumors with echography: IV. Diagnosis of orbital tumors. Current Concepts in Ophthalmology, Vol 4. F.C. Blodi (ed). St. Louis: Mosby: 313.
5. Ossoinig KC, Trier HG, Sawada A, Till P, Hillman JS, Blackwell WL, Bryan PJ, Byrne SF, Dallow RL, Green RL, Kerman BM, Skalka HW. 1983. SIDUO Round-Table: The role of echography in the diagnosis and management of orbital and periorbital disorders. Ultrasound '82. R.A. Lerski and P. Morley (eds). Oxford: Pergamon: 369.

Differential diagnosis of orbital neurolemmoma (schwannoma) with standardized echography

SANDRA FRAZIER BYRNE[1] and BARRY M. BYRNE[2]

[1] Miami; [2] San Antonio, USA

Abstract

Neurolemmoma (schwannoma) is a rare orbital tumor, comprising less than 2% of all orbital tumors. [3, 4] We report two cases of neurolemmoma where standardized echography [9] was performed just prior to surgical removal. This paper will address the acoustic characteristics of these two neurolemmomas to provide criteria for differentiating these lesions from other orbital tumors.

Introduction

Standardized echography combines specific equipment and examination techniques to reliably detect and differentiate orbital lesions. Essential instrumentation includes the standardized A-scan (Kretztechnik 7200 MA/Sonokretz); contact, real-time B-scan and Doppler instrumentation. Since the late 1960s, Ossoinig has described the acoustic characteristics of most orbital lesions [5–10] but little has been written about neurolemmoma. Therefore, this paper provides echographic criteria for differentiating these tumors from other more common orbital lesions.

Report of cases

Case 1. A forty-one year old white male presented with a one to two year history of painful, progressive proptosis of the right eye. CT-scan demonstrated a large orbital mass (Fig. 1).

This study was supported in part by the Florida Lions Eye Bank and by a research development grant from the Research to Prevent Blindness, Inc., New York.

K.C. Ossoinig (editor), *Ophthalmic Echography*, ISBN 978-94-010-7988-4

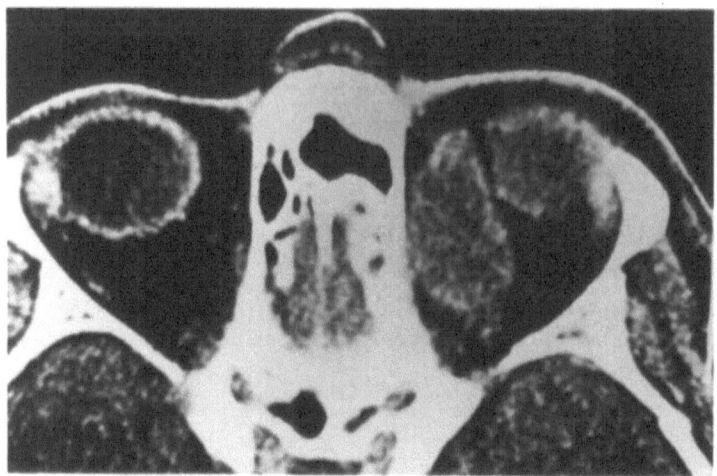

Fig. 1. Axial CT-scan performed with contrast media shows spindle-shaped mass in the superior medial aspect of the right orbit.

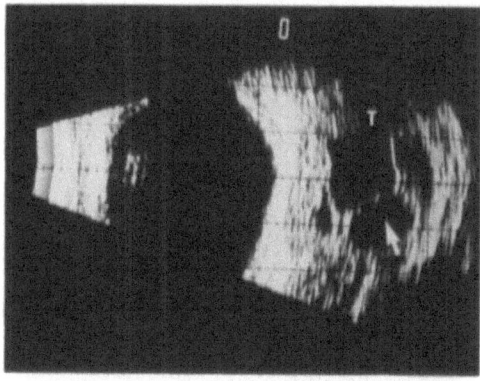

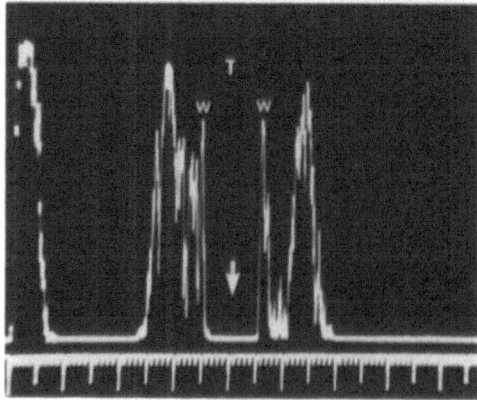

Fig. 2. Transocular B- and A-scans show large tumor (T) with cystic spaces centrally (arrows). Contents of the cystic cavities are extremely low reflective on A-scan (note baseline between steeply rising spikes produced from the smooth cavity walls [W]).

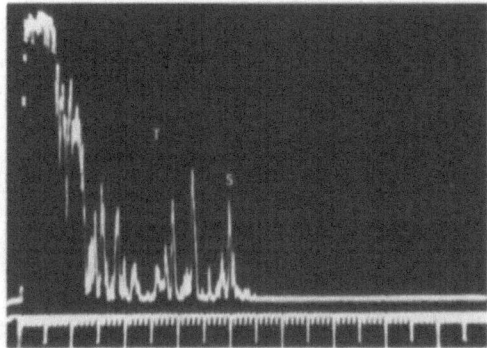

Fig. 3. Paraocular A-scan of tumor (T) shows low angle kappa and low reflectivity with long spikes indicative of coarse internal structure. S = distinct posterior border spike.

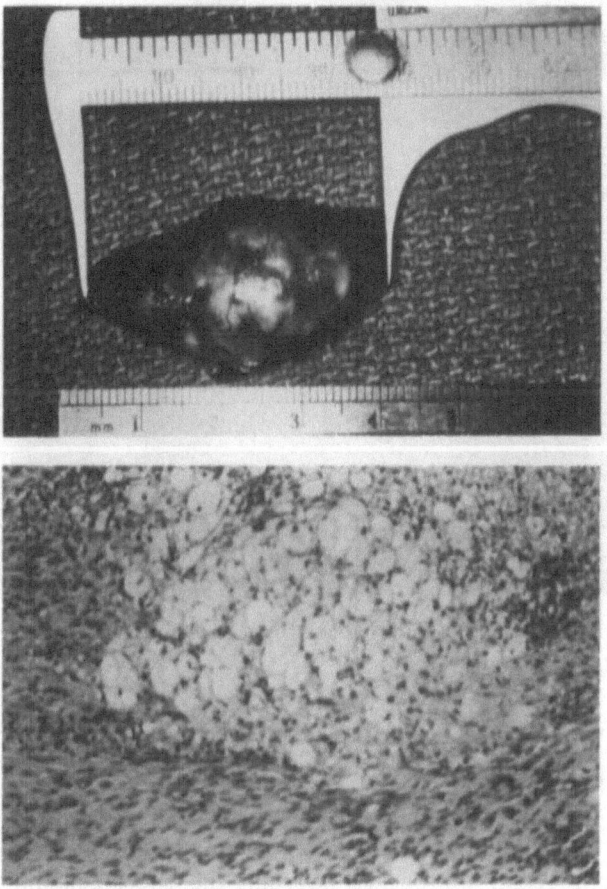

Fig. 4a 4 cm ovoid shaped mass is well encapsulated.

Fig. 4b. Histopathology reveals Schwann cells with palisading of nuclei, loose fibrous tissue and marked infiltration of foamy histiocytes. Chronic inflammatory cells and blood vessels were seen in some areas.

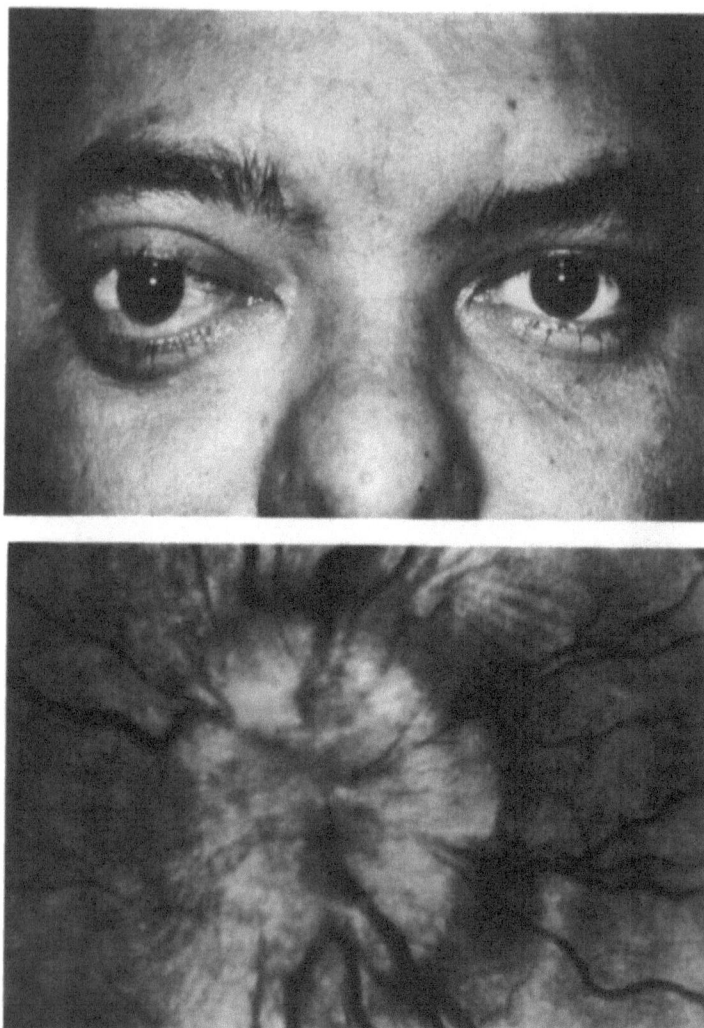

Fig. 5a. Examination revealed 9 mm of proptosis of the right eye. The patient had motility restriction in superior and temporal gaze.

Fig. 5b. Fundus photograph of right eye shows mildly hyperemic and swollen optic disc. Visual acuity pinholed to 20/25–2 in the right eye and 20/15–2 in the left eye. A central scotoma was present on the right.

The lesion was examined with standardized echography using both transocular and paraocular approaches according the 'special examination techniques' developed by Ossoinig. [1, 2] Transocular echograms demonstrated a predominantly low reflective lesion with very large central cystic cavities (Fig. 2). During the dynamic examination, the mass was moderately vascularized on

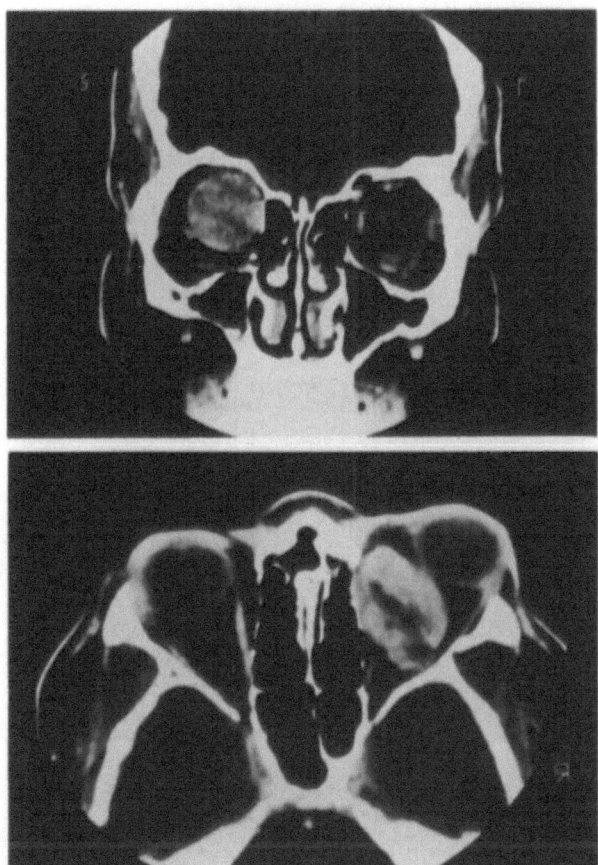

Fig. 6. Coronal (6a) and axial (6b) CT-scans with contrast media indicate a moderately enhancing mass with a central lucency in the axial view. The mass shows slight erosion of the bone into the ethmoidal sinus. The optic nerve was not visualized.

Doppler echography, but no vascularity was noted on standardized A-scan examination. The lesion's consistency was firm to hard and there was questionable mobility within the anterior aspect of the tumor.

Paraocular examination indicated low reflectivity with long spikes indicative of coarse internal structure. A low angle kappa signified minimal sound attenuation and a distinct posterior border spike denoted a well outlined, possibly encapsulated lesion (Fig. 3).

The well encapsulated tumor was excised; neurolemmoma was diagnosed histopathologically (Fig. 4).

Case 2. A thirty-two year old white male complained of progressive proptosis and blurred vision in the right eye of four years duration (Fig. 5a). Fundus

488

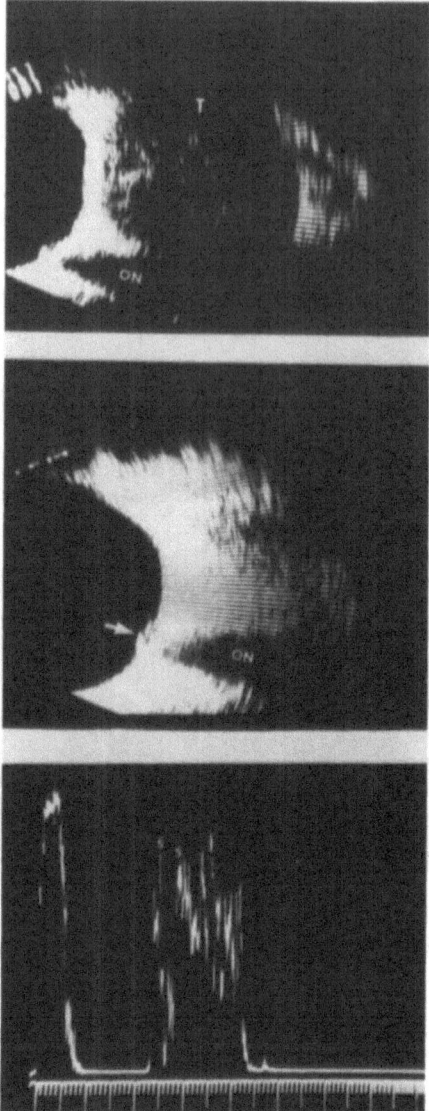

Fig. 7. Top, B-scan shows large tumor mass (T) adjacent to the optic nerve (ON). Center, B-scan through optic nerve next to tumor shows elevation of optic nerve head (arrow) corresponding to disc edema and retrobulbar optic nerve (ON). Bottom, standardized A-scan cross section of optic nerve shows normal width (2.4 mm) between perineural sheath spikes (S).

examination disclosed right optic disc swelling (Fig. 5b). CT-scan showed a well defined right orbital mass which was eroding the medial orbital wall (Fig. 6). Although the optic nerve was not clearly visualized on CT-scan, it could be easily identified in relationship to the tumor echographically (fig. 7).

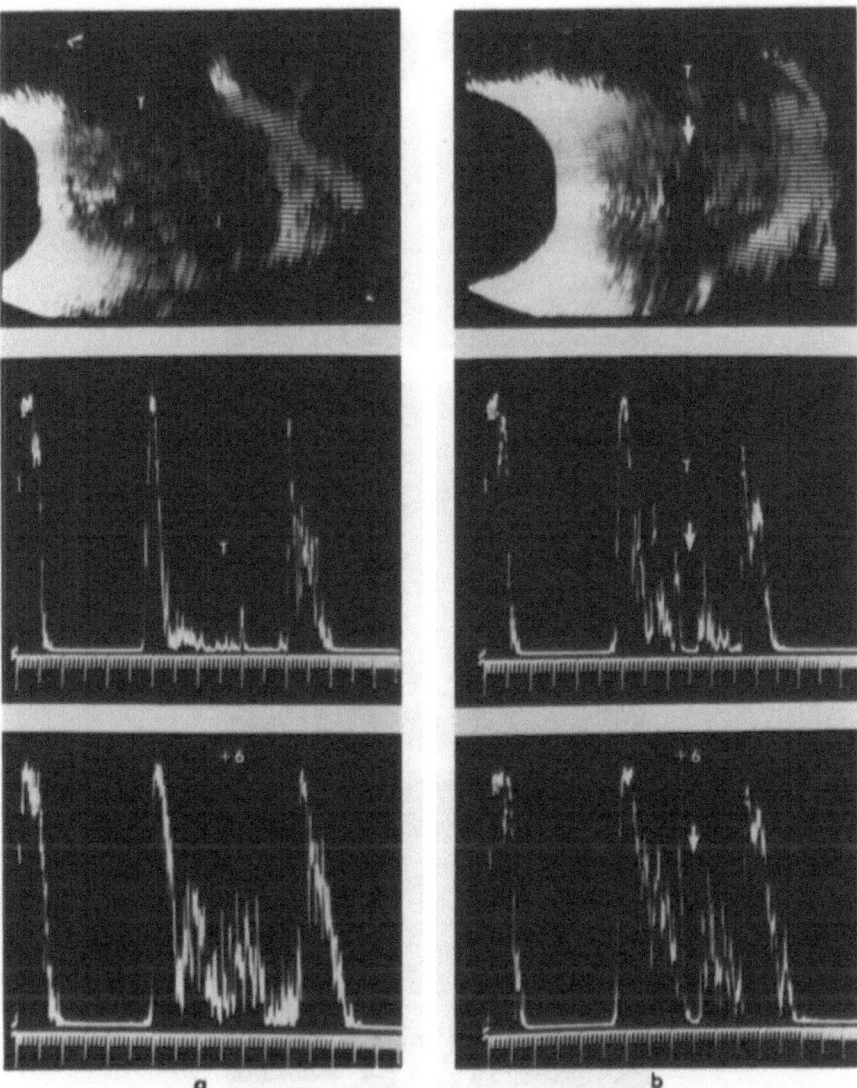

Fig. 8. Transocular B- and A-scans show tumor (T) in area peripheral to cystic degeneration (8a) and through center of cystic degeneration (8b). Arrows = cystic cavity. Notice more homogeneous appearance of center A-scan echogram in 8a as compared to 8b. Bottom, standardized A-scans at tissue sensitivity plus six decibels indicate low to variable angle kappa.

In transocular view, the lesion showed slightly irregular internal structure with predominantly low reflectivity and a large cystic cavity centrally. The angle kappa was judged to be mainly low but was somewhat variable, due in part to the cystic degeneration (Fig. 8). The lesion was diffusely vascularized on A-scan, but Doppler examination was negative. On paraocular examin-

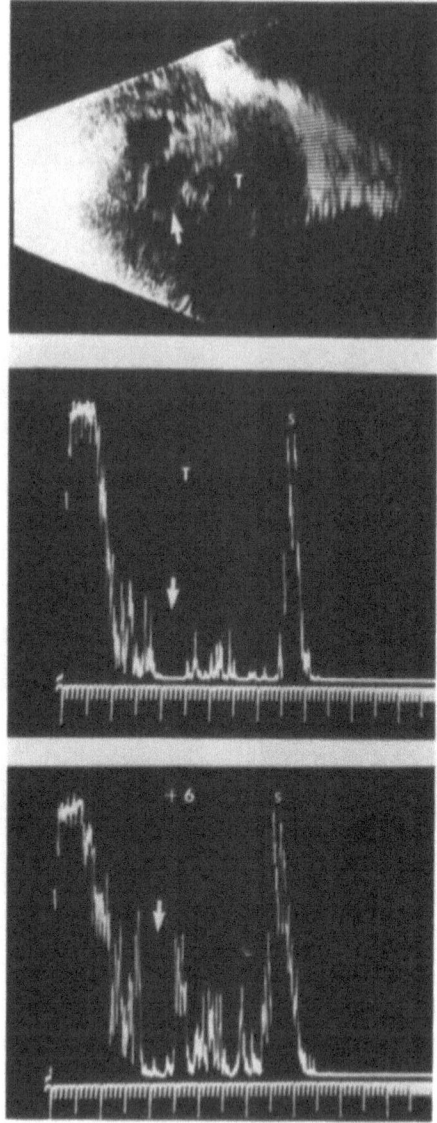

Fig. 9. Paraocular views of tumor (T) show central cystic degeneration (arrow). Cystic space is better appreciated on standardized A-scan using tissue sensitivity plus six decibels (bottom). Note double-peaked posterior surface spike(s) corresponding to encapsulation.

ation, the tumor was well encapsulated with a high, steeply rising, smooth double-peaked posterior border spike (Fig. 9).

The tumor was debulked through an anterosuperior orbitotomy; A large cavity filled with liquid was noted within the lesion at surgery. The diagnosis of neurolemmoma was confirmed histopathologically (Fig. 10).

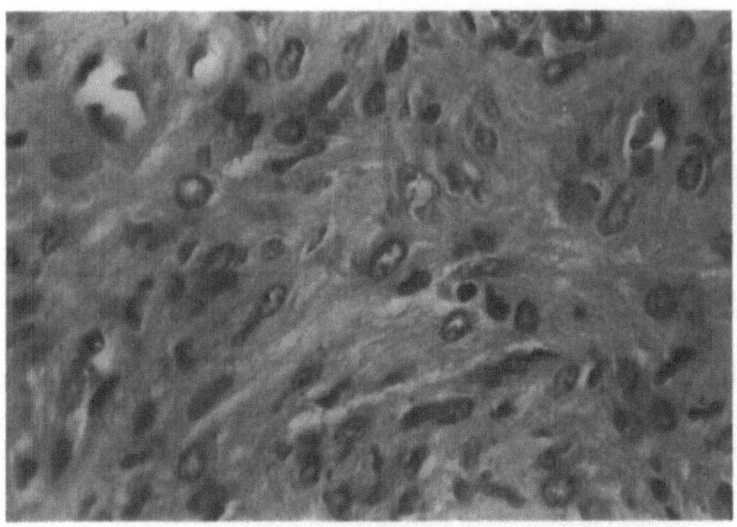

Fig. 10. Histopathology of neurolemmoma in area devoid of cystic degeneration.

Conclusion

These two cases of neurolemmoma were located superonasally and involved both the periocular and retrobulbar spaces. Other significant findings include large cystic cavities and diffuse vascularity of moderate intensity. Table 1

Table 1. Acoustic criteria for neurolemmoma*.

Topographic:	
1. Location:	Superonasal orbit (B, A**)
2. Shape:	Oval (B, A)
3. Borders:	Well-outlined (A)
Quantitative:	
4. Structure:	Coarse with cystic spaces (A, B)
5. Reflectivity:	Low with medium high septi (A)
6. Angle kappa:	Low/variable (A)
Kinetic:	
7. Vascularity:	Diffuse (moderate intensity) (A, D)
8. Compressibility:	Firm (A)
9. Mobility:	May have internal mobility (A)

* Based on instrumentation and techniques of standardized echography. Criteria based on two cases of orbital neurolemmoma.
** A: Standardized A-scan; B: Contact, Real-time B-scan; D: Doppler.

492

summarizes the acoustic criteria of neurolemmoma using the special examination techniques.

Reliable differentiation of neurolemmoma from other lesions requires that standardized echography be used. Standardized echography calls for the use of appropriate instrumentation and examination techniques by an echographic diagnostician.

Acknowledgement

The authors are grateful to Michele L. Fagin for typing this manuscript and for editorial assistance. Additional thanks are extended to the other Echography personnel: J. Randall Hughes, Eileen K. Novinski and Maria L. Rivera.

References

1. Byrne SF. 1979. Standardized echography. Part 1: A-scan examination procedures. Int Ophthalmol Clin; 19(4): 267–81.
2. Byrne SF, Glaser. 1983. Orbital tissue differentiation with standardized echography. Ophthalmology; 90(9): 1071–1090.
3. Henderson JW. 1973. Orbital Tumors. Philadelphia, W.B. Saunders Co.: 308.
4. Jones IS, Jackobiec FA. 1979. Diseases of the Orbit. Hagerstown, Harper & Row: 375.
5. Ossoinig KC. 1968. Echography of orbital tumors – examinations with A- and B-scan techniques. (Ger.) Albrecht Von Graefes, Arch Klin Ophthalmol; 172: 364.
6. Ossoinig KC. 1974. Quantitative echography – the basis of tissue differentiation. J Clin Ultrasound: 2: 33–46.
7. Ossoinig KC. 1978. The role of clinical echography in modern diagnosis of periorbital and orbital lesions. In: Proceedings of the 3rd International Symposium on Orbital Disorders, Amsterdam, September 5–7,1977. The Hague: Junk; 496–540.
8. Ossoinig KC. 1978. Orbital disorders. In: deVlieger M, ed. Handbook of Clinical Ultrasound. New York: John Wiley & Sons: 884–904.
9. Ossoinig KC. 1979. Standardized Echography: Basic Principles, Clinical Applications and Results. Int Ophthal. Clin.; 19(4): 127–210.
10. Ossoinig KC. 1981. Echographic differentiation of vascular tumors in the orbit. Doc Ophthalmol Proc Ser; 29: 283–91.

An unusual periorbital pathology: the neuroma. Clinical-surgical and anatomical-pathological aspects

G. CASCIO, S. GIULIANO and A. DI LIBERTO
Palermo, Italy

An amputation neuroma is a scattered regeneration similar to the simple regeneration of nerve stumps. It can arise as a result of laceration or traumatic crushing of a nerve. The principal components of neuromas are formed by an exuberant proliferation of nerve fibers and connective tissue of the endo-, peri- and epineurium. There are few cases of amputation neuromas of the orbit; however, they may appear after enucleation of the eye or after exenteration of the orbit.

The first case was reported by A. Bietti in 1900. He described the regeneration of the ciliary nerve after a neurectomy. Later on, Loehlein (1910) histologically examined a series of patients upon whom a resection of the ciliary nerve had been performed. In two cases he discovered an amputation neuroma behind the eyeball. Adamantiadis (1935) described an amputation neuroma which appeared after an operation for a hydative cyst of the orbit. Babel and Valerio (1945) reported the first case of neuroma after enucleation. Four years later, Blodi (1949) verified and described an amputation neuroma in a male child enucleated for retinoblastoma of the right eye.

Much more recent is the case reported by Sutula and Weiter (1980). The rarity of this type of pathology prompted us to describe a case under our observation.

Clinical case

An eight-year-old girl was admitted to our Institute in May, 1983. She presented a small swelling in the superonasal area of the periorbital region of the right eye. The tumor manifested itself after a blunt facial trauma that had occurred six months before admittance. The swelling was the dimension of a pea. The tumor had an elastic consistency and was not adherent to the upper and lower levels. The X-ray examination did not show any appreciable alterations. The echographic examination of the orbit only demonstrated the pre-

K.C. Ossoinig (editor), Ophthalmic Echography, ISBN 978-94-010-7988-4

494

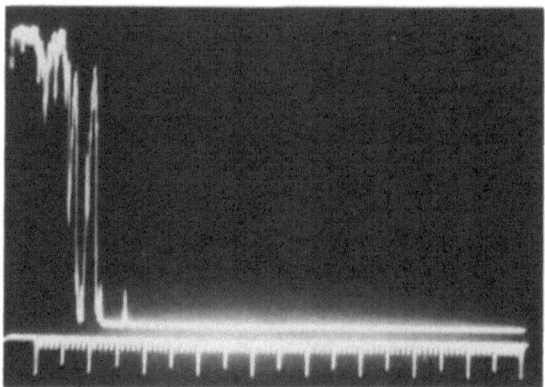

Fig. 1

sence of a very small lesion characterized by high boundaries and low reflectivity which vaguely resembled a cyst (Fig. 1). We did not take a picture of the patient because her lesion was very small. The patient was then discharged because of a temporary tonsillar infection.

By January 1984 the tumor had shown substantial growth (Fig. 2). It was now the size of a large bean, moderately sensitive to manipulation, of a soft elastic consistency, and scarcely movable with respect to the upper and lower levels. The X-ray examination was unchanged, while echography of the orbit revealed a well-defined mass showing a medium reflectivity and moderate compressibility (Fig. 3). A CT scan of the orbit revealed an expansive formation of heterogeneous density in the subcutaneous region of the superonasal angle of the periorbital area of the right eye. The bone adjacent to the mass

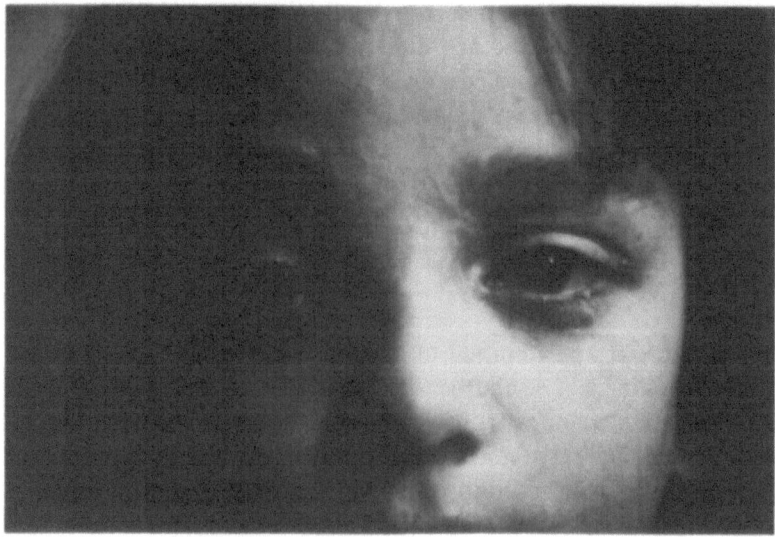

Fig. 2

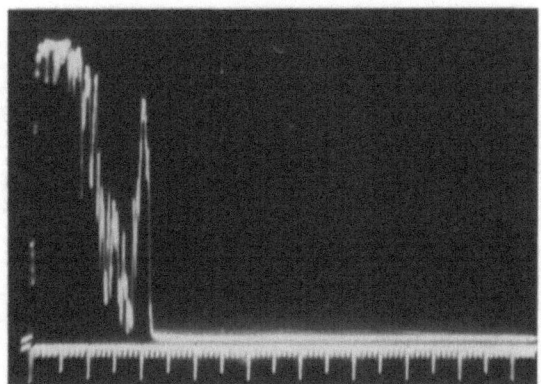

Fig. 3

seemed regular (Fig. 4). Surgery was then performed under general anesthesia. It revealed an easily bleeding, friable tumor. It was whitish and plurilobular. The surgeon removed it completely.

Histological report

The histological examination revealed the presence of numerous, regularly distributed nerve bundles whose morphology varied with respect to the different strata of the section. Each of these structures resulted from the mostly disorganized proliferation. At times it was organized in parallel fascicles of axons, Schwann cells, and fibroblastic elements of the endo- and perineural types. The latter frequently formed a pseudocapsular barrier which delimited

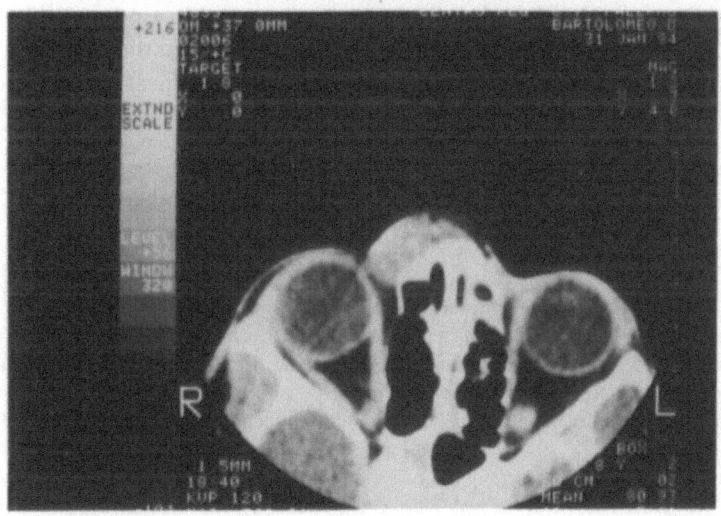

Fig. 4

496

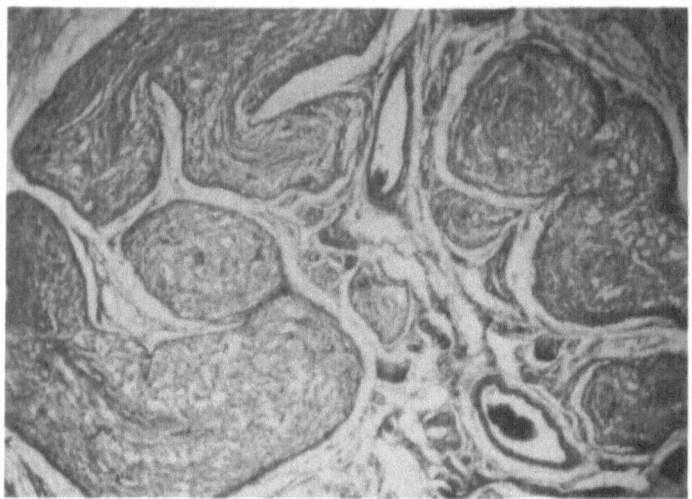

Fig. 5

peripherally the single fibrillary bundles. They seem to be separated by loose connective tissue discretely vascularized by the bundles of striated muscle cells (Fig. 5).

A diagnosis of amputation neuroma was formulated on the basis of his report.

Discussion

All of the known orbital neuromas follow from orbital surgery. But a neuroma can appear after a blunt facial trauma that caused brusque crushing of one nerve. Our case is peculiar in that it is the first time, in the ophthalmological literature, that it has been possible to have echographical and CT images.

References

Adamantiadis B. 1935. Névrome de l'orbite. Arch. Ophthal Paris 52: 582–585.
Babel J and Valerio M. 1945. Névrome d'amputation de l'orbite. Ophthalmologica 109: 317–323.
Blodi FC. 1949. Amputation neuroma in the orbit. Amer. J. Ophth. 32: 929–932.
Gallone L. 1979. Patologia chirurgica. Vol. 1°: 265–272 Casa Editrice Ambrosiana Milano.
Harking JC and Reed RJ. 1969. Non-neoplastic masses. In 'Peripheral nervous system'. Washington Armed Forces Institute of Pathology: 19–23.
Hogan MJ and Zimmerman LE. 1962. Ophthalmic Pathology. Philadelphia, W.B. Saunders CO.: 753–755.
Loehlein W. 1910. Zur Bewertung der resectio optico-ciliaris. Arch. Ophthal. 75: 291–332.
Reese AB. 1951. Tumors of the eye. New York, Paul B. Hoeber: 188–189.
Sutula FC and Weiter JJ. 1980. Orbital socket pain after injury. Amer. J. Ophth. 90: 692–696.

Orbital aerocele

K.C. OSSOINIG and C. TAMBURRELLI
Iowa City, USA

Abstract

Orbital mucoceles produce a classical picture in Standardized Echography, and are readily diagnosed using this method (the accuracy was 98% in 50 cases seen in the Eye Department at the University of Iowa). Occasionally, an orbital mucocele may drain spontaneously through the nasal cavity and consequently fill up with air. This changes the acoustic appearance entirely and may cause diagnostic confusion. The echographic findings in one such case that we experienced were similar to fibrous dysplasia of the bony orbital wall: the orbital roof (the orbital wall of the aerocele) protruded clearly into the orbit, and no signals were obtained from the cavity of the aerocele itself as the air blocked the ultrasound from entering the aerocele (similar to the blockage of the ultrasound by thickened, calcified bone in fibrous dysplasia). In contrast to fibrous dysplasia, multiple signals from the outer and inner surfaces of the cyst wall were noted; protrusion of the lesion was more circumscribed and pronounced than in fibrous dysplasia where the protrusion is more diffuse.

References

1. Ossoinig KC. 1979. Standardized Echography: Basic Principles, Clinical Applications and Results. In: Ophthalmic Ultrasonography: Comparative Techniques (Dallow R.L. ed.) Int. Ophthal. Clin., 19/4: 127–210. Little, Brown & Co., Boston.
2. Hasenfratz G, Ossoinig KC. 1983. The Diagnosis of Orbital Mucoceles and Pyoceles with Standardized Echography. In: Ophthalmic Ultrasonography, J.S. Hillman and M.M. LeMay (eds.), The Hague: Dr W. Junk Publishers: pp. 407–415.

K.C. Ossoinig (editor), Ophthalmic Echography, ISBN 978-94-010-7988-4
© 1987, Martinus Nijhoff/Dr W. Junk Publishers, Dordrecht.

Ultrasonographic and clinical characteristics of orbital pseudotumors

F. GOES
Ghent, Belgium

In the Ghent University Eye Clinic, we examined 239 patients with unilateral exophthalmos. Diagnosis could be verified in 196 patients.

1. *Dysthyroid Orbitopathy* was responsible for 21% of the cases (41) and exophthalmos was the first manifestation of the disease in over 50% of the cases.
2. *Non-tumorous lesions* were responsible for the exophthalmos in 13% (26) of the patients.
3. *Tumorous lesions* were present in 52% (101); malignant tumors in 54% and benign tumors in 46% of the cases.
4. *Orbital pseudotumor* was present in 14%. This disease covers a heterogeneous category of lymphoid infiltrations in the orbit with a wide spectrum of pathological conditions and intraorbital locations. The clinical appearance includes the sudden onset of pain, eyelid edema and, in varying percentages unilateral exophthalmos, diplopia and visual loss. Most cases resolve spontaneously or respond well to steroid treatment.

An orbital pseudotumor is one of the *most common* causes of unilateral exophthalmos. In large series it was responsible for the exophthalmos in 4.7% to 28% of the cases (Table 1): Henderson and Farrow, 1980; M. Wright, 1981; Ossoinig and Hermsen, 1983. In the literature *no sex difference* (134 females, 131 males in the combined series of Blodi and Gass, 1968; Heersinck et al.,

Table 1. Pseudotumor etiology of orbital pathology.

Exophthalmos pseudotumour		N		%
Janev et al. 1979	:	776	–	6.7%
Wright 1981	:	1.041	–	8.4%
Till and Hauff 1981	:	316	–	28% (+ lymphoma)
Rootman and Nugent 1982	:	484	–	4.7%
Henderson and Farrow 1980	:			10%

K.C. Ossoinig (editor), Ophthalmic Echography, ISBN 978-94-010-7988-4

500

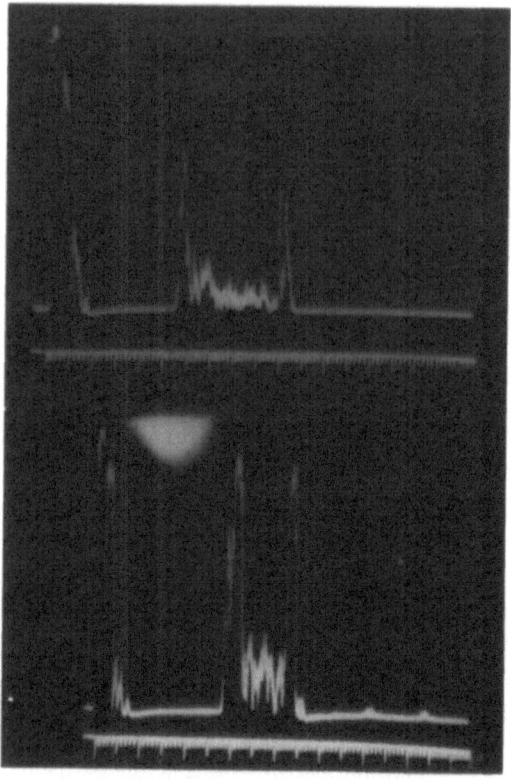

Fig. 1. Regression of pseudotumor after cortisone treatment (above: before; below: after).

1977; Mottow and Jakobiec, 1978; Chairs et al., 1978; Diaz et al., 1980; and Sergott et al., 1981), and *no side difference* could be observed (83 right, 81 left, 16 bilateral) in the combined series of Blodi and Gass, 1969; Heersinck et al., 1977; and Mottow and Jakobiec, 1978. In 96 cases of the three series (Heersinck et al., 1977; Chairs et al., 1978; and Sergott et al., 1981), the mean *age* was 54 years old with extremes between 10 and 83 years.

Most of the pseudotumors are anteriorly situated in the orbit. In combined series of 82 cases (Heersinck et al., 1972; Nugent et al., 1981; Rootman and Nugent, 1982; and Hara and Ohnishi, 1983), 46% were situated anteriorly, 17% posteriorly and 36% at the lacrymal gland.

Symptoms are linked with the localization. Pain is the primary and most important symptom in anteriorly situated tumors (Rootman and Nugent, 1982), and is usually combined with a palpable mass, swelling of the eyelid and signs of inflammation (50% Henderson and Farrow, 1980). Posteriorly situated lesions produce greater exophthalmos, visual loss and motility disturbances. The visual prognosis is poor in cases with marked visual loss (Hender-

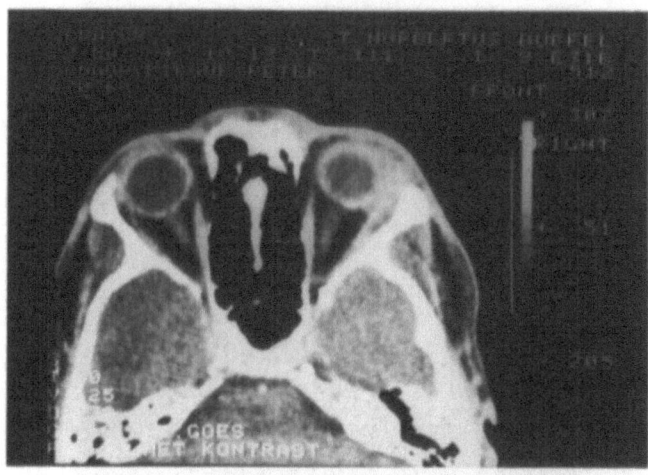

Fig. 2. C.T. scan with uveo-scleral tickening and solid tissue mass in the region of the lacrymal gland (granuloma).

son and Farrow, 1980) and in bilateral cases (Mottow and Jakobiec, 1978). In orbital pseudotumor, exophthalmos may be present in 60% (Blody and Gass, 1968) to 90% (Henderson and Farrow, 1980) of the cases.

Different *therapeutic* approaches exist. Oral steroid treatment is effective in the acute cases (Rootman and Nugent, 1982; Fig. 1). In chronic cases (Heersinck et al., 1977, Nugent et al., 1981), posteriorly-situated pseudotumors (Rootman and Nugent, 1982), and in sclerosing pseudotumors (Abramovitz et al., 1983) this treatment is less effective and small doses of radiotherapy should be applied. Complete surgical excision is proposed by other authors (Henderson and Farrow, 1980).

Because of the varied character (infiltrative, diffuse, circumscribed) and different localization in the orbit, neither ultrasound nor CT show a specific *diagnostic* image. CT-scan is especially useful in detecting apical lesions and bony wall changes and in the follow-up of the lesion. It is, however, not pathognomonic (Bernardino et al., 1977; Nugent et al., 1981; Edwards et al., 1982). It may show a soft tissue mass with variable density dimensions, form and localization. Sclero-uveal thickening is found in 53% of pseudotumors, especially in the anteriorly situated forms (Bernardino et al., 1977; Rootman et al. 1977). Inflammatory thickening of the muscle as well as the adjacent sclera is more indicative of pseudotumor, while localized muscle thickening points more toward myositis (Fig. 2).

In 1975 Ossoinig and Till stated that lymphoma and pseudotumor form a group that could not be differentiated, and were characterized by homogeneity (1), low reflectivity (2), hard consistency (3), and the absence of vas-

502

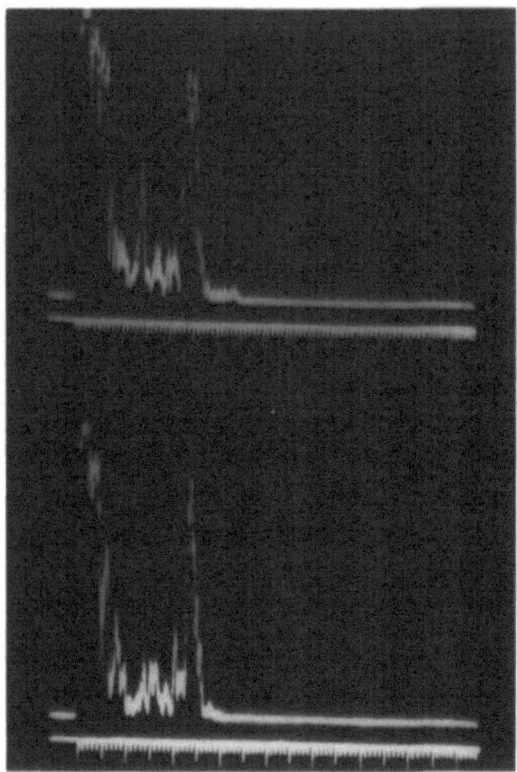

Fig. 3. Low reflective echogram of orbital pseudotumor.

cularity (3). In 1977 Coleman described the irregular outline (1), the high
sound absorption (2), the eventual indentation of the orbital fat pattern (3)
and the possible edema of the orbital structures in tenonitis (4). In 1981 Poujol
stressed the fact that orbital pseudotumors could not always be differentiated
from real tumors, but that on the whole they were more heterogeneous and
had more irregular borders.

Ultrasound examination may show irregular borders, a homogeneous internal structure, rather low-reflective interfaces and low-sound attenuation.
Because of their regular internal structure (homogeneous cellular infiltrate
without significant connective tissue interfaces), lymphomas and pseudotumors form a group that can be separated only with difficulty upon ultrasound
examination (Fig. 3).

Different *histological* classifications are proposed for orbital pseudotumors.
Reese (1963) grouped his cases into five categories, while Blodi and Gass
(1968) divided their cases into nine types. Henderson and Farrow (1973)
described two types: type I with necrosing vasculitis and diffuse polymorphous

infiltrate, and type II with lymphocytic infiltrations. Both types can be either acute, subacute or chronic. In 1980 the same authors reserved the term 'pseudotumor' for lesions with unknown etiology. Zimmerman and Sobin (1980) described 11 pseudotumor types.

Association of orbital pseudotumor with choroidal osteoma (Katz and Gass, 1983), myasthenia (Van De Mosselaer et al. 1980), Crohn's disease (Weinstein, 1984), thyroiditis (Anderson et al. 1963) and sinusitis (Heersinck et al. 1977) is mentioned.

Personal observations

We had the occasion to examine 32 orbital pseudotumors in 28 patients (M12–F16), 4 of which were recurrences. Fourteen cases were situated on the right side and 18 were situated on the left. The mean age was 49 years with extremes between 13 and 85 years: 4 were over 70 years of age and 2 were younger than 20 years.

Roentgenography, when performed, was invariably negative (24).

Gammagraphy showed a hyperactivity in 6 of 15 examined cases.

Angiography showed a pathology in 8 of 13 examined cases. *CT-scan* examination was performed in 18 cases. It remained negative in two cases and was doubtful in 1 case. In the other 16 cases, it showed a soft tissue infiltrate, enlargement of muscles and/or a soft tissue mass along the muscles (Table 2). *Ultrasound* demonstrated the lesion in all but one case, the mean diameter of the lesions being 14 mm with extremes between 5 and 30 mm (only 4 cases above 20 mm). The reflectivity was rather low (10–15%) except in two cases (30–50%).

The majority of the lesions had a hard consistency. We could not make a differential diagnosis only from the ultrasound appearance but, in more than 90% of the cases, ultrasound together with the clinical characteristics pointed towards the right diagnosis. In 90% of our cases we obtained a low-reflective, rather homogeneous echogram with irregular borders (Fig. 4, Fig. 5). The

Table 2. Positive diagnosis in 32 orbital pseudotumour cases.

Diagnosis	
R.X.	: 0% +
Gammagraphy	: 40% +
Angiography	: 60% +
CT	: 90% +
Ultrasound	: 97% +

504

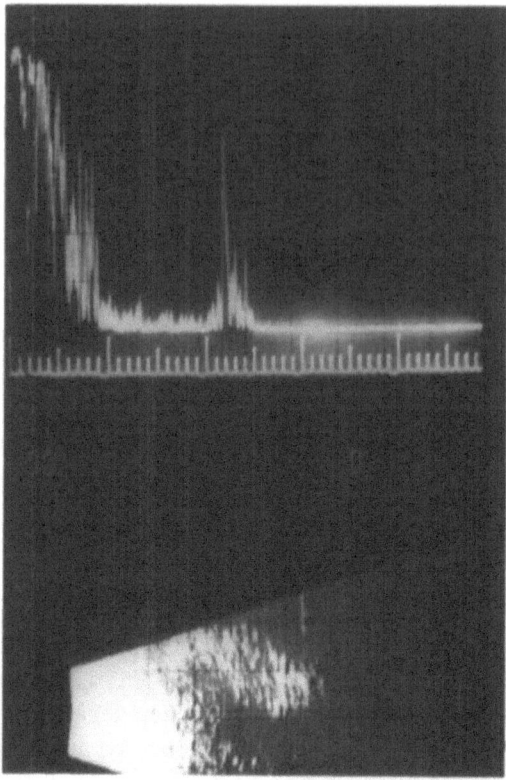

Fig. 4. Typical echogram with low reflectivity and homogeneity (orbital granuloma).

diagnosis of pseudotumor was *confirmed* by histology in 19 cases (inflammatory pseudotumor in 18 cases; sclerosing type in 4 cases; sarcoid in 1 case), by
surgery in 7 cases, and by the response to steroid treatment in 6 cases.

Table 3 shows the *clinical characteristics*. In most cases the onset of the
pathology was acute and the exophthalmos moderate. *Motility disturbances*
were present in most of the cases with immobilization of the eye in 9 cases.
Pain and inflammatory changes of the anterior eye segment (redness,
episcleral congestion) were present in the majority of the cases.

In 10 cases a *palpable mass* was situated in the lacrimal fossa (5 cases, usually
with pain) or inferiorly (5 cases). A temporal superior localization was most
frequent (9) but, on the whole, inferior lesions were as frequent as superior
lesions. One case was bilateral from the beginning, and three cases recurred
after tapering of the steroids.

Treatment consisted of systemic steroids in 20 cases, and surgical resection
and decompression in 6 cases. Follow-up was lost in 1 case and short (<6
months) in 7 cases. Of the other cases, 11 remained without symptoms, 5 had

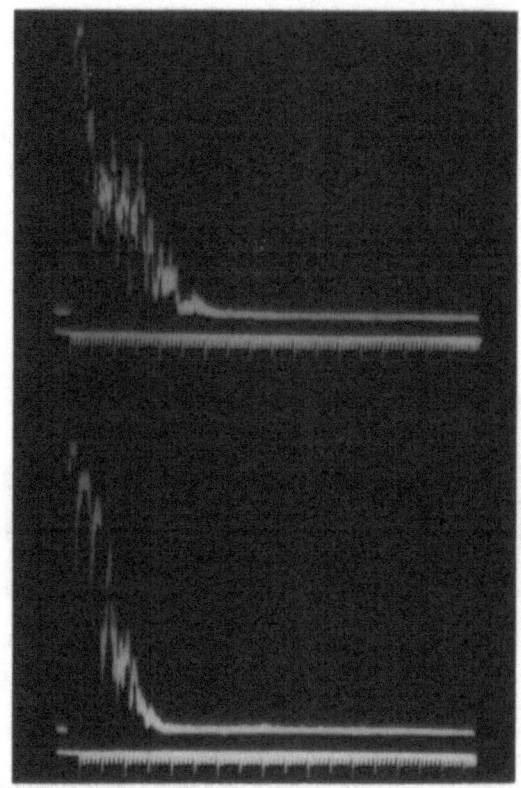

Fig. 5. Regression of pseudotumor in a patient with Crohn disease (above; before, below; after).

Table 3. Clinical characteristics of orbital pseudotumours.

Pseudotumor		
Onset: acute	<1 month	: 13/32
slow	>3 month	: 3/32
Exophthalmos:	<3 mm	: 13/32
	>6 mm	: 4/32
Visual loss		: 10/32
Motility ↓		: 23/32
Pain		: 22/32
Inflammation		: 21/32
Ptosis		: 9/32
Edema eyelid		: 14/32

one or two recurrences in the same eye, and 6 had a recurrence in the other eye after a period of from six weeks to 13 years.

In *conclusion,* neither ultrasonography nor computer tomography are specific in diagnosing an orbital pseudotumor, but they give us helpful diagnostic information. They outline the extent of the pathology prior to surgery and they demonstrate the regression of the lesion during treatment.

The associated signs of fast onset, unilaterality, pain, and inflammatory changes, as well as the age of patient and the reaction on steroid therapy, give helpful clinical information for the diagnosis.

References

Abramovitz JN, Kasdon DL, Sutula F, Post KD, Chong FK. 1983. Sclerosing orbital pseudotumor. Neurosurgery 12: 463–468.

Anderson et al. 1963. Thyroiditis with myxedema and orbital pseudotumor. Aeta Ophthal, K b h., 41: 120.

Bernardino ME, Zimmerman RD, Citrin CM, Davis DO. 1977. Scleral thickening: A CT sign of orbital pseudotumor. Am J Roentgenol 129: 703–706.

Blodi FG, Gass JDM. 1968. Inflammatory pseudotumor of the orbit. Br J Ophthalmol 52: 79–93.

Chairs RM, Garner A, Wright JE. 1978. Inflammatory orbital pseudotumor. A clinicopathologic study. Arch Ophthalmol 96: 1817–1822.

Coleman DJ, Lizzi F, Jack R. 1977. Ultrasonography of the eye and the orbit. Lea and Febiger, Philadelphia: 334–335.

Diaz AG, Lopez AS, Perres MJA, Zorrilla MYF, Gozalvez TM, de la Fuente, Gomez M. 1980. Orbital pseudotumor. Ophthalmologica, Basel, 181: 181–187.

Edwards MK, Zanel DW, Gilmar RL, Muller J. 1982. Invasive orbital pseudotumor CT demonstration of extension beyond orbit. Neuroradiology 23: 215–217.

Hara Y, Ohnishi Y. 1983. Orbital inflammatory pseudotumor: clinicopathologic study of 22 cases. Jpn J Ophthalmol 27: 80–89.

Harr DL,Quencer RM, Abrams GW. 1982. Computed tomography and ultrasound in the evaluation of orbital infection and pseudotumor. Radiology 142: 395–401.

Heersinck B, Rodriguez MR, Flanagan JD. 1977. Inflammatory pseudotumor of the orbit. Ann of Ophthalmol: 17–29.

Hendersen JW, Farrow GM. 1980. Orbital tumors. Georg Thieme Verlag, Stuttgart, New York: 513.

Janev KG, Ossoinig K, Frazier SW, Fish G. 1979. Ultrasound in diagnosis of orbital diseases. Diagnostica ultrasonica in ophthalmologia. Siduo VII, 159–165. R.A. Remky Verlag Munster.

Katz RS, Gass DM. 1983. Multiple choroidal osteomas developing in association with recurrent orbital inflammatory pseudotumor. Arch Ophthal 101: 1724–1727.

Mottow LS, Jakobiec FA. 1978. Idiopathic Inflammatory Orbital pseudotumor in childhood I. Clinical characteristics. Arch Ophthalmol 96: 1410–1417.

Nugent RA, Rootman K, Robertson WD, Lapointe JS, Harrison PB. 1981. Acute orbital pseudotumors: classification and CT features. Amer Journ Radiology, 137: 957–962.

Ossoinig KC, Hermsen V. 1983. Myositis of extraocular muscles diagnosed with standardized echography. In Hillman JS, LeMay MM: Ophthalmic Ultrasonography, Dr. W. Junk Publ., The Hague, Boston, Lancaster: 381–391.

Poujol J. 1981. Echographie en Ophthalmologie, 6065, Masson Paris.

Reese AB. 1963. Tumors of the eye. Harper and Row, New York: 538–541.

Rootman J, Nugent R. 1982. Classification and management of acute orbital pseudotumors. Ophthalmol 89: 1040–1048.

Till P, Hauff W. 1983. Differential diagnostic results of clinical echography in orbital tumors. In Hillman JS, LeMay MM: Ophthalmic Ultrasonography, Dr. W. Junk Publ. The Hague, Boston, Lancaster: 277–282.

Van De Mosselaer, Van Deuren H, DewolfPeeters C, Missotten L. 1980. Pseudotumor orbita and myasthenia. Arch Ophthal, 98: 1621–1622.

Weinstein JM, Koch K, Lane S. 1984. Orbital pseudotumor in Crohn's colitis. Ann Ophthal 16: 275–278.

Wright JE. 1981. The role of ultrasound in the investigation and management of orbital disease. Docum Ophthal Proc Series, vol. 29: 273–276. Ed. J.M. Thyssen and M. Verbeek Dr. W. Junk Publ. The Hague.

Zimmerman LE, Sabin LH. 1980. Types histologiques des tumeurs de l'oeil et de ses annexes. Class Int tumeurs, Genève 24: 46.

Retrobulbar pseudotumor with ultrasonically empty orbit

H.C. FLEDELIUS
Hillerød, Denmark

Introduction

A case of orbital pseudotumour is presented because of its striking discrepancy between CT and ultrasound findings. From earlier comparative studies of the two diagnostic methods in orbital disease (Gyldensted et al. 1977, Fledelius & Gyldensted 1978) similar experience has been gained. In the latter report, pseudotumour was the diagnosis in 17 out of 126 orbital cases sent for evaluation. In six of the 17, however, the orbital lesion could be demonstrated only by CT-scanning while ultrasound showed normal orbital echopatterns (at that time evaluated by Kretztechnik 7000, A-mode).

The present case of verified orbital pseudotumour was examined with a Sonometrics 400 Ocuscan equipment, which showed 'empty orbit' instead of the expected tumourpattern. Further it is discussed whether a 'thick eye wall' by CT-scan might be a sign of orbital pseudotumour.

Case report

In 1977, a 46-year old male immigrant from Turkey came to the University Eye Clinic of Rigshospitalet, Copenhagen, due to diplopia and 5–6 mm painful proptosis of the right eye. There was a slight upwards and lateral displacement of the eye (Fig. 1), with restricted eye motility, in particular downwards. A mass lesion could be palpated in the lower nasal orbital quadrant. The overlying skin was unaffected, and the eye showed no redness or other signs of inflammation. Visual acuity was 6/6, ophthalmoscopy normal.

Thorough laboratory investigation gave no evidence of immune (or other systemic) disease. Roentgenogrammes showed intact orbital walls and no sign of sinusitis.

A solid or semisolid lesion was demonstrated by ultrasound (A-mode), consistent with the CT-scanning shown in Fig. 1.

K.C. Ossoinig (editor), Ophthalmic Echography, ISBN 978-94-010-7988-4

© 1987, Martinus Nijhoff/Dr W. Junk Publishers, Dordrecht.

510

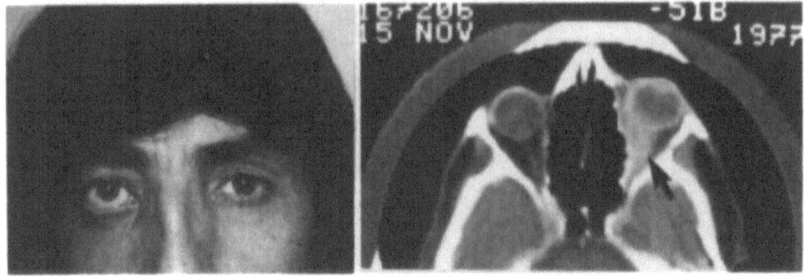

Fig. 1. Clinical photo and CT-scan when first examined. Proptosis of right eye without redness. A solid lesion in the nasal part of right orbit (arrow).

Bioptic specimens were taken by way of an anterior approach. Tumour tissue was hard, with no apparent relation to external eye muscles. PAD: dense collagen connective tissue with unspecific chronic inflammatory reaction (lymfocytes and plasmacells), so-called pseudotumour. Thick-walled vessels stained positive for PAS (Copenhagen University Eye Pathology Institute 1159/77 a–e).

On general prednisone treatment he recovered over months, but after 6 years there was clinical relapse, with proptosis and moderate pain, but this time without diplopia and restricted eye motility; visual acuity and ophthalmoscopy still normal. There was no indication of thyroid dysfunction, TRH-stimulation and other tests being normal. CT-scanning indicated diffuse mass lesions especially in the posterior orbit and upwards (Fig. 2), and prednisone therapy was started, again with some improvement clinically, but with persistance of the changes on CT-scanning when repeated after two months.

I then saw him for ultrasound examination, now performed with Sono-metrics 400 Ocuscan A + B, with the findings shown in Fig. 3. The retrobulbar pattern of the right side was short and 'motheaten' as compared to the pattern of the healthy left orbit. Ultrasound gave no indication of enlarged external eye muscles.

Discussion

When first examined, there was good accordance between ultrasound, CT-scanning, and clinical picture. This did not hold for the relapse 6 years later where examining results differed markedly. CT-scanning now showed rather dense, somewhat diffuse mass lesions, with obvious relation to the posterior part of the muscle cone, however without the typical features of dysthyroid myopathy (usually appearing as well demarcated thick external eye muscles on coronal scan). Nor were there restrictions of eye movement.

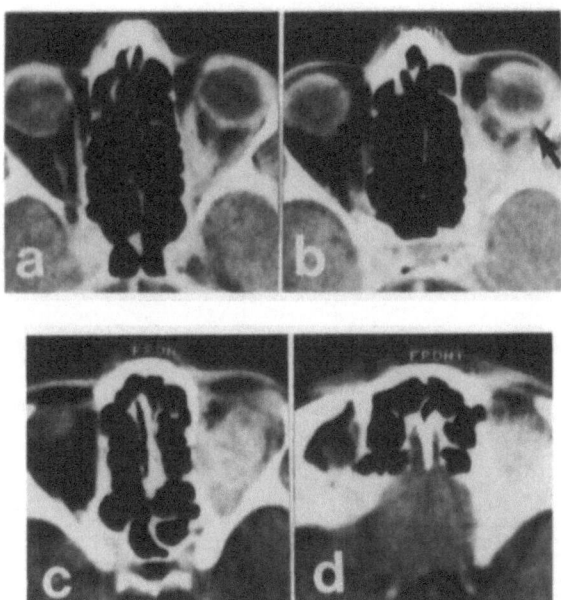

Fig. 2. Differently located CT-changes 6 years later, now predominantly upwards and far back in the right orbit, with some relation to the muscle cone. CT-sections from orbital midlevel and upwards (a through d), after telebrix contrast. Thick eye wall best seen on b (arrow).

Clinical findings thus seemed in better accord with the negative ultra-sonogramme, which however was not normal either. As compared with the healthy orbit, the retrobulbar echopattern was too short and irregularly delineated. With the moth-eaten boundary it gave the appearance of an 'empty orbit', in particular because there was no final spike as seen for example in cysts and in most solid tumours, to mark the posterior boundary of abnormal tissue.

Keeping in mind the variability of lesions comprised under the collective term of pseudotumour, it is no wonder that ultrasound may give varying and

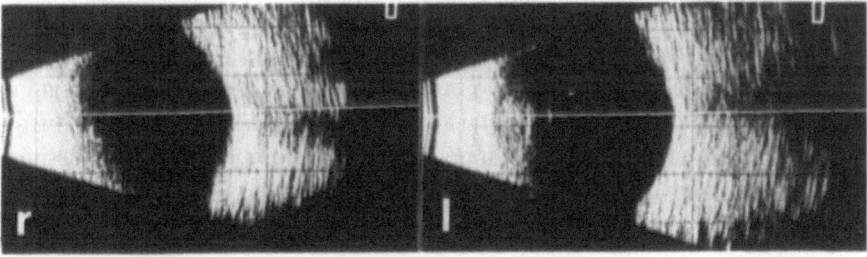

Fig. 3. Ultrasound B-scan of right and left orbits. Moth-eaten foreshortened retrobulbar echopattern on the right side (r).

512

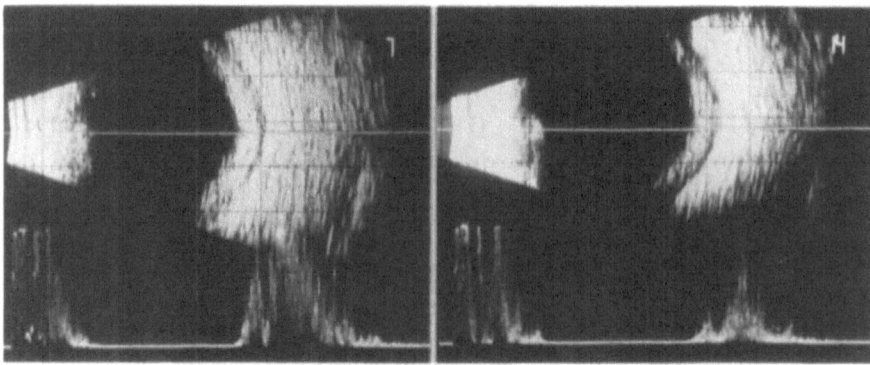

Fig. 4. Ultrasonographically demonstrated thick eyewall in another patient with presumed orbital pseudotumour. Sensitivity settings reduced 7 and 14 db.

inconsistent echopatterns. Nevertheless, a typical pattern has been forwarded, showing mostly a rather uniform tissue of low reflectivity, ultrasonically resembling what is seen in orbital lymfoma (e.g. Ossoinig & Till, 1975). The diffuse character of the present orbital lesion, as apparent by CT-scanning, may explain the lack of a final tumour spike on the echogrammes, but not the empty appearance. Nor was this found in our previous ultrasonically falsely negative pseudotumour cases (Fledelius & Gyldensted, 1978).

A final remark on the CT description of a thick eye wall as being typical in orbital pseudotumour cases, usually most evident as enhancement after contrast injection. A thick eye wall may be demonstrated also by ultrasound (Fig. 4, from another pseudotumour case) but to my knowledge, ultrasound literature has no indication of this feature being an added pseudotumour characteristic.

Summary

According to previous personal experience with ultrasonography in orbital pseudotumour, there is a certain amount of patients with normal orbital echopatterns, inconsistent with the positive CT-scans. On this background a case is presented where ultrasound shows a moth-eaten foreshortened retrobulbar echogramme, giving the appearance of an 'empty orbit'. A possible CT-scanning indicator of orbital pseudotumour, 'thick eye wall', is further discussed.

References

Fledelius HC, Gyldensted C. 1978. Ultrasonography and computer tomography in orbital diagnosis. Acta Ophthalmol 56: 751–762.

Gyldensted C, Lester J, Fledelius HC. 1977. Computed tomography of orbital lesions. Neuroradiology 13: 141–150.

Ossoinig KC, Till P. 1975. Ten year study on clinical echography in orbital disease. Bibl Ophthal 83: pp. 200–216, Karger, Basel.

Echographic diagnosis of posterior scleritis

R.L. GREEN
Los Angeles, USA

Introduction

Diagnosis of posterior scleritis is often difficult and is commonly made on the basis of exclusion. The clinical diagnosis is often made indirectly from signs and symptoms, including pain, proptosis, chemosis, serous retinal detachment and vitreous inflammation (Watson and Hayreh, 1976, Cleary, 1975). It is also not uncommon for posterior scleritis to be included in the overall diagnosis of orbital pseudotumor. We have studied a series of patients with inflammation of the posterior sclera who were referred for echography. It was found that these inflammatory entities could be divided into three general categories: posterior episcleritis, posterior inflammatory scleritis and posterior nodular scleritis.

Subjects and methods

Twenty-eight patients with inflammation of the posterior sclera were examined by standardized echography using both the Kretz 7200 A scan and a contact B scan.

Results

Seventeen of the patients were found to have posterior episcleritis. The echographic examination showed a thin area of decreased reflectivity between the normally highly reflective sclera with orbital signals on both the A scan and the B scan (Fig. 1). This area of decreased reflectivity often extended back to the optic nerve. Posterior episcleral infiltration was seldom seen as a primary disorder but, rather, was usually secondary to some other inflammatory disease of the orbit, such as pseudotumors, inflammatory myositis and optic neuritis.

K.C. Ossoinig (editor), Ophthalmic Echography, ISBN 978-94-010-7988-4

516

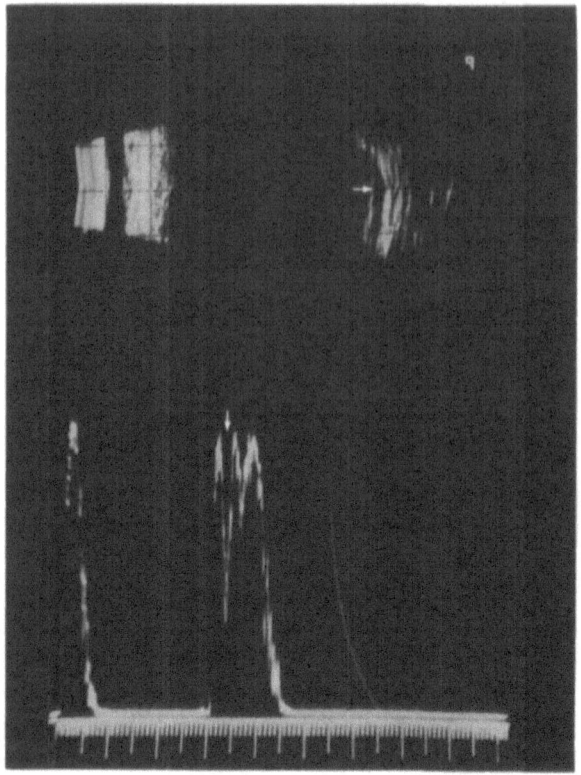

Fig. 1. B scan and A scan echograms of posterior episcleritis. Note the episcleral infiltration indicated by decreased reflectivity posterior to the scleral signal (arrows).

Seven of the patients were found to have simple posterior inflammatory scleritis. In contrast to posterior episcleritis, this entity often represents the primary inflammatory process, which may, in turn, be associated with second-ary myositis, optic neuritis, or inflammation of the lacrimal gland. These patients often present with severe ocular pain, although this is not invariably present (Benson, 1979). The typical echographic findings consist of episcleral infiltration with thickening of the retina and choroid. Typically, the normally highly reflective scleral signal on standardized A scan shows a decrease (Fig. 2). The echogram often shows serous retinal detachments and choroidal effusion; mild thickening of the sclera is also often seen accompanying inflam-matory scleritis.

Four of the patients were found to have marked thickening of the posterior sclera, indicative of posterior nodular scleritis. In standardized A scan, the reflectivity of these lesions was usually quite high with a regular internal structure (Benson, 1979) (Fig. 3). The B scan revealed the lesions to extend

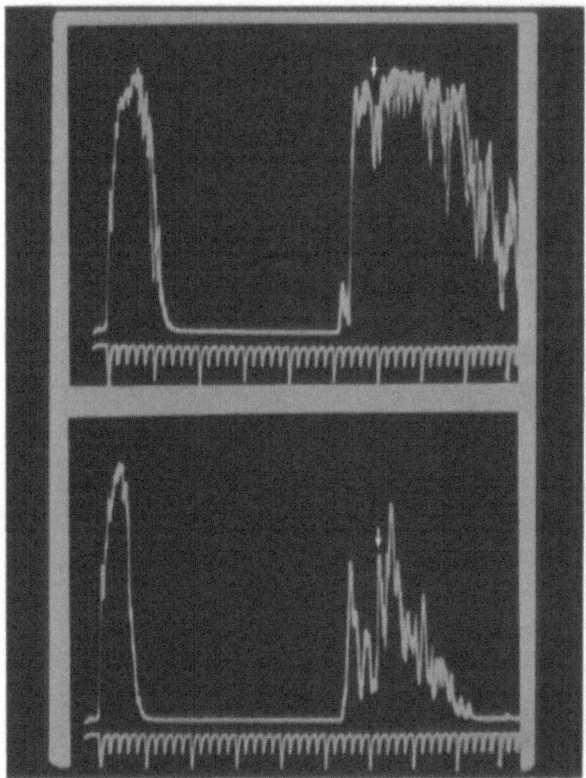

Fig. 2. A scan echograms of posterior inflammatory scleritis. Note episcleral infiltration (arrow) at tissue sensitivity (top) and thickening of retina – choroid at lower sensitivity (bottom). Arrow = scleral signal on bottom echogram. Note decreased reflectivity of scleral signal typically seen when the sclera is inflamed.

both within and outside the contour of the globe (Fig. 4). These patients rarely had the thickened retinal choroid layer, serous retinal detachments or choroidal effusion seen in inflammatory posterior scleritis.

Discussion

Inflammation of the posterior sclera can usually be differentiated by standardized echography (Ossoinig, 1979) into one of three groups. These are posterior episcleritis, posterior inflammatory scleritis and posterior nodular scleritis. Occasionally, these diagnoses will overlap, when the patient show signs of more than one of these categories. Generally, however, most patients can be placed into one of these three groups.

Posterior episcleritis is usually secondary to some other primary orbital

518

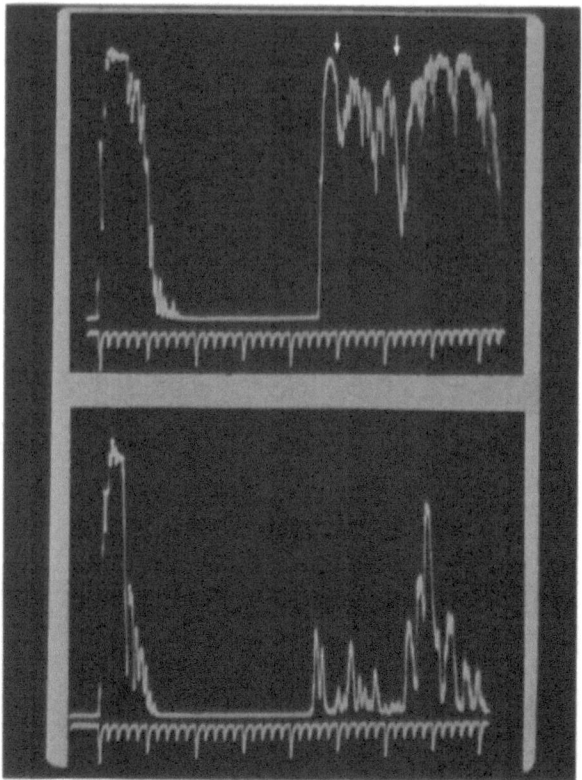

Fig. 3. A scan echograms showing marked thickening of sclera in posterior nodular scleritis. At tissue sensitivity (top) note high reflective spikes (between arrows) from thickened sclera.

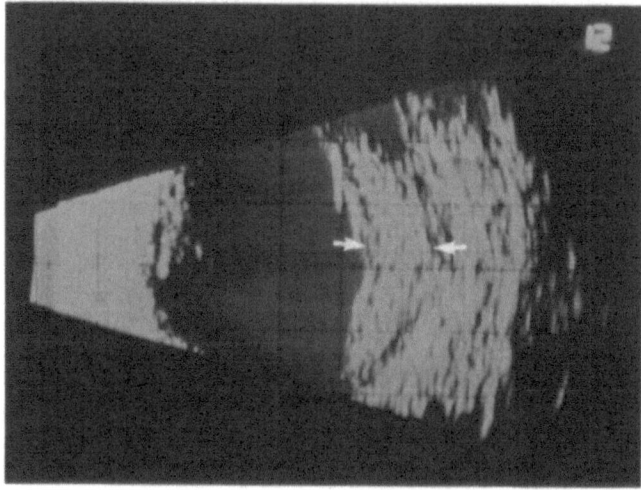

Fig. 4. B scan echogram showing marked thickening of sclera in posterior scleritis (between arrows).

inflammatory disease, such as orbital pseudotumor, inflammatory myositis, and optic neuritis.

On the other hand, posterior inflammatory scleritis is a primary entity that often results in a secondary orbital disorder, such as myositis or optic neuritis. Clinically, inflammatory scleritis is often associated with severe ocular pain, which, if severe enough, is diagnostic. This disorder usually responds dramatically to steroids, with rapid abatement of the pain and more gradual resolution of the echographic signs. As the objective echographic signs usually take longer to resolve than do the symptoms, we feel that ultrasound is the better way of monitoring results of therapy in these cases.

Posterior nodular scleritis is associated with marked thickening of the sclera and often the patient does not complain of severe ocular pain, such as is seen with inflammatory scleritis. The ultrasound does not reveal the choroidal effusion or serous retinal detachment so commonly seen in inflammatory scleritis. Nodular scleritis often responds dramatically to steroids (Feldon, 1978), with a melting away of the thickened sclera.

Conclusions

Twenty-eight patients with inflammation of the posterior sclera were evaluated by echography. In general we were able to differentiate these inflammatory processes into three diagnostic categories: posterior scleritis, posterior inflammatory scleritis, and posterior nodular scleritis. Standardized echography thus proved to be a very effective method for diagnosing and following-up these disorders, which are often quite difficult to diagnose on a clinical basis; in addition, ultrasound is more effective in monitoring results of treatment than are purely subjective symptoms.

References

1. Benson WE, Shields JA, Tasman W, Crandall AS. 1979. Posterior Scleritis: A Cause of Diagnostic Confusion. Arch Ophthalmol 97: 1482–1486.
2. Cleary PE, Watson PG, McGill JI, Hamilton AM. 1975. Visual Loss Due to Posterior Segment Disease in Scleritis. Trans Ophthalmol Soc UK 95: 297–300.
3. Feldon SE, Sigelman J, Albert DM, Smith TR. 1978. Clinical Manifestations of Brawny Scleritis. Am J Ophthalmol 85: 781–787.
4. Ossoinig KC. 1979. Standardized Echography: Basic Principles, Clinical Applications and Results, in Dallow RL (ed.): Int Ophthalmol Clin 19/4, Boston: Little Brown and Co., pp. 127–210.
5. Watson PG, Hayreh SS. 1976. Scleritis and Episcleritis. Br J Ophthalmol 60: 163–191.

Standardized echography in orbital myositis

J.R. MACNEILL
Halifax, Canada

Abstract

It is only within the past few years that acute orbital myositis has received much attention in world ophthalmic literature. A major reason for this is that until recently techniques were not available to demonstrate the enlarged extra-ocular muscle of acute orbital myositis.

Standardized echography has proven to be an extremely useful technique both to diagnose acute orbital myositis, and to provide a useful working differential diagnosis. Several cases are presented to demonstrate this diagnosis and its differential.

References

1. Ossoinig KC. 1979. Standardized Echography: Basic Principles, Clinical Applications and Results. In: Ophthalmic Ultrasonography: Comparative Techniques (Dallow RL, ed.) Int Ophthal Clin, 19/4 (1979), 127–210. Little, Brown & Co., Boston.
2. Ossoinig KC. 1982. Advances in Diagnostic Ultrasound. ACTA: XXIV International Congress of Ophthalmology, (San Francisco), Paul Henkind, ed. Philadelphia: J.B. Lippincott Co., Vol. 1, pp. 89–114.
3. Ossoinig KC, Hasenfratz G. 1983. Die Rolle der standardisierten Echographie in der Diagnose und Behandlung der orbitalen Myositis [Ger., 'The Role of Standardized Echography in the Diagnosis and Treatment of Orbital Myositis']. Ophthalmologie, 80: 475–481.
4. Ossoinig KC, Hermsen V. 1983. Myositis of Extraocular Muscles Diagnosed with Standardized Echography. In: Ophthalmic Ultrasonography. Hillman JS, LeMay MM (eds.), The Hague: Dr. W. Junk Publishers, pp. 381–392.

Standardized echography in C.C. fistulas

J.R. MACNEILL
Halifax, Canada

The clinical diagnosis of intracranial A.V.M. with orbital manifestations can sometimes be uncertain. Standardized echography has proved to be a very rapid and useful screening technique to identify both the 'fast-flow' (C.C. fistula with rapid orbital drainage) and 'slow-flow' (usually dural shunt with orbital congestion) types of this entity.

The purpose of this report is to describe the standardized echographic characteristics of this entity. For information on other aspects of this entity one is referred to the recent literature including excellent papers by Phelps, Thompson, and Ossoinig [1], and Grove [2].

Fast-flow type (Fig. 1)

The most outstanding feature of this type is the greatly dilated and arterialized superior ophthalmic vein coursing from nasally in the anterior orbit and extending more laterally as it progresses posteriorly to exit the orbit through the superior orbital fissure. This vein lies in the superior orbit above the level of the optic nerve. Occasionally one may also observe other dilated orbital veins in direct communication with the superior orbital vein. Generalized congestion within the orbit is not a typical feature of this type, although muscles adjacent to the S.O. vein may be slightly thick. Doppler reveals reversal of the normal venous flow within the orbit.

Slow-flow types (Figs. 2–4)

As one approaches this end of the entity, the dilated superior ophthalmic vein is no longer seen. The important echographic feature is generalized swelling of orbital fat, extra-ocular muscles, and the optic nerve sheath, due to orbital congestion. This type is impartant to recognize because many of these patients are elderly, the group in whom arteriography is especially dangerous.

K.C. Ossoinig (editor), Ophthalmic Echography, ISBN 978-94-010-7988-4

522

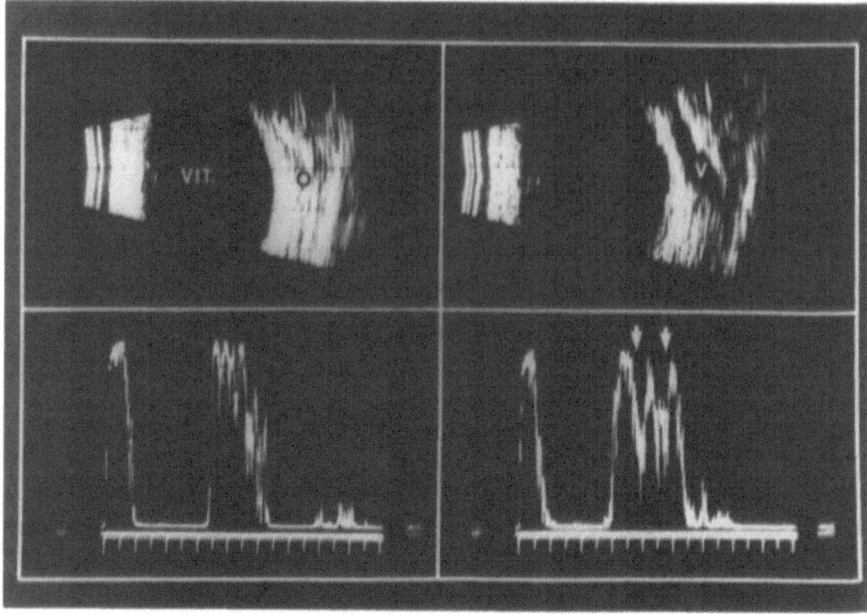

Fig. 1. (left top) Normal trans-ocular B-scan produced by placing the horizontally held probe against the 6 o'clock limbus and aiming into the superior orbit. The normal vitreous (VIT) and orbital (O) patterns are displayed. Contrast this with *(right top)* the B-scan pattern seen in a patient with C.C. fistula. Here the meandering dilated superior ophthalmic vein is seen coursing from antero-medially (TOP *of picture*) to a more postero-lateral position within the orbit in a longitudinal vein. B-scan provides good topographic documentation of this orbital lesion.

(left-bottom) Normal trans-ocular standardized A-scan (through same region as above B-scans) with Kretz 7200 MA at 'Tissue Sensitivity'. Contrast this with *(right bottom)* the standardized A-scan through the same region in a patient with C.C. fistula. Here we note two adjacent cross-sections (arrowheads) of the dilated superior ophthalmic vein, appearing as well – outlined defects in the orbital pattern. The low to mid-reflective pattern within the vein walls is blurred due to flickering produced by the continous fast flowing arterial blood.

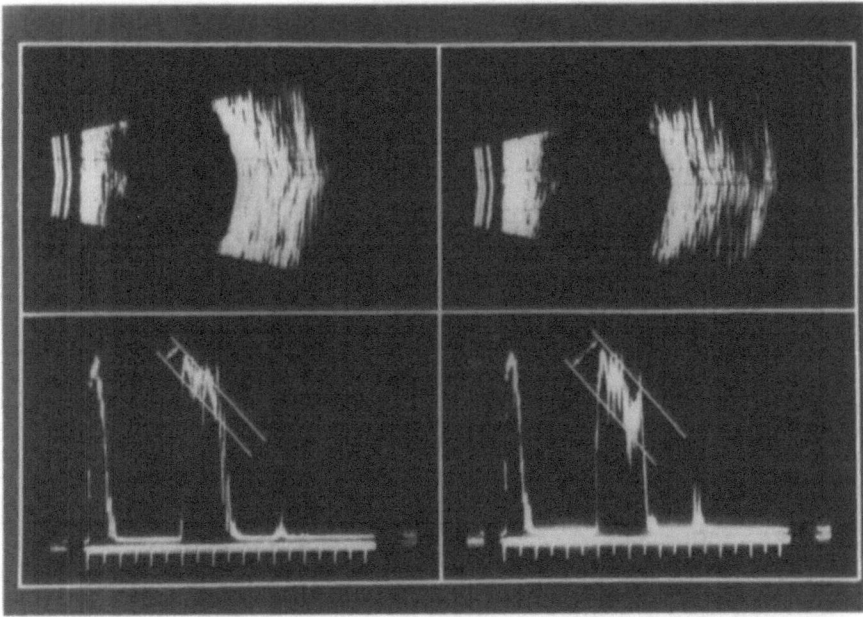

Fig. 2. (left top) Normal trans-ocular B-scan produced by placing the horizontally held probe against the 6 o'clock limbus and aiming into the superior orbit. Note that the orbital pattern is wider *(right top)* in this patient with 'slow-flow' fistula. Also note the absence of a dilated superior ophthalmic vein. *(left bottom)* Normal trans-ocular standardized A-scan (through same region as above B-scans) with Kretz 7200 MA at 'Tissue Sensitivity'. Contrast this with *(right bottom)* the standardized A-scan through the same region in a patient with 'slow-flow' fistula. Note that the vertical amplitude of the fat echoes is higher, and that the fat thickness is greater in the congested (right bottom) orbit.

524

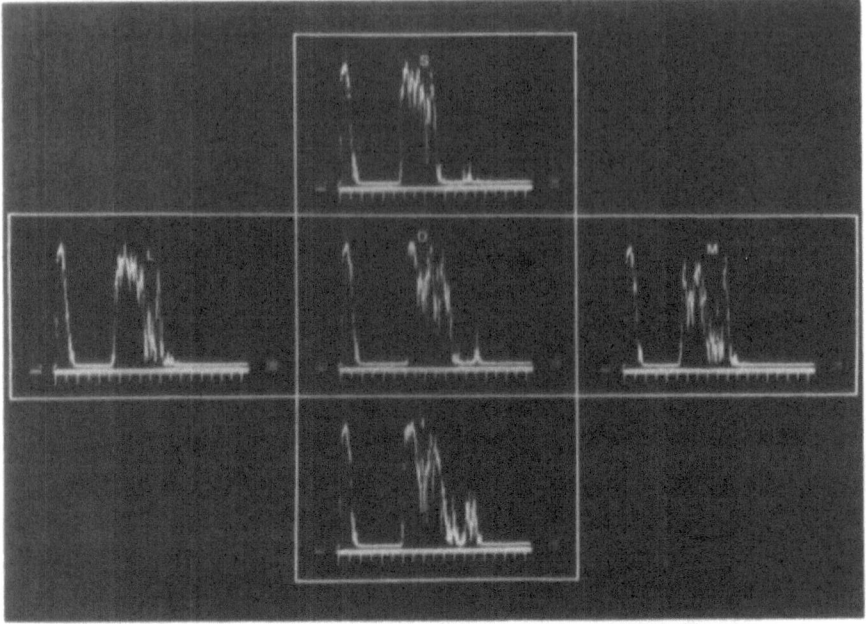

Fig. 3. Trans-ocular standardized A-scan echograms of maximum thickness of medical (M), superior (S), lateral (L), and inferior (I) rectus muscles, and optic nerve (O). These structures are demonstrated as sharply outlined defects in the orbital pattern and are wider in this orbit with 'slow-flow' fistula, than in the normal fellow orbit as demonstrated in Fig. 4.

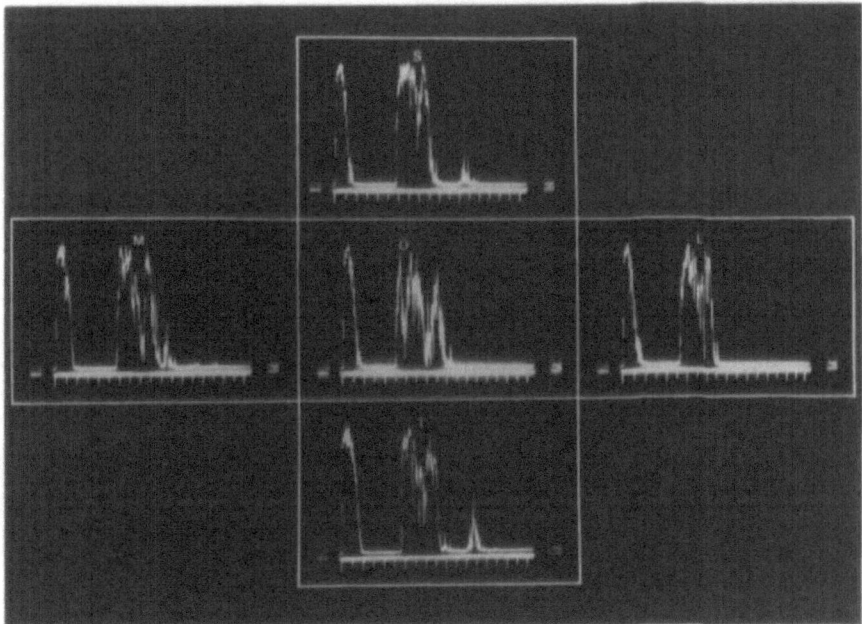

Fig. 4. See Fig. 3 for explanation.

References

1. Phelps CD, Thompson HS, Ossoinig KC. 1982. The diagnosis and prognosis of atypical carotid – cavernous fistula (Red – Eyed Shunt Syndrome) AJO 93: 423–436.
2. Grove AS JR. The dural shunt syndrome, pathophysiology and clinical course. Reprint request to Arthur S. Grove, JR. M.D., Massachusetts Eye and Ear Infirmary, 243 Charles St., Boston, MA 02114.

Superior ophthalmic vein thrombosis – an echographic diagnosis

K.C. OSSOINIG, E. FRIELING, C. TAMBURRELLI and L. WARNER
Iowa City, USA

Introduction

The echographic findings of a dilated superior ophthalmic vein, which contains fast blood-flow, have long been recognized as being specific for intracranial arteriovenous fistulas [1, 2, 3]. More recently, such fistulas were classified as 'fast-flow' or 'high-flow' fistulas [3, 4], draining blood from the cavernous sinus through an orbit anteriorly toward the angular and facial veins, and/or inferiorly into the inferior ophthalmic vein. The faster the blood flows through an orbital vein, the faster the blood spikes move on the screen in a vertical flickering mode, and the lower is the reflectivity of this blood. This kinetic and quantitative A-scan evaluation together with Doppler echography allows a fairly accurate judgment of the severity of a fistula. As long as there is blood flow noticeable by kinetic A-scan and Doppler echography, and the blood spikes are lower than 40% of the display height at Tissue Sensitivity of the standardized A-scan instrument, the intracranial fistula is classified as fast-flow and draining.

The intracranial A-V fistulas of the type which congests an orbit by not allowing normal drainage of the orbital blood through the superior ophthalmic vein into and through the cavernous sinus, and which subsequently thicken all extraocular muscles as well as the optic-nerve sheaths rather than dilating the superior ophthalmic vein and its anastomosing vessels, have been termed 'slow-flow' or 'low-flow' fistulas [3, 4] causing the red-eye shunt syndrome [5]. Between these two extremes of orbital involvement in intracranial arteriovenous fistulas, a wide spectrum of patients has been noted to present more of either the draining or the congestive signs of the disease.

In recent years, another type of congestion of the orbit has been observed in 6 patients suffering from thrombosis of the superior ophthalmic vein. The echographic signs of such a thrombosis are presented and discussed in this report.

K.C. Ossoinig (editor), Ophthalmic Echography, ISBN 978-94-010-7988-4
© 1987, Martinus Nijhoff/Dr W. Junk Publishers, Dordrecht.

528

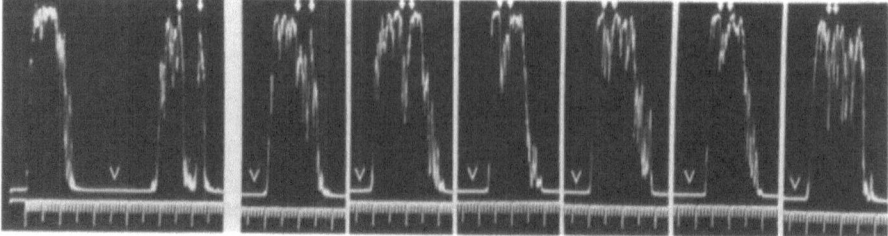

Fig. 1. Series of A-scans (photomontage) obtained during a scan along the superior ophthalmic vein in a patient with thrombosis of this vein. The sequence of echograms from left to right illustrates cross-sections of the vein from its most anterior medial portion (left) to increasingly more posterior sections. The defects in the orbital echograms, which represent slowly moving blood (approximately 10% high, slightly blurred spikes) and thrombus (60–80% high spikes), are outlined by very high, steeply falling or rising surface spikes from the vessel walls on each side (arrows). Note the decreasing width of the vessel and the suddenly increased reflectivity (increased spike height) of its contents as the sound beam glides to more posterior sections of the vein (from left to right in the photomontage). V = vitreous cavity.

Echographic signs

Six patients with thrombosis of the superior ophthalmic vein have been studied using Standardized Echography. In 2 of the cases the thrombosis was caused by cerebral abscesses in the region of the cavernous sinus. In 4 of the patients thrombosis of the superior ophthalmic vein resulted in a complication of cavernous sinus arteriovenous fistulas. In each case sudden onset or worsening of proptosis was accompanied by marked lid swelling, engorgement of the epibulbar vessels, and other signs and symptoms of acute orbital congestion. In all cases the clinical signs and symptoms as well as the echographic findings, discussed below, improved after several weeks following antibiotic therapy (2 infectious cases), or ceased spontaneously after several months duration (4 A-V fistulas).

1. Superior ophthalmic vein

As in fast-flow arteriovenous fistulas, the superior ophthalmic vein is dilated when thrombosed; however, dilatation is only moderate and is seen mostly anteriorly. The more posterior portions of the vein are much less dilated and are high-reflective (Fig. 1). Even the low-reflective anterior portion shows very little movement during kinetic evaluation, indicating fluid but slow-moving blood. The high reflectivity of the contents of the vein in its posterior portion is consistent with thrombosis. Doppler studies of thrombosed superior ophthalmic veins are negative. Because of the high reflectivity of the thrombus, the vein is difficult or impossible to display in B-scan echograms. Even

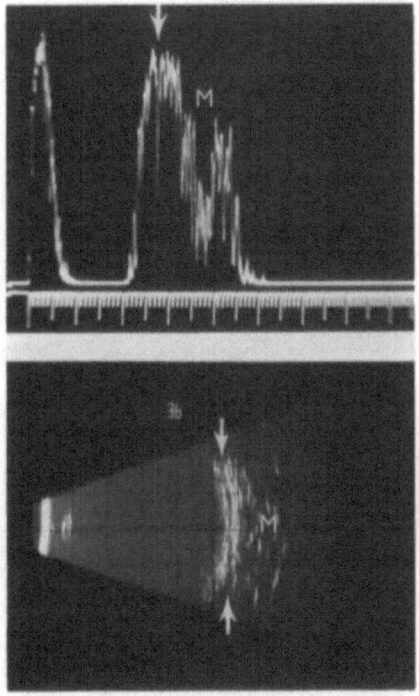

Fig. 2. Echograms from a thin vertical vein (arrow) in a normal orbit. M = medial rectus muscle.

using A-scan echography only the most anterior, low-reflective portion of the vein is easy to detect. In contrast to fast-flow arteriovenous fistulas, the dilatation of the superior ophthalmic vein is a secondary echographic finding in a thrombosed vein. The echographic key to the diagnosis of superior ophthalmic vein thrombosis is the detection and evaluation of another vessel: the so-called vertical vein.

2. Vertical vein

A medial orbital vein is one of the anastomoses between the superior and inferior ophthalmic veins in the mid-orbit. This vessel branches from the superior ophthalmic vein before that vein crosses over the optic nerve, and takes a vertical and slightly forward course between the optic nerve and the anterior portion of the medial rectus muscle before communicating with the inferior ophthalmic vein. Because of its almost straight, vertical course this vessel is termed the 'vertical vein'; it can be found echographically even in normals (Fig. 2).

In order to display the vertical vein on B-scan, the probe is placed vertically

530

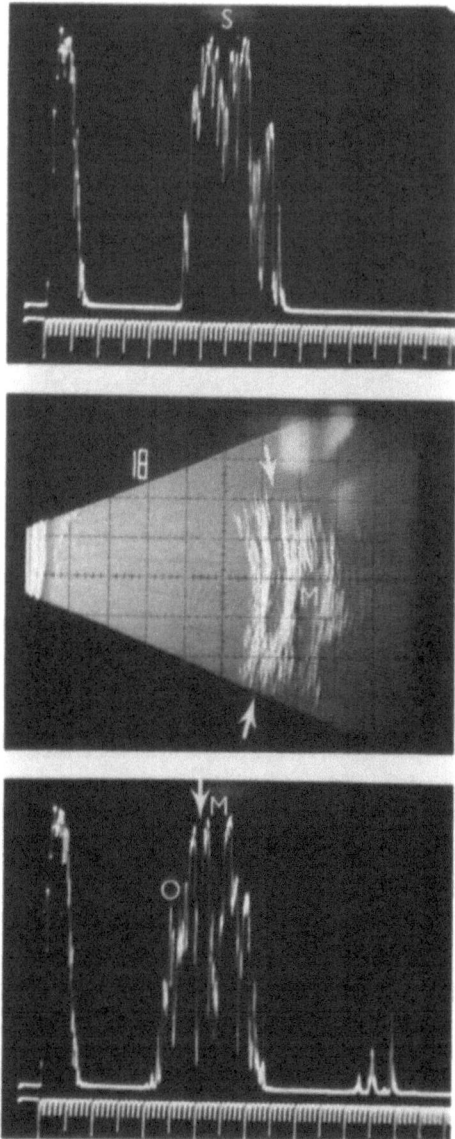

Fig. 3. Transocular echograms from a thrombosed superior ophthalmic vein (S in top A-scan), and a markedly dilated vertical vein (arrows in B-scan and bottom A-scan) in a patient with a cerebral abscess near the cavernous sinus). M = medial rectus pattern; O = optic nerve reached by an oblique beam.

across the lateral horizontal meridian (9 o'clock when examining the right orbit, 3 o'clock on the left side). After displaying the inserting tendon of the medial rectus muscle, the acoustic section is angled posteriorly until the most anterior portion of the optic nerve is displayed. Then the probe and acoustic

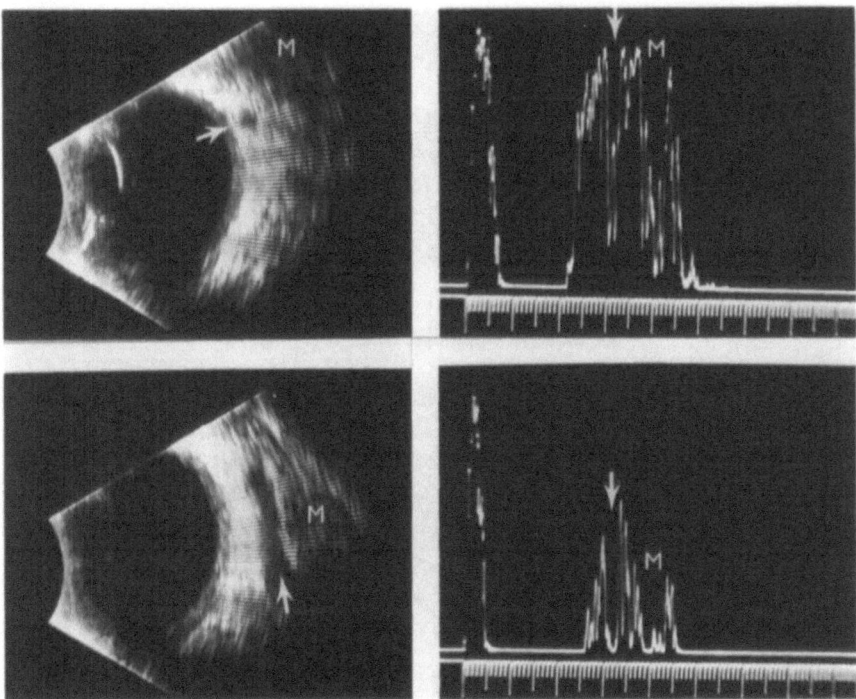

Fig. 4. Transocular echograms from a markedly dilated vertical vein (arrows) in a patient with fast-flow arteriovenous fistula. The top B-scan displays a horizontal section through the eye and orbit slightly above the insertion of the optic nerve. The bottom B-scan represents a vertical, slightly tilted (see text) section through the medial mid-orbit. The top A-scan was obtained at Tissue Sensitivity (technique described in text), whereas the bottom A-scan was documented with low Measuring Sensitivity. The width of the vertical vein may be measured by correlating the horizontal distance between the peaks of the surface spikes representing the vessel wall on either side of the low-reflective 'defect' marked by the arrow with the electronic measuring scale (at Measuring Sensitivity). M = pattern of the medial rectus muscle.

section are angled minimally forward again until the optic-nerve pattern disappears. At this point the probe is slightly tilted (superior end of probe posteriorly, inferior end anteriorly) and minimally angled until the vertical vein becomes visible as a thin, dark line. Care must be taken to optimize resolution by significantly decreasing the system sensitivity (Fig. 2).

On A-scan examination, the probe is placed as it is for an examination of the medial rectus muscle [3]. The inserting tendon of this muscle is displayed at Tissue Sensitivity. Then the probe and sound beam are angled posteriorly until a tiny, well-outlined depression is displayed on the left side of the medial-rectus pattern (arrow in Fig. 2). The vertical vein pattern appears before the optic-nerve is reached by the beam.

When blood flow through the superior ophthalmic vein is blocked by a

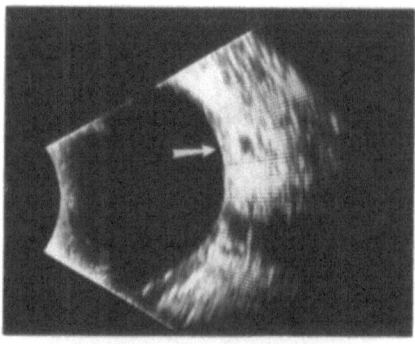

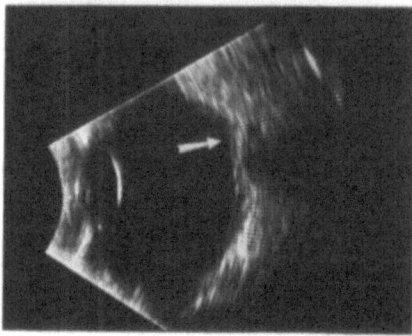

Fig. 5. Horizontal axial B-scan echograms from the dilated vertical vein in the case described in Figure 4. Both B-scans display the insertion of the optic nerve together with a cross-section of the vertical vein (arrow). The bottom echogram was obtained in straight gaze with both structures in close approximation; the top echogram was displayed with nasal gaze direction, the optic nerve remote from the vein.

thrombus the blood backs up and congests the orbit, thereby opening up and widening the vertical vein. Then the blood slowly drains through the vertical vein and other anastomoses leaving the orbit through other channels such as the inferior ophthalmic vein, the angular vein and the ethmoidal veins. A dilated vertical vein is readily displayed by both the A-scan and the B-scan with the techniques described above (Fig. 3–9).

The reflectivity of the blood within a dilated vertical vein is low to medium (less than 50% spike height at Tissue Sensitivity as shown in Figs. 3 and 4). Neither A-scan nor Doppler echography reveal a significant flow of blood. These quantitative and kinetic findings indicate that the blood is fluid, but that it is stagnant, or flows slowly within the dilated vertical vein.

3. Other anastomosing vessels

In orbits with obstructed or decreased outflow facilities, other veins too

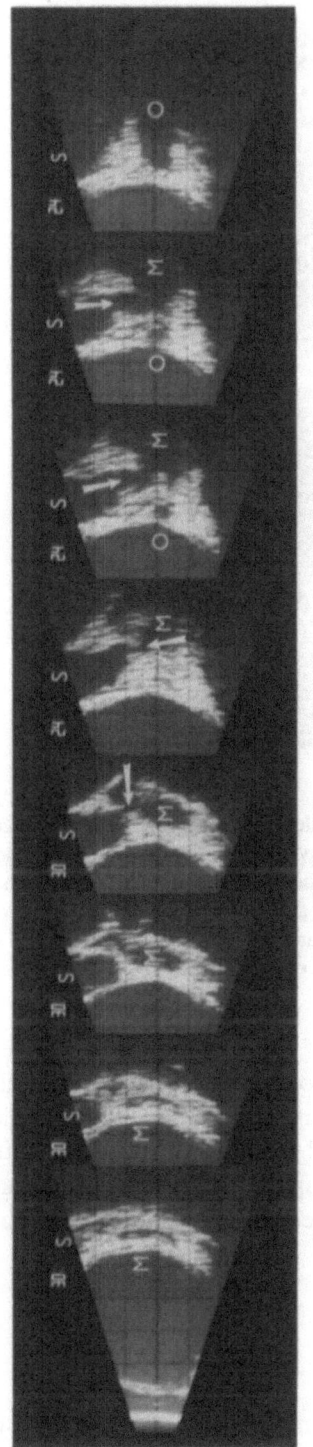

Fig. 6. Series of vertical (transverse) B-scans (photomontage) from the markedly dilated (ampulla-like) anterior portion (S) of an otherwise thrombosed superior ophthalmic vein, and from the largely dilated vertical vein (arrows) in a patient with intracranial fast-flow arteriovenous fistula. The initial left echogram shows a cross-section of the inserting tendon of the medial rectus muscle (M), and a tangential cut through the most anterior part of the ampulla-like dilatation. As the probe and acoustic section are continuously angled to the posterior (echograms from left to right), the muscle pattern gets wider and shifts toward the medial orbital wall; the ampulla-like distension of the superior ophthalmic vein then increases in size and opens up toward the large vertical vein (arrows). Finally, the optic nerve (O) comes into the picture.

534

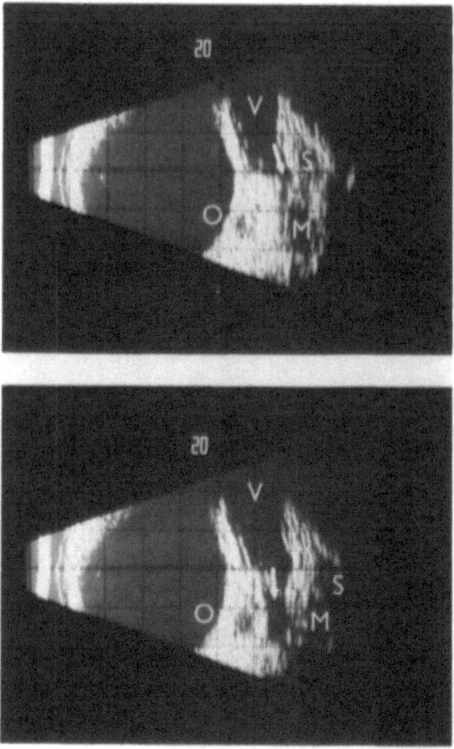

Fig. 7. Vertical B-scan echograms from the same case as illustrated in Fig. 6. The acoustic sections were aimed at the nasal edge of the inserting optic nerve (O). The acoustic sections also cut through the ampulla-like distension of the anterior portion of the superior ophthalmic vein (V), the medial rectus (M), the superior oblique (S) muscles, and through the vertical vein (arrows). The top echogram represents a peripheral cut along the antero-nasal margin of the vertical vein, whereas the bottom echogram shows the maximal width of this vessel.

become widened. This is particularly true of the anterior ethmoidal veins, which can be seen as multiple, small, low-to-medium reflective cavernous spaces in both the A-scans and the B-scans from that area (Fig. 9). While blood flow may not be detected within the ethmoidal veins in either fast-flow fistulas or in orbits with superior ophthalmic vein thrombosis by kinetic A-scan or Doppler, this blood flow is usually documented within the angular vein in all cases (Fig. 9).

The difference

A widening of the superior ophthalmic vein, the vertical vein and other anastomosing vessels within the orbit is seen in patients with fast-flow ar-

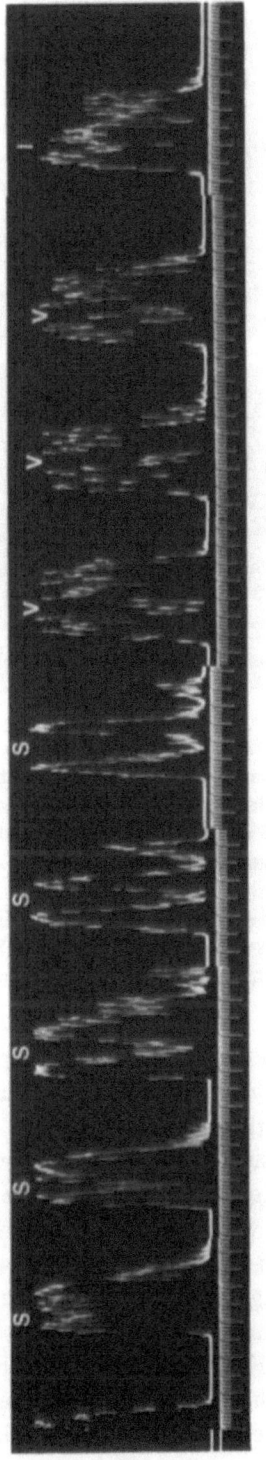

Fig. 8. Series of transocular A-scans (photomontage) from the right orbit of the case, also shown in Figures 6 and 7, tracing the anterior half of the superior ophthalmic vein (S) and the vertical vein (V) as it courses down toward the inferior ophthalmic vein (I). The left echogram shows a cross-section of the thrombosed part of the superior ophthalmic vein (high reflectivity). The second to fifth echograms (from left) display the ever-widening, most anterior portion of the superior ophthalmic vein. The fourth echogram (from right) represents a cut through the vertical vein near its upper end. The echograms following toward the right show lower cross-sections of the vertical vein, and the last echogram on the right displays a cross-cut through the inferior ophthalmic vein. During this scanning procedure, the probe was initially placed at 7 o'clock and the beam was aimed into the mid-to-posterior orbit at 1 o'clock (left echogram); then the beam was angled and shifted in a circular fashion following the course of the vessels, toward the anterior and inferior, and again to the posterior. The right echogram was obtained from the inferior ophthalmic vein with the probe placed at 10 : 30 o'clock and the beam aimed into the mid-to-posterior orbit at 4:30 o'clock.

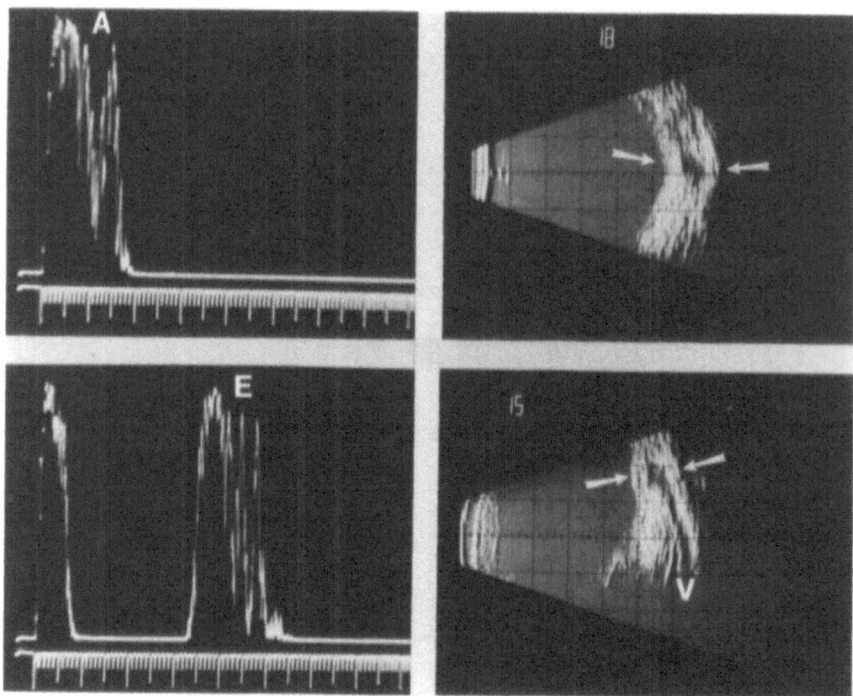

Fig. 9. Echograms from a patient with thrombosis of the superior ophthalmic vein caused by cerebral abscess. The top A-scan was obtained from the angular vein (A) by placing the probe over it. The bottom A-scan represents an area of engorged and dilated ethmoidal veins (low-reflective cavernous spaces separated by high spikes from the vessel walls; E). The top B-scan shows a longitudinal cut along the horizontal medial meridian in front of the optic nerve; it displays a cross-section of the dilated vertical vein (V), and on its nasal side (above the vein pattern in the echogram) an area of cavernous spaces representing dilated and engorged ethmoidal veins (E). The bottom B-scan represents a vertical cut along the course of the dilated vertical vein (V) as it emerges from the slightly more dilated, most anterior end of the superior ophthalmic vein (arrow).

teriovenous fistulas as well as in patients with thrombosis of the superior ophthalmic vein. The difference between these two conditions, and a clear-cut one for that matter, lies in important details of the widening:

In cases of superior ophthalmic vein thrombosis, the widening of this vessel is minor and much less prominent than that of the vertical vein. However, the most anterior portion of the superior ophthalmic vein always widens markedly (Fig. 1), often in an ampulla-like fashion (Figs. 6–8). This wide portion of the superior ophthalmic vein is low-reflective, though not as low-reflective as in arteriovenous fistulas when the blood moves much faster; in contrast, the posterior portion of the vein is high-reflective (Fig. 1) because of the thrombosis. Blood flow is not fast in the superior ophthalmic vein, in the vertical vein, or in any other widened anastomosing vessel. Occasionally, minimal movement of blood may be observed with Standardized A-scan; no abnormal Doppler signals are obtained. In contrast, the A-scan displays fast and extensive blood flow and the Doppler response is overwhelmingly strong in fast-flow fistulas. In fast-flow fistulas, the superior ophthalmic vein remains extremely low-reflective right into the superior orbital fissure.

References

1. Ossoinig KC. 1966. Die Ultraschalldiagnostik der Orbita (A-Bildverfahren) [Ger. – Orbital Echography]. Klin Mbl Augenheilk 149: 817.
2. Ossoinig KC, Blodi FC. 1974. Preoperative Differential Diagnosis of Tumors by Echography: IV. Diagnosis of Orbital Tumors. Curr Conc Ophthal 4/17: 313.
3. Ossoinig KC. 1979. Standardized Echography: Basic Principles, Clinical Applications, and Results. Int Ophthal Clin 19/4: 127.
4. Ossoinig KC. 1981. Echographic Differentiation of Vascular Tumors in the Orbit. Proc SIDUO VIII (J.M. Thijssen and A.M. Verbeek, eds.), Docum Ophthal Proc series, 29: 283.
5. Phelps CD, Thompson HS, Ossoinig KC. 1982. The Diagnosis and Prognosis of Atypical Carotid-Cavernous Fistula (Red-Eyed Shunt Syndrome). Am J Ophthal 93: 423.

From the Echographic Service of the Department of Ophthalmology, University of Iowa Hospitals and Clinics. This research was supported in part by an unrestricted grant from Research to Prevent Blindness.

Reprint requests to Karl C. Ossoinig, M.D., C.S. O'Brien Library, Department of Ophthalmology, University of Iowa Hospitals, Iowa City, Iowa 52242, U.S.A.

Results of ophthalmodynamometry and directional Doppler ultrasound in ophthalmic diseases

H.G. TRIER, H.G. LÜNEBORG and R. ROTHE
Bonn, West-Germany

Macroangiopathies of the ophthalmic artery and its branches can cause a number of eye diseases. Most often, the vascular pathology is confined to those segments of the common and internal carotid artery which are located proximally to the ophthalmic artery, although sometimes the changes can be confined only to the branches of the ophthalmic artery, which are the central retinal artery and the ciliary arteries. Accordingly, organs distal to these diseased vascular segments are affected. More than 75% of patients with stroke have preceeding ischemic attacks with vision related symptoms, so that quite often the patient with underlying carotid vascular disease will first present to the ophthalmologist.

A number of non-invasive techniques can be used by the ophthalmologist to detect carotid vascular diseases (Table 1). The techniques we concentrated on in this study were Doppler ultrasound and measurement of ophthalmic artery pressure by means of ophthalmodynamometry.

The purpose of this retrospective study was first, to investigate if routine Doppler ultrasound examination techniques alone enable a precise diagnosis and second, to determine the value of supplementing the Doppler examination with ophthalmodynamometry and/or i.v. or i.a. angiography.

Table 1. Non-invasive examination methods.

- Oculoplethysmography
- Oculosphygmography (e.g. Mackay-Marg; Stepanik)
- Ophthalmodynamometry (impression/suction)
- Combined methods
    Ocular pneumoplethysmography (Gee)
    Ocular oscillodynamography (Ulrich)
- Doppler ultrasound
    directional CW-Doppler
    Doppler-imaging
    Duplex-scanning

K.C. Ossoinig (editor), Ophthalmic Echography, ISBN 978-94-010-7988-4

Table 2. Clinical symptoms and findings.

Transient
- amaurosis fugax
- other intermittent disturbances of monocular or binocular vision
- vascular headache

Permanent
- decrease in vision
- visual field loss
- optic disk edema or atrophy
- unilateral cataract
- unilateral rubeosis iridis
- retinal vascular occlusions

The patients examined had been refered to the Bonn University Eye Clinic with a variety of symptoms and pathological findings as shown in Table 2. All patients were examined using compression ophthalmodynamometry according to Weigelin and Lobstein, and continuous-wave Doppler ultrasound (Table 3). Ophthalmodynamometry (ODM) was performed by two experienced examiners. One of the examiners compressed the eye on the temporal sclera with a dynamometer, while the other examiner observed the pulsation phenomena of the retinal vessels on the optic disc with an ophthalmoscope. At the same time, blood pressure was measured in the brachial artery. Findings were graded as pathological according to Weigelin and Lobstein if the difference in mean ophthalmic artery pressure on both sides was greater than 3 mm Hg or deviated more than 9 mm Hg from the nominal value derived from the ipsilateral brachial artery pressure.

Prior to Doppler examination, the common carotid and superficial temporal artery were palpated. Then, direct Doppler examination of the vessels of the neck was performed in the following sequence: common carotid, external carotid, and internal carotid artery. The audio signal was evaluated and recorded in a number of cases.

Next, indirect Doppler examination was performed by placing the flow-

Table 3. Examination methods.

---

1. Ophthalmodynamometry – compression method – (Weigelin & Lobstein, 1962)

2. Directional CW-Doppler (Delalande. 4 MHz)
   with: audio output
         flow velocity meter
         strip chart recorder

Table 4. Results.

	n
Patients examined	50
Doppler and ODM normal	35
Doppler and/or ODM pathological	15
Angiography findings known	8

probe over the supratrochlear artery at the medial angle of each orbit. Direction and velocity of flow were noted. Compression tests of the facial and superficial temporal artery were then performed. By means of a strip chart recording with Doppler shift calibration marks, quantitative flow evaluation according to Reuter and Trier is enabled.

A total of 50 patients were examined (Table 4). Of these, 35 had normal Doppler and ODM findings, 15 had pathological Doppler and/or ODM findings. These 15 patients were refered to angiography: to date 8 angiography reports have been obtained. We compared the conformity of ODM findings with the Doppler ultrasound findings (Table 5). It was remarkable that Doppler and ODM findings did not coincide. Of the 41 patients with normal Doppler findings, 35 patients also had normal, but 6 had pathological ODM findings. Of the 9 patients with pathological Doppler findings, 4 also had pathological, but 5 had normal ODM findings.

We also compared the conformity of angiography findings with Doppler and ODM (Table 6). In 3 out of 8 patients conformity of angiography, Doppler and ODM was present. In 4 other patients there was conformity of the angiography with the ODM, but not with the Doppler results. In one patient the normal angiography could not explain the pathological Doppler and ODM findings. So, we can see that the Doppler examination alone, as we performed it, does not offer a solution to all ophthalmological problems related to carotid vascular disease.

Table 5. Conformity of ODM with Doppler.

		Doppler	
		normal	pathol.
ODM	normal	35	5
	pathol.	6	4
Total number of patients: 50			

Table 6. Conformity of angiography findings with Doppler and ODM findings.

		n
Conformity of	Doppler and ODM	3
angiography with:	ODM only	4
	Doppler only	0
No conformity	Doppler and ODM	1
Total no. of patients n = 8.		

Schoop and *Neuerburg-Heusler* compared arteriography with Doppler and were able to show that by using a combination of direct and indirect Doppler examination a sensitivity of 80 to 90% and a specifity of 98% could be achieved.

Even though Doppler technique has been refined and has become more and more sophisticated, for example: spectral analysis and flow-imaging combined with B-scan imaging of the carotid vessels, we believe that an isolated Doppler approach seems not to be an ideal method for the ophthalmologist. The combination of Doppler ultrasound and measurement of the ophthalmic artery pressure seems to be more reliable. ODM as one of these methods has not only proven to be quite sensitive in detecting carotid disease but also offers a potential for quantitative assessment of peripheral intracranial flow resistance.

In conclusion, it has to be reflected on why Doppler and ODM findings do not always coincide. In carotid stenosis, for example, the Doppler will usually be pathological, whereas ODM can be normal. Probably, the normal pressure in the ophthalmic artery is maintained by collateral blood flow from the circle of Willis at the base of the brain. Therefore, this normal ODM result should not be put off as a false negative finding, but valued as additional information on the potential collateral capacity of the involved cerebral hemisphere (Weigelin et al., Imre et al.). The prognosis of carotid stenosis for the patient and the indication for surgery can thus be judged not only by the location and degree of the stenosis, but also by the potential for collateral compensation (Eikelboom).

Another point worth mentioning is that a pathological Doppler over the supratrochlear artery does not always mean that carotid artery disease is present, but can be due to localized disease, for example trauma or inflammation of the supratrochlear artery itself.

Furthermore, if the ophthalmic or central retinal artery are occluded, ODM cannot rule out disease of the internal carotid artery.

Why did the angiography results not always coincide with the Doppler and

ODM findings? This could be due to the fact that, at our clinic, classic arteriography is being replaced more and more by intravenous digital subtraction angiography. We believe that this technique does not always allow adequate evaluation of the intracranial vessels and, therefore, intracranial lesions can be missed. In this way, we believe that angiography should not be regarded as the absolute 'gold'-standard for verifying the presence of carotid artery disease.

Acknowledgement

We acknowledge the skilled assistance of the nurses Elli Matern and Alla Purer and of Roland Müller-Breitenkamp, M.D. in examining the patients and evaluating the material.

References

Eikelboom BC. 1981. Evaluation of carotid artery disease and potential collateral circulation by ocular pneumoplethysmography. Proefschrift (Diss.) Leiden.

Imre G, Mesko E, Salacz G, Bögi J. 1978. Carotis-kerimgészavarok okozta szemtünetekröl és azok eredetének non invasiv kimutatásáról. (Carotis-kreislaufbedingte Augenerkrankungen. Ätiologie und Nachweis durch nicht-invasive Untersuchungsmethoden.) Orvosi Hetilap 119: 1349–1353.

Reuter R, Trier HG. 1983. Der Doppler-Simulator DS 81. Eine neue Kalibriermethode für Ultraschall-cw-Doppler-Blutfluß-Meßgeräte. Ultraschall 4: 188–192.

Schoop W, Neuerburg-Heusler D. 1980. Ann Radiol 23: 265–267.

Weigelin E, Lobstein A. 1962. Ophthalmodynamometrie (Karger, Basel/New York).

Weigelin E, Iwata K, Halder M. 1964. Fortschritte auf dem Gebiet der Blutdruckmessung am Auge. Fortschr Augenheilk 15: 44–184 (Karger, Basel/New York).

Echographical diagnosis of lacrimal sac tumors

R. ROCHELS, U. SCHERER, A. NOVER and W. LIEB
Mainz, FRG

Introduction

Tumors of the lacrimal drainage system are rare (Duke-Elder and MacFaul, 1974; Busse and Hollwich, 1978); in the literature there are only 282 reported cases until 1984. They can be devided into epithelial tumors (benign: squamous cell papilloma, transitional papilloma; malignant: squamous cell, transitional cell and adeno-carcinoma), those of the melanogenic system (benign: nevi; malignant: melanoma) as well as cysts and tumor-like lesions (Zimmerman, 1980). The clinical course of lacrimal sac tumors is almost uniform: epiphora, swelling of the medial canthus, stenosis of the drainage system with consecutive dacryocystitis, sometimes bloodstained discharge as a diagnostic sign and finally ulceration through the skin and/or infiltration of the ethmoidal or maxillary sinus (Duke-Elder and MacFaul, 1974; Busse and Hollwich, 1978; Royer et al., 1982). The early diagnosis of lacrimal sac tumors is rarely achieved: dacryocystography may show partial or complete occlusion of the duct with consecutive dilation of the sac, filling defects and wall irregularities (Gulotta and v. Denffer, 1980). Echography has proved to be a very useful method in the examination of the drainage system (Rochels and Hackelbusch, 1982; Montanara et al., 1983; Rochels et al., 1984 a); in 1982 we detected the first sac tumor by sonography.

Materials and methods

Since then we have done A- and B-scan echography in eight patients with primary lacrimal sac tumors (4 transitional cell carcinomas, 1 squamous cell carcinoma, 1 papilloma, 1 squamous cell papilloma, 1 pyogenic granuloma) and in further six patients with tumors of the ethmoidal sinus secondarily invading the sac (2 transitional cell carcinomas, 2 fibrosarcomas, 1 adenocystical carcinoma, 1 mucoepidermoidal tumor). Standardized A-scan sonography

K.C. Ossoinig (editor), Ophthalmic Echography, ISBN 978-94-010-7988-4

© 1987, Martinus Nijhoff/Dr W. Junk Publishers, Dordrecht.

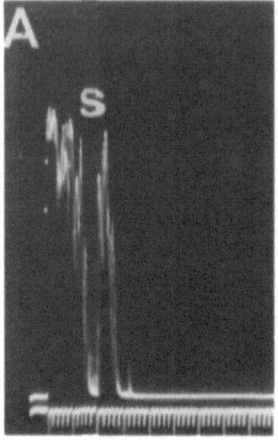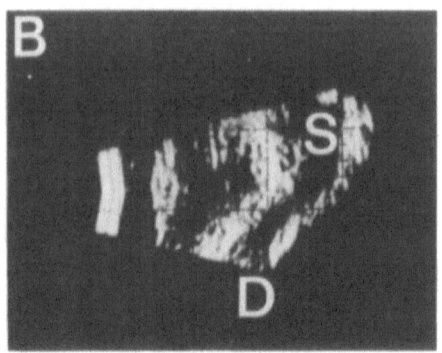

Fig. 1. A- and B-scan of the normal drainage system. *Fig. 1A*. A-scan: the lacrimal sac (S) is outlined by two high, doublepeaked spikes following an echochain from the skin; the contents of the sac is echofree. *Fig. 1B*. B-scan: the vertical section shows the sac (S) and duct (D).

was done with the Kretz-Technik machine 7200 MA using a probe with a frequency of 8 MHz, B-scan sonography with the Bronson-Turner, Xenotec- and Ocuscan 400 machine (probe frequency 10 MHz). The drainage system can either be evaluated by directly placing the probe on the medial lid region or through the globe (transocular examination) with the probe being placed on the anesthesized conjunctiva in the lateral palpebral fissure.

Normal findings

In A-scan (Fig. 1A) the *lacrimal sac* is characterized by two very high spikes following the initial signal and some overloaded spikes from the skin. Between the two separate spikes from the external and internal wall there is a short zero-line caused by the aqueous contents of the sac. Mild pressure of the probe against the sac causes its collapse. In vertical B-scan sections (Fig. 1B) the contours of the sac are sharply outlined; the *sinus of Arlt* and the passage to the *duct* are clearly displayed. In horizontal sections the sac causes a roundish, echo-free area.

Clinical findings

Small tumors of the sac can be argued if in the A-scan picture (Fig. 2A) it is dilated and presents with areas of low reflectivity from the inflammatory

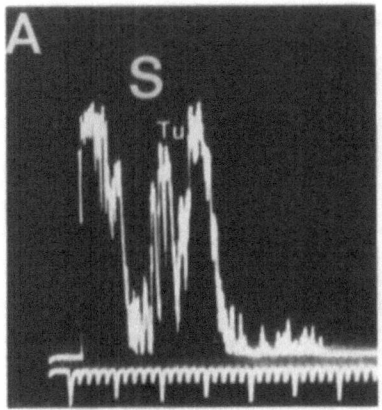
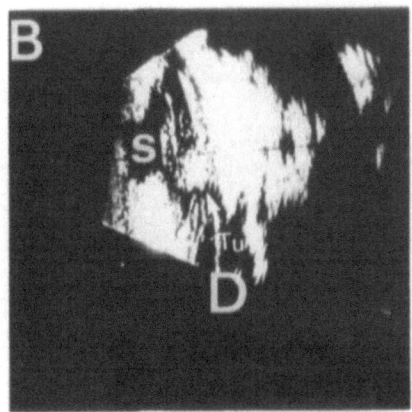

Fig. 2. A- and B-scan of a small sac tumor (histology: pyogenic granuloma) emanating from the inner sac wall. *Fig. 2A.* A-scan: the echogram of the sac (S) is widened and consists of a low reflective (inflammation, I) and an irregular, high reflective part (tumor, Tu). As a sign of infiltration, the internal wall is multipeaked. *Fig. 2B.* B-scan: the mushroom-shaped tumor (Tu) at the border of the sac (S) to the duct (D) is clearly visible.

contents and some steeply rising, high spikes from a solid mass. This medium to high reflectivity of the tumor can be explained by histology with a mixture of extensive tumor cell and stromal formations. The B-scan picture (Fig. 2B) shows a roundish, sometimes mushroom-shaped solid lesion emanating from the outer or inner wall of the dilated sac.

Large tumors completely filling the lacrimal sac are characterized in A-scan (Fig. 3A) by a broad chain of medium to high echospikes in the dilated sac. Kinetic echography shows some blurred spikes as a sign of blood-stream in tumor-vessels and accounts for a hard, immobile and incompressible lesion. If the sac wall is already infiltrated by the tumor, the external and internal wall-spikes are no longer steeply rising and falling but widened and multipeaked. In the B-scan (Fig. 3B) a dilated, completely filled sac can be displayed in such cases. The tumor itself presents as a more or less homogeneous mass, the sac wall can no longer be clearly visualized as a sign of infiltration.

Tumors of the ethmoidal or maxillary sinus secondarily affecting the lacrimal drainage system can be recognized (Fig. 4) by impression and/or infiltration of the sac, bony defects in the medial canthal region and furthermore by the pathognomonical criteria of periorbital malignancy such as irregular structure, reflectivity and borders, hard consistency, immobility, extraorbital location and varying sound attenuation.

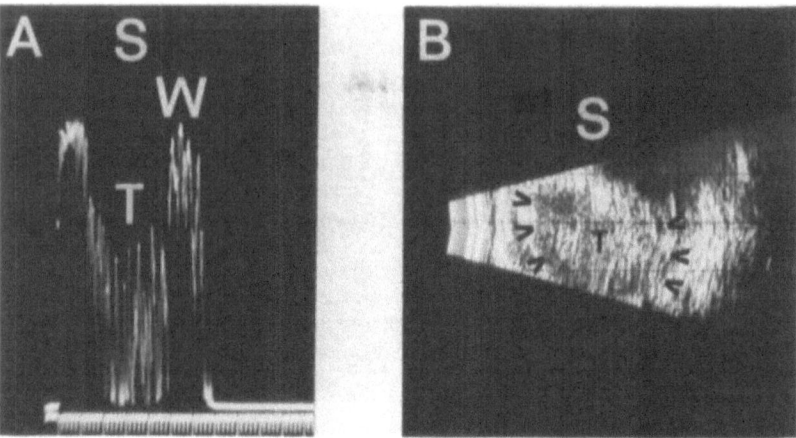

Fig. 3. A- and B-scan of a tumor (histology: squamous cell carcinoma) completely filling the sac. *Fig. 3A.* A-scan: the echogram of the sac (S) is widened, the tumorous contents (T) is of medium reflectivity; the sac wall (W) is multipeaked as a sign of infiltration. *Fig. 3B.* B-scan: the sac (S) is completely filled with a homogeneous tumor (T).

Differential diagnosis

The differential diagnosis of primary and secondary tumors of the lacrimal sac has to take into account acute and chronic dacryocystitis, dacryocystoceles and muco(pyo)celes.

Dacryocystitis is characterized in the A-scan (Fig. 5A) by dilation of the sac and a low to medium regular echogram between the external and internal wall spikes that are not as steeply rising and falling as usual but multipeaked and broadened as a sign of inflammatory wall infiltration. The B-scan picture (Fig. 5B) shows a dilated sac filled with a homogeneous echo pattern. Additionally, the initial echochain is widened in the A- and B-scan by inflammatory thickening of the skin overlying the sac area.

In *dacryocystoceles* the A-scan (Fig. 6A) presents with two zero-lines from the cele and the sac respectively, separated and outlined by three steeply rising and falling, overloaded, doublepeaked echospikes. The B-scan (Fig. 6B) clearly shows the dilated sac, the cele and the communication between them.

The echographical findings in orbital *muco(pyo)celes* such as regular internal structure, low reflectivity, bony defect, sharply outlined borders, roundish shape have been published in detail by Hasenfratz and Ossoinig (1984) and by Rochels et al. (1984b).

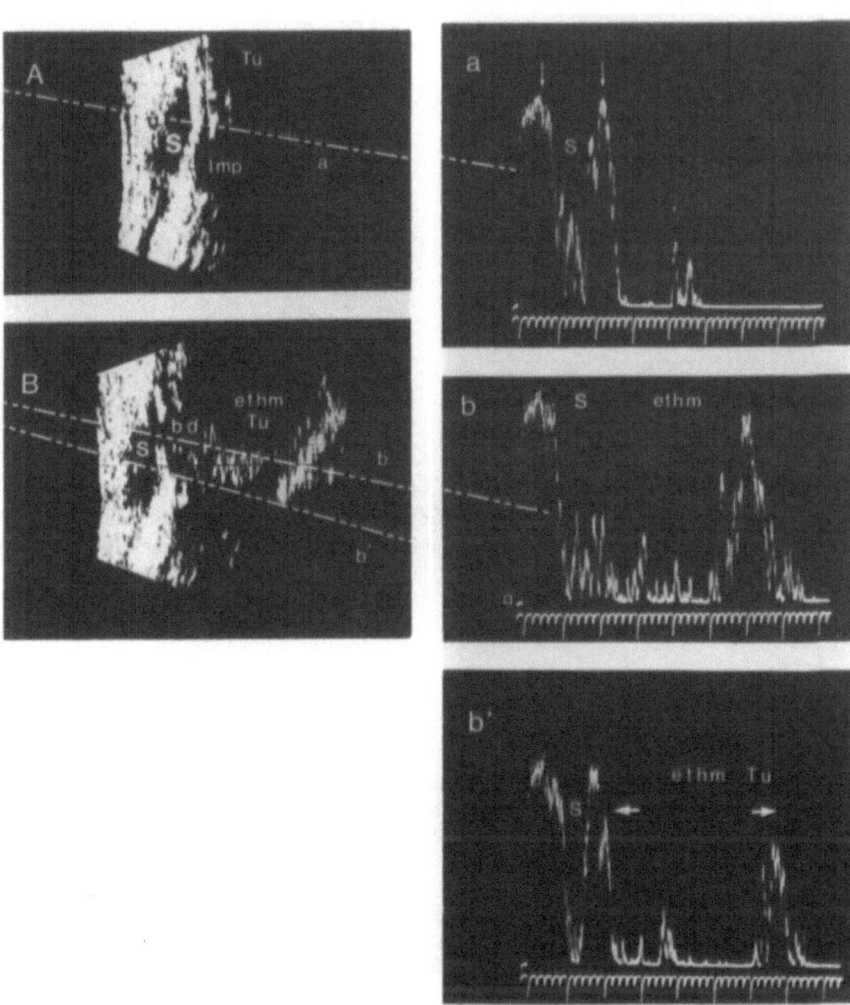

Fig. 4. A- and B-scans of an ethmoidal tumor (histology: transitional cell carcinoma) secondarily invading the drainage system. *Fig. 4A.* B-scan (frontal section): the sac (S) is impressed (Imp) by the tumor (T). *Fig. 4a.* Corresponding A-scan (dotted line a): dilation of the sac (S); low internal echos from mucus. *Fig. 4B.* B-scan (oblique vertical section towards the ethmoidal sinus) displaying a bony defect (bd), infiltration of the internal sac wall and echos from the ethmoidal tumor (ethm Tu). *Fig. 4b.* Corresponding A-scan through the bony defect (dotted line b): irregular echochain from the sac (S) and ethmoid (ethm). The internal sac wall is destroyed causing a homogeneous transition of the irregular echos from the sac to the tumor. *Fig. 4b'.* Corresponding A-scan (dotted line b'): the sac (S) with the intact medial wall and irregular tumor echospikes (ethm Tu) are displayed.

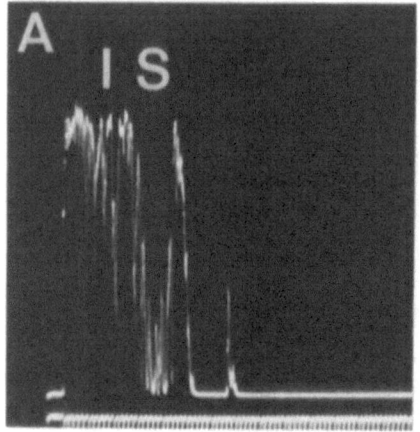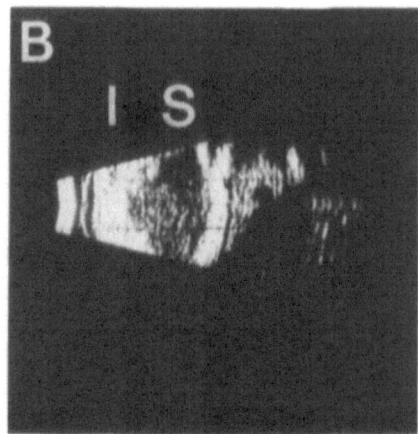

Fig. 5. A- and B-scan in dacryocystitis. *Fig. 5A.* A-scan: extremely high echochain from the infiltrated (I) and thickened skin overlying the dilated sac (S) with low to medium reflective contents (pus). *Fig. 5B.* B-scan: thickened and infiltrated skin (I), dilated sac (S) with heterogeneous contents.

Discussion

A- and B-scan sonography have proved to be a very predicatory and reliable method in the examination of the lacrimal drainage system (Rochels et al., 1984a); malformations such as persistence of the membrane of Hasner and

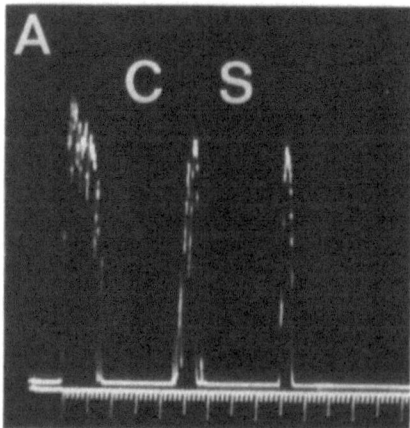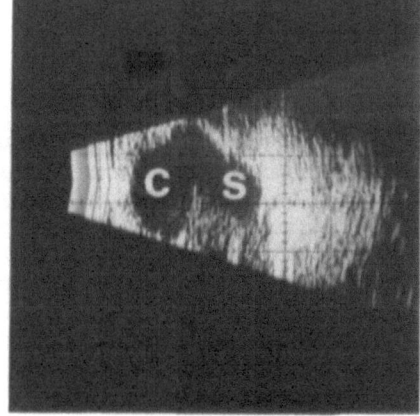

Fig. 6. A- and B-scan of a dacryocystocele. *Fig. 6A.* A-scan: both the cele (C) and the sac (S) without internal echos, delineated by steeply rising, doublepeaked high spikes. *Fig. 6B.* B-scan showing the cele (C), the sac (S) and their communication.

congenital cystoceles as well as inflammatory conditions and their complications (fistula, membrane-formation, stenosis) can easily be detected and differentiated. Furthermore echography helps in the clinical follow-up of surgery of the drainage system. Our first results in eight patients with primary tumors of the lacrimal sac and in six further patients with ethmoidal tumors secondarily invading it have shown that echography is also a very useful method in the early diagnosis of such neoplasias. In contrast to dacryocystography, sonography can display the whole drainage system and not only parts of it above a stenosis or an obstruction caused by a tumor. The A-scan criteria of periorbital malignancy (Ossoinig, 1977) can be used to distinguish between primary and secondary lacrimal sac neoplasias. Thus, standardized A- and B-scan sonography should always be used as a screening method to clarify any suspicious swelling of the medial lid region.

Abstract

The echographical findings of eight lacrimal sac tumors and six ethmoidal neoplasias secondarily affecting the drainage system are reported. In the first group, A-scan sonography displays a medium to highly reflective solid lesion, whereas B-scan presents with a roundish mass obstructing the sac or duct. In ethmoidal tumors an irregular extraorbital echopattern from the paranasal sinus and bony defects can be detected. Furthermore sonography helps in the differential diagnosis of all suspicious swellings in the medial lid region and is thus recommended as a predicatory screening method.

References

Busse H, Hollwich F. 1978. Erkrankungen der ableitenden Tränenwege und ihre Behandlung. Enke, Stuttgart.

Duke-Elder SS, MacFaul PA. 1974. Tumours of the lacrimal sac. In: S.S. Duke-Elder (ed.): System of Ophthalmology, Vol. XIII, Part II, 738–759. Kimpton, London.

Gullotta U, v. Denffer H. 1980. Dacryocystography. An atlas and textbook. Thieme, Stuttgart.

Hasenfratz G, Ossoinig KC. 1984. The diagnosis of orbital mucoceles and pyoceles with standardized echography. In: J.S. Hillman, M.M. LeMay (eds.): Ophthalmic ultrasonography, 407–415. Junk, The Hague.

Montanara A, Mannino G, Contestabile MT. 1983. Macrodacryocystography and echography in diagnosis of disorders of the lacrimal pathways. Surv Ophthalmol 28: 33–41.

Ossoinig KC. 1977. Echography of the eye, orbit, and periorbital region. In: P.H. Arger (ed.): Orbit roentgenology, 224–269. Wiley, New York.

Rochels R, Hackelbusch R. 1982. B-Bild-Echographie bei Erkrankungen der ableitenden Tränenwege. Klin Mbl Augenheilk 181: 181–183.

552

Rochels R, Lieb W, Nover A. 1984a. Echographische Diagnostik bei Erkrankungen der ableitenden Tränenwege. Klin Mbl Augenheilk 185: 243–249.

Rochels R, Geyer G, Bleier R. 1984b. Echographische Diagnostik bei orbitalen Mukozelen.
Laryng. Rhinol. Otol. 64: 181–184.

Royer J, Adenis JP, Bernard JA, Métaireau JP, Rény A. 1982. L'apparail lacrymal. Masson,
Paris.

Zimmerman LE. 1980. Tumours of the lacrimal drainage system. In: L.E. Zimmerman, L.H.
Sobin (eds.): Histological typing of tumours of the eye and its adnexa, 37–38. WHO, Geneva.

Echography in the lacrimal apparatus diagnosis

A. REIBALDI, T. AVITABILE, G.L. SCUDERI and V.V. LORUSSO
Bari, Italy

Introduction

The lacrimal apparatus comprises two components:
- The lacrimal gland, and
- The lacrimal passages.

Obviously the two components are affected by different types of pathology: mainly inflammatory or neoplastic in the gland, inflammatory and consequently obstructive in the passages. The semiological methods of studying this region are multiple and continuously increasing, but only a few of them succeed in going beyond the experimental phase and into everyday practice. They can be grouped as follows:
- Instrumental clinic investigations;
- Radiological investigations (scintigraphy; roentgenocinematography; dacryocystography);
- Echographical investigations.

Of all these techniques echography affords several advantages: easy execution, innocuousness and repeatability. It permits, within certain limits, a tissue diagnosis which, in the case of gland pathology, makes possible the differentiation between an inflammation and a tumor; and in the case of lacrimal passages, the studying of the sac and the nasolacrimal duct before and after a surgical procedure.

Materials and methods

Our aim has not been to show a case report of the different forms of lacrimal passage pathology, but rather to point out their different echographical aspects considering the lack of literature. We will not dwell upon the lacrimal gland aspects since that subject has already been widely examined (Ossoinig 1978). A-scan and B-scan equipment have been used in this study. The

K.C. Ossoinig (editor), Ophthalmic Echography, ISBN 978-94-010-7988-4

following types of pathology have been differentiated by echography:
- Presence or absence of the sac
- Acute dacryocystitis
- Chronic dacryocystitis
- Tumors of the sac
- Congenital dacryocystitis
- Dacryocystectomy
- Dacryocystorhinostomy
- Prosthesis implantation

Presence of absence of the sac

An unusual problem is the presence or absence of the sac, both in young subjects where a congenital lack is suspected, and in older patients in whom the sac was removed but who are unable to explain the operation. The echographical diagnosis is rather simple with the A-scan where, instead of showing an entry and an exit peak through the sac, we can note a series of peaks rapidly decreasing due to the presence of the bone.

Acute dacryocystitis

Echographically in the A-scan we can see a swelling of the sac, and inside the sac a series of low peaks is visible due to the presence of pus. In the B-scan the sac results are dilated and full of echographically dishomogeneous material. The A-scan echography is very useful not only for diagnosis, but also for discovering an eventual extension of the phlogistic process to the paranasal cavities. In fact, in this case we note an enormous extension of the echo pattern.

Chronic dacryocystitis

In both the A- and B-scans the sac swells (although not as it swells in the acute phase) with thicker material, and shows some difficulty in being compressed although peaks heighten in the A-scan. Sometimes the sac is atrophied (Montanara; et al. 1979).

Congenital dacryocystitis

From the echographical point of view it does not differ from the adult form. The role of echography is important in the discovery of the probable presence of congenital anomalies (sac absence or atrophy – stenoses of the first part of the nasolacrimal duct) and the eventual phlogosis extension to the adjacent paranasal cavities. This extension is very dangerous and easily appears in young patients due to the bone thickness.

Sac tumors

Echographically in the A-scan we note a series of irregular peaks often not compressible in an echogram extention due to the bone erosion. Topographically, the B-scan better characterizes the presence of a dishomogeneous mass.

Dacryocystectomy

Refers to what was previously stated in the 'Presence or absence of the sac' paragraph.

Dacryocystorhinostomy

In the A-scan, an echogram extension with a series of very high peaks showing the ultrasonic beam passing through the bone resection can be seen. In the B-scan the bone wall is interrupted by the resection, in which the dimensions and perviousness may be noted.

Prosthesis implantation

Our study concerns the Thorthon's prosthesis exclusively. In the A-scan we noted two high peaks in the sac corresponding to the prosthesis walls. Reduced reflectivity in B-scan prosthesis presence appears as two parallel hyper-reflecting bands inside the sac corresponding to the longitudinal section of the prosthesis. The position and its previousness can be better seen in the B-scan by considering the reduced dimensions of its section and the reflection among the walls.

Conclusion

Lacrimal passage pathology occurs rather frequently and often can be diagnosed by a simple clinical exam. Instrumental investigations, excluding syringing, are not simple procedures to carry out, and nearly always require the use of x-rays (scintigraphy, roentgenocinematography, serial dacryocystography). Echography, on the other hand, can certainly be considered among these diagnostic procedures the easiest and safest to carry out, in addition to its repeatability and low cost. The various pathological types able to be isolated by echography are the following:

556

- Presence or absence of the sac
- Acute dacryocystitis
- Chronic dacryocystitis
- Congenital dacryocystitis

Furthermore, from surgery patients we have singled out the following operations and their function as related to echography:

- Dacryocystectomy
- Dacryocystorhinostomy
- Prosthesis implantation

Besides the aforementioned innocuousness and ease of execution, echography offers the possibility of receiving information about the adjacent paranasal cavity. In the case of surgical patients, echography provides (in addition to an evaluation of the surgical procedure), its functionality, the perviousness of the bone resection in rhinotomy, and determines the correct position and perviousness of a prosthesis. It is limited, on the other hand, due to its inability to investigate the small lacrimal passages, such as the lacrimal canaliculi and the distal part of the nasolacrimal duct. Also, echography is not useful in studying functional lesions, which requires complex radiological methods.

References

1. Avitabile T, Vinci L, D'Ambrosio V, Acquaviva A. 1983. L'ecografia nella patologia delle vie lacrimali di deflusso'. Relaz. VIII Congr. Naz SISUM Bologna 13–15, Nov.
2. Callahan WP, Forbath PG, Besser WDS. 1965. A method of determining the patency of the naso-lacrimal apparatus. Amer J Ophthalm 60: 476.
3. Mazzeo V. 1981. Indicazioni cliniche non comuni della ultrasonografia. Minerva Oftalmologica 23: 65–74.
4. Montanara A, Rizzo P. 1979. Il ruolo delle indagini cliniche e radiologiche nella dimostrazione delle alterazioni lacrimali di tipo funzionale. Analisi critica dei vari procedimenti. Parte I. Boll Ocul 58: 167–185.
5. Montanara A, Rizzo P. 1979. Il valore della dacriocistografia nella diagnosi radiologica delle alterazioni lacrimali organiche e funzionali. Part II. Boll Ocul 58: 187–199.
6. Montanara A, Mannino G, Scorcia G, Fiorillo M, Contestabile MT. 1981. Studio ecografico del sacco lacrimale. Quadri normali. Clinica Oculistica e Patologia Oculare n° 4: 377.
7. Oksala A. 1959. Diagnosis by ultrasound in acute dacryocystitis. Acta Ophthalmol 37: 176.
8. Ossoinig KC. 1978. The Role of Clinical Echography in Modern Diagnosis of Periorbital and Orbital lesions. In G. Bleeker (Ed.), Proceedings of the third International Symposium on Orbital Disorders (Amsterdam, 1977). Amsterdam: Junk, Pp. 496–540.
9. Peyman GA, Sanders DR, Goldberg MF. 1981. Oftalmologia principi e pratica Vol. III, 2254–2255, Verduci Editore Roma.
10. Rochels R, Nover A, Lieb W. 1984. Aussagemöglichkeiten und Grenzen der Echographischen Diagnostik bei Erkrankungen der Ableitenden Tränenwege. VIIth Congress of the European Society of Ophthalmology. Helsinski: 21–25 May.
11. Scorcia G, Montanara A, Mannino G, Martelli M. 1982. Utilità della indagine ecografia nella semeiotica chirurgica delle vie lacrimali di deflusso. Relazione XVI Congresso SOM Viterbo.
12. Scott WE, Fabre JA, Ossoinig KL. 1979. Congenital Mucocele of the Lacrimal Sac. Arch Ophthalmol (Chicago) 97/9 (1965–1658).

Standardized echography in graves' disease

G. HASENFRATZ
Munich, FRG

In major clinical surveys Graves' disease (thyroid ophthalmopathy) is the most common cause of exophthalmos – in about 50% in cases of unilateral and in about 90% in cases with bilateral proptosis [5, 7]. Clinical signs and symptoms are defined and summarized in a number of classifications and modifications (Table 1) [6, 15]. Besides clinical and endocrinologic diagnosis, both of which can be difficult particularly in hypothyroid and euthyroid patients, standardized echography has become very valuable and effective in the diagnosis of Graves' disease [9, 12, 13].

Standardized echography is based on the use of standardized A-scan (specific design for tissue differentiation) complemented by a real-time contact B-scan and, for orbital disorders, by Doppler echography together with specific and standardized examination techniques [8, 9].

Since – besides exact measurements of the thickening of the extraocular muscles that are the predominant sites in orbital involvement in Graves' disease – specific acoustic signs of the thickened muscles were found and other pathologic changes in the orbit and periorbit in this disorder could be demonstrated echographically with this method, standardized echography became the most important and effective additional diagnosing method after clinical

Table 1. Abridged classification of eye changes of graves' disease ('no specs'). ATA (American Thyroid Association) – or Werner – Classification 1977.

Class	Definition
0	No physical signs or symptoms
1	Only signs, no symptoms (signs limited to upper eyelid retraction, stare, and eyelid lag)
2	Soft-tissue involvement (symptoms and signs)
3	Proptosis
4	Extraocular muscle involvement
5	Corneal involvement
6	Sight loss (optic nerve involvement)

K.C. Ossoinig (editor), Ophthalmic Echography, ISBN 978-94-010-7988-4

examination to confirm or rule out thyroid ophthalmopathy (Table 2) [8, 11, 13]. This has also improved the differential diagnosis of thickened extraocular muscles caused by other conditions [3, 11].

Histopathologic correlations

Echographic findings in Graves' disease using standardized echography correlate very closely to the histopathologic changes in the orbit.

Five pathologic changes within the orbital tissues are known: increase in fat content, increase in mucin content, increase in water content, fibrosis and lymphocytic infiltration. The extraocular muscles are predominantly affected and though all muscles show histopathologic changes to a certain degree there seems to be a predominance of these changes in the inferior and medial rectus muscle, to a lesser degree in the lateral rectus muscle [4, 5]. The tendons of the affected muscles are not involved. Exudate and fibroblastic proliferation usually first occur in the inferior rectus muscle. The pathophysiologic features that are responsable for the mentioned changes are an infiltration with mononuclear cells and fibroblasts. Predominantly those infiltrates are in the endomysium of the affected muscle. After an early stage with only sparse infiltrations and perivascular mast cells, lymphocytes and plasma cells increase in number and stimulate fibroblasts in the interstitium to proliferate and secrete collagen and acid mucopolysaccharides. This leads to an increased and over time changing water content (edema) of the muscle and to a separation and a

Table 2. Acoustic signs of Graves' ophthalmopathy as evaluated with standardized A-scan (Ossoinig 1982).

1   Absence of tumors
2   Diffuse swelling of orbital fat tissues (mostly in anterior orbit; coarser structure than in normal tissues)
3   Thickened extraocular muscles
    – most often both orbits
    – inserting tendons poorly visible in echograms
    – thickening more pronounced in posterior orbit
    – muscle thickness varies greatly over time
    – different muscles affected over time
4   High reflectivity (must be evaluated in anterior one-third of muscle) and pronounced heterogeneity of thickened muscles
5   Thickened optic nerve sheaths (markedly distened by increased subarachnoidal fluid in compressive optic neuropathy)
6   Thickened periorbit
7   Enlarged lacrimal glands

compression of bundles of muscle fibers which show atrophy. This separation, as it will be shown later, enhances the acoustic interfaces that are the surfaces of the bundles of fibers within the muscle and thus causes a changed echogram of the muscles. In a late stage the chronic edema and activation of fibroblasts leads to fibrosis, lipomatosis and sclerosis of the endomysium [5].

Acoustic criteria

Thickened extraocular muscles

Standardized echography with the dynamic examination technique allows clearly to identify and display all – straight and oblique – extraocular muscles [8, 13]. Though a pronounced thickening of extraocular muscles can be displayed by contact B-scan, CT or NMR standardized A-scan is most effective in detecting and measuring the thickness of all extraocular muscles particularly if there is only a slight increase. To achieve exact measurements it is important to maximize the width of the muscle-pattern in the echogram and to maximize the height and steepness of both surface spikes from the muscle-sheaths. This technique guarantees true cross sections of the muscle while examining in a dynamic scanning way. To diagnose a thickening of muscles comparison of both orbits is important. During the course of Graves' disease different muscles in both orbits are affected to a different degree over time as it is explained by the histopathologic changes. The tendon of the affected muscle is – in contrast to e.g. acute myositis – not involved, the most pronounced thickening occurs in the area of the muscle belly that is in the middle or more posterior orbit (Figs 1 and 2).

Specific acoustic signs

Thickened extraocular muscles in Graves' disease show an increased reflectivity and heterogeneity. These are specific acoustic signs caused by the described changes in histopathologic sections and allow a clear differentiation from thickened muscles in other diseases, e.g. acute and chronic myositis, lymphoma, hypertrophy and congestion, metastatic carcinoma in extraocular muscles or hematoma [11, 13]. The evaluation of these specific acoustic criteria is a dynamic procedure as well. They should be judged in the anterior third of the muscle where the muscle can be displayed with a perpendicular sound beam and the sound attenuation is minimalized. In the posterior part of the muscle the reflectivity tends to become low regardless to the disorder since the sound beam is attenuated by an increasing oblique angle when passing the ocular wall.

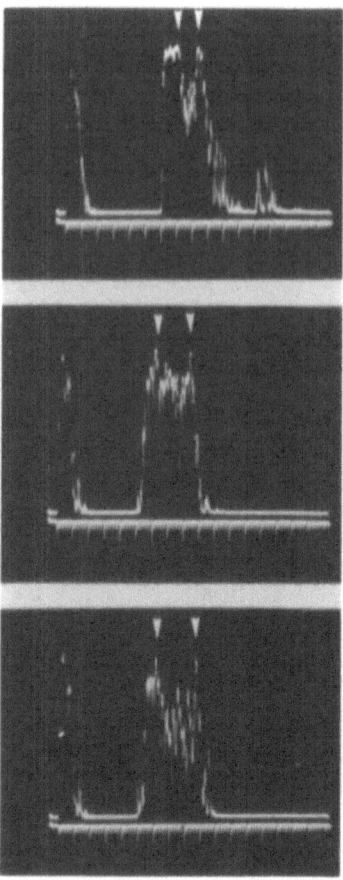

Fig. 1. A-scan cross sections from (top) normal medial rectus muscle, (middle) thickened medial rectus muscle in Graves' disease / anterior segment, (bottom) thickened medial rectus muscle / more posterior segment. Arrows indicate the surface spikes representing the inner and outer sheaths of the muscle. Note the differences in spike heights of the muscle pattern as well as the differences of the internal structure: short spikes in the normal muscle pattern, longer more different sized spikes in the thickened muscles. (see also Figs 3, 4 and 5).

The specificity of these acoustic criteria was stressed by clinical surveys [12, 13]. Thus thickening and increased reflectivity and heterogeneity of the extraocular muscles are objective acoustic key criteria for the diagnosis of endocrine ophthalmopathy (Figs 3, 4 and 5).

Other acoustic findings

According to the histopathology in Graves' disease a diffuse swelling of the orbital fat tissues occurs echographically. This can be evaluated best in the

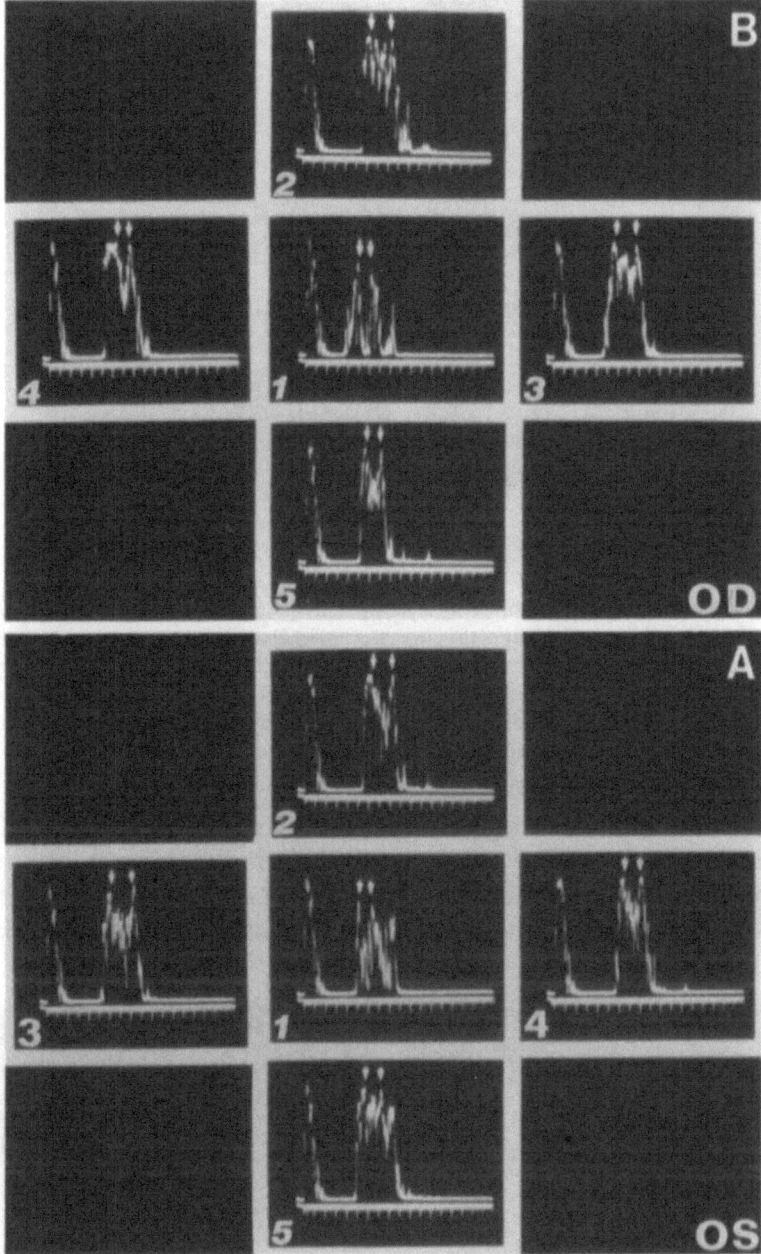

Fig. 2. A-scan cross sections of the straight extraocluar muscles and the optic nerve of both eyes in Graves' disease. 1 – optic nerve, 2 – superior rectus muscle, 3 – medial rectus muscle, 4 – lateral rectus muscle, 5 – inferior rectus muscle. Arrows indicate the surface spikes representing the inner and outer muscle sheaths and the dural sheath of the optic nerve. Note the differences in the widths, the spike height and the internal structure of the corresponding muscle patterns of both eyes.

562

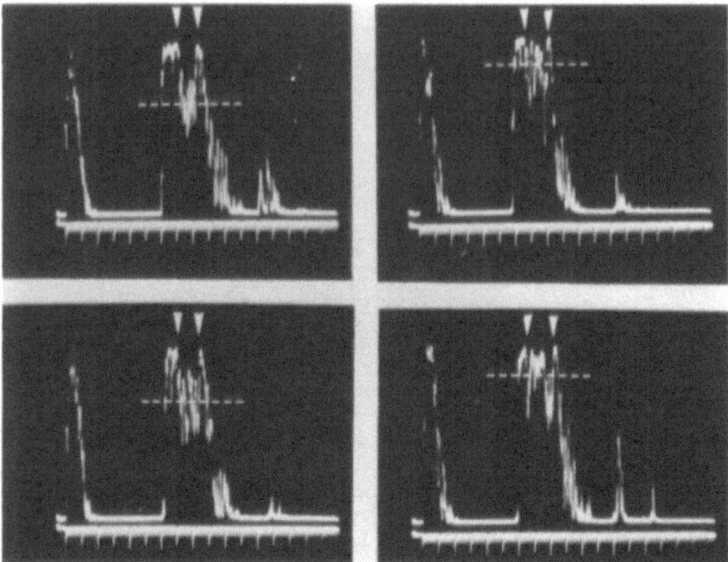

Fig. 3. A-scan cross sections of a normal medial (top, left) and a normal superior (bottom, left) rectus muscle with normal reflectivity of the internal echo signals of the muscle pattern. A-scans of a medial (top, right) and a superior (bottom, right) rectus muscle in Graves' disease showing an increased reflectivity. The echograms were obtained from muscle segments anterior to the muscle belly and were recorded at standardized tissue sensitivity setting of the A-scan instrument (Kretz 7200 MA). The arrows indicate inner and outer surface spikes of the muscles.

more anterior orbit, the echogram shows a widening and a coarser structure than in normal orbital tissues. Occasionally the periorbit becomes thickened and prominent and the lacrimal glands appear swollen. These acoustic signs are additional to the key criteria and although not specific support the diagnosis (Fig. 6).

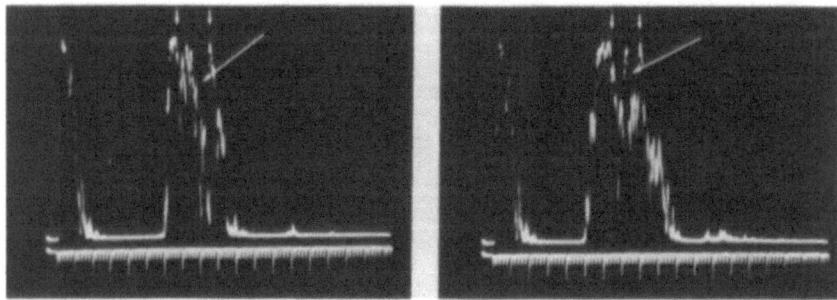

Fig. 4. A-scan cross sections of a thickened medial rectus muscle in Graves' disease. Left echogram: more anterior segment near the inserting tendon. Right echogram: more posterior segment near the muscle belly. Note the heterogeneity of the muscle pattern (longer arrows). Small arrows outline the surfaces of the muscle.

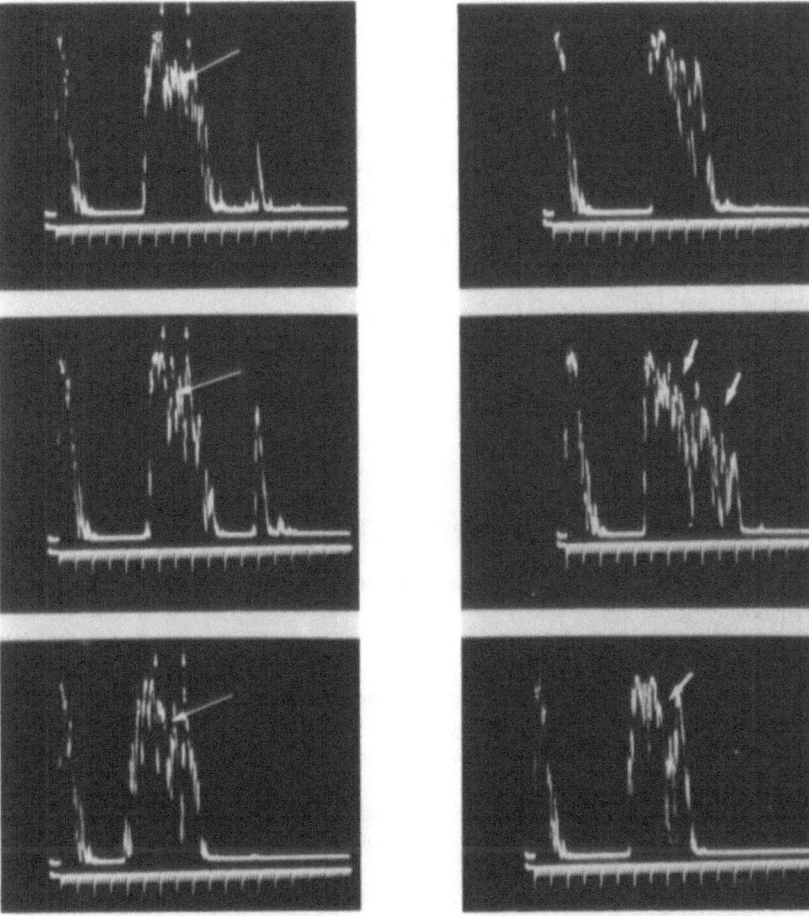

Fig. 5. Comparison of normal internal structure of a superior rectus muscle (top) with pronounced heterogeneity in a superior rectus muscle in Graves' disease. Note that the spikes within the two surface spikes (small arrows) show same height and same length in the normal muscle whereas the echograms of muscles in Graves' disease are heterogeneous thus the muscle pattern shows an overall higher reflectivity with different high and variable long spikes.

Fig. 6. Orbital echograms in a transocular examination technique of normal (top) and as in Graves' disease thickened (middle) orbital fat tissue. The echogram appears wider and shows a coarser structure (arrows). Both echograms (top, middle) display the temporal superior more posterior orbit. The third echogram (bottom) displays a thickened temporal superior – anterior periorbit (arrow).

Optic neuropathy

Optic nerve involvement is associated with thyroid dysfunction in about 5% [2, 14]. As it is true for the measurement of the extraocular muscles the

564

thickening of the optic nerve sheaths and – in compressive optic neuropathy – the widening of the subarachnoidal space by an increased amount of subarachnoidal fluid as it is present in thyroid neuropathy can be detected, displayed and exactly measured with standardized A-scan [13]. It must be stressed that the proof of optic nerve involvement echographically, even though there is no relationship between the incidence of this finding and the severeity of the ophthalmopathy or the decrease of visual acuity, standardized A-scan became very helpful in judging the prognosis and the management of Graves' disease [2].

References

1. Boergen KP, Hasenfratz G, Markl A. 1985. Zur Klinik verdickter, äußerer Augenmuskeln. Z. prakt. Augenheilkd. 6: 231–238.
2. Bouzas AG. 1980. Endocrine ophthalmopathy. The Montgomery Lecture. Trans Ophthal Soc UK, 100: 511–520.
3. Byrne SF, Glaser JS. 1983. Orbital tissue differentiation with standardized echography. Ophthalmology 90: 1071–1090.
4. Campbell RJ. 1984. Pathology of Graves' ophthalmopathy. In: The eye and orbit in thyroid disease. Gorman CA et al. (eds.), pp. 25–31. Raven Press, New York.
5. Daicker B. 1979. Das gewebliche Substrat der verdickten äußeren Augenmuskeln bei der endokrinen Orbitopathie. Klin Mbl Augenheilk, 174: 843–847.
6. van Dyk HJL. 1983. Orbital Graves' disease. A modification of the 'NOSPECS' classification. Ophthalmology, 88: 479–483.
7. Jones IS, Jakobiec FA, Nolan BT. 1983. Patient examination and introduction to orbital disease. Vol. 2, Chap 21 in: Clinical ophthalmology. Duane TD (ed.), Harper and Row, Philadelphia.
8. McNutt LC, Kaefring SL, Ossoinig KC. 1977. Echographic measurement of extraocular muscles. In: Ultrasound in medicine, Vol. 3A. White D, Brown RE (eds.), pp. 927–932. Plenum Press, New York.
9. Ossoinig KC. 1979. Standardized echography: basic principles, clinical applications and results. Int Ophthalmol Clin 19: 127–210.
10. Ossoinig KC. 1982. Ein neues echographisches Merkmal zur verläßlichen Differentialdiagnostik des endokrinen Exophthalmus. Klin Mbl Augenheilk, 180: 189–197.
11. Ossoinig KC, Hasenfratz G. 1983. Die Rolle der standardisierten Echographie in der Diagnose und Behandlung der orbitalen Myositis. Fortschr Ophthalmol, 80: 475–481.
12. Ossoinig KC. 1983. Advances in diagnostic ultrasound. In: Acta: XXIV Int Congr of Ophthalmology. Henkind P (ed.), pp. 89–114. Lippincott, Philadelphia.
13. Ossoinig KC. 1984. Ultrasonic diagnosis of Graves' ophthalmopathy. In: The eye and orbit in thyroid disease. Gorman CA et al. (eds.), pp. 185–211. Raven Press, New York.
14. Trobe JD, Glaser JS, Laflamme P. 1978. Dysthyroid optic neuropathy. Arch Ophthalmol, 96: 1199–1209.
15. Werner SC. 1983. Orbital changes in Graves' disease. Vol. 2, Chap 36 in: Clinical ophthalmology. Duane TD (ed.), Harper and Row, Philadelphia.

Echographic criteria of endocrine exophthalmos

W. BUSCHMANN, W. HAIGIS and B. WALLNER
Würzburg, FRG

Graves' disease is the most common origin of bilateral and unilateral exophthalmos. An analysis of the literature has yielded numerous echographic criteria for the detection and differentiation of endocrine orbitopathy. The criteria depend partially on equipment and examination techniques.

A- and B-scan criteria are summarized in Table 1 and 2. Enlarged muscle spaces as well as increased width and inhomogeneity of the fat echogram were mentioned most often. Some authors described changes in the optic nerve echogram, enhanced orbital bone wall echoes or pathologic echoes within external eye muscles.

Würzburg material. Table 3 demonstrates our material and the grade groups according to Werner and the American Thyroid Association scheme. We analyzed the echograms of 63 orbits (48 patients, endocrine orbitopathy) retrospectively for all the recommended criteria (Table 4).

Marked enlargement of muscle diameters was found in 87%, including sand-glass shaped fat echo displacement. Reliable data on normal diameters and their physiologic variations are still lacking, so that only crude enlarge-

Table 1. Endocrine orbitopathy, A-scan.

Echographic criteria	number of authors
	Enlarged width or orbital
Echogram	10
Number and intensity of orbital echoes increased	6
Convex-shaped decrease of echo complex without final spike/peak?	2

Literature: Buschmann, Coleman, Dallow, Fledelius, François, Hodes, Mann, McNutt, Ossoinig, Schoener, Shammas, Skalka.

K.C. Ossoinig (editor), Ophthalmic Echography, ISBN 978-94-010-7988-4

Table 2. Endocrine orbitopathy, B-scan.

Echographic criteria	number of authors
Echo-free, enlarged muscles	9
Fat echogram alterations	5
Optic nerve or sheath echo changes	4
Pathologic echoes in muscle area	4
Enhanced orbital wall echoes	3

Literature: Buschmann, Coleman, Dallow, Hilal, Hodes, Hurwitz, Purnell, Reis, Rochels, Skalka, Sutherland, Werner, Yamamoto.

ments could be counted. Many authors reported on a much lower rate of swollen muscles – doubtless a result of different examination techniques and patient selection.

Enhancement of bone wall echoes and fat tissue edema were seen in 54% of the orbits, optic nerve sheath edema in 24%.

Quantitative analysis of echograms

The volume increase of external eye muscles and orbital fat, as well as changes of the fat tissue echo pattern were predominant and should, therefore, be analysed quantitatively. Yamamoto's muscle index and muscle-fat-volume measurements are probably most suitable to quantify the volume increase. However, the opposite orbital bone walls must be shown simultaneously (i.e., medial and lateral wall in one scan), and the technique should be applied in vertical scans as well. We could use this evaluation method in 29 orbits (of 25 patients) examined with the Ophthalmoscan immersion technique (Table 5).

Table 3. Würzburg material (48 patients).

Grade of endocrine orbitopathy	number of patients
0	6
I	4
II	4
III	20
IV	12
V	2
VI	1
Total:	48

Table 4. Endocrine orbitopathy, A- and B-scan, Würzburg material.

Echographic criteria	positive	
	number	%
Muscle enlargment, fat displacement	55	87
Enhancement of bone wall echo, fat edema	34	54
Sheath edema of optic nerve	15	24
Total number of orbits	63	100

The marked increase of the muscle-fat-volume with higher grades of the disease could be demonstrated (and was statistically significant).

The contact scanners available nowadays are not optimum for ultrasonography of the most common orbital disease. They do not facilitate the application of Yamamoto's volume or muscle index measurement. Suitable scanning techniques for time-saving volume determination should be preferred. This means wide-angle sector or arc scans in meridional or horizontal plus vertical scanning planes. Oblique planes must be used to measure the inferior oblique muscle.

The quantitative analysis of fat and muscle structure echo amplitudes has a high impact on treatment decisions, because corticosteroid therapy as well as orbital decompression surgery should be applied – if indicated – before marked fibrosis develops (and causes immobility of the orbital tissues).

Measurement-based ultrasonography provides reproducible, comparable data on muscle and fat structure echo amplitudes. Reference to the W38 test reflector echo or any IEC-resp. AIUM-accepted reference reflector, to the working frequency (IEC definition), and to the beam profile has to be made. Flat-stalked transducer probes proved indispensable for proper quantitative A-scan analysis of muscle structure echoes, especially from inferior and lateral rectus muscle and inferior oblique muscle.

Table 5. Endocrine orbitopathy, muscle-fat-volume (Yamamoto's technique), B-scan (Ophthalmoscan).

Grade	0	I	II	III	IV	V	VI
volume (mean, cm³)	8.9	–	12.2	13.4+	12.9+	–	14.1
number of orbits	4	0	2	18	4	0	1
Total:	29 orbits (25 patients)						

+) = statistically significant difference to grade 0, p<1%.

Conclusion

For progress,
- equipment and examination technique should be developed further to facilitate the quantitative analysis of the volume increase according to Yamamoto's muscle index and fat plus muscle volume measurement, and
- measurement-based A- and B-scan ultrasonography, corresponding to the IEC draft on performance measurement of ultrasonic diagnostic apparatus, should be preferred instead of empirical approaches to get reproducible, comparable echographic data on volumes and tissue echo amplitudes. Then, even in the time of high resolution CT scanning and magnetic resonance imaging, ultrasonography will last to be an extremely helpful, cost-effective examination method for detection, differentiation, and follow-up of endocrine exophthalmos.

References

Yamamoto KKI, Yoshida S, Saito K, Sakamoto Y, Matsuda A, Saito T, Kuzuya T. 1979. A Quantitative Analysis of Orbital Soft Tissue in Graves' Disease Based on B-mode Ultrasonography. Endocrinol Japon 26 (2): 255–261.

Early detection of compressive optic neuropathy in Graves' disease with standardized A-Scan

K.C. OSSOINIG
Iowa City, USA

Abstract

In most cases, Graves' Ophthalmopathy ('Endocrine Exophthalmus') is a self-limiting disease that causes tolerable discomfort to the patient and may require no more than mild symptomatic treatment. Occasionally, Graves' disease may, however, become so severe that the sight of one or both eyes of the patient is threatened and may be lost permanently if prompt and proper treatment is not installed. One such instance is compression of the optic nerve (compromising its blood supply) by markedly thickened and crowded extra-ocular muscles in the orbital apex and, additionally, by severe thickening of the optic-nerve sheaths. It is crucial to detect compressive optic neuropathy early and treat it with high doses of systemic steroids, or decompress the orbit.

Standardized A-scan detects optic-nerve compression early (sometimes even before functional loss occurs), and has become an important diagnostic tool in managing these patients. The role of Standardized A-scan in the detection of compressive optic-nerve disease may be compared to the role of ocular tonometry in the detection of glaucoma: both indicate the respective condition often before functional deficits become evident. The typical echographic findings in compressive optic neuropathy are: increased subarachnoidal fluid in straight gaze (prior to any exercise of the eye such as taking extreme gaze directions which usually squeeze the subarachnoidal fluid out of the orbit); vanishing subarachnoidal fluid during 30 degree examinations and particularly during exercise. The fluid stays out of the orbit (optic nerve remains 'dry') thereafter unless the fluid is pushed back into the orbit through a Valsalva's procedure. Without compression, the optic nerves are either dry or contain only minimal amounts of subarachnoidal fluid. The critical measuring value for the arachnoidal diameter, which indicates beginning compression, is 5.7 microseconds (4.3 mm). In severe compressive optic neuropathy, diameters as large as 8 microseconds (6 mm) have been observed.

K.C. Ossoinig (editor), Ophthalmic Echography, ISBN 978-94-010-7988-4

The echographic measurement and differential diagnosis of optic nerve lesions (review)

SANDRA FRAZIER BYRNE
Miami, USA

Abstract

Because of its compact, homogeneous structure, the optic nerve is well-suited for evaluation by standardized echography. [3, 6, 7] B-scan is useful for evaluating the optic disc and topography (gross size, shape and location) of retrobulbar optic nerve disease. Standardized A-scan supplements B-scan evaluation of the optic disc and is the optimal method for detecting and differentiating retrobulbar optic nerve lesions.

Standardized A-scan provides accurate measurement of retrobulbar optic nerve width, both anteriorly behind the globe and more posteriorly. Furthermore, standardized A-scan differentiates optic nerve disease through the analysis of three primary criteria: (1) degree of optic nerve thickening, (2) internal structure and reflectivity of the nerve echogram, and (3) the 30° test to prove or exclude increased subarachnoid fluid.

Introduction

Both the optic disc and retrobulbar optic nerve may be evaluated with standardized echography (i.e. contact real-time B-scan combined with standardized A-scan* instrumentation). B-scan is the primary modality for assessing status of the optic disc while standardized A-scan is paramount in detecting, measuring and differentiating retrobulbar optic nerve disease.

This work has been supported in part by the Florida Lions Eye Bank.

* Kretztechnik 7200 MA or Ophthascans.

K.C. Ossoinig (editor), Ophthalmic Echography, ISBN 978-94-010-7988-4
© 1987, Martinus Nijhoff/Dr W. Junk Publishers, Dordrecht.

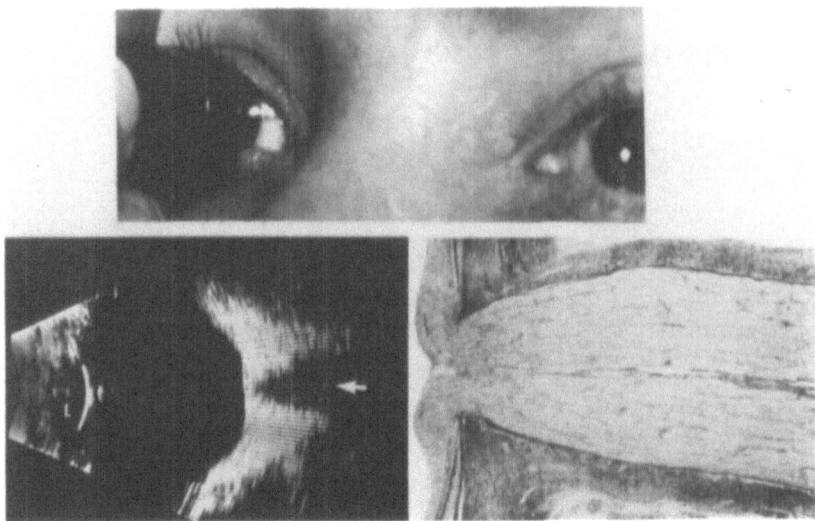

Fig. 1. Axial B-scan approach. The lens (L), optic disc and wedge-shaped optic nerve void (arrow) are centered within the echogram. Pathology shows compact structure of normal optic nerve.

Optic disc evaluation

The two dimensional B-scan is best suited for demonstrating the optic disc to display abnormal excavation, elevation or calcified drusen. The axial approach is optimal with the B-scan probe placed directly on the cornea and the fellow eye fixating a target (Fig. 1). Optic disc elevation and large optic cups may be displayed with B-scan, provided that the B-scan instrument has sufficient resolution (Fig. 2). Both B- and A-scan are useful for proving or excluding the presence of optic disc drusen which clinically may be difficult to distinguish from papilledema. More oblique B- and A-scan sections are used to display these foreign body-like sources (Fig. 3).

Retrobulbar optic nerve evaluation

The optic nerve is initially examined with standardized A-scan (at the tissue sensitivity setting) as the patient fixates in primary gaze. The probe, placed at the lateral equator, is angled posteriorly until a cross-section of the optic nerve appears as a depression or defect behind the globe echogram (Fig. 4). Measurements of optic nerve width are normally made between the steeply rising, smooth, high arachnoid sheath spikes.

The optic nerve as assessable because of its sinuous nasal orbital course and

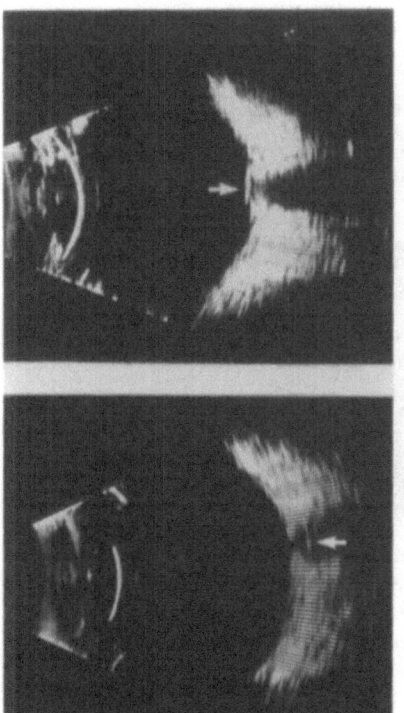

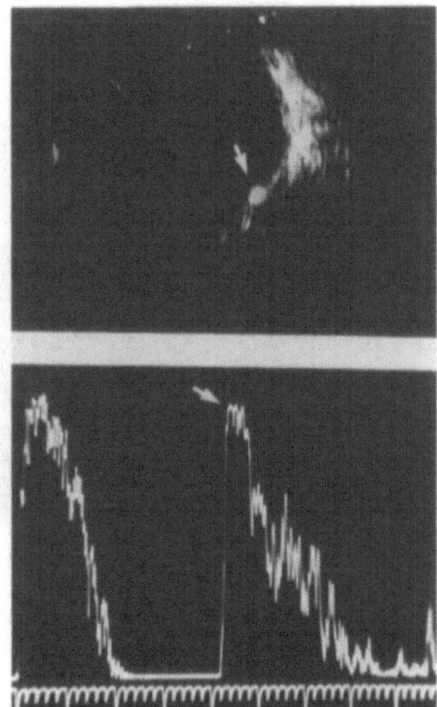

Fig. 2. Echograms obtained with Coopervision contact real-time B-scan instrument. Top, optic disc elevation (arrow) in patient with papilledema. Bottom, totally excavated optic disc in patient with glaucomatous cupping. A low to medium sensitivity setting is used to display the lamina cribrosa (arrow).

Fig. 3. Optic disc drusen. The longitudinal B-scan echogram at low sensitivity setting shows persistence of round foreign body-like echo at optic disc (arrow). The A-scan, at tissue sensitivity with oblique sound beam incidence, shows 100% tall spike from drusen (arrow). Lower orbital spikes behind drusen spike are produced by partial shadowing (strong sound attenuation).

its well defined composition as well as refraction which occurs at the surface of the nerve. [7] The optic nerve may be measured from anteriorly just behind the globe to about two thirds of the distance to the orbital apex; when thickened, it may also be measured in the orbital apex (Fig. 5). Width or thickness of the normal optic nerve may range from 2.3 mm to 3.3 mm in a given patient. When comparing between right and left optic nerves in the same patient, however, differences of less than 0.3 mm anteriorly and 0.5 mm posteriorly are the norm.

574

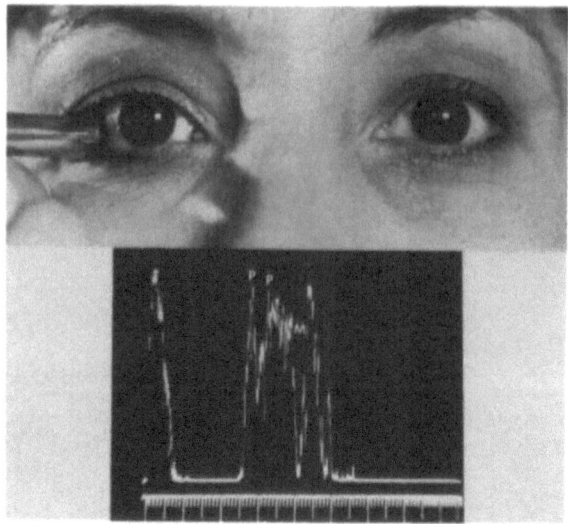

Fig. 4. Top, A-scan technique for displaying cross section of the optic nerve and medial rectus muscle. Bottom, A-scan of normal optic nerve. Note smooth rise and high reflectivity of perineural sheath spikes (P) indicating perpendicularity. Also note low to medium reflectivity of normal optic nerve (between sheath spikes). M = medial rectus muscle.

B-scan is normally applied to document topography of retrobulbar optic nerve disease which has already been detected and differentiated with standardized A-scan. B-scan may demonstrate topographic cross-sections of the optic nerve with techniques similar to that of A-scan. The probe, positioned vertically at the temporal equator, is angled through the periphery of the globe until a circular acoustic void appears behind the globe echogram (Fig. 6).

Another approach is the longitudinal orientation, which allows more perpendicular alignment with the perineural sheaths than with the axial approach (Fig. 7a). Heterogeneities within the optic nerve void (the main B-scan clue of optic nerve disease) may be more readily displayed with this approach (Fig. 7b). [2, 4]

CT-scan vs. standardized echography

CT-scan provides an attractive anatomical display of both orbits and the intracranial space. The optic nerves may be visualized in relation to one another as well as to surrounding orbital structures and periorbital cavities. Even high resolution CT-scan, however, often fails to detect slight optic nerve

575

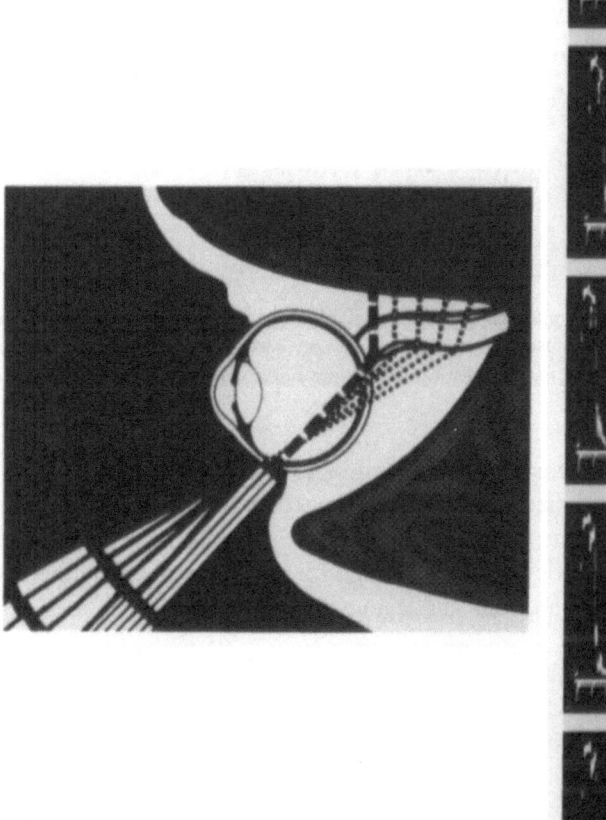
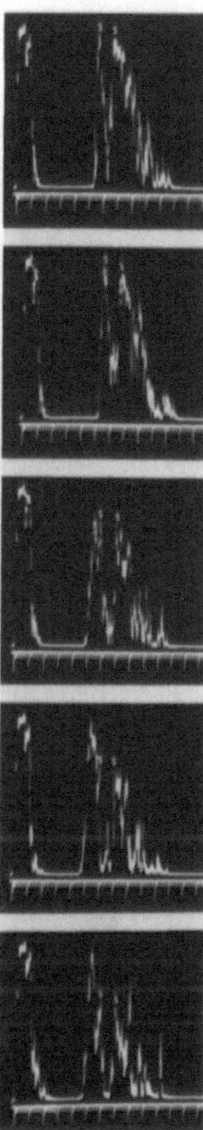

Fig. 5. Schematic representation and echograms showing dynamic A-scan technique for displaying optic nerve crosssections both anteriorly and posteriorly. A-scan montage shows normal optic nerve echograms beginning anteriorly (Top) to posteriorly (Bottom). Note smooth rise of perineural sheath spikes (S), maintained throughout this dynamic examination. Height of the sheath spikes decreases posteriorly mainly because of sound attenuation by normal orbital tissue. There is little difference in thickness of the normal optic nerve anteriorly and posteriorly. [Drawing reprinted with permission of KC Ossoinig, M.D.]

576

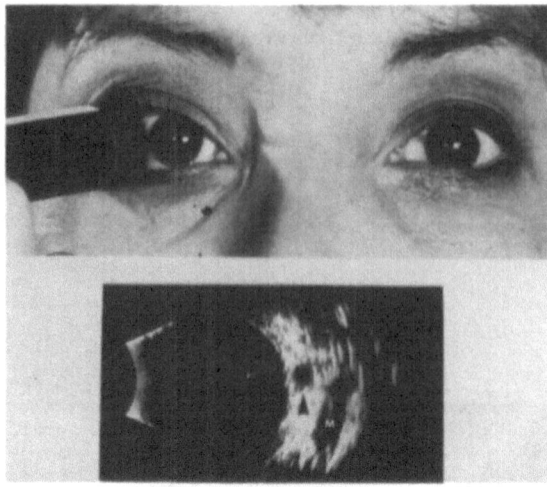

Fig. 6. Vertical (transverse) approach. B-scan cross section of normal optic nerve. Arrow = optic nerve, M = medial rectus muscle. A constant sensitivity setting should be maintained when comparing contralateral optic nerves since size of the optic nerve void changes in proportion to the sensitivity used.

widening or narrowing and is frequently unable to differentiate detected optic nerve disease. Standardized echography (especially the standardized A-scan) on the other hand, has the high resolution and sensitivity necessary for detecting very small optic nerve lesions and for reliably differentiating a wide range of optic nerve conditions and lesions.

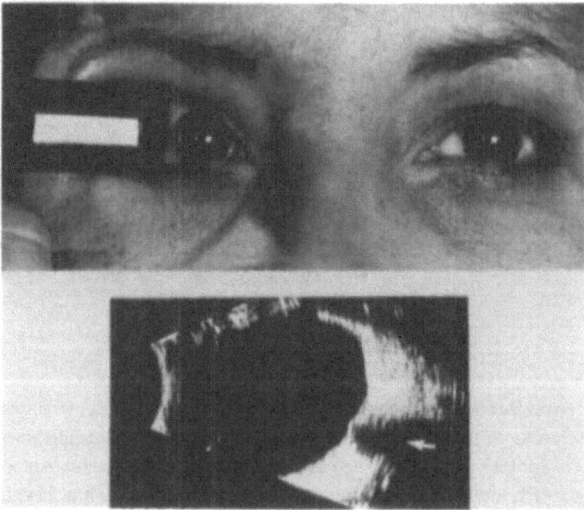

Fig. 7a. Longitudinal approach. Probe is held so that sound beam strikes perineural sheaths in more parallel fashion. Arrow = optic nerve.

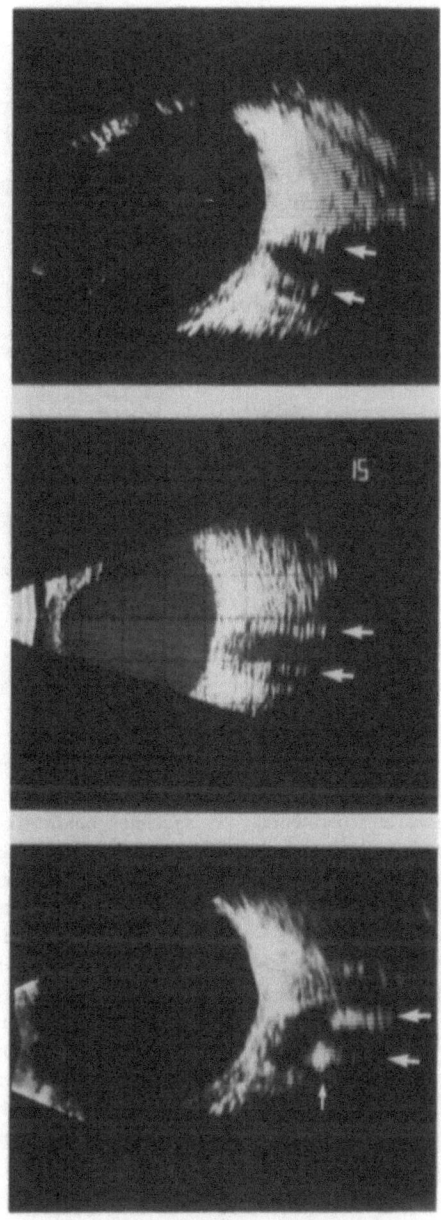

Fig. 7b. Sheath accentuation is the best B-scan indicator of disease but is not reliable for lesion detection or differentiation. Top, normal optic nerve. Center, increased subarachnoid fluid. Bottom, optic nerve sheath meningioma. Small arrow = focus of calcium.

578

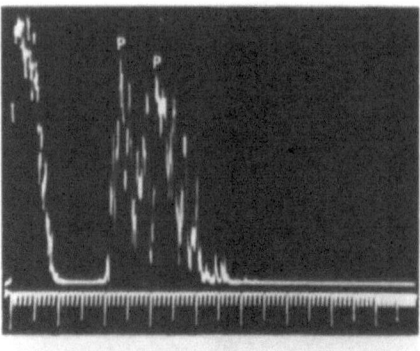

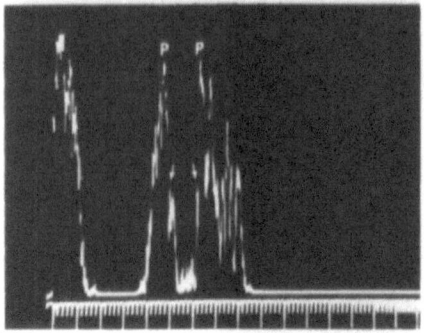

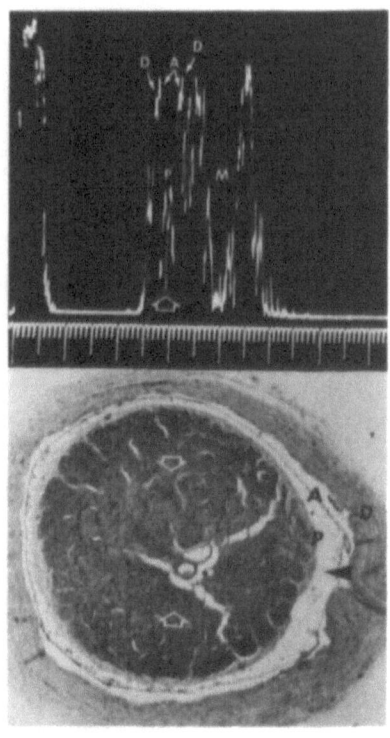

Fig. 8. Irregular structure and reflectivity (Top) and regular structure with low reflectivity (Bottom). P = perineural sheath spikes. Top echogram indicates perineural disease (increased subarachnoid fluid or perineural sheath thickening). The 30° test is necessary to differentiate between the two. Bottom echogram indicates thickening of optic nerve proper. Arrows = pia mater surfaces which are abutting the perineural sheath spikes.

Fig. 9. A-scan cross section of normal optic nerve with ideal sound beam incidence to various optic nerve structures shown on path specimen below. Top, double-peaked perineural sheath spikes are produced by the smooth inner arachnoid (A) and more coarse outer dural (D) sheaths. Two lower reflective spikes are produced by the pia mater (P), open arrow = optic nerve proper. Tiny defect on either side of pial spikes is from normal subarachnoid fluid. M = medial rectus muscle. Bottom, normal optic nerve cross section. Open arrows = optic nerve proper, P = pia mater, Black arroq = subarachnoid space, A = arachnoidal sheath, D = dural sheath.

Retrobulbar optic nerve disease

Width and reflectivity (i.e. spike height) of the anterior and posterior optic nerve are first evaluated with standardized A-scan. Reflectivity of the normal optic nerve echogram is low to medium. The echographic diagnostician[1] observes the optic nerve echogram during the dynamic examination in search of abnormal width or reflectivity. Optic nerve disease generally falls into one of two basic reflectivity categories: (1) *regular structure* with low to medium reflectivity indicative of nerve proper disease and (2) *irregular structure* with variable reflectivity indicative of perineural disease (Fig. 8).

Increased subarachnoid fluid

The normal optic nerve substance (optic nerve proper bordered by pia mater) is surrounded by a small amount of serous fluid. The nerve substance and subarachnoid fluid is enveloped by the smooth arachnoid and dural sheaths (Fig. 9). The elastic perineural sheaths become distended by increased subarachnoid fluid in a variety of conditions [3] (Table 1). Such fluid accumulation may be unilateral or bilateral, usually depending upon whether the predisposing condition is systemic or local.

Because increased subarachnoid fluid is a perineural condition, the optic nerve echogram is irregular when viewed in primary gaze with standardized A-scan. Since irregular echograms are produced by both increased subarachnoid fluid and perineural sheath thickening, the 30° test must be implemented to differentiate these two conditions.

The 30° test

This maneuver allows differentiation of increased subarachnoid fluid from perineural sheath thickening by measuring and evaluating the optic nerve in primary gaze and again at gaze at least 30° toward the probe. [1–3, 5–7] When the perineural sheaths are distended by increased subarachnoid fluid, the echogram significantly narrows when remeasured at 30° due to stretching of the elastic sheaths and redistribution of the fluid (Fig. 10). Conversely, if the

Table 1. Conditions where subarachnoid fluid may be found with standardized A-scan.

Increased intracranial pressure
Arachnoid cyst
Optic neuritis
Secondary to optic nerve tumor
Secondary to compression by orbital mass
Trauma (presumably subarachnoid hematoma)
Uveal effusion syndrome
Optic pits and optic disc colobomas

580

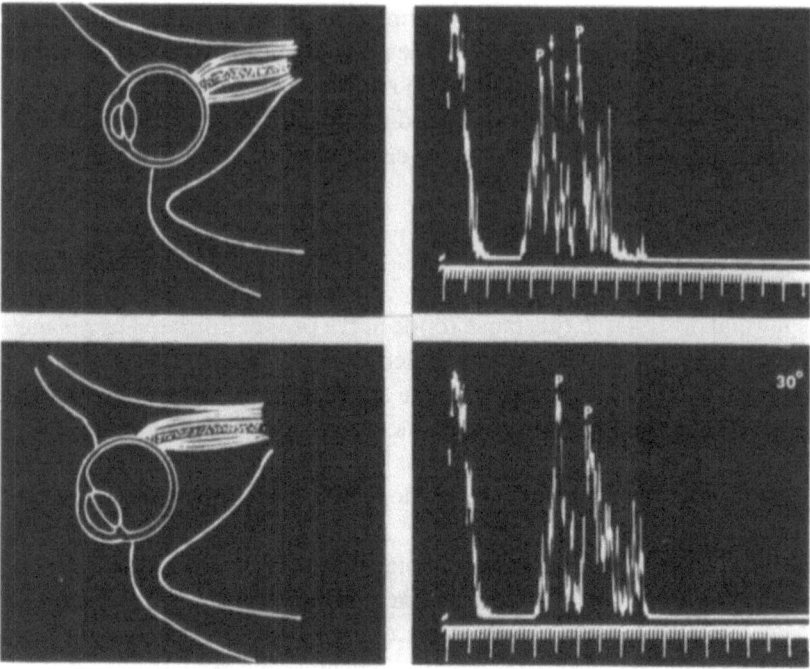

Fig. 10. 30° Test. Top, schematic representation with corresponding A-scan of distended perineural sheaths by increased subarachnoid fluid. A-scan shows irregular structure and reflectivity indicative of perineural disease and maximal width corresponding to maximal fluid accumulation in primary gaze. P = perineural sheath spikes, arrows = pia mater. Depression on either side of pia mater = increased subarachnoid fluid. Since perineural sheath thickening may produce this same appearance when the patient is fixating in primary gaze, the 30° test is used for differentiation. Bottom, patient rotates eye at least 30° toward the probe. The elastic perineural sheaths contract and stretch, thus redistributing the subarachnoid fluid and decreasing width of the space. Corresponding A-scan shows significant narrowing between perineural sheath spies which proves increased subarachnoid fluid.

perineural sheaths are thickened and there is no increased subarachnoid fluid, there will be no significant change in echogram width with the 30° remeasurement.

Perineural sheath thickening

The perineural sheaths may become thickened in some forms of optic neuritis as well in optic neuropathies such as in advanced thyroid eye disease and perineural sheath meningiomas. Optic nerve meningiomas, which infiltrate the perineural sheaths rather than the nerve proper, are diagnosable once the

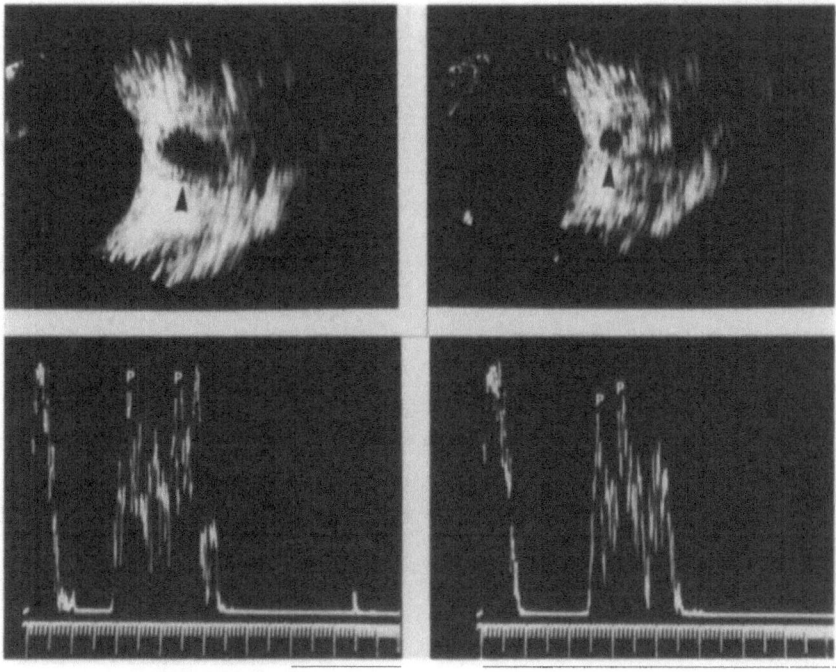

a

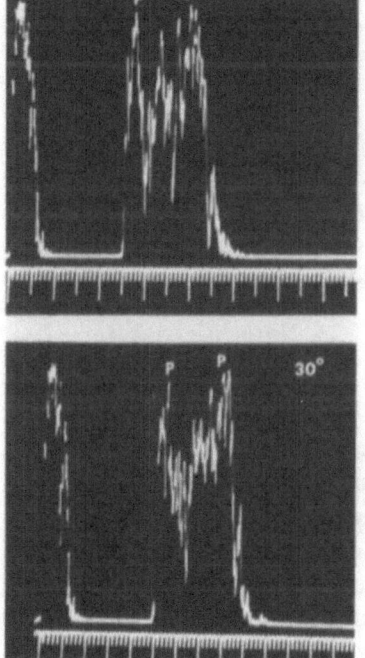

b

Fig. 11a. Typical optic nerve meningioma (left) and normal contralateral optic nerve (right). Top, vertical B-scan (transverse) cross sections show gross widening of optic nerve void on left (arrow). Bottom, optic nerve sheath meningioma produces irregularly structured A-scan echogram measuring more than twice the width of the normal contralateral optic nerve. P = perineural sheath spikes.

Fig. 11b. 30° test of the optic nerve meningioma. Top, maximal width of echogram in primary gaze. Bottom, remeasurement in gaze at least 30° towards the probe shows no significant change in echogram width.

582

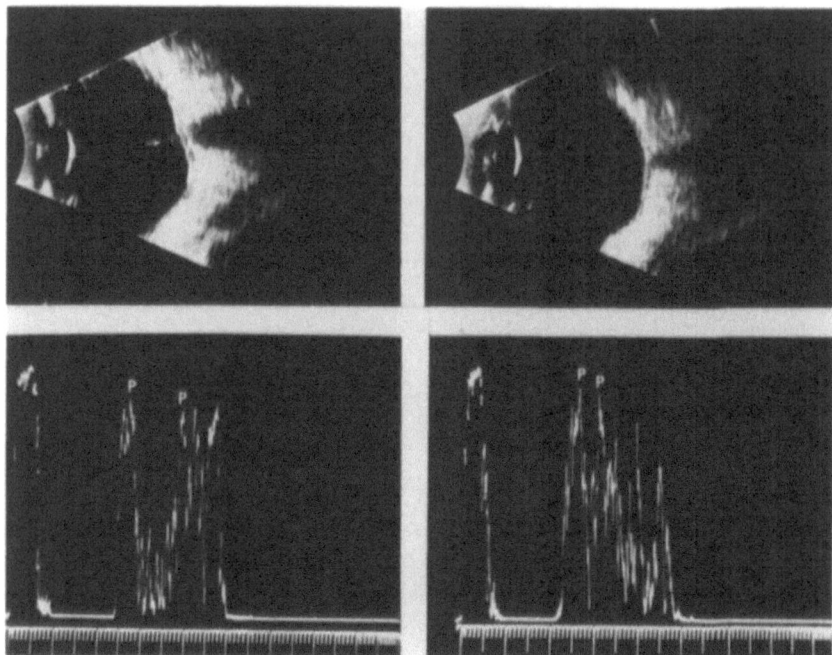

Fig. 12a. Optic nerve glioma (left) and normal contralateral optic nerve (right). Top, axial B-scans show elevated optic disc (arrow) of glioma and slight widening of retrobulbar optic nerve void compared to the normal right optic nerve. Bottom, glioma produces regularly structured, low to medium reflective A-scan echogram which measures more than twice the width of the normal contralateral optic nerve. P = perineural sheath spikes.

irregular, widened echogram measures more than twice as wide as the normal contralateral optic nerve and the 30° test is negative (Fig. 11). Smaller optic nerve meningiomas are more difficult to diagnose. However, their tendency to thicken the optic nerve unevenly gives a clue as to their presence and helps differentiate them from more benign conditions.

Optic nerve proper thickening

Thickening of the optic nerve proper may occur in optic neuritis as well as in optic nerve glioma. In contrast to the irregular echograms produced by increased subarachnoid fluid and perineural sheath thickening, thickened optic nerve proper produces regularly structured echograms with low to medium reflectivity (Fig. 8). Therefore, optic nerve gliomas (which are primarily tumors of the optic nerve proper) normally produce regularly structured, low to medium reflective echograms. Typically, optic nerve glioma produces

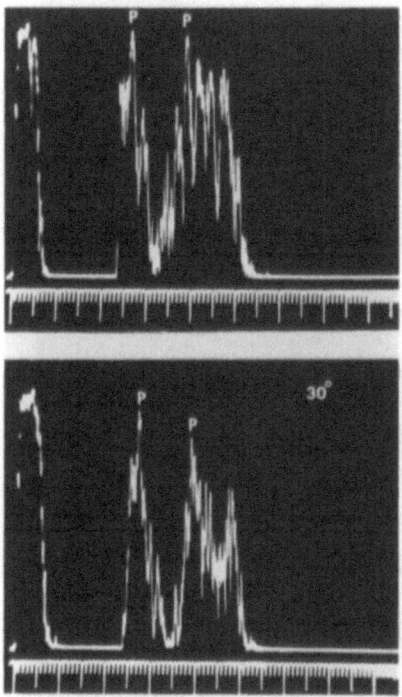

Fig. 12b. 30° test of the optic nerve glioma. Top, maximal width of echogram in primary gaze. Bottom, remeasurement at gaze at least 30° towards the probe indicates no significant change in echogram width. P = perineural sheath spikes.

marked widening of the echogram compared to the normal contralateral optic nerve (more than twice the size of the contralateral optic nerve) and the 30° test is negative (Fig. 12). If very large, the glioma may totally replace the optic nerve void on B-scan and the lesion may be displayed from other sound beam approaches with standardized A-scan (Fig. 13).

Optic atrophy

Optic atrophy produces optic nerve echograms which normally measure the same width as the contralateral fellow optic nerve echogram but have more irregular internal structure and higher reflectivity. This is explained by shrinkage of the optic nerve proper, resulting in more prominent pial spikes within the echogram (Fig. 14). Another explanation of the higher reflectivity may be cavernous optic atrophy. The importance of identifying optic nerve atrophy is not so much for diagnosis since this is usually clinically observable, but is rather

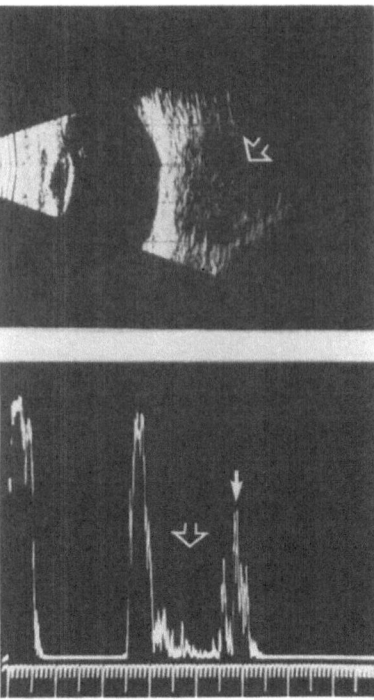

Fig. 13. Very large optic nerve glioma (open arrows). B-scan shows huge mass replacing normal wedge-shaped optic nerve void. A-scan taken with probe positioned next to the limbus inferotemporally allows alignment of sound beam with axis of tumor. This shows regular structure and low reflectivity with distinct, double-peaked posterior border spike (closed arrow).

in the exclusion of other optic nerve lesions as the etiology of the optic atrophy.

Conclusion

Standardized echography is a viable means of detecting and differentiating disease of the optic disc and retrobulbar optic nerve. Contact B-scan is optimal for evaluating the optic disc and for documenting gross topography of retrobulbar optic nerve disease. Standardized A-scan, however, is extremely sensitive in detecting, measuring and differentiating retrobulbar optic nerve lesions. As in all aspects of ophthalmic echography, appropriate instrumentation, examination technique and examiner skill are prerequisites for optimal results.

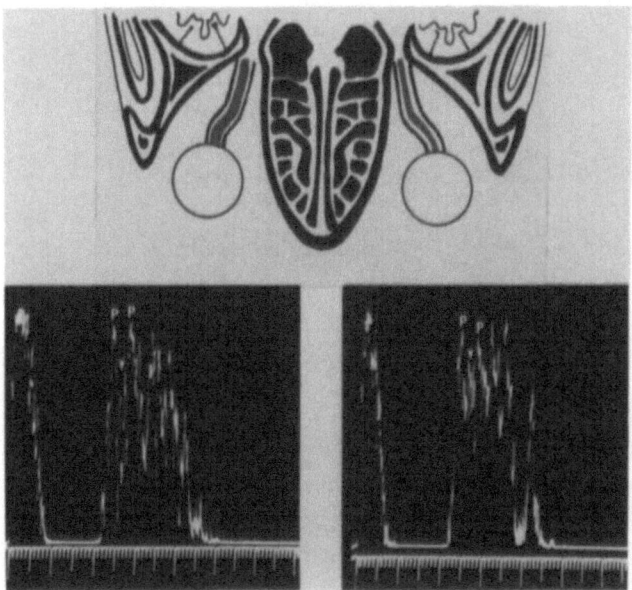

Fig. 14. Schematic representation and echograms of normal optic nerve (left) and optic atrophy (right). Note low to medium reflectivity of normal optic nerve echogram on left and high reflectivity atrophic optic nerve on right. P = perineural sheath spikes, arrows = pia mater and optic nerve proper.

Acknowledgement

The author is grateful to Michele L. Fagin for typing this manuscript and for editorial assistance. Additional thanks are extended to the other Echography personnel: J. Randall Hughes, Eileen K. Novinski and Maria L. Rivera.

References

1. Byrne SF, Saclarides EE. 1982. Standardized ophthalmic echography and the health care professional. J Ophthalmic Nurs Technol 1: 21.
2. Byrne SF, Glaser JS. 1983. Orbital tissue differentiation with standardized echography. Ophthalmology 90: 1088.
3. Byrne SF. 1985. Evaluation of the optic nerve by standardized echography. Neuro-ophthalmology update; in press.
4. Coleman DJ, Lizzi FL, Jack RL. 1977. Ultrasonography of the Eye and Orbit. Philadelphia: Lea & Febiger: 331.
5. Hupp SL, Buckley EG, Byrne SF, et al. 1984. Posttraumatic venous obstructive retinopathy associated with enlarged optic nerve sheath. Arch Ophthalmol 102: 254–56.
6. Ossoinig KC. 1979. Standardized echography: basic principles, clinical applications and results. Int Ophthalmol Clin 19(4): 127–210.
7. Ossoinig KC, Cennamo G, Byrne SF. 1981. Echographic differential diagnosis of optic-nerve lesions. Doc Ophthalmol Proc Ser 29: 327–31.

Experimental studies on the display of the optic nerve

G. HASENFRATZ
Munich, FRG

After introduction of standardized A-scan in 1971/72 the display and the measurement of the optic nerve became possible. [5] For measurements of the width of the optic nerve as well as for the detection and differential diagnosis of optic nerve lesions standardized echography and particularly standardized A-scan proofed to be the most sensitive and accurate echographic method. [8, 9]

Using this method the optic nerve is displayed in a cross-sectional echogram within the orbital tissues. Usually the procedure for evaluation of the optic nerve is performed with the transducer placed on the temporal conjunctiva between corneal limbus and temporal equator of the globe while the patient is asked to gaze straight forward. The medial rectus muscle serves as a landmark. Display and measurements of the nerve are done dynamically thus shifting the sound beam along the optic nerve from the retrobulbar area of the orbit towards the orbital apex. Other positions of the transducer with or without different directions of the gaze of the patient with thus different sound beam directions are described and possible. [7, 9, 12, 13]

When evaluating the optic nerve within the orbital tissues it is represented by a clear defect. Corresponding to the histologic section of the optic nerve (less numerous and smaller acoustic interfaces than in the surrounding orbital tissues) the optic nerve fibers show a lower reflectivity with a more homogeneous internal structure than the high reflective, irregularly structured orbital tissues. This area of lower reflectivity is limited by steeply falling and rising spikes on each side which represent the surfaces of the optic nerve. Both surface spikes are usually double (sometimes triple) peaked, very high and steeply rising.

Such steeply falling and rising, very high surface spikes in the A-scan echograms indicate a perpendicular approach of the sound beam. With the specific technical design of standardized A-scan steeply rising signals – as they occur as surface spikes in the display of the optic nerve – only can be obtained when the sound beam is directed to acoustic interfaces in a perpendicular

K.C. Ossoinig (editor), Ophthalmic Echography, ISBN 978-94-010-7988-4

588

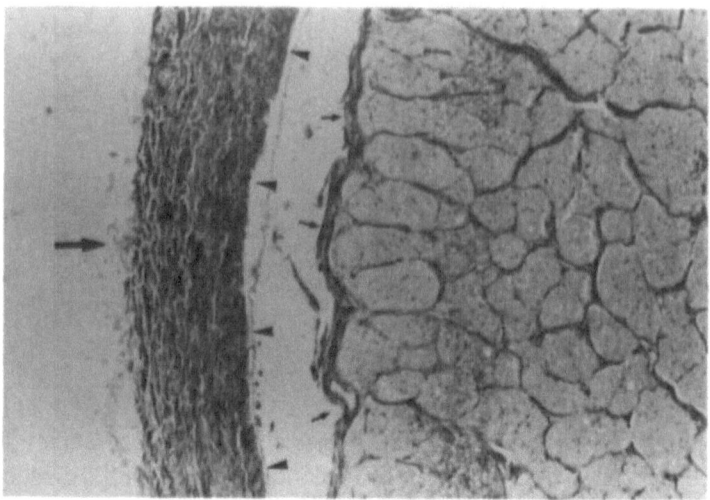

Fig. 1. Histologic cross section of a normal human optic nerve. Large arrow indicates the outer dural surface, smaller arrows indicate the inner dural surface towards the subdural/subarachnoidal space. The arachnoid is represented by the fine trabeculae within the subdural space. Little arrows indicate the pia mater which tightly encloses the optic nerve substance and shows a somewhat scalloped interface with the subdural/subarachnoidal space.

direction. Oblique sound beam incidence would result in a widened and lower reflective signal. [9]

Two questions were discussed – sometimes controversially – in various publications:

– What are the histological correlations of the two, in some cases three surface spikes at each side of the optic nerve, and – when considering the topography of the orbit with the optic nerve surrounded by orbital tissues as well as the examination techniques –:
– How can it be achieved to get a perpendicular approach of the sound beam to the optic nerve.

Histology

Histopathologic sections show the dura mater as a layer of dense connective tissue sheaths containing thick bundles of collagen and a fair amount of elastic tissue. The inner surface is lined by flattened cells, so called meningoendothelial cells. The arachnoid lies underneath the dura mater, closer to the dura than to the pia mater. It commences a rather ill defined layer under the dura from which very thin trabeculae extend in a branching fashion to the pia

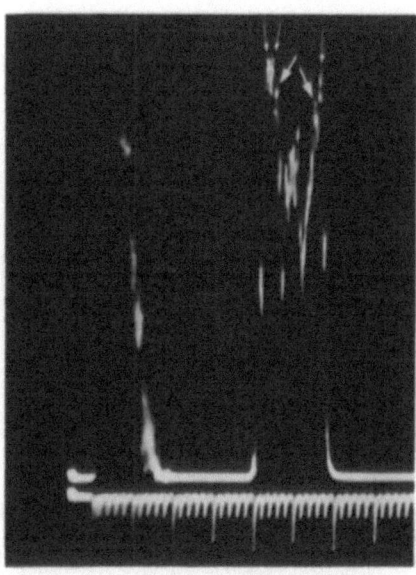

Fig. 2. A-scan cross section of a human optic nerve in-vitro (see section: 'material and method') with a perpendicular sound beam incidence, the orbital fat tissue was removed. Small arrows indicate the dura mater (outer and inner surface, left surface), larger arrows indicate the pia mater/optic nerve surface. When the double peaked spike from the dura mater may be observed during in-vivo examinations the outer dural surface (interface between fat and dura) usually shows – in contrast to the display in-vitro (interface between water and dura) – a lower reflectivity.

mater. [3] The dura mater/arachnoid-complex has a thickness of 0.3–0.5 mm [3]. The pia mater is represented by a layer of connective tissue with numerous small blood vessels which encloses tightly the intraorbital part of the optic nerve and divides the nerve fibers into bundles by sending numerous septa into the nerve substance. [3] (Fig. 1).

Experimental studies [13] as well as the observations of changes of the optic nerve in various pathologic conditions have shown that it is the dura mater which corresponds to the first steeply rising surface spike on both sides of the nerve. [9, 10, 11, 14] In our understanding, the surface between the dura mater and the subarachnoidal fluid/subarachnoidal space is both regular and rather smooth and produces a high and distinct (steeply falling or rising) echo-signal on either side of the optic nerve pattern. The outer surface between orbital fat tissues and the dura mater is less distinct and less regular thus less reflective, but it may produce another and to some degree lower echo-signal which can be displayed in in vitro experiments but may be distinguished in vivo in some echograms of the optic nerve as well. (Fig. 2). Thus the first spike of the surface signals of the optic nerve may be seen double-peaked. The second

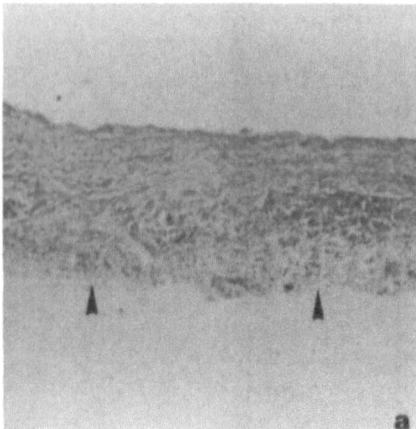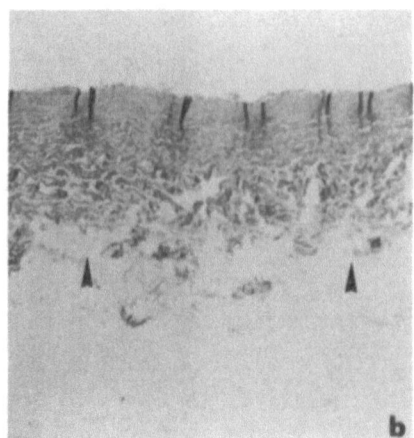

Fig. 3. a: Histologic section of the dura mater of a human optic nerve. Arrows indicate the outer surface of the dura. Note the difference of the type of interface between this surface and the more smooth and distinct inner surface towards the subdural/subarachnoidal space. b: Histologic section of the dura mater of the optic nerve from the eye of a cow. Arrows indicate the outer surface of the dura. Note the irregularity and not clearly defined interface between dura and orbital fat tissue (removed in this specimen). Also note the difference of this interface compared to that of the human dura (a). The inner dural surface appears similar to the conditions in human optic nerves.

spike that limits the echographic area of the optic nerve substance corresponds to the interface between subarachnoidal fluid and the pia mater. This surface usually is less high reflective. The fact that the in vivo display of the optic nerve together with the optic nerve sheaths with distinct and high reflective borders is possible postulates – in regard to the orbital topography as well as to the in vivo examination technique – refraction of the sound beam towards the optic nerve and/or special effects to the sound beam by reflection and scattering at the interfaces of the different surfaces: orbital tissues – outer surface of the dura mater, dura mater/arachnoid – subarachnoidal fluid and subarachnoidal fluid – pia mater/optic nerve substance. As it was stated already in earlier publications [11] – though in the 'pre-standardized A-scan' time – the sound beam can not be directed perpendicularly to the nerve in vivo. Because of the lack of a clear distinction between tissues of different reflectivity, which became possible by standardized A-scan that was developed for tissue differentiation, these earlier experiments could not display the optic nerve within the orbital tissues – or at least the optic nerve could not be distinguished, measured and examined exactly. [4]

To achieve other and new findings on this problem we performed an experimental display of the optic nerve under defined conditions in vitro. First results and their discussion will be presented in this paper.

Material and method

The standardized A-scan we used was the KRETZ 7200 MA unit with a 8 MHz non-focused transducer. [8, 15] In two series the human optic nerve (from eyes enucleated for keratoplasty) and the optic nerve from the eyes of cows (the eyes were enucleated from newly slaughtered cows) were examined. The experimental work-up was performed at the day of enucleation.

The optic nerve of eyes from cows in our opinion served as a good model for comparison since the overall thickness is about the same as that of human optic nerves and the dural/arachnoidal sheath is less thick and shows a less distinct and even coarser outer surface. (Fig. 3).

The eyes as well as the transducer were fixated in stands and brought into a waterbath (room-temperature). By a sutured string at the most proximal end of the optic nerve it could be hold in different positions in correlation to the sound probe while the globe was fixated. Three different preparations of the optic nerve were made:
- display of the optic nerve with surrounding orbital fat tissue
- display of the optic nerve with the fat tissue removed
- display of the optic nerve without the dura/arachnoid-complex. (Fig. 4).

Control of the experimental preparations was done by histologic work-up of the used specimen.

The display in each category of preparation was done by angling the nerve (by pulling the string upwards) so that the sound beam incidence was
+/− 90 degrees
+/− 75 degrees
+/− 60 degrees. (Fig. 5)

Polaroid pictures were taken at tissue sensitivity and at reduced sensitivity (−12 dB/−20 dB) for evaluation and measurements. The total number of experiments was 21 (12 human eyes, 9 cows's eyes, at least three measurement pictures were taken per category of preparation and angle of sound beam incidence).

Results

Display of the optic nerve with surrounding orbital fat:

Angle 90/75/60 degrees

Optic nerve of human eyes
Optic nerve of cows's eyes

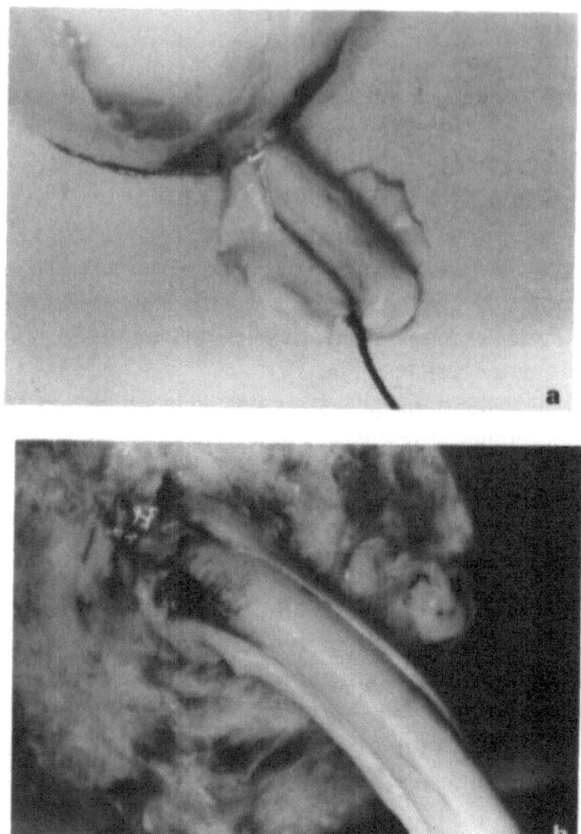

Fig. 4. a: Human optic nerve, the dura mater and arachnoid partly removed; b: Optic nerve and globe from a cow, the dura mater and arachnoid partly removed.

As it can be observed in vivo when evaluating a patient the first spike that limits the optic nerve sometimes is displayed double peaked. In vitro this was only true for the perpendicular sound beam incidence, not at oblique angles. (Fig. 2).

When the optic nerve was brought into the sound beam with an angle of about 75 and about 60 degrees there was a decrease of the height of the surface spikes as well as of the echosignals from the optic nerve substance. Though the decrease of reflectivity occured at the oblique angles of soundbeam incidences the surface spikes of the optic nerve still could be displayed steeply rising. There was no increase in the diameter at these oblique angles of incidence. (Fig. 6, Table 1).

When examining the optic nerve of eyes from cows we could not display a double peaked first surface spike, but as in human optic nerves two steeply

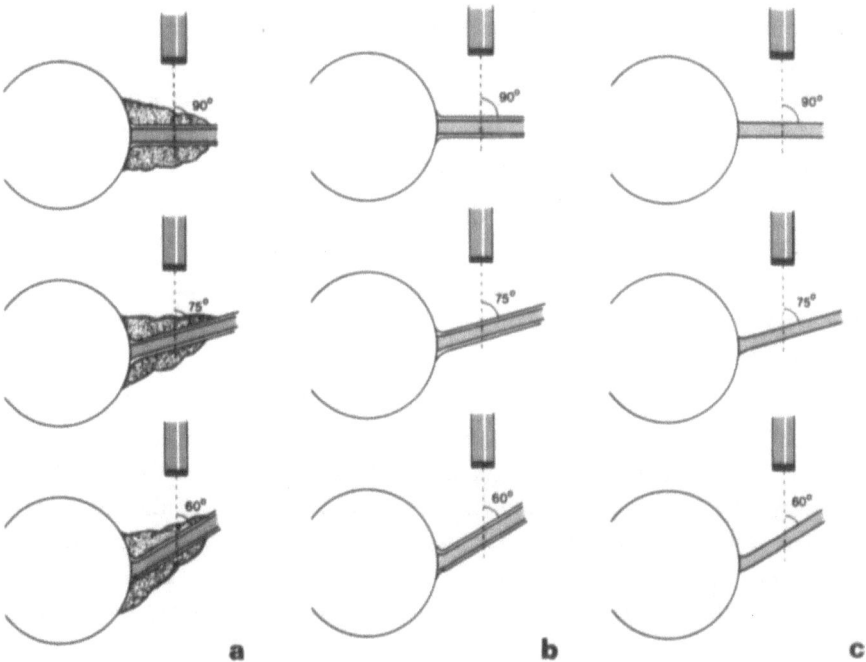

Fig. 5. Schematic drawings of the different types of preparation and sound beam approaches. (a) Optic nerve with surrounding orbital fat, (b) optic nerve without orbital fat, (c) optic nerve without dura/arachnoid sheaths.

rising spikes on each side of the nerve (see Fig. 3). As it could be observed in the experiments with the human optic nerve the spike height – surface spikes and internal spikes of the nerve substance – were decreasing but still steeply rising at 75 and 60 degrees and there was no increase in diameter at these transducer positions. (Fig. 7, Table 1).

Display of the optic nerve without surrounding orbital fat:
Angle 90/75/60 degrees

Optic nerve of human eyes
Optic nerve of cows's eyes

When removing the orbital fat tissue carefully and repeating the above described evaluations (angles at about 90/75/60 degrees) we basically got the same results regarding the surface spikes and the echosignals from the optic nerve substance. Even at the oblique angles between sound beam and optic nerve the display of steeply rising surface spikes was possible. (Figs. 8 and 9).

For both types of preparation – with and without orbital fat tissue around

594

the optic nerve – additional effects caused by our experimental set-up could be observed: because we had no occlusion of the subarachnoidal space at the proximal end there was an increase of this space – thus a distinct separation of the surface spikes – over time. This was due to an inflow of water into the subarachnoidal space during the evaluation.

Display of the optic nerve without dura mater/arachnoid
Angle 90/75/60 degrees

Optic nerve of human eyes
Optic nerve of cows's eyes

In this category of preparation – in both human and animal optic nerves the removal of the dura/arachnoid complex can be done rather easily – we definitely saw only one single peaked surface spike. At the perpendicular transducer position they were still rather high reflective and steeply rising. When angling the optic nerve to oblique angles we saw – in contrast to the equivalent situations when the dura/arachnoid was not removed – a more rapid decrease

Table 1. Diameters (microseconds).

Human optic nerve

---

with/without surrounding fat tissue:
+/– 90 degrees: 5.75   (n = 18)
+/– 75 degrees: 5.6   (n = 15)
+/– 60 degrees: 5.65   (n = 15)

without dura mater/arachnoid:
+/– 90 degrees: 4.8   (n = 9)
+/– 75 degrees: 4.9   (n = 6)
+/– 60 degrees: 5.0   (n = 9)

Optic nerve from cows' eyes

---

with/without surrounding fat tissue:
+/– 90 degrees: 5.7   (n = 9)
+/– 75 degrees: 5.5   (n = 7)
+/– 60 degrees: 5.55   (n = 7)

without dura mater/arachnoid:
+/– 90 degrees: 5.75   (n = 5)
+/– 75 degrees: 5.8   (n = 5)
+/– 60 degrees: 6.0   (n = 3)

(n = number of measurements)

of the height of these surface spikes. But as we could observe in the two previous experimental models also here the surface spikes representing the interface between pia mater/optic nerve substance and the water were steeply rising at oblique sound beam incidences. This was true for both human and cows's optic nerve. Regarding the diameters we found in this type of preparation a slight increase (max. 0.7 microseconds) (Figs. 10 and 11) (Table 1).

Discussion

As in previous publications and descriptions about the evaluation of the optic nerve the different layers (optic nerve sheaths, optic nerve substance) could be distinguished in the experimental display. The facts that even at oblique angles of sound beam incidences the signals of the different layers could be displayed as steeply rising signals and that the cross-sectional measurements did not increase in the experimental model with surrounding fat and/or with the dura/arachnoid complex in situ (as it would be suggested by mathematical and geometrical calculations) only leaves the explanation that the sound beam underlies refraction when passing the dura mater. Considering the cylindric shape of the nerve and the different types of interfaces – coarse indistinct surface of the fat/outer dura mater interface, rather smooth and distinct interface between the dura and the subarachnoidal fluid and the again more coarse and scalloped surface of the pia mater – and since refraction depends on the different acoustic properties of the two media on each side of an interface [2, 6], the dura mater most likely represents a very outstanding tissue layer.

When the dura was removed a slight increase of the nerve diameter – though not as much as it would result from calculation – was observed. With regard to differences in sound velocities (water/subarachnoidal fluid/optic nerve substance) and in case that all surfaces surrounding the optic nerve would be specular the observed displays of the nerve – particularly at the oblique angles – would not have been possible. [1, 2, 6] Specular reflection would have resulted in a disappearance of the echograms when angling the sound beam incidence in another direction besides the perpendicular position. The third spike (that is a second peak of the outer, first limiting surface spike) in some observations is due to scattering at the interface between orbital fat and the outer dural surface. Most likely scattering also is responsible for the at oblique angles observed steeply rising and – at least at perpendicular sound beam incidence – still high spikes from the surface of the pia mater/optic nerve substance. The proof of the influences of the dura mater on the propagation of sound waves, that may depend on the histopathologic structure with its high content of bundles of collagen and elastic tissue, will be subject of further investigations.

596

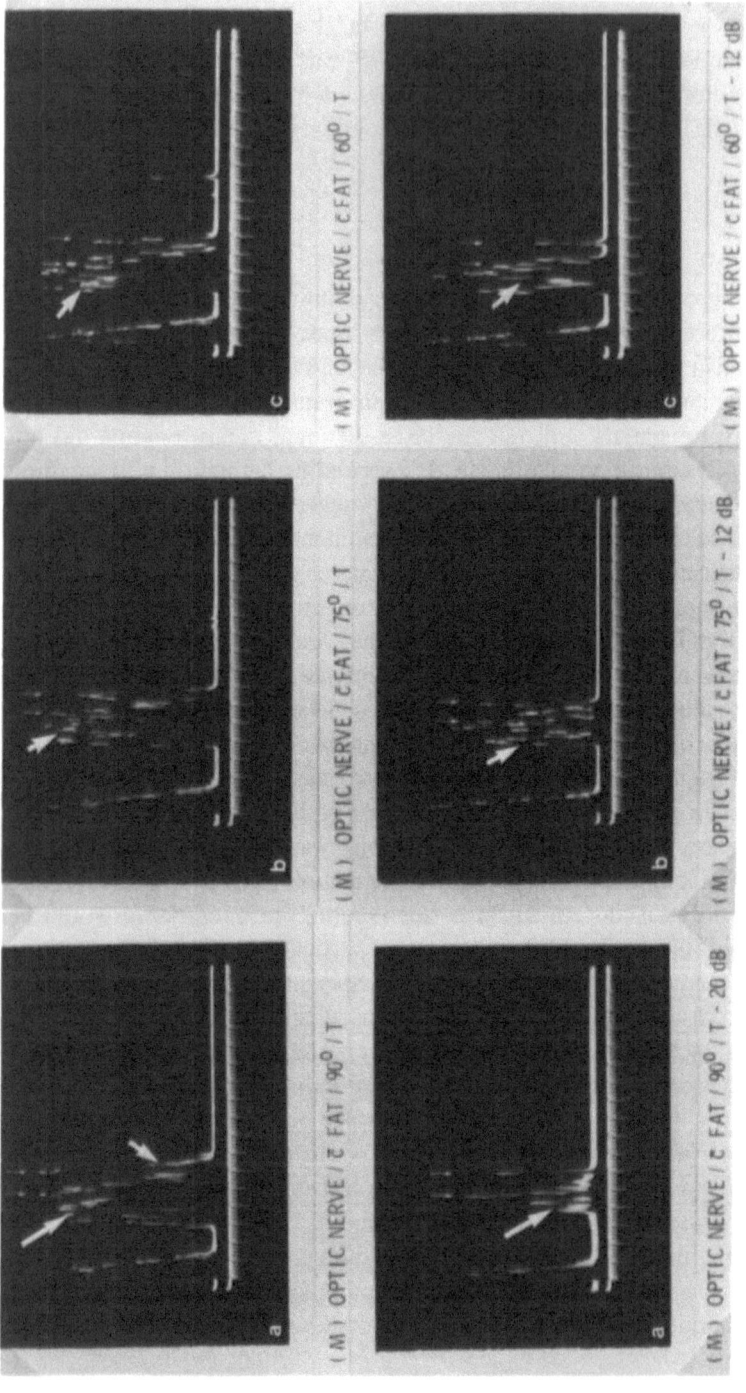

Fig. 6. Displays of the human optic nerve with surrounding orbital fat in-vitro. a: +/− perpendicular sound beam incidence, b: +/− 75 degrees sound beam incidence, c: +/− 60 degrees sound beam incidence. Large arrows indicate the echo signals from the fat tissue, small arrows indicate the optic nerve surfaces (dura mater). The bottom echograms were obtained at reduced system sensitivity. (a: T–20 dB, b and c: T–12 dB).

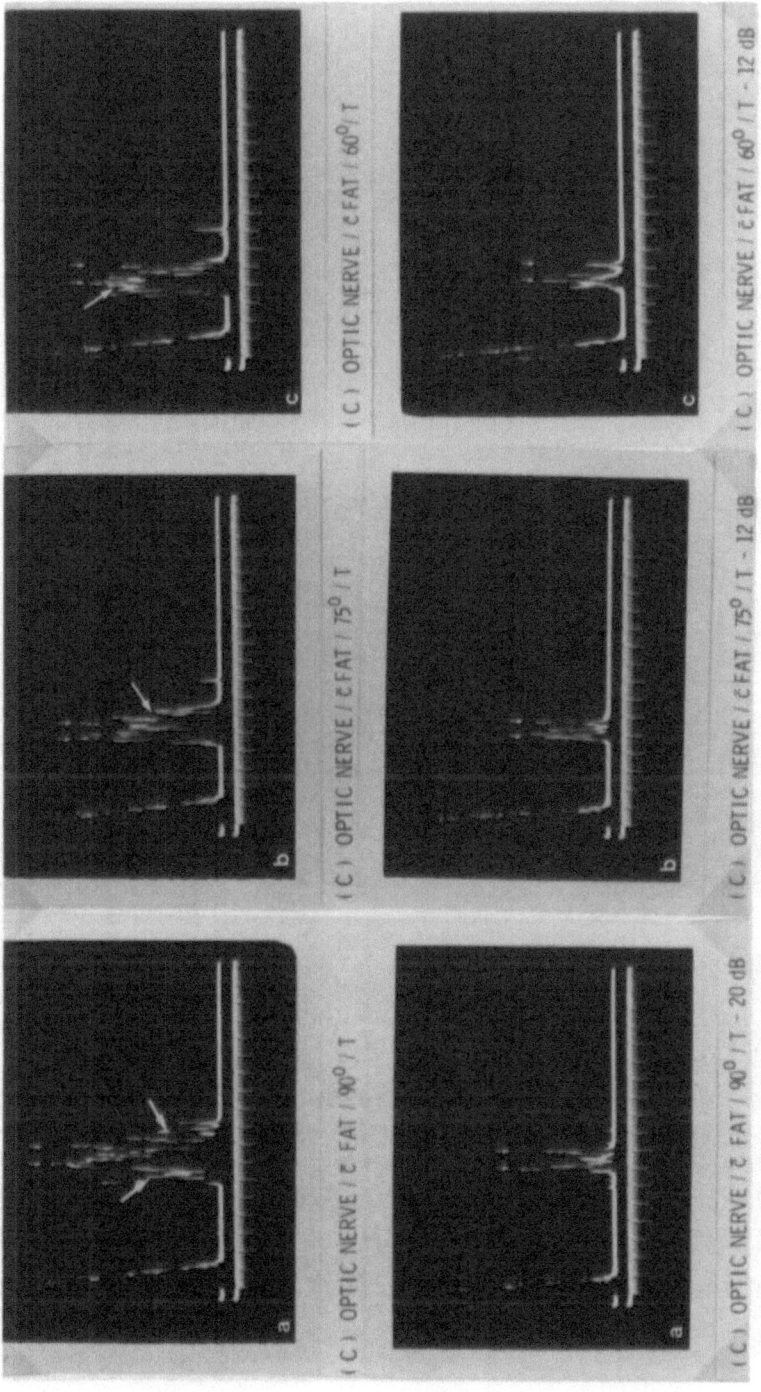

Fig. 7. Displays of the optic nerve from a cow with surrounding orbital fat in-vitro. (for explanation see Fig. 6).

598

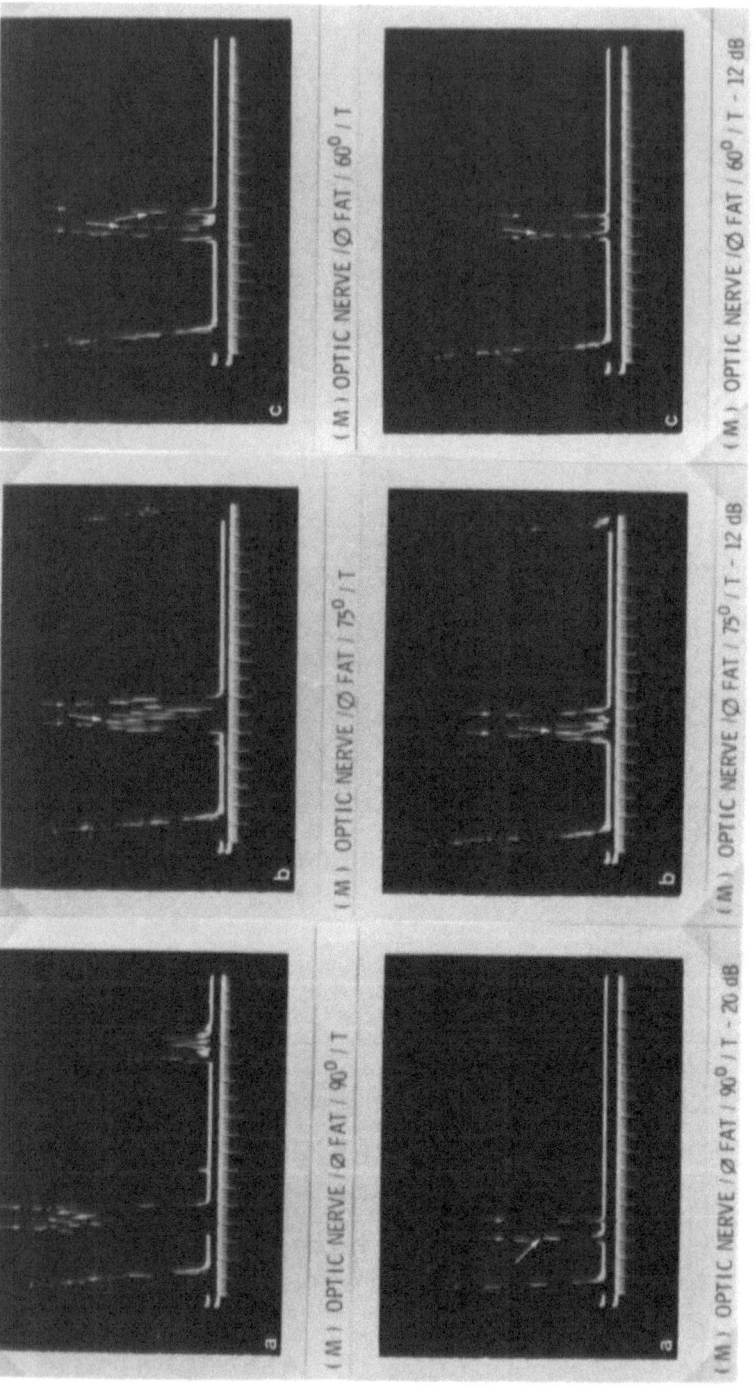

Fig. 8. Displays of the human optic nerve without surrounding orbital fat in-vitro. a: +/– perpendicular sound beam incidence. b: +/– 75 degrees sound beam incidence, c: +/– 60 degrees sound beam incidence. Bottom echograms at reduced sensitivity (see Fig. 6). Small arrows indicate the dura mater (inner interface towards the subdural space; the – in some displays observed – second dural spike is not displayed in these echograms). Particularly in the echograms at reduced system sensitivity the spike corresponding to the pia mater/optic nerve substance more clearly is displayed (longer arrows). The spikes that appear in some echograms in front of the dura at 75 and 60 degrees sections are explained by time differences at both sides of the sound beam.

599

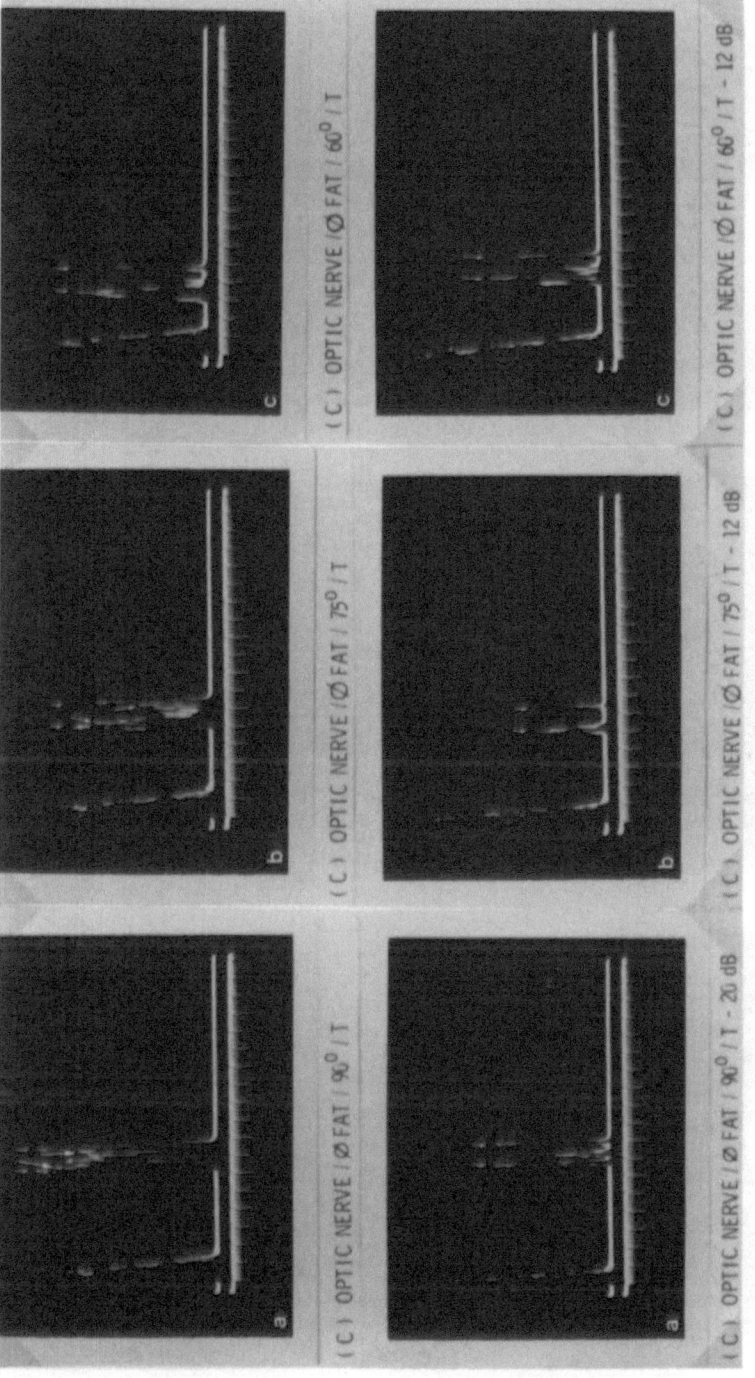

Fig. 9. Displays of the optic nerve from a cow without surrounding orbital fat in-vitro. (for explanation see Fig. 8).

600

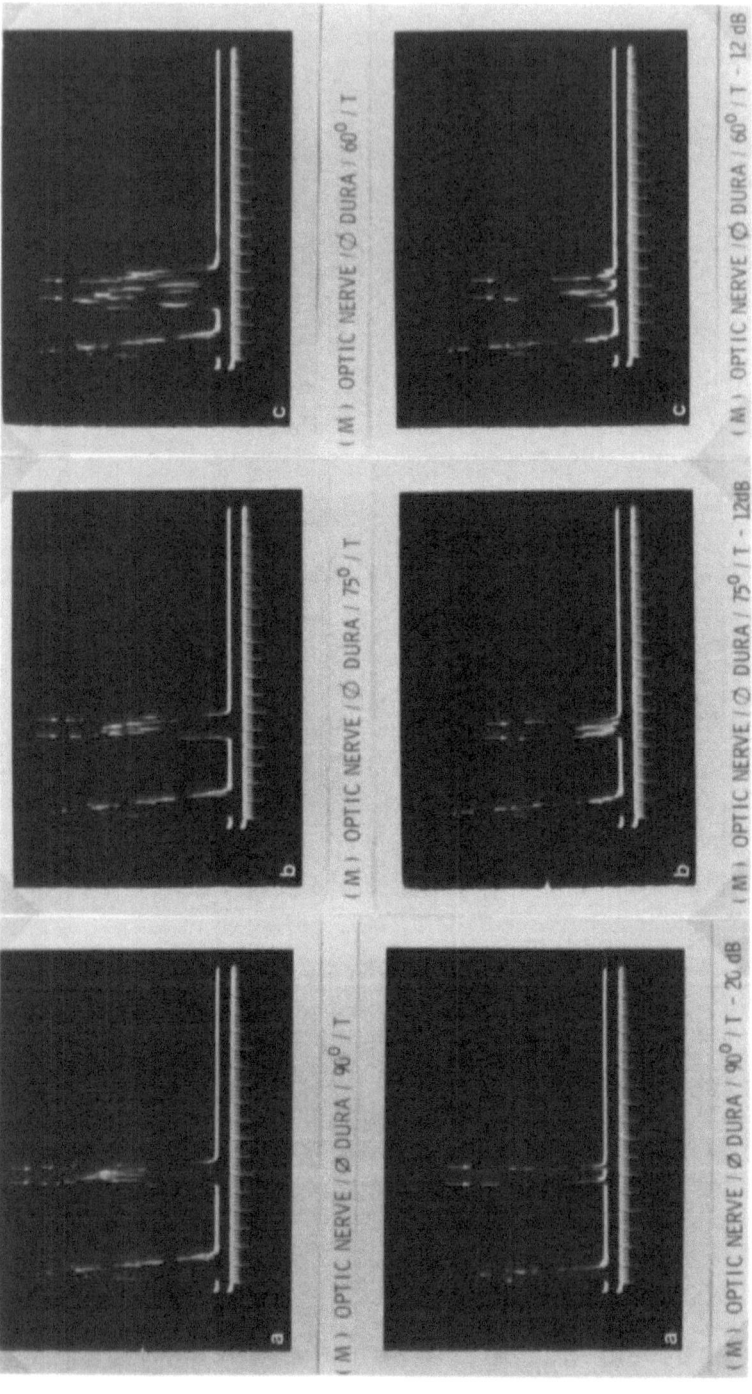

Fig. 10. Displays of the human optic nerve without the dura mater/arachnoid in-vitro. a: +/− perpendicular sound beam incidence, b: +/− 75 degrees sound beam incidence, c: +/− 60 degrees sound beam incidence. Arrows indicate the surface of the optic nerve substance with the enclosing pia mater. Bottom echograms at reduced system sensitivity (see Fig. 6). (For explanation of the in some echograms displayed signals in front of the pia mater see Fig. 8).

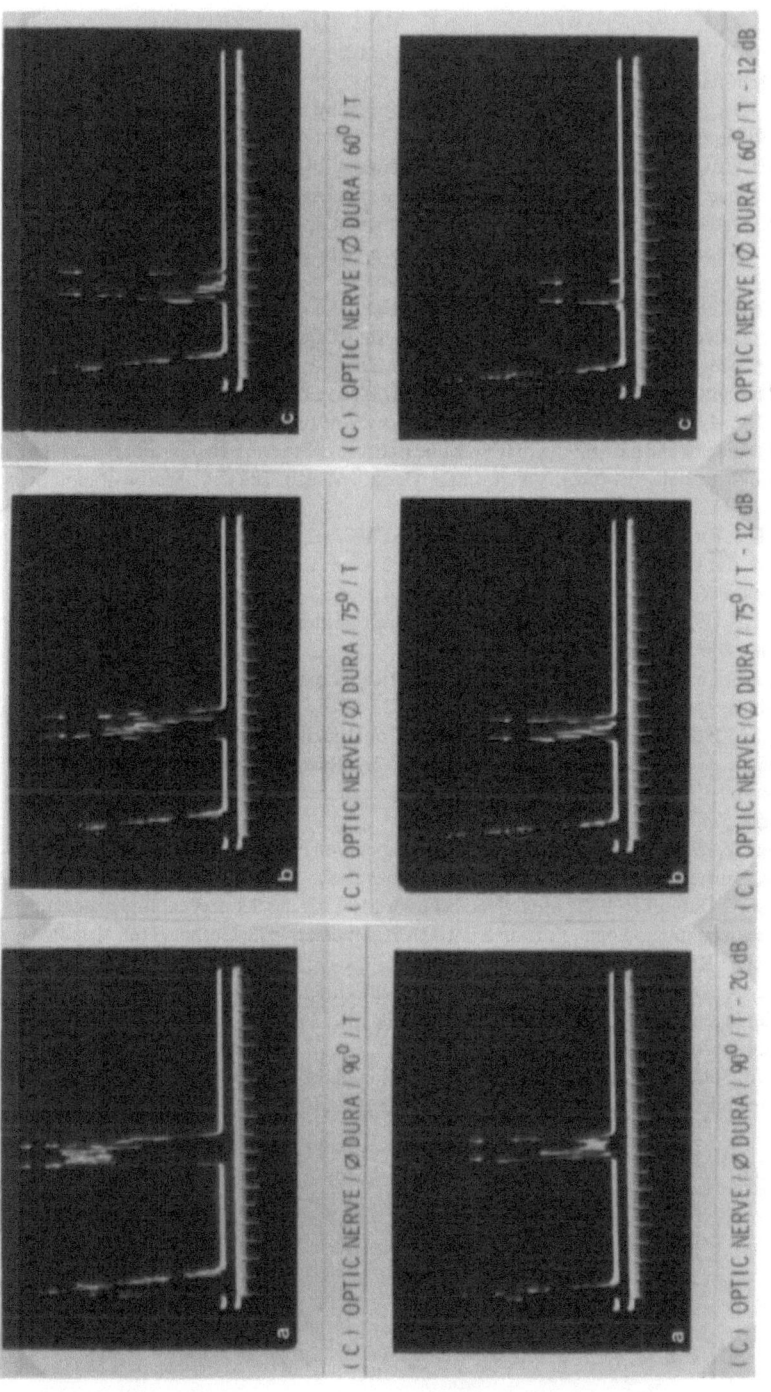

Fig. 11. Displays of the optic nerve from a cow without the dura mater/arachnoid in-vitro. (for explanation see Fig. 10).

602

References

1. Buschmann W, Voss M, Kemmerling S. 1970. Acoustic properties of normal human orbit tissues. Ophthalmol. Res., 1: 354–364.
2. Coleman JD, Lizzi FL, Jack RL. 1977. Ultrasonography of the eye and orbit. Lea and Febiger, Philadelphia.
3. Hogan MJ, Alvarado JA, Weddell JE. 1971. Histology of the human eye. An atlas and textbook. Chap. X: Optic nerve. pp. 523–606. W.B. Saunders Comp., Philadelphia.
4. Oksala A, Hadidi MA, Jääslahti SL. 1972. Experimental observations on the echograms of the optic nerve and on the effects of some tissues upon them. Acta Ophthalmologica, 50: 360–366.
5. Ossoinig KC. 1973. Ein neues Gerät für die klinische Echo-Ophthalmographie. Vorschläge zur Standardisation wichtiger Geräte-Parameter. In: Diagnostica ultrasonica in ophthalmologia. Proceedings of SIDUO IV, Paris, 1971. Massin M, Poujol J. (eds.). Paris: Centre National d'Ophthalmologie des Quinze-Vingts, 1973, pp. 131–137.
6. Ossoinig KC. 1974. Preoperative differential diagnosis of tumors with echography. Part I: Physical principles and morphologic background of tissue echograms. In: Current concepts in ophthalmology. Blodi FC. (ed.). Vol. 4, Chap. 17, pp. 264–280. The C.V. Mosby Comp., St. Louis.
7. Ossoinig KC, Kaefring SL, McNutt L, Weinstock SJ. 1977. Echographic measurements of the optic nerve. In: Ultrasound in medicine. White D, Brown RE (eds.). Vol. 3a, pp. 1065–1066. Plenum, New York.
8. Ossoinig KC. 1979. Standardized echography: Basic principles, clinical applications, and results. Int. Ophthalmol. Clin., 19/4: 127–210.
9. Ossoinig KC, Cennamo G, Frazier-Byrne S. 1981. Echographic differential diagnosis of optic nerve lesions. Doc. Ophthalmol. Proc. Ser., 29: 327–332.
10. Ossoinig KC. 1984. Ultrasonic diagnosis of Graves' ophthalmopathy. In: The eye and orbit in thyroid disease. Gorman CA et al. (eds.), pp. 185–211. Raven Press, New York.
11. Schroeder W. 1976. Schallaufzeitmessungen im distalen Sehnervenquerschnitt. Klin. Mbl. Augenheilk., 169: 743–745.
12. Schroeder W. 1978. Ultrasonography of the optic nerve. Proc. 3rd Int. Symp. on orbital disorders, Amsterdam, 1977. pp. 71–77. The Hague: Junk.
13. Schroeder W, Guthoff R. 1979. Modellversuche zur Messung des Sehnerven. In: Diagnostica ultrasonica in ophthalmologia. Proc. of SIDUO VII, Münster, 1978, Gernet H (ed.), pp. 166–172. Münster: Remy.
14. Stanowsky A, Kreissig I. 1984. Hat die echographische Untersuchung des Nervus opticus und seiner Meningen eine Bedeutung in der Diagnostik eines Pseudotumors cerebri? Fortschr. Ophthalmol., 81: 604–607.
15. Till P. 1976. Solid tissue model for the standardization of the echoophthalmograph 7200 MA (Kretz-Technik). Doc. Ophthalmol. Proc. Ser., 41: 205–240.

The correlation between endocranial pressure and optic nerve diameter: an ultrasonographic study

G. CENNAMO, M. GANGEMI and L. STELLA
Naples, Italy

Summary

Measurements of optic nerve diameter with standardized A-scan echography were made in a group of patients with cerebral diseases. Intracranial pressure was monitored at the time of the optic nerve diameter measurements. This study indicates that optic nerve sheath distension completely disappears as soon as intracranial pressure is normalized.

Introduction

In recent years, the measurement of intracranial pressure (ICP) has assumed an increasingly important role in neurosurgical pathology. This is due not only to progress regarding the technical aspects of measurement, but also to increased knowledge of the biological and physiological parameters that comprise ICP readings.

ICP measurements may be obtained either directly or indirectly: the former by placement of the transducer in cerebrospinal fluid, and the latter may be obtained through a membrane; for example, the dura mater. Both techniques involve surgery, but the former (although more precise) exposes the patient to an increased risk of infection (Brock & Coll, 1972; De Rougemont 1974; Lacombe 1980).

The purpose of this study is to establish any eventual correlation, in real time, between endocranial pressure readings and the diameter of the optic nerve (ON) along its length as it passes through the orbit.

Materials and methods

The echographic examination of the ON was carried out by standardized

K.C. Ossoinig (editor), Ophthalmic Echography, ISBN 978-94-010-7988-4

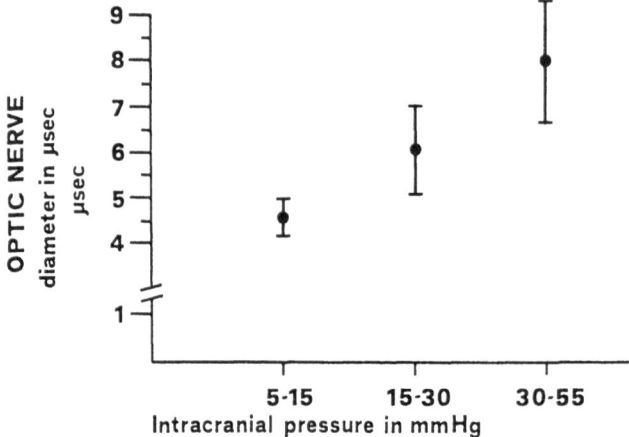

Fig. 1. Correlation between intracranial pressure and optic nerve diameter in the first group of ten patients showing an immediate variation of intracranial pressure and optic nerve diameter during anesthesia.

The echographic examination of the ON was carried out by standardized A-scan echography. ICP monitoring was carried out by the intraventricular insertion of a catheter and transducer. ON diameter measurements and IC readings were taken simultaneously in the right eyes of 10 patients who were to undergo neurosurgery for various intracranial pathologies. These measurements were taken prior to, during and following the induction of anesthesia for a 30-minute period. In fact, during this phase it is possible to obtain a variation of ICP's according to the anesthetic administered prior to intubation for general anesthesia. In some patients, the ON diameter was measured during the intraventricular infusion test.

Finally, these measurements were taken in a second group consisting of 10 patients with a normal ICP in order to show any eventual absence of correlation between the two groups of values. In these cases the optic nerve diameter was normal.

Results and discussion

In a comparison of the data obtained from the two methods in the first group (Fig. 1), the following was noted:
– the existence of a direct relationship between the degree of endocranial hypertension and the thickness of the optic nerve.
– any modification of the optic nerve thickness in relation to variations of endocranial pressure was immediate.
On the contrary, in the second group, whose ICP readings did not vary from

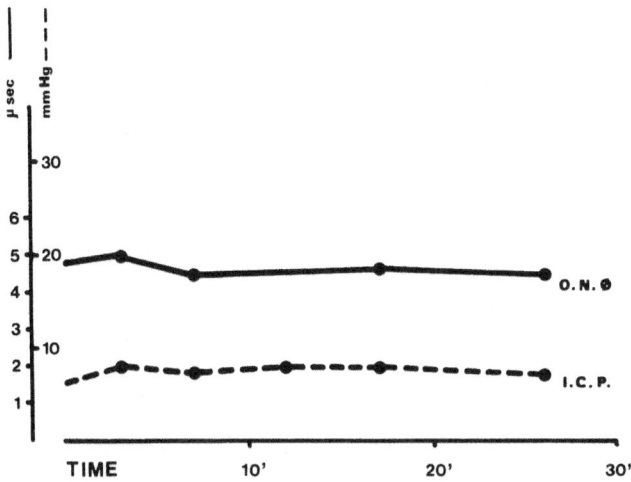

Fig. 2. Correlation between optic nerve diameter and intracranial pressure in the second group of ten patients. There is no variation of intracranial pressure and optic nerve diameter during anesthesia.

physiological values, there was no evidence of abnormal values of ON diameter measurements (Fig. 2). These data are substantiated by the particular anatomic situation that exists in the orbit surrounding the ON. In fact, the ON is enveloped by meninges. The posterior continuance of these involucres are the cerebral meninges. Moreover, the subarachnoid space contains cerebrospinal fluid which, via the optic canal, communicates directly with the cerebrospinal system.

It is therefore evident that even slight variations in ICP may influence the diameter of the ON. In fact, as opposed to the brain, the ON is not surrounded by a rigid structure, but by orbital fat which is easily compressible. Thus, any increasing pressure variations of cerebrospinal fluid will provoke swelling of the ON sheaths owing to the increase in the quantity of internal fluid which subsequently increases the diameter of the ON. It is therefore evident that echographic examination of the ON and, in particular, the measurement of its diameter by means of A-scan can furnish an immediate valuation, in real time, of endocranial pressure.

In conclusion, these data are all the more relevant if one considers that the appearance of a papilledema caused by endocranial hypertension or its disappearance when pressure is once again normalized is not immediate, but necessitates an interval of several days for both its manifestion and its regression.

References

Brock M, Deitz H. 1972. Intracranial pressure – experimental and clinical aspects. Springer-Verlag, New York.

Cennamo G. 1981. L'orbita l'esame ecografico in assenza di data patologici. Radiol. Med., 67, suppl. 1.

Cennamo G, Gangemi M, Stella L, Falivene R. 1984. Correlazione fra la pressione endocranica ed il diametro del nervo ottico: studio ecografico. Clinica Oculistica e Patologia Oculare, Suppl. Vol. V: 39.

De Rougemont J. 1974. Méthode de mesures de la pression intracranienne. Neurochirurgie, 20: 473.

Gallenga R, Bellone G, Gallenga PE, Pasquarelli A. 1971. Ultrasonografia clinica dell'occhio e dell'orbita. 53° Congr. S.O.I. Malta.

Lacombe J. 1980. Méthodes de mesure de la pression intracranienne. Rev. Ped. 9: 553.

Ossoinig KC. 1978. The Role of Clinical Echography in Modern Diagnosis of Periorbital and Orbital Lesions. Proc. 3rd Int. Symp. on Orbital Disorders, Amsterdam, 1977, Dr. Junk W. Publishers.

Ossoinig KC, Cennamo G, Frazier-Byrne S. 1981. Echographic differential diagnosis of optic nerve lesions. Documenta Ophthalmologica Proceedings Series 29, Ultrasonography in Ophthalmology: 327, Dr. Junk W. Publishers, London.

Echographic examination of the optic nerve and its meninges in the diagnosis of a pseudotumor cerebri

A. STANOWSKY and I. KREISSIG
Tübingen, FRG

Summary

We used standardized A-scan echography [8] to examine the optic nerve and its meninges 4 to 6 mm behind the lamina cribrosa in 16 patients with pseudotumor cerebri. The examinations took place between December, 1980 and September, 1984. The following pathological changes were present with the eye in a lateral position of 30°:
1. The echographic diameter of the optic nerve with its meninges, except for the dura, averaged 5.9 mm (standard deviation: 0.8 mm) in comparison to 3.5–3.9 mm in the normal eye (standard deviation: 0.8 mm). [12]
2. An enlargement of the subarachnoidal space surrounding the optic nerve to a total average width of 2.6 mm (standard deviation: 1.0 mm).
3. There were signs of a slight optic nerve atrophy. The average diameter of the optic nerve was about 10% less than normal.
4. The changes were bilaterally symmetrical.
5. The optic nerve was 'mobile'; that is, eye movements caused it to shift within the enlarged subarachnoidal space.
In only one of the 16 patients the echogram showed no signs of pathology in the optic nerve or its meninges.

Our findings suggest that standardized A-scan echography is an important adjunct to other methods of-diagnosing a pseudotumor cerebri.

Introduction

Anatomical examinations by Cogan [2], Walsh and Hoyt [15] have shown that in chronic intracranial hypertension, such as that of pseudotumor cerebri, the subarachnoidal space often becomes distended.

Clinically, this situation is very difficult to detect. Various authors have therefore applied echography to the optic nerve and its meninges (pia mater,

K.C. Ossoinig (editor), Ophthalmic Echography, ISBN 978-94-010-7988-4

arachnoidea and dura mater) to detect these pathological changes. In 1972 Coleman and Carroll [3] identified an enlargement of the optic nerve or its meninges [4, 5, 10] with B-scan echography. In 1976 Schroeder [11, 12] reported on echographic detection of unilateral diseases of the optic nerve with standardized A-scan echography. He defined the normal echographic diameter of the optic nerve as being 4.5 to 5.0 μsec (3.5–3.9 mm*) with a standard deviation of 1.0 μsec (0.8 mm*). In 1977 Ossoinig described a 'fluid pattern' within the optic nerve in a patient with pseudotumor cerebri [7]. In 1981 he reported that the boundaries of the enlarged subarachnoidal space surrounding the optic nerve of such patients can be determined echographically by means of surface signals from the pia mater and the arachnoidea [1, 9].

Since 1980 at the University Eye Clinic in Tübingen we [13] have made a practice of echographically examining all patients with papilledema, the object of which is to detect changes in the area of the optic nerve and its meninges. The following is a report on our findings.

Material and methods

From December of 1980 to September of 1984 we examined 137 patients with papilledema of various origins. These patients had been referred to us for echographical diagnosis by Professor Aulhorn (Department for Neuro-ophthalmology and Pathophysiology). Sixteen of these patients suffered from a chronic intracranial hypertension. Thirteen of the 16 patients were female, and 3 were male. The average age was 38 years.

The examinations were conducted wit the Kretz 7200 MA A-scan and the Ocuscan 400 A/B-scan procedure. The Kretz instrument had been standardized according to the guidelines of Ossoinig [8] and Till [14]. After topical anesthesia with Proxymetacain-HCl the ultrasound probe was placed on the temporal conjunctiva of the globe. The patient was first asked to look straight ahead and then to abduct the eye approximately 30°. In both directions of gaze the ultrasound beam was adjusted to hit the opic nerve and its meninges as perpendicularly as possible. The proof that this had succeeded was invariably an echogram in which the opic nerve was defined on both sides by steeply rising amplitudes of equal height and depth (Fig. 1). These inner amplitudes corresponded to the inner layer of the arachnoidea [9], and are here defined as the 'outer boundary amplitudes' of the subarachnoidal space. Within these outer boundary amplitudes were 2 additional amplitudes of equal height – likewise vertical. These originated in the pial sheathing of the optic nerve, and are here designated as the 'inner boundary amplitudes' of the subarachnoidal

---

* at ultrasound speeds of 1550 m/sec.

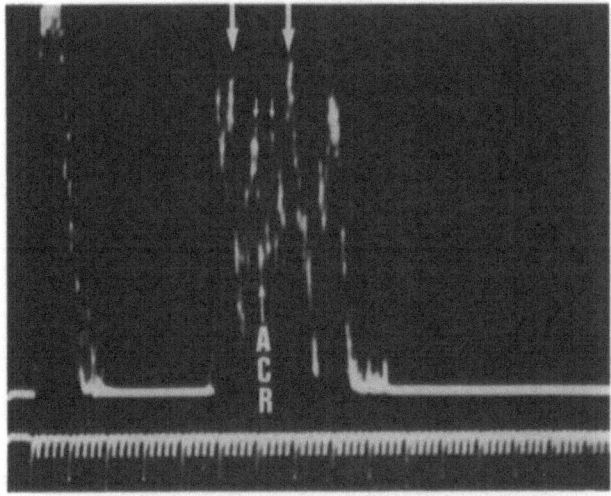

Fig. 1. Widening of the meninges surrounding the optic nerve in a 40-year-old female patient with pseudotumor cerebri (standardized A-scan echography). Patient is looking straight ahead. The *large arrows* point to the outer boundary amplitudes; the *small arrows* to the inner boundary amplitudes of the enlarged subarachnoidal space on either side of the optic nerve. The arteria centralis retinae (ACR) is recognizable at the bottom of the V-shaped gap in the area of the optic nerve and appears in the form of an indistinct area due to its rapid pulsation.

space. The maximal reflectivity of the inner boundary amplitudes was lower than that of the outer boundary amplitudes. Echographically, the sub-arachnoidal space appeared between these 2 sets of boundary amplitudes as an area of very low reflectivity.

The diameter of the optic nerve and its surrounding meninges was determined 4–6 mm behind the lamina cribrosa when the eye was abducted at an angle of 30°. A V-shaped gap was seen between the 2 inner boundary amplitudes. A rapid vertical oscillation which appeared at its bottom corresponded to the pulsation of the central retinal artery in this area.

Results

In 15 of the 16 patients with pseudotumor cerebri the echogram showed the following pathological findings in the area of the optic nerve and its meninges when the eye was abducted at an angle of 30° (Fig. 2).

The distance between the outer boundary amplitudes was enlarged to an average of 7.6 μsec (standard deviation: 1.0 μsec). Clinically this is equivalent to:

1. An average increase in the overall diameter of the optic nerve and me-

610

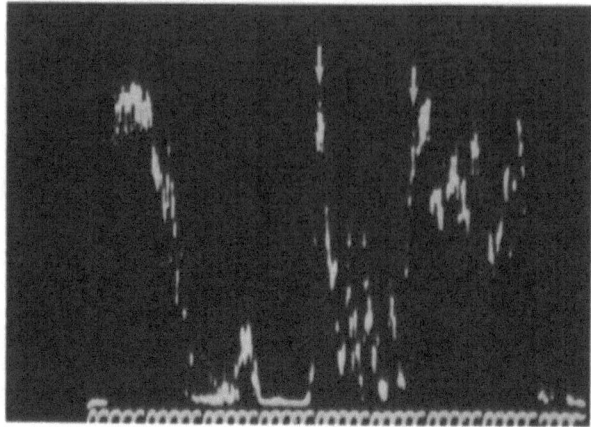

Fig. 2. The phenomenon of the 'mobile optic nerve' in an31-year-old female patient with pseudotumor cerebri (standardized A-scan echography). The patient is looking temporally. Noteworthy here is that the subarachnoidal space (bounded by a *large arrow* and a *small arrow*) is clearly wider nasally than temporally.

ninges (except the dura) to 5.9 mm (standard deviation: 0.8 mm) in contrast to the normal diameter of 3.5–3.9 mm (standard deviation: 0.8 mm).

Between the inner and outer boundary amplitudes was a large area of low reflectivity whose average width was altogether 3.4 μsec (standard deviation: 1.3 μsec). Clinically, this is equivalent to:

2. An enlargement of the subarachnoidal space surrounding the optic nerve to a total average width of 2.6 mm (standard devation: 1.0 mm). The subarachnoidal space in this situation constituted almost half of the total diameter of the optic nerve and its meninges.

In addition, the distance between the two inner boundary amplitudes decreased on the average from 4.7 μsec to 4.2 μsec (standard deviation: 1.0 μsec), which is clinically equivalent to:

3. Atrophy of the optic nerve.

4. The changes were bilaterally symmetrical.

A shift in the position of the optic nerve within the enlarged subarachnoidal space was observed in the echogram when the eye was moved. When the eye was maxially abducted, the echogram of the optic nerve moved closer to the temporal outer boundary amplitude and further away from te nasal outer boundary amplitude (Fig. 2). As a result, the optic nerve was no longer evenly surrounded by the subarachnoidal space. The subarachnoidal space was on the average twice as wide nasally (2.3 μsec) as temporally (1.1 μsec). We called this changing echographical situation:

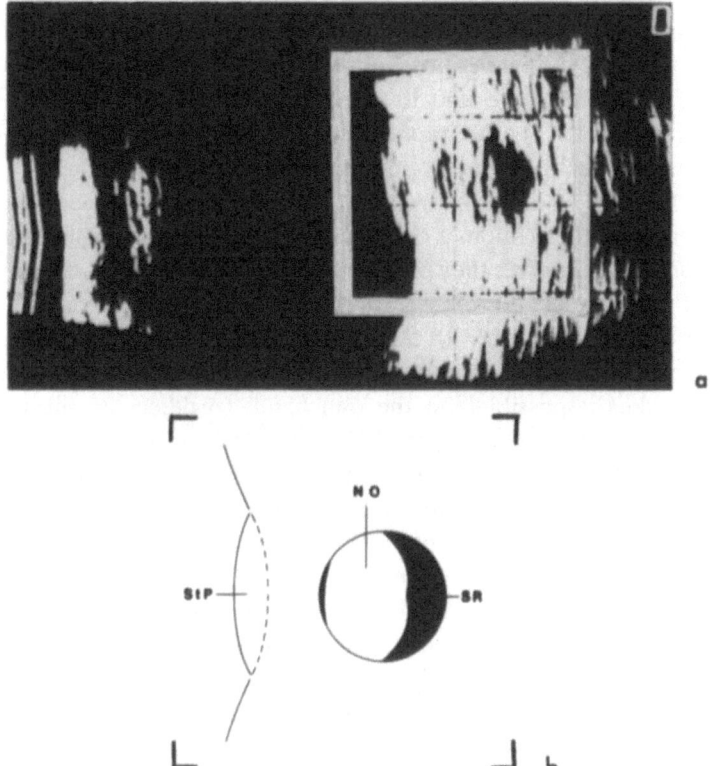

Fig. 3a. The phenomenon of the 'mobile optic nerve' in B-scan echography. Same patient as in Fig. 2. The white square defines the area which is schematically presented in Fig. 3b.

Fig. 3b. Diagram of the echogram shown in Fig. 3a. The patient is looking temporally. In this case, the ultrasonic beam struck the optic nerve (NO) and its meninges at a 90° angle some 5 mm behind the lamina cribrosa. The subarachnoidal space (SR) is larger nasally than temporally. The papilledema (StP) shows up clearly in the echogram.

5. 'Mobile optic nerve.' These changes were confirmed with the B-scan only when the diameter of the optic nerve and its meninges had a minimum width of 7.4 μsec (Fig. 3).

In 1 of the 16 patients we detected no pathological changes in the area of the optic nerve in spite of a clinically certain pseudotumor cerebri.

Discussion

Our echographical studies confirmed 5 different kinds of pathological changes in the area of the optic nerve and its meninges in 15 of the 16 patients. These changes, as shown in the echograms, consisted of (1) an increase in the overall diameter of the optic nerve and its meninges; (2) an enlargement of the subarachnoidal space; (3) echographical signs of a slight atrophy of the optic nerve; (4) involvement of both optic nerves in each patient; and (5) the phenomenon of the 'mobile optic nerve'. It is important to keep in mind, however, that all of these findings confirm only the presence of an intracranial hypertension; by themselves they provide no information on any etiology. An intracranial process must therefore always be excluded by a diligent differential diagnosis in combination with other methods. Nevertheless, the examination using echography is an important tool in the diagnosis of a pseudotumor cerebri. It makes it possible, on the one hand, to detect an intracranial hypertension and, on the other, to differentiate this from other causes of papilledema, such as an opticus tumor, a retrobulbar neuritis, or a vascular process of the optic nerve. Inasmuch as the enlarged subarachnoidal space surrounding the optic nerve can be precisely measured using this method, it is possible to document any changes precisely (e.g., following a lumbar tap), and so have a basis for choosing the most suitable surgical therapy should this become necessary. In 6 of the 16 patients in whom the echograms had indicated a pseudotumor cerebri a fenestration of the optic sheaths was performed [6]. In all 6 patients the preoperative echographical findings, namely enlargement of the subarachnoidal space, were confirmed intraoperatively.

Acknowledgement

The authors wish to thank Thomas Rice for translating and editing the manuscript.

References

1. Byrne SF. 1984. The Echographic Measurement and Differential Diagnosis of Optic-Nerve Lesions (this volume).
2. Cogan DC. 1966. Neurology of the visual system. Thomas, Springfield, 4. Aufl.
3. Coleman DJ, Carroll FD. 1972. A new technique for evaluation of optic neuropathy. Am J Ophthalmol 74: 915–920.
4. Feneis H. 1982. Anatomisches Bildwörterbuch. Thieme, Stuttgart, 5. Aufl.
5. Foos R. 1984. Personal communication.
6. Herzau V, Aulhorn E, Wiethölter H. 1983. Diagnose und Therapie bei Pseudotumor cerebri aus augenärztlicher Sicht. Fortschr Ophthalmol 80: 26–29.
7. Ossoinig KC. 1977. Echography of the eye, orbit and periorbital region. In: Arger PH (Hrsg) Orbit roentgenology. Wily, New York: 224–269.

8. Ossoinig KC. 1979. Standardized echography. Basic principles, clinical applications and results. In: Dallow PL (Hrsg), Ophthalmic ultrasonography: Comparative techniques (Int Ophthalmol Clin). Little, Brown, Boston.
9. Ossoinig KC et al. 1981. Echographic differential diagnosis of optic nerve lesions. Doc Ophthalmol 29: 327–335.
10. Schlote W. 1970. Monographien aus dem Gesamtgebiet der Neurologie und Psychiatrie, Heft 131. Springer, New York.
11. Schroeder W. 1976. Ergebnisse der A-Bild-Echographie bei einseitigen Sehnervenerkrankungen. Klin Mbl Augenheilk 169: 30.
12. Schroeder W. 1976. Schallaufzeitmessung im distalen Sehnervenquerschnitt. Klin Mbl Augenheilk 169: 743.
13. Stanowsky A, Richard G, Kreissig I. 1982. Echographie bei Orbitaveränderungen. 142. VersVerRhein-Westf Augenärzte: 111–119.
14. Till P. 1976. Solid tissue model for the standardization of the echoophthalmograph 7200 MA (Kretz-Technik). Doc Ophthalmol 41: 205–240.
15. Walsh FB, Hoyt WF. 1969. Clinical neuroophthalmology. Williams and Wilkins Co, Baltimore, 3. Aufl.

Optic nerve evaluation by echography and computerized tomography in patients with optic disc drusen

D. DORO, S. PERRONE, D. FIORE, and F. MORO

Padova, Italy

Abstract

Axial and coronal CT sections of the orbital optic nerve appeared normal in four out of five male patients, aged between 39 and 49 years, who had bilateral ophthalmoscopically visible optic nerve drusen. One patient had no clinical signs of increased intracranial pressure, but CT showed bilateral, symmetrical enlargement of the orbital optic nerves with no change after contrast enhancement. X-rays revealed a large sella and normal optic foramina. Orbital optic nerve thickness was also measured with standardized echography and was found to be greater than in the other four patients whose optic nerves measured within normal values. The usefulness of A- and B-scan echography for the evaluation of the optic nerve and the controversial pathogenesis of optic disc drusen are discussed.

A 39-year-old man who had never undergone ophthalmological examination was admitted to our Clinic with cranial trauma and a large lid tear. Ophthalmoscopical and retinal fluorescein angiographic findings and pre-injection autofluorescence evidenced bilateral expsed drusen of the optic nerve head. Both eyes had full vision and inferonasally restricted visual fields.

Skull x-rays revealed a large sella with clear-cut margins and normal optic foramina. Computed axial tomography unexpectedly revealed a bilateral narrow-diffuse symmetrical enlargement of the orbital optic nerve; no change was observed after contrast enhancement (Fig. 1). In the coronal projections, the optic nerve outlines appeared well circumscribed.

No cafe au lait spots were observed at the neurological examination, which was negative. The patient, who complained of moderate transient headache, refused both lumbar puncture and carotid arteriography. During the four-year follow-up, no changes were observed in the optic disc, visual field, visual acuity and CT picture and no proptosis was recorded.

The optic nerves, measured by means of standardized 7200 MA A-scan, were found to be thicker than normal: 6.5 microseconds in the right eye and 6

K.C. Ossoinig (editor), Ophthalmic Echography,

616

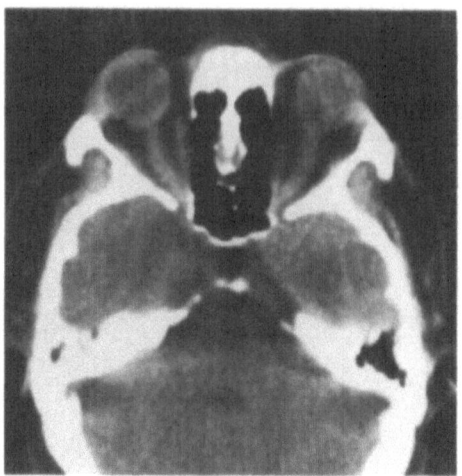

Fig. 1. Axial CT-Scan showing narrow-diffuse enlargement of the optic nerves in patient 1.

microseconds in the left eye (Fig. 2). No distension of nerve sheaths by increased subarachnoidal fluid was observed and no differences were observed between the optic nerve obtained in primary-gaze and abduction positions.

Pseudotumor cerebri was excluded on the basis of fluorescein angiographic and A-scan investigations. CT-scans were inconsistent with the diagnosis of optic nerve glioma or meningioma (Jacobiec et al. 1984). A diagnosis of bilateral astroglial proliferation of the optic nerves associated with optic nerve head drusen was suggested (Doro et al. 1982).

This case prompted us to submit four 39 to 49-year-old male patients with bilateral optic nerve drusen to standardized A-scan echography and CT to

Table 1. Visual acuity and field defects in five patients with bilateral optic disc drusen.

Patient	Age	V.A.		F.D.	
		R.E.	L.E.	R.E.	L.E.
1	39	1	1	lower nasal	lower nasal
2	48	0,3	0,4	lower nasal	lower nasal
3	49	1	hm	lower temporal	mainly inferior irregular narrowing
4	40	1	1	severe irregular narrowing	mild upper temporal
5	39	0,8	0,4	lower nasal	central and upper temporal islet

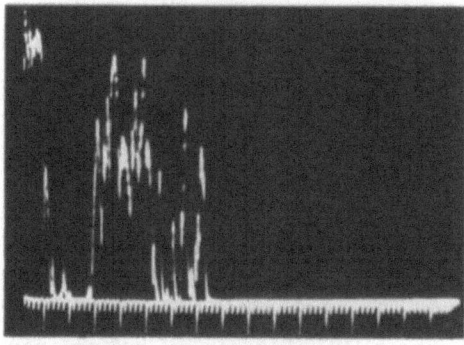

Fig. 2. Standardized A-Scan echogram of thickened right optic nerve in patient 1.

ascertain whether they had optic nerve enlargement.

The visual acuity and field defects of all five patients are summarized in Table 1. The pre-injection autofluorescence and the retinal fluorescein angiograms of the four patients evidenced optic nerve head drusen. Axial and coronal sections of the orbital optic nerves of the four patients appeared normal; in three patients, there were obvious drusen of the optic nerve head. The optic nerve widths measured with standardized A-scan echography, ranged from 4 to 5.5 microseconds (Table 2). In all patients, the optic nerves were higher reflective than in five controls.

Discussion

Retinal fluorescein angiography is necessary for, and usually provides enough evidence to make a diagnosis of drusen of the optic nerve head (Moro et al. 1979). B-scan and CT are useful in the detection of exposed and mostly buried optic nerve head drusen. Standardized A-scan is the most accurate means for

Table 2. Standardized A-scan measurements of optic nerve diameters of five patients with bilateral optic disc drusen.

Patient	Microseconds	
	R.E.	L.E.
1	6,5	6
2	4	4,5
3	5,5	5
4	4,5	5
5	5	5,5

618

measuring the optic nerve width (Ossoinig et al. 1981); a width of 4.7 ± 0.9 microseconds is considered normal (Guthoff et al. 1982) and the optic nerve widths observed in four of our cases may, therefore, be considered normal. In four of our patients, CT images of the retrobulbar optic nerve appeared normal, as did those of the five patients with optic nerve head drusen reported by Frisen et al. (1978). The diameter of the optic nerve was found to be greater than normal in both eyes of our first patient with drusen of the optic nerve head associated with CT evidence of bilateral optic nerve enlargement.

The pathogenesis of drusen of the optic nerve has long been a controversial subject. Recently Spencer (1978) suggested that an axoplasmic transport alteration may be the basic pathogenetic mechanism for formation of drusen in the optic nerve; the mild axonal swelling and the inconstant moderate gliosis observed histologically by Tso (1981) in patients with optic nerve head drusen may account for the increased optic nerve diameter found in our first patient. Further investigations using standardized A-scan are needed to establish how frequently optic disc drusen are associated with increased optic nerve thickness.

References

Doro D, Perrone S, Cardin P, Pardatscher K, Fiore D. 1982. Bilateral optic nerve enlargement associated with optic disc drusen. A case report. Orbit 1: 181.
Frisen L, Schöldström G, Svendsen P. 1978. Drusen in the Optic Nerve head: verification by computerized tomography. Arch. Ophthalmol. 96: 1611-1614.
Guthoff RF, Schroeder W, Hagemann J. 1982. Examination of the optic nerve by ultrasound and CT Scan. Orbit 1: 152.
Jacobiec FA, Depot MJ, Kennerdell JS, Shults WT, Anderson RL, Alper ME, Citrin CM, Housepian EM, Trokel SL. 1984. Combined Clinical and Computed Tomography Diagnosis of Orbital Glioma and Meningioma. Ophthalmol. 91: 137-155.
Moro F, Saraniti G. 1979. Fluorangiografia della papilla ottica. In Maione M. and Moro F. Le otticopatie. Maccari ed. Parma, Italy.
Ossoinig KC, Cennamo G, Frazier-Byrne S. 1981. Echography differential diagnosis of optic-nerve lesions. Docum. ophthal. proc. Series Vol. 29, ed. by J.M. Thijssen and A.M. Verbeek. Dr. W. Junk Publisher The Hague.
Spencer WH. 1978. Drusen of the optic disc and aberrant axoplasmic transport. Am. J. Ophthalmol. 85: 1-12.
Tso MOM. 1981. Pathology and Pathogenesis of Drusen of the Optic Nervehead. Ophthalmol. 88: 1066-1080.

Ultrasonic treatment of choroidal detachment

V. TANEV, R. GOLEMINOVA and M. SJAROV
Sofia, Bulgaria

One of the most frequent complications in intraocular operations, and particularly in fistula-provoking operations, is the choroid detachment. This complication also occurs in contemporary microsurgical operations – trabecolectomy, trepano-trabecolectomy, phakoemulsification, etc. [1, 2, 3].

Ultrasound causes a specific micromassage of the tissues which improves blood circulation, affects the different biomembranes by enhancing their permeability, and stimulates the metabolic processes. On the basis of those principles ultrasonic therapy was applied by the authors on patients with choroidal detachment.

Method

Ultrasonic equipment with a continuous emission at a frequency of 800 KHz and 0,2–0,3 W/cm^2 was used. Ultrasonic treatment was carried out every day. It started with three minutes, and on the fifth treatment we reached the maximum duration time of five minutes in order to check the individual patient's tolerance and to avoid hemorrhage in the freshly operated eye. Distilled water in a bottomless bath was used for a contact medium. The sound was applied through the eyelids without local anesthesia. Ultrasonic wave permeability was guaranteed in the entire bulb and the paraocular zone.

The surface and prominence of the detached choroi was followed by biomicroscopy, ophthalmoscopy, echography, ultrasonic biometry before, during and after the treatment.

The brightening of the detachment area itself is a sign of the starting resorption of choroidal liquid.

K.C. Ossoinig (editor), Ophthalmic Echography, ISBN 978-94-010-7988-4

BEGINING OF TREATMENT

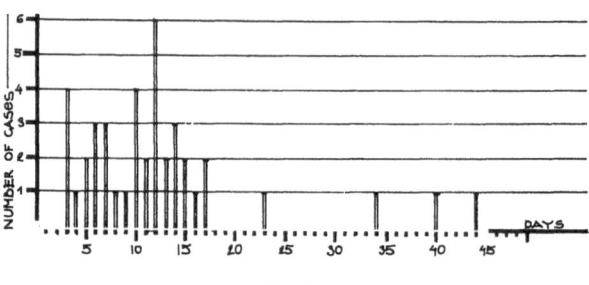

Fig. 1.

Results and discussion

Forty-two patients (43 eyes) were treated. Before commencement of the treatment not even the slightest resorption of the subchoroidal liquid was observed in the patients. Conservative therapy was applied initially to most of the patients without effect. Only three patients were subjected to ultrasonic treatment. One patient was treated after surgical intervention in the detached choroid.

Treatment started between the third and the forty-fourth day following surgery, depending on the clinical state (Fig. 1). In the majority of the cases, treatment was started after the tenth day.

The ultrasonically treated choroid detachments were post-glaucoma operations in 31 cases, post-cataract exraction in 8 cases, and post combined glaucoma and cataract operations in 4 cases.

Excellent effect was observed for 41 of the treated eyes (95.35%). Reattachment of the detached choroid was not observed in only two eyes (one of the cases was a post-glaucoma surgery, and the other a post-cataract extraction).

The full reattachment of the detached choroid occurs on the average at the 7th application ($\bar{x} = 7.25$ days, $\sigma n - 1 = 3.16$). The start of the brightening of the detached choroid occurs, on the average, at the fifth application ($\bar{x} = 5.05$ days, $\sigma n - 1 = 2.35$). From the brightening of the detached choroid to the completereattachment takes, on the average, two applications ($\bar{x} = 2.29$ days, $\sigma m - 1 = 1.38$).

No such correlation was found in the study of the dependence of the prominence of the choroid detachment, measured by means of ultrasonic biometry at the start and end of the reattachment. No complications and no recurrence was observed in any of the patients.

In conclusion, we can state that we recommend ultrasonic treatment of detached choroids as a simple, safe and efficient method.

References

1. Volkov VV. 1953. On the Pathogenesis and Therapy of Post-Operative Choroidal Detachment. Annals of Ophthalmology 5: 31–36.
2. Fechner PU. 1975. Erfahrungen mit der Trabekulektomie bei Glaukom Simplex. – Ber. Dtsch. Ophthal. Ges. 74: Essen, 639–646, Munchen, J.F. Bergmann, 1977.
3. Piffaretti JM, Ramel C u. Gloor BP. 1975. Ergebnisse der Trabekulektomie – Ophthalmologica 170: 2–3, 133–138.

Index of subjects

624

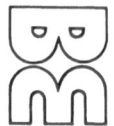

biophysic medical

**International Supplier
of the**

OPHTHASCAN® "S"

**Digital Standardized Ophthalmic
Ultrasound System**

**is proud to be a sponsor
of**

SIDUO X

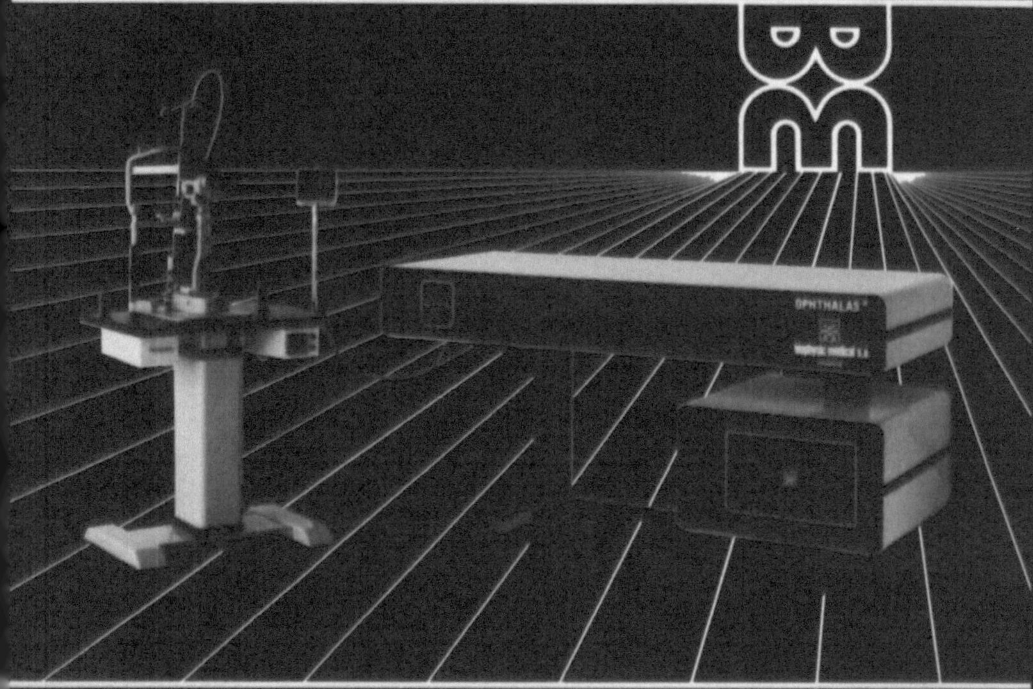

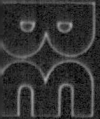

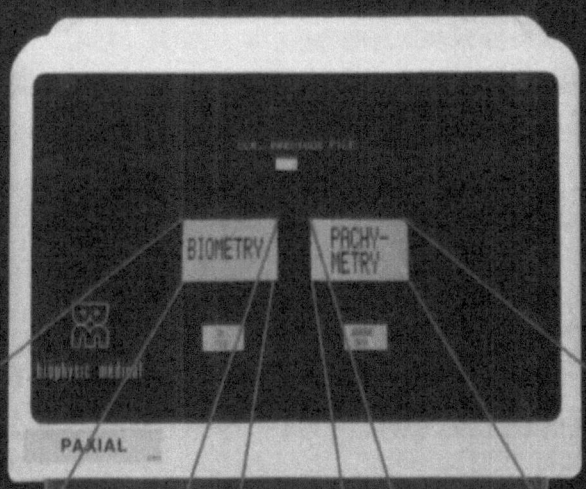
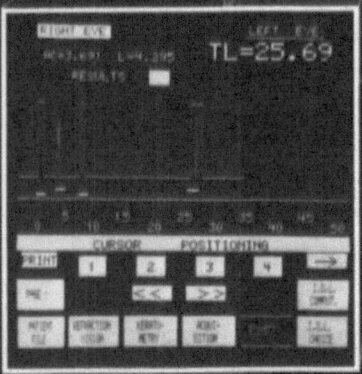
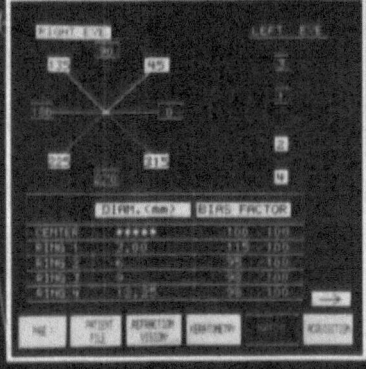
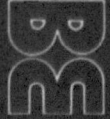

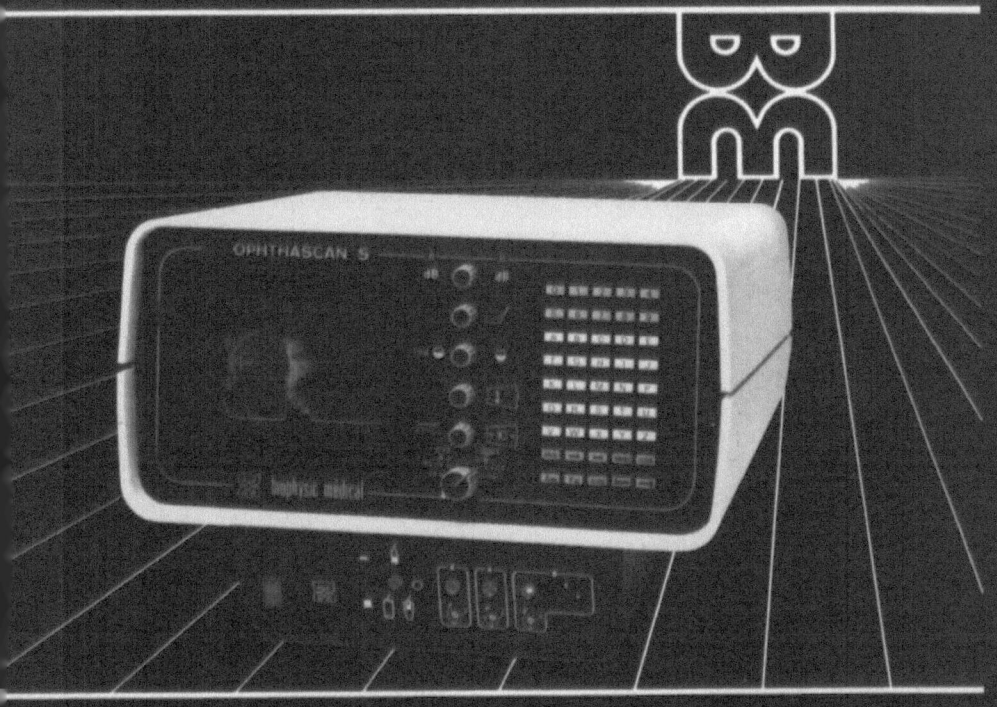